Clinical Neurocardiology

FUNDAMENTAL AND CLINICAL CARDIOLOGY

Editor-in-Chief

Samuel Z. Goldhaber, M.D.

Harvard Medical School
and Brigham and Women's Hospital
Boston, Massachusetts

Associate Editor, Europe

Henri Bounameaux, M.D.

University Hospital of Geneva
Geneva, Switzerland

1. *Drug Treatment of Hyperlipidemia*, edited by Basil M. Rifkind
2. *Cardiotonic Drugs: A Clinical Review, Second Edition, Revised and Expanded*, edited by Carl V. Leier
3. *Complications of Coronary Angioplasty*, edited by Alexander J. R. Black, H. Vernon Anderson, and Stephen G. Ellis
4. *Unstable Angina*, edited by John D. Rutherford
5. *Beta-Blockers and Cardiac Arrhythmias*, edited by Prakash C. Deedwania
6. *Exercise and the Heart in Health and Disease*, edited by Roy J. Shephard and Henry S. Miller, Jr.
7. *Cardiopulmonary Physiology in Critical Care*, edited by Steven M. Scharf
8. *Atherosclerotic Cardiovascular Disease, Hemostasis, and Endothelial Function*, edited by Robert Boyer Francis, Jr.
9. *Coronary Heart Disease Prevention*, edited by Frank G. Yanowitz
10. *Thrombolysis and Adjunctive Therapy for Acute Myocardial Infarction*, edited by Eric R. Bates
11. *Stunned Myocardium: Properties, Mechanisms, and Clinical Manifestations*, edited by Robert A. Kloner and Karin Przyklenk
12. *Prevention of Venous Thromboembolism*, edited by Samuel Z. Goldhaber
13. *Silent Myocardial Ischemia and Infarction: Third Edition*, Peter F. Cohn
14. *Congestive Cardiac Failure: Pathophysiology and Treatment*, edited by David B. Barnett, Hubert Pouleur, and Gary S. Francis
15. *Heart Failure: Basic Science and Clinical Aspects*, edited by Judith K. Gwathmey, G. Maurice Briggs, and Paul D. Allen

16. *Coronary Thrombolysis in Perspective: Principles Underlying Conjunctive and Adjunctive Therapy*, edited by Burton E. Sobel and Désiré Collen
17. *Cardiovascular Disease in the Elderly Patient*, edited by Donald D. Tresch and Wilbert S. Aronow
18. *Systemic Cardiac Embolism*, edited by Michael D. Ezekowitz
19. *Low-Molecular-Weight Heparins in Prophylaxis and Therapy of Thromboembolic Diseases*, edited by Henri Bounameaux
20. *Valvular Heart Disease*, edited by Muayed Al Zaibag and Carlos M. G. Duran
21. *Implantable Cardioverter-Defibrillators: A Comprehensive Textbook*, edited by N. A. Mark Estes III, Antonis S. Manolis, and Paul J. Wang
22. *Individualized Therapy of Hypertension*, edited by Norman M. Kaplan and C. Venkata S. Ram
23. *Atlas of Coronary Balloon Angioplasty*, Bernhard Meier and Vivek K. Mehan
24. *Lowering Cholesterol in High-Risk Individuals and Populations*, edited by Basil M. Rifkind
25. *Interventional Cardiology: New Techniques and Strategies for Diagnosis and Treatment*, edited by Christopher J. White and Stephen R. Ramee
26. *Molecular Genetics and Gene Therapy of Cardiovascular Diseases*, edited by Stephen C. Mockrin
27. *The Pericardium: A Comprehensive Textbook*, David H. Spodick
28. *Coronary Restenosis: From Genetics to Therapeutics*, edited by Giora Z. Feuerstein
29. *The Endothelium in Clinical Practice: Source and Target of Novel Therapies*, edited by Gabor M. Rubanyi and Victor J. Dzau
30. *Molecular Biology of Cardiovascular Disease*, edited by Andrew R. Marks and Mark B. Taubman
31. *Practical Critical Care in Cardiology*, edited by Zab Mohsenifar and P. K. Shah
32. *Intravascular Ultrasound Imaging in Coronary Artery Disease*, edited by Robert J. Siegel
33. *Saphenous Vein Bypass Graft Disease*, edited by Eric R. Bates and David R. Holmes, Jr.
34. *Exercise and the Heart in Health and Disease: Second Edition, Revised and Expanded,* edited by Roy J. Shephard and Henry S. Miller, Jr.
35. *Cardiovascular Drug Development: Protocol Design and Methodology,* edited by Jeffrey S. Borer and John C. Somberg
36. *Cardiovascular Disease in the Elderly Patient: Second Edition, Revised and Expanded,* edited by Donald D. Tresch and Wilbert S. Aronow
37. *Clinical Neurocardiology,* Louis R. Caplan, J. Willis Hurst, and Mark I. Chimowitz

ADDITIONAL VOLUMES IN PREPARATION

Cardiac Rehabilitation, edited by Nanette Kass Wenger, L. Kent Smith, Erika S. Froelicher, and Pat Comoss

Heparin-Induced Thrombocytopenia, edited by Ted Warkentin and Andreas Greinacher

Clinical Neurocardiology

Louis R. Caplan
Beth Israel Deaconess Medical Center
Boston, Massachusetts

J. Willis Hurst
Emory University School of Medicine
Atlanta, Georgia

Marc I. Chimowitz
Emory University School of Medicine
Atlanta, Georgia

MARCEL DEKKER
Marcel Dekker, Inc. New York • Basel

ISBN: 0-8247-1991-3

This book is printed on acid-free paper.

Headquarters
Marcel Dekker, Inc.
270 Madison Avenue, New York, NY 10016
tel: 212-696-9000; fax: 212-685-4540

Eastern Hemisphere Distribution
Marcel Dekker AG
Hutgasse 4, Postfach 812, CH-4001 Basel, Switzerland
tel: 41-61-261-8482; fax: 41-61-261-8896

World Wide Web
http://www.dekker.com

The publisher offers discounts on this book when ordered in bulk quantities. For more information, write to Special Sales/Professional Marketing at the headquarters address above.

Current printing (last digit):
10 9 8 7 6 5 4 3 2 1

PRINTED IN THE UNITED STATES OF AMERICA

Series Introduction

Ten years after Graham Garratt, the late Executive Vice President and Publisher of Marcel Dekker, Inc., first met with me to discuss my being Editor-in-Chief of the Fundamental and Clinical Cardiology Series, it is a privilege to introduce *Clinical Neurocardiology*. This book is long overdue and much needed by practicing cardiologists and neurologists who dread the complications that can occur in each other's chosen discipline. Graham Garratt and I waited nearly a decade to ask Louis R. Caplan, MD, to coordinate this important undertaking. He responded enthusiastically and, along with J. Willis Hurst, MD and Marc I. Chimowitz, MD, has produced a masterpiece.

Like other practicing cardiologists, I regularly consult neurologists for my own patients before and after cardiac and vascular surgery. *Clinical Neurocardiology* will be within arm's reach as I ponder over especially challenging consultative issues or update myself on the latest trends in these closely intertwined disciplines. This volume of the Fundamental and Clinical Cardiology Series as conceived by Graham Garratt is an impressive achievement, and I am certain that he is looking down and nodding with pride and approval.

Samuel Z. Goldhaber

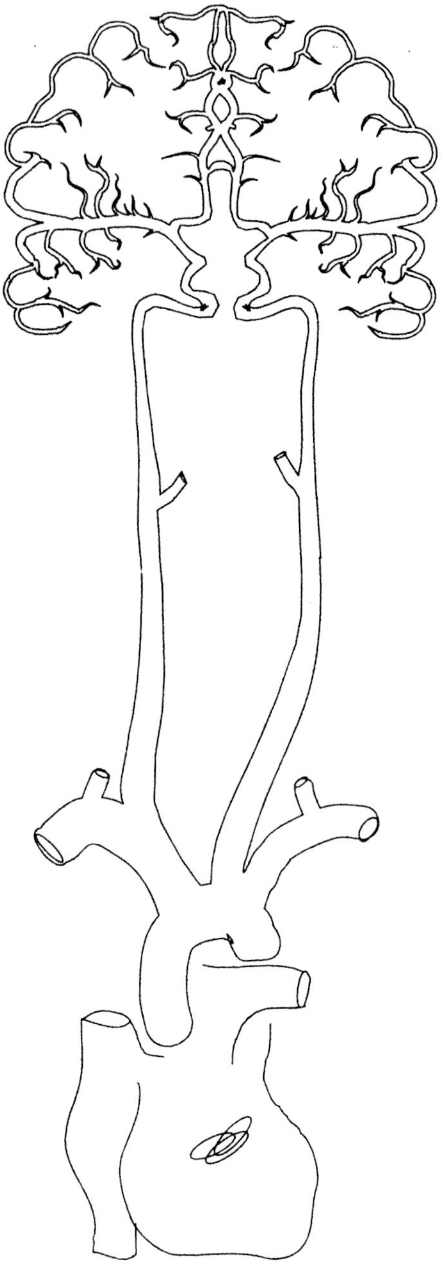

Drawing by Juan R. Sanchez-Ramos, 1999. Reproduced with permission.

Preface

The heart and the brain are arguably the most important organs in the human body. The brain is the organ that makes us what we are. The traits that allow others to recognize and characterize each of us as individuals, including our intelligence, personality, ambition, character, and sense of humor, are all determined by our brains. Intact brain function is necessary for us to move, walk, feel, see, hear, speak, read, and communicate.

The heart is the core, the hub, of the body. The heart is absolutely necessary for life to continue; when our heart dies, we die. The heart's pumping action keeps the other body organs alive. The brain, in turn, exerts some control over cardiac function. Both organs have tentacles that reach the periphery of the body—the blood vessels and the spinal cord and peripheral nervous systems—and carry activity and information to and from all the body's vital regions.

The heart and brain are so interdependent and interrelated that it is impossible to practice first-rate neurology or cardiology without a working knowledge of each specialty. Neurological complications of cardiac disease and cardiac procedures and operations—strokes, seizures, coma, paralysis—are probably among the most feared patient outcomes for cardiologists. Cardiologists are often asked to consult on patients with strokes and neurological diseases to determine the presence of heart abnormalities and their relation to the neurological condition.

This book is aimed at cardiologists, internists, and neurologists. We intend the book to serve them as a practical, clinical, and relatively concise source of information for them about the neurological and cardiological abnormalities relevant to their practices. At present there is no other handy reference source that serves this function.

The first three chapters consider neurological findings in patients with heart disease. Chapter 1 explores the neurology of cardiac arrest and circulatory failure. Coma and brain damage guide prognosis and heavily determine the treatment strategies that cardiologists will choose for these patients. Chapter 2 considers brain embolism. Newer diagnostic techniques such as emboli monitoring using transcranial Doppler ultrasound show that an ever-increasing percentage of brain infarcts are due to embolism from the heart, aorta, and proximal cervicocranial arteries. The effects of various toxic and metabolic disorders that cause neurological symptoms in patients with cardiac disease are discussed in Chapter 3, which also includes a discussion of the neurological side effects of drugs commonly given to cardiac patients.

The next two chapters consider neurological complications of cardiac surgery and cardiac procedures. Unfortunately, neurological symptoms and signs often follow cardiac interventions. The causes and outcomes of neurological complications and their prevention and treatment are considered in these chapters.

Finally, Chapters 6 and 7 describe the cardiac and cardiovascular as well as the neurological findings in patients whose primary disorders are neurological. Chapter 6 discusses the management of patients who have both coronary artery and carotid artery disease. Since occlusive vascular disease is one of the most common causes of both brain disease and heart disease, the topic of coexistent coronary and cerebrovascular disease is an important issue for both cardiologists and neurologists. Chapter 7 describes the cardiac lesions and cardiac findings as well as the common neurological findings in patients with primary neurological diseases such as stroke, muscle dystrophy, hereditary ataxias, etc., and the cardiac and cardiovascular findings in patients with disorders that affect both the heart and the nervous system.

Central nervous system and muscle diseases often have an associated cardiopathy. Cardiologists are frequently asked to consult on patients with a wide variety of neurological conditions, and neurologists often consult on patients with various systemic and cardiac disorders. Many of the neurological diseases are rare. In some patients, a systemic condition such as an endocrinopathy affects both the heart and nervous system. In other patients, the cardiac and neurological conditions are concurrent but not causally related and are each a part of a genetically mediated condition—e.g., a mitochondrial disorder.

Associated cardiac findings are important and often determine prognosis. There is now no ready source of information available for cardiologists, neurologists, or other physicians to look up the cardiac and neurological findings in these diseases, many of which will be unfamiliar to them. We do not discuss hypertension, cerebrovascular disease, or stroke diagnosis or management in any depth in this book, since excellent texts are available on these vast subjects.

The two principal neurologist authors, Drs. Caplan and Chimowitz, each have had, for a very long time, a major interest in both stroke and heart disease. Dr. Caplan is board-certified in internal medicine as well as neurology. In medical school he was a disciple of Drs. Barney Marriott and Leonard Sherlis. He was fortunate at the Beth Israel Deaconess Medical Center and the New England Medical Center in Boston and at the Michael Reese Hospital in Chicago to have worked closely with many outstanding cardiologists, including Paul Zoll, Stafford Cohen, George Kurland, Ivan D'Cruz, Herb Levine, Deeb Salem, Nat Pandian, Mark Estes, Paul Wang, Earl Silber, and Arnold Pick. Dr. Marc Chimowitz was the director of the stroke service at the University of Michigan and now serves in that capacity at Emory University in Atlanta. He developed an interest in heart–brain interactions when, as an intern, he spent 2 months on Professor Christiaan Barnard's cardiac surgery service at the Groote Schur Hospital in Cape Town, South Africa. During his fellowship in stroke at the Cleveland Clinic, he had extensive experience with patients who had cardiac procedures and cardiac surgery. He was fortunate to have been guided by Drs. Tony Furlan and Cathy Sila, neurologists at the Cleveland Clinic who have written extensively on cardiac neurology.

Drs. Caplan and Chimowitz have had extensive experience in writing about stroke and in writing for cardiologists and internists. They enlisted the help of Dr. J. Willis Hurst of Emory University to write about the cardiac findings in patients with primary neurological diseases. Dr. Hurst has always had a wide interest in general internal medicine, including neurology as well as cardiology. His writings are very well known to cardiologists throughout the world. Dr. Hurst has read and commented on all the chapters in this book, which represents the combined experience of the three authors.

We owe thanks to a great many individuals who helped with this book. In Boston, Pauline Dawley was instrumental in ensuring that the references, permissions, and final drafts were prepared speedily and accurately. Susan Marshall and Carol Miller played similar roles in Atlanta. Dr. Rick Schiefe, a neuropharmacologist, reviewed Chapter 3 and offered sage advise. Dr. Roy Freeman, an expert on the autonomic nervous system, reviewed Chapter 7 and offered a number of suggestions. Dr. Frank Sellke, a cardiac surgeon, critiqued Chapter 4. A number of colleagues from the neurology and cardiac services at the Beth Israel Deaconess Medical Center, the New England Medical Center, and Emory University were very helpful in consulting on aspects of the first three chapters and Chapter 7.

Louis R. Caplan
J. Willis Hurst
Marc I. Chimowitz

Contents

1

Cardiac Arrest and Other Hypoxic-Ischemic Insults

BACKGROUND

Sudden loss of the pumping capabilities of the heart is a very common cause of death and an important cause of loss of brain functions. Sudden cardiac death is the leading cause of mortality among middle-aged men. In the United States about 400,000 individuals have sudden cardiac arrests each year, and sudden cardiac death is a major medical and public health problem throughout the world [1–3].

At the time of resuscitation of patients who have had cardiac arrest, ventricular fibrillation is the most common rhythm found, followed by asystole and electromechanical dissociation [3]. Coronary artery atherosclerosis is the predominant pathology leading to the arrhythmias, but younger patients often have hypertrophic cardiomyopathy and congenital anomalies. The etiology of cardiac arrest in many patients remains unexplained even after necropsy.

The ancients tried to resuscitate the dead by physical stimulation, warming, and blowing air into the mouth [2,4]. In the middle of the 18th century, Tossach described the case of a man resuscitated by mouth-to-mouth ventilation, and by the beginning of the 19th century physicians had conceived of using electric shocks to treat abnormal hearts [4]. In 1947, Beck and colleagues reported successful cardiac defibrillation at thoracotomy [5], and 9 years later Paul Zoll and his colleagues at the Beth Israel Hospital in Boston reported the first successful termination of ventricular fibrillation by an externally applied electrical countershock [6]. Dr. Zoll was an esteemed colleague of one of the authors (L.R.C.) when he was a junior staff neurologist; contact with Paul Zoll stimulated an intense interest in cardiac arrest and its neurologic sequellae. In 1958 Safar et al. popularized the present method of mouth-to-mouth respiratory resuscitation [7], and Kouwenhoven, Jude, and Knickerbocker at Johns Hopkins in 1960 described the now popular method of closed-chest cardiac massage [8]. The next year, Safar and colleagues described the currently used method of cardiopulmonary resuscitation (CPR), which combines cardiac massage with mouth-to-mouth respiratory resuscitation [9].

During the last three decades, there have been few important advances in CPR methodology. Attempts at out-of-hospital resuscitation of patients who have had cardiac arrests are now quite commonplace, and many urban centers in the United States and Europe have trained paramedic teams and systems to manage such emergencies. Some communities have attempted to educate bystanders about the initiation of CPR. In-hospital cardiac arrests are an extremely common occurrence and nearly all hospitals have code protocols and training for management of this potentially mortal event. Table 1 shows data from some large studies of out-of-hospital CPR efforts [10–17], and Table 2 contains data from in-hospital resuscitations [18–21]. About one in five out-of-hospital CPR efforts results in survival until hospitalization, but less than one patient in 10 (9%) survives hospitalization.

About twice as many patients who have CPR after in-hospital cardiac arrests survive hospitalization, compared with those resuscitated outside of hospitals. Survival is better when patients are young and have ventricular fibrillation as the cardiac rhythm when first examined, when the arrests are witnessed, and when resuscitative efforts are begun quickly by bystanders [22], paramedics, or physicians. Long-term survival from prehospital or in-hospital cardiac arrests is complex and depends on the age and premorbid health of the patients, the nature and severity of their cardiac and other medical diseases, further complications during the hospitalization, the recurrence of cardiac arrest [1,2,23], and the time of the initiation of CPR and the length of time taken for successful resuscitation.

Few reports discuss in depth the neurological sequelae of the patients who have been successfully resuscitated from cardiac arrest. Many patients are comatose or stuporous when first examined after in-hospital CPR. Alertness and neurological status are important prognostic factors in predicting recovery. Taffet et al. commented that mental function was often severely impaired in survivors, especially in the elderly [20]. About half of the patients in their study under age 70 attained a level at which they were oriented, but only one in five of those 70 or over was ever oriented to person after CPR [20]. Most of the patients with poor neurological survival died in the hospital.

In another study, among 117 patients admitted to a coronary care unit after

Table 1 Large Out-of-Hospital Cardiac Arrest Series

Reference	Area	Years	Arrests	Admit to hospitals	Discharged alive
Longstreth [10]	Seattle	1983–88	3029	860 (28%)	363 (12%)
Becker [11]	Chicago	1987	3221	296 (9%)	55 (2%)
Eisenberg [12]	Seattle	1976–81	1567	557 (36%)	302 (19%)
Eisenberg [13]	Israel	1984–85	3594	531 (15%)	198 (7%)
Cummins [14]	Seattle	1976–83	2043	no data	373 (18%)
Goldstein [15]	Michigan	1975–82	3849	699 (18%)	274 (7%)
Troiano [16]	Milwaukee	1983–85	1660	421 (25%)	138 (8%)
Weaver [17]	Seattle	1984–86	1287	181 (14%)	102 (8%)
Totals			19,651	3545/17,608 (20%)	1805 (9%)

Table 2 In-Hospital CPR Series

Reference	Area	Years	Patients	Successful CPR	Discharged alive
Murphy [18]	Boston[a]	1977–87	259	92 (36%)	17 (6.5%)
Bedell [19]	Boston	1981–82	294	128 (44%)	41 (14%)
Taffet [20]	Houston[b]	1984–85	329 pts (399 CPRs)	161 CPRs (40%)	22 (7%)
Tunstall-Pedoe [21]	U.K.	1985	2838	1277 (45%)	580 (20%)
Totals			3720 pts	1658 (44%)	660 (18%)

[a] Elderly patients (>70 yrs).
[b] Male Veterans Administration Hospital Patients.

successful CPR, four of the 17 (24%) patients who were alert during the first hospital examination died, compared to 60 deaths among the 100 (60%) patients who had reduced levels of consciousness [24]. Among the 17 patients in this series who were alive and were examined 3-1/2 years after cardiac arrest, two were neurologically normal, six were mildly demented, and eight were severely demented, three of whom also had other neurological disabilities; one other patient was aphasic and had a hemiparesis [25]. Troiano and colleagues were able to follow the neurological outcome of 128/138 patients who were successfully resuscitated [16]. Moderate neurological disability was present in 28 (22%); 21 (16%) were severely disabled and dependent, and 7(5%) were left in a persistent vegetative state [16].

Clearly, advances in CPR techniques; widespread dissemination of information to medical, paramedical, and lay persons; and the increasing availability of trained personnel and facilities within many communities, have saved innumerable lives. Unfortunately, in some patients the heart is able to recover from ischemia only to beat within an individual whose brain has been irreversibly damaged by the ischemic-anoxic insult suffered during the period of circulatory failure. Machines are now sometimes able to prolong life indefinitely in patients with severe brain damage. Many such patients survive in a persistent vegetative state even after the machines are disconnected. Other patients survive with varying degrees of loss of mental functions and other neurological handicaps.

Nearly all physicians have experienced the tragedy of performing successful CPR, only to have saved a now brainless soul whose survival is only vegetative. Long-term survival in a senseless or demented state is a disaster for the family and friends of the survivor, and creates untold and incalculable costs to the community in dollars, utilization of resources, and heartache.

The remainder of this chapter will be devoted to describing the neurologic sequelae of cardiac arrest and other disorders that cause general systemic hypoperfusion or anoxia, including the pathology and pathophysiology of the central nervous system damage (so-called hypoxic-ischemic encephalopathy), the resulting clinical syndromes and their neurological findings, the prognostic utility of various neurologic signs at various times after cardiac arrest, the utility of neurological tests for prognostication, and the effects of various treatments on neurologic recovery [26,27].

PATHOPHYSIOLOGY AND PATHOLOGY OF BRAIN DAMAGE

The brain depends for survival on an almost continuous supply of oxygen-rich blood carrying glucose. Brain damage invariably follows any prolonged or severe loss of adequate brain circulation and any persistent period of severe hypoxia.

Because these two conditions, hypoperfusion and hypoxia, almost invariably coexist to some degree, the ensuing brain damage is often called hypoxic-ischemic encephalopathy. Prolonged severe hypoxia, as occurs in carbon monoxide poisoning, strangulation, and drowning, eventually causes cardiac damage and hypotension. Cardiac arrest or severe hypotension and shock causes respiratory insufficiency and secondary hypoxemia. The severity and distribution of hypoxic-ischemic damage depends heavily on the relative ratio of hypoxia to ischemia, and the severity and duration of the hypoxia and of the hypoperfusion [26]. Cardiac arrest produces a different distribution of brain lesions than systemic hypotension.

The pathology of ischemic cell damage is distinctive. Hypoxic-ischemic neurons are usually shrunken; the nuclei are pyknotic and contain course nuclear chromatin; the cytoplasm is typically eosinophilic [27–29]. Although much of the effect of severe hypoxic-ischemic insults are detectable immediately in necropsied brains, some pathological changes develop later, even after circulation and adequate respirations have been restored. For example, microvascular damage with failure of perfusion of regions of brain tissue (the so-called no-reflow phenomenon [30]) can develop after the circulation is restored, and causes persistent regional hypoperfusion. Arterioles and capillaries are plugged by endothelial cell fragments, swollen endothelial cells, polymorphonuclear leukocytes adherent to endothelial cells, platelet-fibrin clumps, and microthrombi [28,30,31]. Brain areas such as the hippocampus [32], cerebral white matter [33,34], and basal ganglia [33–35] can show delayed neuronal necrosis. Controversy still surrounds whether these delayed changes are set in motion by the hypoxic-ischemic insult which initiates a self-perpetuating chain of events that takes time to mature, or restitution of oxygenation and blood flow somehow promote some of the changes. ''Reperfusion injury'' is a theoretical hypothesis [36,37], but the evidence that reperfusion actually causes brain damage in humans is very scanty.

In areas of ischemia there is breakdown of cell membrane functions with intracellular potassium ion release into the interstitial extracellular space and calcium influx into the cells. This process could facilitate further cell death. Edema [38], lactic acid, glutamate, and other ''excitotoxic'' substances [39] and free radicals can be generated by the ischemic process and lead to further cell death [28]. Reperfusion could theoretically (1) enhance ischemic brain damage by precipitating hemorrhages from damaged capillaries; (2) promote edema because of deficient endothelial cell membrane and capillary functions; (3) bring particles such as platelet-fibrin aggregates, cholesterol chrystals, and erythrocyte-fibrin thrombi that had formed during slowed circulation into the region; (4) carry metabolic substrates such as glucose and oxygen into the region (these could be metabolized to lactate and free oxygen radicals which are potentially toxic to neurons); and (5) cause increased circulation of potentially toxic chemicals and ions such as glutamate, calcium, potassium, excitotoxins, and free radicals within ischemic zones [28]. Until further proof of the validity of the concept of "reperfusion injury," doctors should continue to aggressively and rapidly try to restore the circulation and oxygenation in patients with cardiac and circulatory arrest and failure.

Clinical experience and the results of laboratory experiments in animals have shown convincingly that certain brain regions are more susceptible than others to injury from hypoxia and ischemia. This selective vulnerability explains why a systemic insult (hypoxia and ischemia) injures some brain cells more than others. The most vulnerable neurons are those in the cerebral cortex, especially in the middle laminae; pyramidal neurons in the CA1 zone of the hippocampus; neurons in portions of the amygdaloid nucleus; Purkinje cells in the cerebellar cortex; neurons in the caudate nucleus, putamen, globus pallidus, motor nuclei in the brainstem; and neurons in the anterior, dorsomedial, and pulvinar thalamic nuclei [27].

The pattern and distribution of injury also depend on the anatomy of the arterial circulation. Brain regions between arterial territories (so-called border zone, or watershed, regions) show more injury than brain areas in the heart of the major feeding brain arteries. Selective vulnerability and circulatory anatomy plus differential responses to hypoxia and ischemia explain the various patterns of brain damage seen in patients with cardiac arrest and severe hypoxia. The most common patterns are listed in Table 3. The various regions of involvement are also illustrated in Figure 1. A knowledge of the anatomical patterns helps clinicians understand the clinical syndromes and also the utility of some of the investigations used in evaluating patients with hypoxic-ischemic encephalopathy.

TABLE 3 Common Patterns of Hypoxic-Ischemic Injury and Their Causes

1. Diffuse cerebral cortical injury sometimes with laminar necrosis of the middle cortical layers; cardiac arrest or prolonged hypotension
2. Ischemic damage to border zone regions especially between the middle and posterior cerebral artery territories and between the anterior and middle cerebral artery territories; cardiac arrest or prolonged hypotension [40–43]
3. Necrosis of hippocampal neurons especially in the CA1 zone; cardiac arrest or prolonged hypotension [32]
4. Necrosis of basal ganglia and thalamic neurons; delayed necrosis of the basal ganglia and cerebral white matter; severe hypoxia, especially strangulation, hanging, carbon monoxide poisoning, drowning; probably more common in young adults [33–35,44]
5. Necrosis of Purkinje cells in the cerebellum; prolonged ischemia [27,45]
6. Necrosis of brainstem motor and tegmental nuclei (especially cranial nerve nuclei, inferior colliculus, vestibular nuclei, and superior olive); sudden severe hypotension in infants, children, and young adults [46,47]

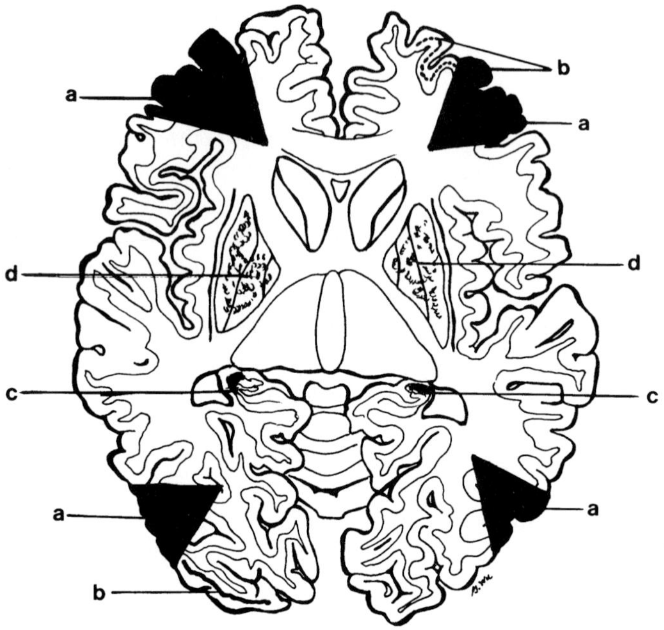

(A)

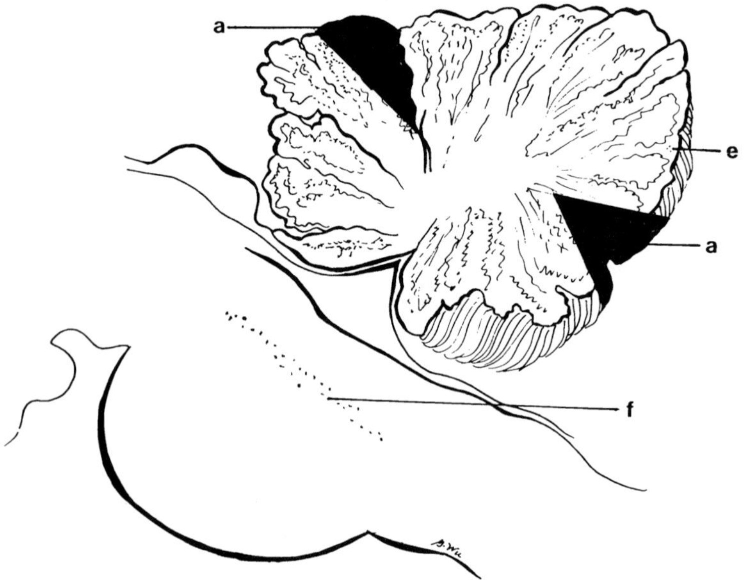

(B)

CLINICAL ABNORMALITIES AND SYNDROMES

Brainstem and Bihemispheral Coma

Consciousness depends upon stimulation of the cerebral hemispheres by neurons within the brainstem tegmentum. Coma occurs after damage to the medial portions of the brainstem tegmentum in the pons and midbrain, or the bilateral cerebral hemispheres. Virtually all patients who have had cardiac arrest have an initial period of coma. When comatose patients are first examined, there are two different patterns of findings, depending on the presence or absence of brainstem reflexes. In patients with severe prolonged hypoxic-anoxic insults, the pupils are dilated, corneal reflexes are absent, and the eyes remain midline and do not move horizontally or vertically to passive head movements (''doll's eyes'' reflex) or react to ice water in the ear canals. Some patients have no spontaneous respirations and must be ventilated mechanically. Spontaneous limb movements, except for low-level decorticate or decerebrate movements, are absent. This state is usually referred to as *brainstem coma* because it indicates injury to brainstem tegmental nuclei. When this state is prolonged, death invariably follows.

Some infants and young children and occasional adults have selective necrosis of their brainstem tegmental nuclei [46,47]. These patients have loss of reflex eye movements; facial, pharyngeal, and tongue weakness; and loss of gag reflex responses. They usually have stiff, immobile limbs and only automatic and autonomic responses to environmental stimuli. Control of respirations may be lost and the pulse and blood pressures may fluctuate widely. This state invariably proves fatal. Imaging may show no cerebral hemispheral abnormalities, and the brainstem may even appear normal on gross inspection at necropsy. Microscopic examination shows selective necrosis of brainstem nuclei.

Some patients with brainstem coma regain their brainstem reflexes and spontaneous respirations and enter a state called *bihemispheral coma*. Other patients have bihemispheral coma when first examined neurologically and have not been recognized to have gone through a stage of brainstem coma. Patients with bihemispheral coma are unresponsive to noise, voice, or bright light. There may be some spontaneous movements of all limbs. The pupils are normal or con-

---

FIG. 1 (A) Drawing of a horizontal section of the cerebrum illustrating common patterns of hypoxic-ischemic damage. (a) Borderzone infarcts; (b) zones of laminar necrosis within the cerebral cortex; (c) hippocampal necrosis; (d) necrosis of nerve cells within the globus pallidus and putamen. (B) Drawing of a sagittal section of the pons and cerebellum showing regions of hypoxic-ischemic damage. (a) Borderzone infarcts; (e) necrosis of Purkinje cells within the cerebellar cortex; (f) necrosis of neurons within the tegmentum of the pons. (Drawings by Gloria Wu, M.D.)

stricted and do react to light. The eyes usually remain in the midline, rove from side to side, or are deviated upward. Passive movements readily elicit horizontal eye movements. Often these "doll's-eyes" movements are hyperactive, indicating lack of cerebral inhibition of the vestibulo-ocular reflex. Vertical eye movements usually can be elicited by flexing and extending the neck. In patients with forced upward eye deviation, it may be difficult to get the eyes to move fully downward on this vertical doll's-eyes maneuver. The gag reflex is usually present. Some patients with bihemispheral coma have their mouths open, and some keep their jaws tightly clenched and "bulldog" down on tubes or sticks placed in their mouths, making it difficult to see the throat or perform the gag reflex. Watching these patients from the foot of the bed shows that they often spontaneously blink, yawn, sneeze, cough, hiccup, protrude their tongue, lick the lips, sigh, and swallow [48]. These spontaneous mouth, face, and tongue movements are mediated through brainstem structures and indicate that the brainstem is working. Coma is due to loss of the normal functions of both cerebral hemispheres.

Spontaneous limb movements and responses to pinch in the limbs vary considerably. Patients who have dysfunction of the corticospinal tracts often have preserved adduction and flexion movements of the shoulders, arms, and wrists. When pinched on either the flexor or extensor surface of the arm, forearm, or hand, they will flex and adduct the arm and shoulder irrespective of the site of stimulation. The flexion response brings the arm into stimuli on the flexor surface. Spontaneous or reactive extension or abducting movements of the arm or forearm, preserved movements of individual fingers, and limb withdrawal from pinch appropriate to the site of stimulation (flexion or adduction when pinched on the extensor surface, and extension or abduction when pinched on the flexor surface, movements which move the upper limb away from the stimulus) show that the corticospinal tracts are preserved and functioning. Similarly, loss of corticospinal tract function leads to extension and adduction of the lower limbs. Flexion and abduction movements, spontaneously or in response to pinch, usually indicate corticospinal tract preservation. The ability to remove or react to pinch with either the same or contralateral arm indicates that the stimulus has been perceived. Use of the arm contralateral to the pinch to ward off the noxious stimulus almost always indicates weakness of the ipsilateral arm. Major asymmetries of motor or sensory function usually mean asymmetrical brain damage.

Patients with bihemispheral coma may remain in a vegetative state poorly responsive to environmental stimuli, or they can become more alert and responsive. A number of clinical patterns of dysfunction can ensue from the bihemispheral coma stage. Figure 2 shows these patterns.

Myoclonic Jerks and Myoclonic Seizures

Some patients with bihemispheral coma have frequent abnormal movements in the form of muscle twitching or jerks of various groups of muscles, referred to

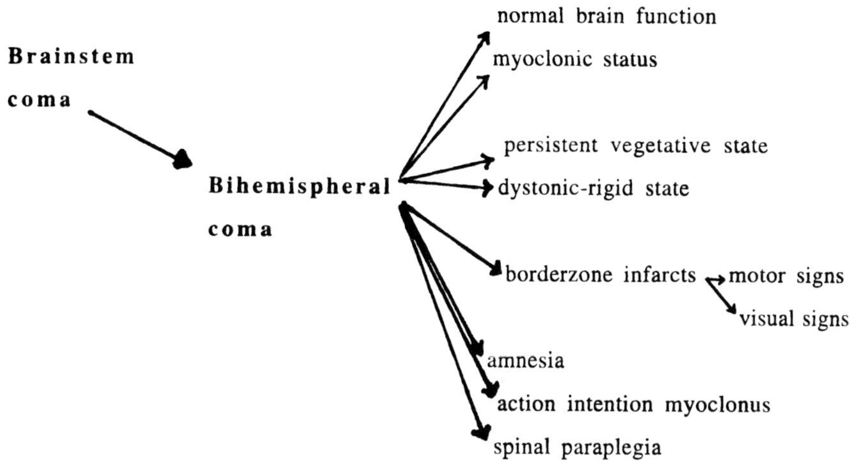

FIG. 2 Clinical patterns of function in patients with hypoxic-ischemic central nervous system injury.

as *myoclonus*. The eyelids, jaw, and facial muscles are often involved and can lead to rhythmic eye opening, jaw clenching, facial grimacing, platysma contractions, and neck movements. The limbs and trunk muscles also jerk. The movements occur spontaneously but are often increased by painful stimuli, insertion of catheters, suctioning, and movement of parts of the body during examinations. In some patients with myoclonic jerks there are also synchronous bilateral generalized jerks which are referred to as *myoclonic seizures*. When the myoclonic jerks and seizures are nearly constant, the disorder has been referred to as *myoclonic status epilepticus*. Myoclonic jerks and myoclonic seizures are found in patients with relatively severe hypoxic-ischemic damage to the cerebral cortex. Usually laminar necrosis of the larger cell layers of the cerebral cortex is present and may be quite diffuse. When myoclonic jerks are widespread and accompanied by frequent myoclonic seizures or status, the prognosis for recovery is dismal [49–51].

Persistent Vegetative State

Vegetative state is a term used to describe patients who awaken from coma and retain reflex functions but show no signs of cognition or meaningful responses to their environments [52–54]. These patients have sleep-wake cycles and preserved brainstem reflexes (oculovestibular, corneal, pupillary, gag, swallowing). The limbs are usually stiff and move spontaneously but do not locate objects accurately or remove painful stimuli such as a pinch. Orofacial movements, sweating, tachycardia, tachypnea, and elevated blood pressure may occur in response to painful stimuli. The eyes usually rove but may seem to fixate transiently on an object or person; the eyes do not show sustained visual pursuit of objects or people. Vegetative patients do not utter words or understandable speech or gesture meaningfully with their limbs, face, or body, and they do not obey commands or show responses to queries; they may emit groans or other noises. The electroencephalograms (EEGs) of these patients usually show low-amplitude, severe delta slowing. Necropsy shows extensive cortical laminar necrosis and infarction [53], sometimes with necrosis of thalamic nuclei [44]. The persistent vegetative state is a manifestation of extensive damage to the cerebral cortex with preservation of the brainstem. Outlook for recovery after months in this state is very poor.

Dystonic, Rigid State

Some patients awaken from bihemispheral coma but have delayed worsening of brain functions and become stiff and immobile. The first reported patients with delayed deterioration after hypoxic-ischemic insults were described by Plum, Posner, and Hain in 1962 [33]. Three of the five patients reported had deterioration after exposure to noxious gases and had predominantly hypoxic injuries. The other two patients worsened after surgery and had both documented hypotension and hypoperfusion, and anoxia [33]. The patients were all in deep coma when first examined after the insult but awakened within 24 hours and resumed relatively normal activities and functions for 4 to 10 days. They then developed cognitive and behavioral abnormalities characterized mostly by apathy, irritability, agitation, restlessness, and confusion. Walking then became quite clumsy and the limbs became rigid and stiff. Outcome varied from full recovery to severe disability to death. Necropsy in the two patients that died showed extensive white matter demyelination in the cerebral hemispheres, and one patient also had cystic necrosis in the medial globus pallidus bilaterally [33].

Subsequent reports have confirmed the existence of a leukoencephalopathy, often with basal ganglionic damage that follows hypoxic-ischemic events [34,35]. The white matter damage involves rather diffuse injury to the white matter that ranges from patchy demyelination to hemorrhagic white matter necrosis [34]. Most reported patients are young and the insult has most often been predominantly hypoxic—e.g., carbon monoxide intoxication, strangulation, drowning, gas inhalation. When initially examined after the insult, the patients were in coma often with loss of muscle tone, quadriparesis, or involuntary movements of the limbs. Most patients who developed severe limb dysfunction with rigidity, abnormal movements, and dystonia never improved after the initial hypoxic-ischemic event, but some have had delayed deterioration as was first reported by Plum et al. [33,34]. The dystonic rigid state is a manifestation of extensive damage to deep subcortical basal gangionic and white matter tracts, usually with relative preservation of the cerebral cortex. The pathological substrate of this syndrome presents a sharp contrast to the cerebral cortex necrosis with usual preservation of subcortical structures found in patients with the persistent vegetative state.

In recent reports, two patients with delayed hypoxic leukoencephalopathy have shown a reduction of arylsulfatase-A activity to $<50\%$ of normal [55,56]. Although this degree of reduction does not ordinarily cause symptoms, hypoxia could cause tissue acidosis, which might potentiate myelin damage. Arylsulfatase-A is a lysosomal enzyme active in the lipid metabolism of myelin. In the presence of local tissue acidosis, this enzyme deficiency could make patients vulnerable to demyelination. Proton MR spectroscopy of the white matter lesions helped to identify one reported patient [56] and might be helpful in evaluating other patients with hypoxic-ischemic ensephalopathies.

Border Zone Infarction

Some patients who have had cardiac arrest or other causes of systemic hypotension and hypoperfusion have discrete zones of infarction located in regions of the cerebrum, cerebellum, and brainstem that are in areas between the usual main supply territories of brain arteries. These regions are usually referred to as border zones, watersheds, or distal fields [40]. The distribution of ischemia in the brain has been compared to damage to a lawn or a farm crop related to disruption of its water supply. Visualize a field fed by three hoses. The hoses are attached to a water supply and a pump. If one of the hoses, the middle one, is blocked and the water supply and pump continue to function as before, then the damage to the field will lie in the direct center of the blocked hose. The amount of water that formerly went into the middle hose would now go into the two lateral hoses which would extend their supply zones medially.

The brain corollary of this instance would be an occluded middle cerebral artery. The infarct would lie in the center of supply of this vessel. Suppose, however, the hoses remained open but there was insufficient water in the tank or the water pressure declined dramatically. Any residual water supply would trickle out of each of the hoses and would supply the center area fed by the individual hoses. The watershed (border zone) between the centers of supply would now be injured. The brain corollary would be damage to the cerebrum in the zones between the supply areas of the middle, anterior, and posterior cerebral arteries, and damage in the cerebellum between the supply areas of the posterior inferior, anterior inferior, and superior cerebellar arteries. This analogy is illustrated in Figure 3.

The most common regions of border zone infarction are in the temporal-parietal-occipital regions between the supply zones of the middle and posterior cerebral arteries and in the frontal lobe in the regions between the anterior and middle cerebral arteries. Cerebellar damage is less common and almost always occurs only in patients who also have important cerebral hemisphere border zone

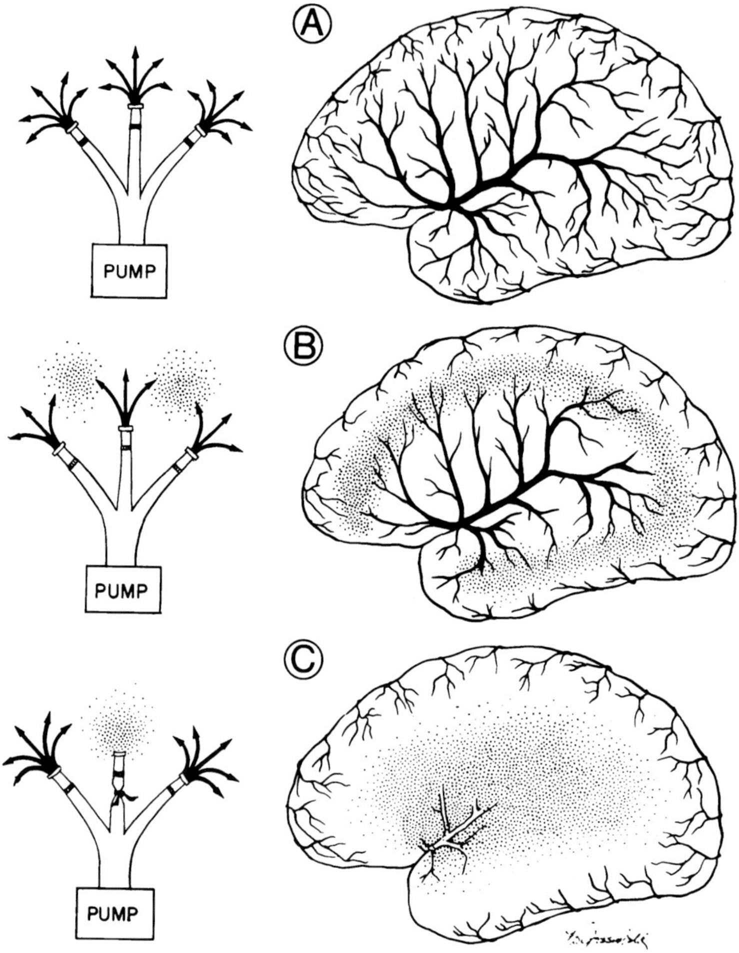

FIG. 3 Cartoon illustrating border zone infarction. The cartoon shows the analogy between a pump system with three hoses drawn in the left figures and the brain and its circulation shown on the right. (A) Normal pump and arterial circulation. (B) Reduced pump pressure causing underperfusion between the hoses and in the arterial border zones (gray speckled regions). (C) Blocked hose. The middle hose is blocked and so is the middle cerebral artery. The resulting underperfusion is in the middle of the hose and the core supply of the middle cerebral artery (gray speckled region). (From Ref. 105.)

infarcts. The pattern of damage is most often a triangular wedge that includes the cortex and subcortex, but in some patients the white matter border zone regions are most involved. Figure 4 illustrates the different patterns of border zone injury. These visual patterns are useful to keep in mind when viewing neuroimaging scans of patients who have had hypoxic-ischemic insults.

Posterior border-zone infarcts in the temporo-parieto-occipital regions between the middle and posterior cerebral artery territories cause predominantly visual abnormalities. Because the calcarine visual cortex is in the heart of the posterior cerebral artery territory and is not included in the infarction, the patients usually do not have unilateral or bilateral hemianopias or frank cortical blindness. Most patients report difficulty seeing clearly, but they often can identify single objects, can read individual letters, and their pupillary reaction to light is normal.

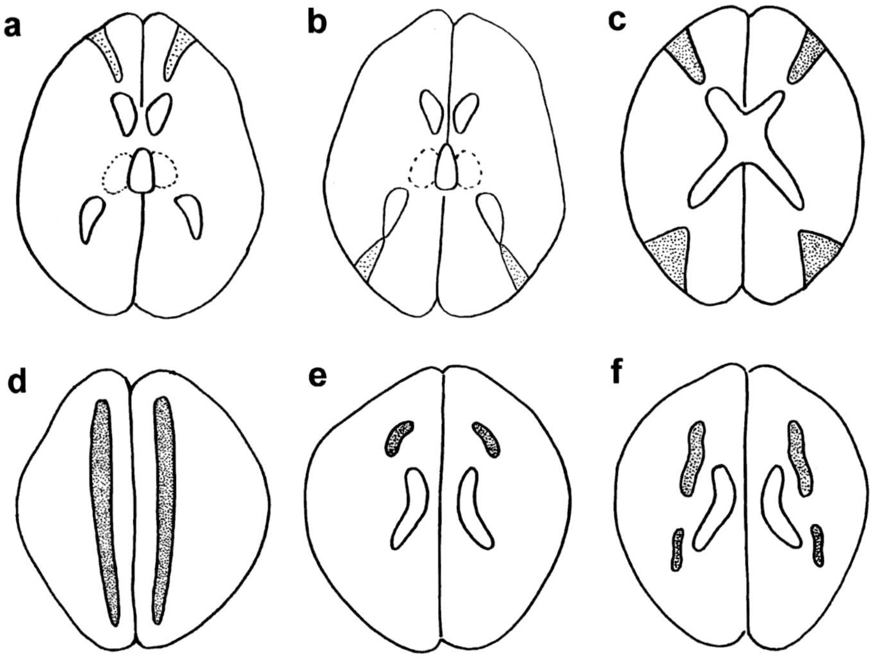

FIG. 4 Montage of cartoons showing various patterns of border zone infarction as they would appear on CT scans. All lesions are bilateral. (a) Anterior border zones between anterior cerebral (ACA) and middle cerebral (MCA) arteries; (b) Posterior border zones between MCAs and posterior cerebral arteries (PCAs); (c) Anterior and posterior border zones; (d) Anterior white matter border zones on a high CT scan cut; (e) White matter anterior border zones on a cut through the lateral ventricles; (f) Anterior and posterior white matter border zones on a lower CT scan cut. (Cartoons drawn by Gloria Wu, M.D.)

The visual abnormalities often conform to what has been called Balint's syndrome after the Hungarian ophthalmologist who first described the findings in 1909 [57,58]. There are three main features of this syndrome: (1) an inability to see and perceive multiple objects at one time (''asimultagnosia''); (2) poor visually directed hand movements (''optical ataxia''); and (3) difficulty directing gaze at desired targets (''optical apraxia''). When patients are shown a picture, or are asked to look at a scene from the window, they will often see only one object or person out of many. In order to see and understand a picture they may have to move the paper or continue to shift gaze. They may also fail to read because they omit letters and words and cannot follow the lines. They have difficulty reaching and grasping objects and cannot accurately focus on objects within their vision [58]. Asking patients to read, describe a picture or a scene, and trace lines or figures with a pencil or a finger are effective screening tests for Balint's syndrome [58].

Anterior border zone lesions in the frontal lobes in territory between the anterior and middle cerebral arteries cause predominantly motor abnormalities. The lesions often involve or undercut the arm regions of the homunculus located within the precentral gyrus and can also extend to fibers which control thigh movements. The syndrome that results has been referred to as the ''man-in-the-barrel'' syndrome [40,59]. Both arms, and sometimes the proximal lower extremities are weak, but the face, hands, and feet are spared. The homunculus portion controlling hand and face movements lies in the heart of the middle cerebral artery supply as does speech while the leg and foot lie in the center of the anterior cerebral artery supply. The findings are reminiscent of a person whose arms and trunk and upper thighs are constrained in a barrel, hence the term man-in-a-barrel syndrome [59]. Some patients whose infarcts extend more toward the frontal pole also have difficulty directing gaze when commanded to and cannot accurately follow moving objects with their eyes [60]. The clinical, imaging, and pathological findings in patients with border zone infarcts are bilateral. Asymmetries may occur when there has been previous arterial occlusions; e.g., hypotension in a patient with an old right carotid artery occlusion could cause more extensive infarction in the right cerebral hemisphere than in the left.

Amnesia

After awakening from coma, some patients have a profound memory disorder. They cannot make new memories (''anterograde amnesia'') and seem to have forgotten memories made in the recent past (''retrograde amnesia'') [61]. Cognitive functions are normal except for the memory loss. In many such patients, the amnesia is temporary and recovers in days, weeks, or a few months [62]. In other patients, the memory deficit persists. At times the loss of memory is patchy and can be specific for some categories of information [63] or for some time periods.

A patient may be completely unable to recall events that occurred during the single past year but have no difficulty remembering events from other time periods. The amnesia that follows hypoxic-ischemic injuries is most likely attributable to the selective vulnerability of the hippocampus and amygdaloid nucleus [32].

Action Myoclonus

In 1963, Lance and Adams described a novel syndrome characterized mostly by clumsiness, ataxia, and abnormal limb movements that followed recovery from hypoxic-ischemic coma [45]. The distinctive feature of this syndrome is involuntary limb movements that the authors dubbed "action myoclonus." When patients reached for objects, or otherwise used their arms, the action would be interrupted by jerking, involuntary movements. The movements were often coarse and chaotic. At times the limb jerks could also be brought on by startle or unexpected noises. Voluntary movements were slow, irregularly halted, and unpredictably varied in force and direction. Patients were unable to eat, dress, write, or perform any fine hand movements because of the jerks and cerebellar-type incoordination and intention tremor. Jerking movements were also present in the lower limbs and abdominal muscles. Anticonvulsants and alcohol sometimes reduced the involuntary myoclonic jerks. During standing and walking, the legs would buckle and jerk. Gait ataxia made it nearly impossible for patients to walk alone. Dysarthria was another prominent finding. None of the patients described by Lance and Adams died, so the neuropathology underlying this syndrome is not known. No subsequent reports have clarified the anatomic basis for the findings. Most likely, ischemic damage to cerebellar Purkinje cells and various thalamic neurons is responsible for this unusual but characteristic syndrome.

Spinal Paraplegia

Occasional patients have recovered from coma without obvious cerebral damage but instead have paraplegia related to hypoxic-ischemic damage to the spinal cord [62,64]. The most vulnerable spinal regions are the upper and lower thoracic and lumbar spinal cord segments. The cervical cord is usually not involved, so the arms function normally despite severe weakness of the lower limbs. The localization of the spinal cord ischemic necrosis relates to the anatomy of the arterial supply of the spinal cord. Although there are arteries from each side that feed into the paired posterior spinal arteries at each spinal segment, the segmental arteries that supply the single unpaired midline anterior spinal artery originate at variable levels and one supply artery can be mostly responsible for nourishing four or five segments.

The largest and most well known artery, the artery of Adamkiewicz, originates anywhere between the ninth thoracic and the second lumbar segment and

ments such as blinking, yawning, coughing, sneezing, gagging, and swallowing utilize brainstem reflex functions. The presence of these movements indicates preservation of brainstem functioning.

In the series of Snyder et al. [68], all patients who at 3 hours after cardiopulmonary arrest had no corneal reflexes or absent pupillary light reflexes died [68]. In that series, by 6 hours, no survivors had absence of the three brainstem reflexes studied (pupillary light response, corneal reflex, and reflex eye movements) [68]. By 24 to 48 hours only three of 25 survivors (12%) had any abnormality of brainstem reflexes [68]. In another series 52 of 210 (25%) patients who had hypoxic-ischemic coma had absent pupillary light reflex when first examined, and none of the 52 had a final outcome better than severe disability [66].

The size of the pupils during the initial hours after the insult is another useful prognostic indicator [65]. The pupil diameter widens and light responses are lost within a few minutes of cardiac arrest. In one series, cardiac resuscitation was more successful in patients who had persistently constricted pupils from the onset of resuscitation or in those in whom the pupils were constricted after initial pupillary dilatation [74]. Pupillary dilatation throughout resuscitation carried a poor prognosis in this series [74]. Drugs used during resuscitation, especially catecholamines and atropine, can affect pupillary size, so clinicians should be cautious about using pupillary size as a prognostic sign in patients who have received drugs that affect pupillary diameter. Persistent dilatation of the pupils is of course an ominous sign.

The depth of coma is another important early indicator during the first hours after cardiac arrest. Deep coma usually means either extensive brainstem dysfunction or injury to the cerebral hemispheres bilaterally. In the great majority of adults, when the hypoxic-ischemic insult is severe enough to injure the brainstem and cause deep coma and loss of brainstem reflexes, the cerebral hemispheres are even more severely damaged. Remember that structures in the cerebrum are more vulnerable to hypoxia than brainstem structures.

During the early hours, analysis of spontaneous movements of the limbs and the motor responses of the limbs to sensory stimuli is useful in prognosis. No movement of flaccid limbs even after pinching is an unfavorable sign. The presence of only automatic decorticate (flexion of the upper limbs and extension of the lower limbs) or decerebrate (extension of the upper and lower limbs) responses to pinch or other painful stimuli also is an unfavorable sign for survival and good recovery. Spontaneous varied limb movements and normal withdrawal of limbs in response to pain is a favorable sign.

The presence of frequent myoclonic movements is also a useful prognostic indicator during the first hours after resuscitation. Sudden jerks of the limbs, face, jaw, eyelids, and limbs are common after cardiac arrest [49–51]. The jerks are often bilateral and synchronous and can be accompanied by upward movement of the eyes and twitching of the eyelids. The jerks are often precipitated by touch, tracheal suctioning, insertion of catheters, or noise. They can also be precipitated by a loud clap. Three studies have shown that frequent myoclonic jerks (''myoclonic status'') predicts nonsurvival or at best a persistent vegetative state [49–51].

In one series, among 114 patients who survived cardiac arrest for at least 24 hours, 50 (44%) had either myoclonus (40; 35%), seizures (41; 36%), or both myoclonus and seizures (31; 27%) [51]. Among the 50 with myoclonus or seizures, only 9 (18%) survived hospitalization. Seizures without myoclonus did not predict a bad outcome [51]. In another large series, 40 of 107 (37%) who failed to awaken quickly after cardiac arrest had myoclonic status [50]. All 40 had either no motor response to pain or abnormal posturing, but only eight had any abnormal brainstem reflexes. None of the patients with myoclonic status awakened, improved in motor responses, or survived hospitalization [50]. In a smaller series, nine patients with myoclonic status died [49]. At necropsy, they had extensive necrosis in all lobes of the cerebral cortex, especially the large cell laminae, and extensive hippocampal and thalamic damage [49]. Myoclonic status implies extensive cerebral cortical injury incompatible with good recovery.

The prognostic importance of seizures was also analyzed by Roine among 155 patients who survived out-of-hospital cardiac arrest in Helsinki [2]. Seizures during the first 24 hours were not very helpful in prognosis since 53% of patients who had seizures during the first day survived, compared to 70% survivors among those who had no first-day seizures. However, seizures after the first day indicated a poor outlook because only three of 15 (20%) patients with seizures after the first day recovered consciousness, and only one (7%) lived for 1 year [2]. Status epilepticus at any time after cardiac arrest was a dire sign since all nine patients with epileptic status died [2].

After the patient has survived the first 24 hours, prognostic indicators are somewhat different during the next few days. Absence of the normal brainstem pupillary, corneal, oculovestibular, and pharyngeal reflexes at 24 hours indicates a poor prognosis. Persistent brainstem dysfunction means brainstem and severe hemispheral damage because the hemispheres are almost always more damaged than the brainstem reflexes. Most patients who will eventually survive, at 24 hours have bihemispheral coma or have become alert. The duration and depth of coma is probably the most important prognostic indicator during the first days. Prolonged bihemispheral coma is a poor prognostic indicator. In one series, day 2 was the most common time for patients to emerge from coma, and most patients who would survive awakened by the end of day 2 [67]. Only 2/27 (7%) in deep coma through day 2 survived. In another series no patient in postanoxic coma after the third day survived [70]. In another series, five of 12 (42%) patients with good outcome remained in coma for 2 days or more, but all but one of the 12 patients awakened and reached their best level of function within the first week after resuscitation [75].

Eye opening, eye movements, and motor responses are also useful prognostic indicators during the first few days. By the end of the first day, the absence of spontaneous eye opening indicates a poor prognosis. Most patients who will have a good recovery begin to open their eyes and have at least intermittent visual fixation movements. However, the presence of eye opening does not always indicate a good outcome. In one large series, spontaneous eye opening was often seen by 48 hours in patients with both good and bad outcomes [75]. Persistence of roving eye movements without visual fixation usually means severe bilateral cerebral hemispheral damage and indicates a poor outcome. Sustained upgaze also carries a poor prognosis [76]. The absence of withdrawal limb movements when painful stimuli are given is also a sign of a poor prognosis as is the retained presence of obligatory reflex decorticate or decerebrate posturing. Most patients who will have good recovery begin to obey commands during the first few days.

The results of some series have found that the score on the Glasgow Coma Scale (GCS) is a very good predictor of prognosis. The GCS yields a score of 3 (worst) to 15 (best), with five points each scored for each of three simple patient responses to various stimuli: eye opening, best verbal response, and best motor response [77]. In one reported series the neurological outcome was accurately predicted 2 days after out-of-hospital cardiac arrest using the GCS with two cutoff points—4 or less, and 10 or higher [77]. A GCS of 3 or 4 after 2 days predicted permanent unconsciousness in all but one of 54 patients [78]. In another series, the GCS during the first 24 hours ranged between 3 and 14 in patients with good outcome and was between 3 and 9 in those who had poor outcomes [75]. Seven of nine patients with a GCS > 8 at 48 hours had good outcomes, but all 20 patients with a GCS of <5 at 48 hours had poor outcomes [75].

Caution must always be used in prognostication even when prolonged coma or a persistent vegetative state is present. Occasional patients improve dramatically despite long-term unresponsiveness [79].

Imaging, Electrophysiologic, and Biochemical Investigations

Unfortunately, investigations have added little to information about neurological recovery gained from the clinical neurological examination. I agree fully with Wijdicks, who stated, "Many clinicians believe that further diagnostic assessment of acute anoxic ischemic coma provides little benefit for prognostication and adds nothing more to a detailed neurological examination" [65].

Brain Imaging

There are scanty data regarding the results of computed tomography (CT) or magnetic resonance imaging (MRI) performed during the acute period after cardiac arrest. Many patients are too unstable to be transported to the scanners. Kjos et al. studied early CT findings in 10 patients [80]. Nine of the patients had some evidence of diffuse cerebral edema and six patients had poor discrimination between the gray and white matter [80]. Watershed infarcts in the cerebrum and cerebellum and bilateral basal ganglia and thalamic hypodensities are also found in some patients. Diffuse mass effect with obliteration of basal cisterns has been described but is rare [81]. In some patients, brain edema and discrete infarcts are seen after several days [65].

Roine analyzed MRI findings among 155 patients who were resuscitated after out-of-hospital cardiac arrest and compared the findings with 88 controls [2,82]. Brain infarcts were more common after cardiac arrest but the difference was significant only for deep infarcts; 25% had cortical infarcts, 14% cerebral watershed infarcts, 21% deep cerebral infarcts, and 4% had deep watershed infarcts. Infarcts and multiple infarcts were more common in the resuscitated group [2,82]. Two patients had diffuse hypointensity of the cerebral white matter. Severe edema on MRI or CT scans was a dire prognostic sign [2]. Repeated MRI examinations during the course of patients with severe neurological deficits may show high signal intensity cortical lesions compatible with laminar necrosis [83].

Single-photon emission computed tomography can show changes in cerebral blood flow after cardiac arrest but the changes are quite nonspecific. In one study regional blood flow was almost invariably abnormal after cardiac arrest [2]. The commonest abnormality was hypoperfusion in the frontal lobes. Regional blood flow improved over time in some patients but often remained abnormal. There was no consistent correlation between blood flow and outcome [2].

Electrophysiologic Brain Studies

Electroencephalography (EEG) was the first investigation available to study patients with global brain ischemia. In general, the degree of rhythm slowing does correlate with the severity of cerebral damage. However, in the 1970s a number of investigators began to report that some comatose patients had 9 to 12-Hz rhythmic activity (alpha rhythms) that had previously been generally correlated with wakefulness [84,85]. In normal awake individuals alpha rhythms are altered by sensory input, eye opening, and other stimuli but in patients with alpha-coma, the alpha rhythms were transient and not responsive to stimuli [84,85].

EEG patterns in patients with hypoxic-ischemic encephalopathy characteristic of increasing severity of brain damage are: diffuse slowing; frontal intermittent severe delta slowing; frequent spikes, especially followed by suppression of the background rhythm; nonreactive rhythms, including transient alpha activity; very low voltage activity; and absence of activity. Isoelectric EEGs with no definite brain activity reflect irreversible damage and brain death in the absence of hypothermia or severe drug intoxications [2]. Table 5 lists the classification most commonly used to describe electroencephalograms in patients with hypoxic-ischemic encephalopathy. This classification is based on a 1965 report by Hockaday

TABLE 5 EEG Classification of Patients with Hypoxic-Ischemic Encephalopathy

EEG class		Outcome prognosis
Grade I	Normal reactive alpha activity; may contain scattered theta	Excellent prognosis
Grade II	Dominant theta and delta rhythms; some reactive alpha	Uncertain prognosis[a]
Grade III	Dominant delta and theta rhythms; no normal alpha	Uncertain prognosis[a]
Grade IV	Nonreactive alpha (alpha-coma) or periodic epileptiform discharges or burst suppression pattern	Poor prognosis
Grade V	Isoelectric, flat EEG	Incompatible with survival[b]

[a] Compatible with survival but unpredictable.
[b] In the absence of severe hypothermia, or hypotension, or high levels of sedative or intoxicating drugs.
Source: Ref. 86.

and colleagues [86]. The classification is reliable in the best (grade I) and worst (grades IV and grade V) grades. The prognosis in patients with these grades of electroencephalograms is usually obvious from the clinical findings. The bulk of patients in whom the prognosis is less clear clinically have grade II and III EEGs in which the prognosis is indeterminate. In summary, the EEG is most useful in confirming a poor clinical state and identifying seizure activity not evident clinically. Recognition of seizure activity is an indication to use anticonvulsant drugs.

Evoked response determinations may have more prognostic utility than standard EEGs. Evoked responses are measured by subtracting the baseline EEG activity from activity after a sensory (visual, auditory, or somatosensory) stimulus. Auditory stimuli are transmitted through the auditory nerves, through the brainstem, to the medial geniculate body of the thalamus, to the auditory cortex in the temporal lobes. Visual stimuli are transmitted through the optic nerves to the lateral geniculate body of the thalamus to the occipital lobe visual cortex. Somatosensory stimuli are usually given through nerves in the limbs and are transmitted to the somatosensory nuclei in the thalamus to the sensory cortex in the parietal lobes. More recently, physicians have studied motor responses after magnetic stimulation of the brain's motor cortex. The presence, number, contour, and duration of various waves and the reaction times in patients with hypoxic-ischemic encephalopathy are compared to those found in normal, age-matched controls.

The most commonly studied evoked responses in hypoxic-ischemic encephalopathy have been the somatosensory evoked responses. Usually the median nerve is stimulated electrically and the waves are recorded over the cerebral cortex. A number of studies have shown that absent responses, delayed or low-voltage responses, and prolonged reaction and central conduction times carry a poor prognosis while relatively normal responses are most often associated with good recovery [75,87–89].

Biochemical Measurements

Physicians have sought simple blood or spinal fluid tests that would identify severe brain damage in the same way that cardiologists use the levels of cardiac enzymes to quantitate cardiac injury after myocardial infarction. Unfortunately, testing to quantitate brain damage has not been nearly as extensive or routine as measurement of cardiac enzymes. To date the utility of measuring five different substances has been explored. These measurements include: spinal fluid lactate and lactate/pyruvate ratios; serum and spinal fluid creatine kinase brain-type isoenzymes (CK-BB); serum and spinal fluid neuron-specific enolase; ionized calcium in arterial blood; and serum levels of the S100 protein.

During brain ischemia and reperfusion, adenosine triphosphate is produced by glycolysis with lactate formation from pyruvate. Presence of elevated lactate levels in the spinal fluid and a high lactate/pyruvate ratio theoretically indicates increased anaerobic brain metabolism and indicates brain damage. Values of lactate above 3 mmol/L seem to be associated with poor outcomes, but the predictive value of spinal fluid lactate has not been well established by prospective testing. Also the finding is not very specific because elevated levels are found in diabetic patients and those with lactic acidosis of any cause [2,91,92].

Brain-type creatine kinase isoenzyme is present in neurons and astrocyte. Unfortunately, the peak of CK-BB in the serum is very transient after cardiac arrest and the radioimmune assay method used doesn't reliably always seperate CK-BB from CK-MB, and many patients with cardiac arrest have elevated CK-MB bands because of myocardial damage [2].

Enolase is an enzyme that is a dimer composed of alpha and gamma units; the gamma-enolase is known as neuron-specific enolase because it is found mostly in neurons and neuroectodermal cells [2,90]. The theoretical advantages of neuron-specific enolase are that it is found only in low concentrations outside the nervous system and that it has little cross-reactivity. Other diseases that raise the neuron-specific enolase levels such as small-cell lung cancer and neuroblastoma are rare enough in patients with cardiac arrest that they should cause little practical problem [2]. Blood ionized calcium levels have been posited to be low in patients after cardiac arrest, but this hypothesis has not been extensively studied [75,93].

Roine and colleagues have studied the use of neuron-specific enolase and CK-BB measurements in patients after out-of-hospital cardiac arrest [2,90]. The spinal fluid level of neuron-specific enolase at 24 hours in patients who did not recover consciousness was more than eight times higher than the level in those patients that awakened [2]. At 24 hours after cardiac arrest, the spinal fluid CK-BB and the serum neuron-specific enolase levels also had high predictive values since elevations meant poor outcome [2]. Unfortunately, the results were not reported until 3 months later, so enzyme levels could not be used for acute decision making.

Among 351 patients with cardiac arrest, Tirschwell et al. found in a retrospective review that the values of spinal fluid CK-BB reliably separated the patients with good prognosis from those that did poorly [94]. The median CK-BB level in 61 patients who awakened was 4 U/L and for those that never awakened 75% were >86 U/L. Only nine patients who awakened had spinal fluid levels >50 U/L and none improved enough to be able to be independent in daily activities [94].

The astroglial protein S100 is specific for brain tissue and has been shown to be a marker for brain injury. Rosen and colleagues measured the serum S100 levels among 41 patients during the first three days after out-of-hospital cardiac arrest using a radioimmunoassay [95]. The highest S100 protein levels were found during the first day after cardiac arrest and were higher than controls. Levels correlated with the degree of coma and the duration of arrest before resuscitation. All patients with an S100 level of >0.2 on day 2 after cardiac arrest died within 14 days, and 89% of patients with levels below 0.2 survived [95]. In this single study the S100 levels were useful in predicting survival and severity of brain damage after cardiac arrest.

The utility of the various investigations is far from clear. Brain imaging, electrophysiologic studies, and blood and spinal fluid analysis can identify patients with little likelihood of survival. But are the patients whose laboratory investigations predict poor outcome the individuals that such a prediction would be highly likely from the clinical examination? More testing needs to be geared to those patients in whom the prognosis after the clinical examination is indeterminate. Would the investigations help in those patients? Bassetti and colleagues favor the use of multiple clinical, radiologic, electrophysiologic, and biochemical data since they believe that the prognostication is better than using any single data item [75].

Outcome depends on both the neurological and cardiological status of the patient [73]. The incidence of acute coronary artery occlusion is high in patients with cardiac arrests. In one study, 60 of 84 (71%) consecutive patients who had out-of-hospital cardiac arrest had clinically significant coronary artery disease on angiography which was performed immediately after hospital admission [96]. Echocardiography, cardiac rhythm monitoring, and electrophysiologic tests of the heart are also very important in predicting long-term outcome [23]. Measurement of end-tidal carbon dioxide levels during and after cardiac resuscitation can also yield important prognostic information [97]. In cardiac arrest patients, the level of end-tidal carbon dioxide is determined by the cardiac output generated during cardiopulmonary resuscitation. A level of 10 mm Hg or less measured 20 minutes after the initiation of advanced cardiac life support predicts a fatal outcome in cardiac arrest patients who have electrical activity but no pulse [97]. A full discussion of cardiac investigations is beyond the scope of this chapter.

TREATMENT

Although many strategies and many different treatments have been tried, none has been judged to be unequivocably useful in improving eventual outcome. The single most important predictor of survival and severity of brain damage is the severity, nature, and duration of the hypoxic-ischemic insult. The brain damage has mostly been done by the time help arrives. A number of different strategies have been or are being tried to minimize the brain damage. Unfortunately, either these treatments have been proven to be ineffective, or there are insufficient data to come to a conclusion about efficacy. The following approach seems reasonable at present.

Reduction of Brain Edema and Increased Intracranial Pressure

Some patients with hypoxic-ischemic injuries develop brain edema which can be severe and can lead to an increase in intracranial pressure. Hyperventilation, osmotic agents, and corticosteroids have been tried in attempts to control the edema. Two retrospective studies failed to show any benefit for corticosteroid treatment [98,99]. Brain edema and increased intracranial pressure probably occur to an important extent only in patients with severe hypoxic-ischemic insults. Furthermore, most of the edema may be inside the cells (cytotoxic edema) and is resistant to corticosteroid and osmotic treatment.

Delivery of More Nutrient-Rich Blood to the Ischemic Brain

Induced hypertension and hypervolemia could increase the amount of brain blood flow. Hemodilution could also theoretically increase blood flow by reducing serum viscosity. The two major nutrients used by brain cells are oxygen and glucose. Elevating the blood sugar level by giving glucose has been shown in experimental animals to worsen outcome. The glucose is metabolized to lactate, and increases tissue acidosis. Hyperoxygenation, e.g., with a hyperbaric chamber, has not been extensively studied. In most patients, blood pressure and oxygen saturation do return to normal quickly. High oxygen levels can be toxic and can cause vasoconstriction, thus reducing cerebral blood flow. Most authorities believe that blood glucose levels should not be raised. The effectiveness of the other therapies mentioned have not been well studied, but there is little enthusiasm that they would work.

"Neuroprotection" Therapies

Can something be done to make the brain more resistant to ischemic-hypoxic damage? Agents that have the theoretical capacity to perform that function have recently been classified as putative neuroprotective agents. There has been great interest in neuroprotection in both focal brain infarcts and global brain ischemia. *Barbiturates*, other *anesthetic agents*, and *hypothermia* all have the potential of decreasing the brain's metabolism. When metabolism is decreased there is a proportionate decrease in the need for nutrients. When thiopental loading was studied in comatose patients after cardiac arrests in a controlled trial, there was no benefit of the treatment [100]. Barbiturates and some other anesthetic agents often have adverse cardiovascular effects such as hypotension, tachycardia, and respiratory suppression. Hypothermia could theoretically severely reduce brain metabolism, although potential adverse cardiovascular effects and susceptibility to infection are potential problems. Hypothermia is now used by many surgeons as a neuroprotective strategy during some surgeries. Hypothermia warrants further clinical study.

Clinicians and researchers have recently become very interested in *calcium channel blockers* as potential neuroprotective drugs. Entry of calcium into cells is a major mechanism of cell death, and calcium channel blockers could theoretically reduce this reaction. Trials of two calcium channel blockers, nimodipine [2,101] and lidoflazine [102], have proven negative. Calcium entry blockers also have hypotensive effects. Trials in patients with focal brain ischemia have also proven negative, and interest in calcium channel blockers as neuroprotective agents has waned. Some interest has surrounded the use of *phenytoin and phosphenytoin, lidocaine*, and *"lazaroids"* in patients with brain ischemia, but none has been studied adequately to test efficacy and safety. Phenytoin and phosphenytoin are potential synaptic inhibitors that could decrease brain metabolic function. Lidocaine is an antiarrhythmic, membrane-stabilizing agent. Nonsteroidal "lazaroids" are antioxidants and inhibitors of iron-catalyzed lipid peroxidation of brain tissue. Free oxygen radicals are known to form in ischemic tissue, especially after reperfusion, and can lead to further brain damage. "Lazaroids" could theoretically dimish damage from free radical formation.

Recent basic research on brain metabolic changes in ischemic neurons has focused on the role of excitotoxins in potentiating cell death of ischemic neurons. Glutamate and aspartate are the two major excitotoxic substances. Levels of these substances are increased in experimental animals with brain ischemia. The two major receptors are the N-methyl-d-aspartate (NMDA) receptor, and the kainate-alpha-amino-3-hydroxy-5-methyl-4-isoxazole proprionate (AMPA) receptor. The action of the NMDA receptors enhances the intracellular entry of calcium, which ultimately kills nerve cells. AMPA receptors utilize sodium channels. A number of agents that diminish the excitotoxic reaction by decreasing the action of glutamate or aspartate, antagonizing the NMDA and AMPA receptors, or blocking calcium entry into nerve cells have been synthesized and are in various stages of research. MK-801, an NMDA receptor antaganist, has been tried both alone [103] and with calcium channel blockers [104] in experimental animals with some success. Some of the receptor blockers have important neurologic side effects such as hallucinations and psychosis, and may also have cardiovascular toxicity. Clinical trials are planned, or in progress, for many of these agents but to date there are no conclusive data on their efficacy or safety for either focal or global brain ischemia patients.

Until there is more definitive information from trials, treatment involves maintenance of normal blood pressure and oxygenation; treatment of cardic arrhythmias and congestive heart failure when present; and prevention, early recognition, and treatment of any complications of coma such as pulmonary and urinary infections, thrombophlebitis, and pulmonary embolism.

REFERENCES

1. Brooks, R, McGovern BA, Garan H, Ruskin JN. Current treatment of patients surviving out-of-hospital cardiac arrest. JAMA 1991; 265:762–768.
2. Roine RO. Neurological outcome of out-of-hospital cardiac arrest. Doctoral thesis, Helsinki, 1993.
3. Myerburg R, Castellanos A. Cardiac arrest and sudden cardiac death. In: Braunwald E, ed. Heart Disease: A Textbook of Cardiovascular Medicine. Philadelphia: W.B. Saunders, 1988:742–777.
4. Liss PL. A history of resuscitation. Ann Emerg Med 1986; 15:65–72.
5. Beck CS, Pritchard H, Feil SH. Ventricular fibrillation of long duration abolished by electric shock. JAMA 1947; 135:985.
6. Zoll PM, Linenthal AJ, Gibson W, Paul MH, Norman LR. Termination of ventricular fibrillation in man by externally applied electric countershock. N Engl J Med 1956; 254:727–732.
7. Safar P, Escarraga LA, Elam JO. A comparison of the mouth-to-mouth and mouth-to-airway methods of artificial respiration with the chest pressure arm-lift methods. N Engl J Med 1958; 258:671–677.
8. Kouwenhoven WB, Jude JR, Knickerbocker GG. Closed chest cardiac massage. JAMA 1960; 173:1064–1067.
9. Safar P, Brown TC, Holtey WJ, Wilder RJ. Ventilation and circulation with closed chest cardiac massage in man. JAMA 1961; 176:574–580.
10. Longstreth WT, Cobb LA, Fahrenbruch C, Copass MK. Does age affect outcomes of out-of-hospital cardiopulmonary resuscitation. JAMA 1990; 264:2109–2110.

11. Becker LB, Ostrander MP, Barrett J, Kondos GT. Outcome of CPR in a large metropolitan area—where are the survivors? Ann Emerg Med 1991; 20:355–361.
12. Eisenberg MS, Hallstrom A, Bergner L. Long-term survival after out-of-hospital cardiac arrest. N Engl J Med 1982; 306:1340–1343.
13. Eisenberg MS, Hadas E, Nuri I, Applebaum D, Roth A, Litwin PE, Hallstrom AP, Nagel E. Sudden cardiac arrest in Israel: factors associated with successful resuscitation. Am J Emerg Med 1988; 6:319–323.
14. Cummins RO, Eisenberg MS, Hallstrom AP, Litwin PE. Survival of out-of-hospital cardiac arrest with early initiation of cardiopulmonary resuscitation. An J Emerg Med 1985; 3:114–118.
15. Goldstein S, Landis JR, Leighton R, Ritter G, Vasu CM, Wolfe RA, Acheson A, Medendorp SV. Predictive survival models for resuscitated victims of out-of-hospital cardiac arrest with coronary heart disease. Circulation 1985; 71:873–880.
16. Troiano P, Masaryk J, Stueven HA, Olson D, Barthell E, Waite EM. The effect of bystander CPR on neurological outcome in survivors of prehospital cardiac arrests. Resuscitation 1989; 17:91–98.
17. Weaver WD, Hill D, Fahrenbruch CE, Copass MK, Martin JS, Cobb LA, Hallstrom AP. Use of the automatic external defibrillator in the management of out-of-hospital cardiac arrest. N Engl J Med 1988; 319:661–666.
18. Murphy DJ, Murray AM, Robinson BE, Campion EW. Outcomes of cardiopulmonary resuscitation in the elderly. Ann Intern Med 1989; 111:199–205.
19. Bedell SA, Delbanco TL, Cook EF, Epstein FH. Survival after cardiopulmonary resuscitation in the hospital. N Engl J Med 1983; 309:569–576.
20. Taffet GE, Teasdale TA, Luchi RJ. In-hospital cardiopulmonary resuscitation. JAMA 1988; 260:2069–2072.
21. Tunstall-Pedoe H, Bailey L, Chamberlain DA, Marsden AK, Ward ME, Ziderman DA. Survey of 3765 cardiopulmonary resuscitations in British hospitals (the BRESUS study): methods and overall results. Br Med J 1992; 304:1347–1351.
22. Cummins RO, Eisenberg MS. Prehospital cardiopulmonary resuscitation. Is it effective? JAMA 1985; 253:2408–2412.
23. Wilber DJ, Garan H, Finkelstein D, Kelly E, Newell J, McGovern B, Ruskin JN. Out-of-hospital cardiac arrest. Use of electrophysiologic testing in the prediction of long-term outcome. N Engl J Med 1988; 318:19–24.
24. Earnest MP, Breckinridge JC, Yarnell PR, Oliva PB. Quality of survival after out-of-hospital cardiac arrest: predictive value of early neurologic evaluation. Neurology 1979; 29:56–60.
25. Earnest MP, Yarnell PR, Merrill SL, Knapp GL. Long-term survival and neurologic status after resuscitation from out-of-hospital cardiac arrest. Neurology 1980; 30: 1298–1302.
26. Ames A III, Nesbett FB. Pathophysiology of ischemic cell death. I. Time of onset of irreversible damage: importance of the different components of the ischemic insult. Stroke 1983; 14:219–226.
27. Adams JH, Brierley JB, Connor RCR, Treip CS. The effects of systemic hypotension upon the human brain: clinical and neuropathological observations in 11 cases. Brain 1966; 89:235–268.
28. Garcia JH. Mechanisms of cell death in ischemia. In: Caplan LR, ed. Brain Isch-

emia, Basic Concepts and Clinical Relevance. London: Springer-Verlag, 1995: 7–18.
29. Miller JR, Myers RE. Neuropathology of systemic circulatory arrest in adult monkeys. Neurology 1972; 22:888–904.
30. Ames A III, Wright LW, Kowada M, Thurston JM, Majors G. Cerebral ischemia: II. The no-reflow phenomenon. Am J Pathol 1968; 52:437–453.
31. Ginsberg MD, Myers RE. The topography of impaired microvascular perfusion in the primate brain following total circulatory arrest. Neurology 1972; 22:998–1011.
32. Petito CK, Feldmann E, Pulsinelli W, Plum F. Delayed hippocampal damage in humans following cardiorespiratory arrest. Neurology 1987; 37:1281–1286.
33. Plum F, Posner JB, Hain RF. Delayed neurological deterioration after anoxia. Arch Intern Med 1962; 110:18–25.
34. Ginsberg MD, Hedley-White T, Richardson EP. Hypoxic-ischemic leukoencephalopathy in man. Arch Neurol 1976; 33:5–14.
35. Hori A, Hirose G, Kataoka S, Tsukada K, Furui K, Tonami H. Delayed postanoxic encephalopathy after strangulation. Arch Neurol 1991; 48:871–874.
36. Babbs C. Reperfusion injury of postischemic tissues. Ann Emerg Med 1988; 17: 1148–1157.
37. Caplan LR. Reperfusion of ischemic brain: why and why not. In: Hacke W, del Zoppo GJ, Hirschberg M, eds. Thrombolytic Therapy in Acute Ischemic Stroke. Berlin: Springer-Verlag, 1991:36–45.
38. O'Brien MD. Ischemic cerebral edema. In: Caplan LR, ed. Brain Ischemia, Basic Concepts and Clinical Relevance. London: Springer-Verlag, 1995:43–50.
39. Choi DW. Excitotoxicity and stroke. In: Caplan LR, ed. Brain Ischemia, Basic Concepts and Clinical Relevance. London: Springer-Verlag, 1995:29–36.
40. Mohr JP. Neurological complications of cardiac valvular disease and cardiac surgery including systemic hypotension. In: Vinken P, Bruyn G, eds. Handbook of Clinical Neurology, Vol. 38. Neurological Manifestations of Systemic Disease. Part I. Amsterdam, North Holland, 1979:143–171.
41. Romanul F, Abramowicz A. Changes in brain and pial vessels in arterial border zones. Arch Neurol 1974; 11:40–65.
42. Caplan LR. Hypoxic-ischemic encephalopathy. In: Caplan LR, ed. Stroke, a Clinical Approach, 2nd ed. Boston: Butterworth-Heinemann, 1993:377–388.
43. Marti-Vilalta JL, Arboix A, Garcia JH. Brain infarcts in the arterial border zones: clinical-pathological correlations. J Stroke Cerebrovasc Dis 1994; 4:114–120.
44. Kinney HC, Korein J, Panigrahy A, Dikkes P, Goode R. Neuropathological findings in the brain of Karen Ann Quinlan. The role of the thalamus in the persistent vegetative state. N Engl J Med 1994; 330:1469–1475.
45. Lance JW, Adams RD. The syndrome of intention or action myoclonus as a sequel to hypoxic encephalopathy. Brain 1963; 86:111–133.
46. Gilles F. Hypotensive brainstem necrosis. Arch Pathol 1969; 88:32–41.
47. Roland EH, Hill A, Norman MG, Flodmark O, MacNab AJ. Selective brainstem injury in an asphyxiated newborn. Ann Neurol 1988; 23:89–92.
48. Fisher CM. The neurological examination of the comatose patient, Acta Neurol Scand 1969; 45(suppl 36):1–56.

49. Young GB, Gilbert JJ, Zochodne D. The significance of myoclonic status epilepticus in postanoxic coma. Neurology 1990; 40:1843–1848.
50. Wijdicks EFM, Parisi JE, Sharbrough FW. Prognostic value of myoclonic status in comatose survivors of cardiac arrest. Ann Neurol 1994; 35:239–243.
51. Krumholz A, Stern BJ, Weiss HD. Outcome from coma after cardiopulmonary resuscitation. Relation to seizures and myoclonus. Neurology 1988; 38:401–405.
52. Jennett B, Plum F. Persistent vegetative state after brain damage: a syndrome in search of a name. Lancet 1972; 1:734–737.
53. Dougherty JH, Rawlinson DG, Levy DE, Plum F. Hypoxic-ischemic brain injury and the vegetative state: clinical and neuropathologic correlation. Neurology 1981; 31:991–997.
54. Multi-Society Task Force on PVS. Medical aspects of the persistent vegetative state. N Engl J Med 1994; 330:1499–1508.
55. Weinberger LM, Schmidley JW, Schafer IA, Raghaven S. Delayed postanoxic demyelination and arylsulfatase-A pseudodeficiency. Neurology 1994; 44:152–154.
56. Gottfried JA, Mayer SA, Shungu D, Chang Y, Duyn JH. Delayed posthypoxic demyelination: association with arylsulfatase-A deficiency and lactic acidosis on proton MR spectroscopy. Neurology. 1997; 49:1400–1404.
57. Husain M, Stein R. Rezso Balint and his most celebrated case. Arch Neurol 1988; 45:89–93.
58. Caplan LR. Visual perceptual abnormalities (cerebral). In: Bogousslavsky J, Caplan LR, eds. Stroke Syndromes. New York: Cambridge University Press, 1965:57–67.
59. Sage JI, van Uitert RL. Man-in-the-barrel syndrome. Neurology 1986; 36:1102–1103.
60. Pierrot-Deseilligny C, Gautier J-C, Loron P. Acquired ocular motor apraxia due to bilateral frontoparietal infarcts. Ann Neurol 1988; 23:199–202.
61. Volpe BT, Hirst W. The characterization of an amnesic syndrome following hypoxic ischemic injury. Arch Neurol 1983; 40:436–440.
62. Caronna J, Finkelstein S. Neurologic syndromes after cardiac arrest. Stroke 1978; 9:517–520.
63. Alexander M. Specific semantic memory loss after hypoxic-ischemic injury. Neurology 1997; 48:165–173.
64. Silver JR, Buxton PH. Spinal stroke. Brain 1974; 97:539–550.
65. Wijdicks E. Neurological complications of cardiac arrest. In: Wijdicks EFM, ed. Neurology of Critical Illness. Philadelphia: E.A. Davis, 1995:86–103.
66. Levy DE, Caronna JJ, Singer BH, Lapinski RH, Frydman H, Plum F. Predicting outcome from hypoxic-ischemic coma. JAMA 1985; 253:1420–1426.
67. Snyder BD, Loewenson RB, Gumnit RJ, Hauser A, Leppik IE, Ramirez-Lassepas M. Neurologic prognosis after cardiopulmonary arrest: II. Level of consciousness. Neurology 1980; 30:52–58.
68. Snyder BD, Gumnit RJ, Leppik IE, Hauser WA, Loewenson RB, Ramirez-Lassepas M. Neurologic prognosis after cardiopulmonary arrest: IV. Brainstem reflexes. Neurology 1981; 31:1092–1097.
69. Bates D, Caronna J, Cartlidge NEF, Knill-Jones RP, Levy DE, Shaw DA, Plum F. A prospective study of nontraumatic coma: methods and results in 310 patients. Ann Neurol 1977; 2:211–220.

70. Bell JA, Hodgson HJF. Coma after cardiac arrest. Brain 1974; 97:361–372.
71. Longstreth WT, Diehr P, Inui TS. Prediction of awakening after out-of-hospital cardiac arrest. N Engl J Med 1983; 308:1378–1382.
72. Shewmon DA, DeGiorgio CM. Early prognosis in anoxic coma: reliability and rationale. Neurol Clin 1989; 7:823–843.
73. Plum F. Vulnerability of the brain and heart after cardiac arrest. N Engl J Med 1991; 324:1278–1280.
74. Steen-Hansen JE, Hansen NN, Vaagenes P, Schreiner B. Pupil size and light reactivity during cardiopulmonary resuscitation. A clinical study. Crit Care Med 1988; 16:69–70.
75. Bassetti C, Bomio F, Mathis J, Hess CW. Early prognosis in coma after cardiac arrest: a prospective clinical, electrophysiological, and biochemical study of 60 patients. J Neurol Neurosurg Psychiatry 1996; 61:610–615.
76. Keane JR. Sustained upgaze in coma. Ann Neurol 1981; 9:409–412.
77. Teasdale G, Jennett B. Assessment of coma and impaired consciousness. A practical scale. Lancet 1974; 2:81–83.
78. Mullie A, Verstringe P, Buylaert W, et al. Predictive value of Glasgow Coma Score for awakening after out-of-hospital cardiac arrest. Lancet 1988; 1:137–140.
79. Rosenberg GA, Johnson SJ, Brenner RP. Recovery of cognition after prolonged vegetative state. Ann Neurol 1977; 2:167–168.
80. Kjos BO, Brandt-Zawadzki M, Young RG. Early CT findings of global central nervous system hypoperfusion. AJNR 1983; 4:1043–1048.
81. Morimoto Y, Kemmotsu O, Kitami K, et al. Acute brain swelling after out-of-hospital cardiac arrest: pathogenesis and outcome. Crit Care Med 1993; 21:104–110.
82. Roine RO, Raininko R, Erkinjuntti T, et al. Magnetic resonance imaging findings associated with cardiac arrest. Stroke 1993; 24:1005–1014.
83. Sawada H, Udaka F, Seriu N, et al. MRI demonstration of cortical laminar necrosis and delayed white matter injury in anoxic encephalopathy. Neuroradiology 1990; 32:319–321.
84. Chokroverty S. ''Alpha-like'' rhythms in electroencephalograms in coma after cardiac arrest. Neurology 1975; 25:655–663.
85. Westmoreland BF, Klass DW, Sharbrough FW, Reagan TJ. Alpha-coma. Electroencephalographic, clinical, pathologic, and etiologic correlations. Arch Neurol 1975; 32:713–718.
86. Hockaday JM, Potts F, Bonazzi A, Schwab RS. Electroencephalographic changes in acute cerebral anoxia from cardiac or respiratory arrest. Electroencephalogr Clin Neurophysiol 1965; 18:575–586.
87. Brunko E, Zegers de Beyl, D. Prognostic value of early cortical somatosensory evoked potentials after resuscitation from cardiac arrest. Electroencephalogr Clin Neurophysiol 1987; 66:15–24.
88. Madl C, Grimm G, Kramer L, et al. Early prediction of individual outcome after cardiopulmonary resuscitation. Lancet 1993; 341:855–858.
89. Madl C, Kramer L, Yeganehfar W, et al. Detection of nontraumatic comatose patients with no benefit of intensive care treatment by recording of sensory evoked potentials. Arch Neurol 1996; 53:512–516.

90. Roine RO, Somer H, Kaste M, Viinikka L, Karonen S-L. Neurological outcome after out-of-hospital cardiac arrest. Arch Neurol 1989; 46:753–756.
91. Bohmer T, Kjekshus J, Vaagenes P. Biochemical indices of cerebral ischemic injury. Scand J Clin Lab Invest 1983; 43:261–265.
92. Edgren E, Hedstrand U, Nordin M, Rydin E, Ronquist G. Prediction of outcome after cardiac arrest. Crit Care Med 1987; 15:820–825.
93. Urban P, Scheidegger D, Buchmann B, Barth D. Cardiac arrest and blood ionized calcium levels. Ann Intern Med 1988; 109:110–113.
94. Tirschwell DL, Longstreth WT, Rauch-Matthews ME, Chandler WL, Rothstein T, Wray L, Eng LJ, Fine J, Copass MK. Cerebrospinal fluid creatine kinase BB isoenzyme activity and neurologic prognosis after cardiac arrest. Neurology 1997; 48: 352–357.
95. Rosen H, Rosengren L, Herlitz J, Blomstrand C. Increased serum levels of the S-100 protein are associated with hypoxic brain damage after cardiac arrest. Stroke 1998; 29:473–477.
96. Spaulding CM, Joly L-M, Rosenberg A, et al. Immediate coronary angiography in survivors of out-of-hospital cardiac arrest. N Engl J Med 1997; 336:1629–1633.
97. Levine RL, Wayne MA, Miller CC. End-tidal carbon dioxide and outcome of out-of-hospital cardiac arrest. N Engl J Med 1997; 337:301–306.
98. Grafton ST, Longstreth WT. Steroids after cardiac arrest: a retrospective study with concurrent, randomized controls. Neurology 1988; 38:1315–1316.
99. Jastremski M, Sutton-Tyrell K, Vaagenes P, Abramson N, Heiselman D, Safar P, Brain Resuscitation Clinical Trial Study Group. Glucocorticoid treatment does not improve recovery following cardiac arrest. JAMA 1989; 262:3427–3430.
100. Brain Resuscitation Clinical Trial I Study Group. Randomized clinical study of thiopental loading in comatose survivors of cardiac arrest. N Engl J Med 1986; 314:397–403.
101. Roine RO, Kaste M, Kinnunen A, Nikki P, Sama S, Kajaste S. Nimodipine after resuscitation from out-of-hospital ventricular fibrillation. A placebo-controlled, double-blind, randomized trial. JAMA 1990; 264:3171–3177.
102. Brain Resuscitation Clinical Trial II Study Group. A randomized clinical study of a calcium-entry blocker (lidoflazine) in the treatment of comatose survivors of cardiac arrest. N Engl J Med 1991; 324:1225–1231.
103. Hattori H, Morin PH, Schwartz PH, Fujikawa DG, Wasterlain CG. Posthypoxic treatment with MK-801 reduces hypoxic-ischemic damage in the neonatal rat. Neurology 1989; 39:713–718.
104. Uematsu D, Araki N, Greenberg JH. Combined therapy with MK-801 and nimodipine for protection of ischaemic brain damage. Neurology 1991; 41:88–94.
105. Caplan LR, Zervas NT. Neurological considerations for the intensive care patient. In: Skillman JJ, ed. Intensive Care. Boston: Little Brown, 1975.

2

Brain Embolism

HISTORICAL BACKGROUND AND OVERVIEW

Knowledge that thrombosis of supply arteries was the cause of necrosis and infarction of the brain, heart, and other body organs developed in the middle of the 19th century. Before then, physicians had known for centuries that coagula could be found in arteries. Vesalius, in 1543, had described unnatural deposits in the left atrium of patients who had limb gangrene [1]. Others found clots in the vascular system at necropsy, but there was controversy about whether the thrombi formed before or after death [2]. During the late 18th and early 19th centuries two important historical figures, John Hunter in Britain and Cruveilhier in France, thought that coagula formed during life and were due to inflammation of the veins. Hunter, writing in 1793, noted the frequency of inflammation of veins after surgery and phlebotomies and thought that clots in the veins formed as exudates from the walls of the blood vessels [3]. Cruveilhier, in 1829, wrote that vein coagulation was the first sign of phlebitis [4]. Thrombi within the arteries and heart, at that time, were attributed to arteritis [2].

The German pathologist Rudolph Virchow deserves the most credit for recognizing that obstruction of arteries caused damage to the organs supplied and that vascular occlusion developed locally (thrombosis) or at a distance (embolism) [5]. Among 76 necropsies that he performed in 1847, Virchow found blood clots in the veins of the extremities in 18, and within the pulmonary arteries in

11. He reasoned that the clots must have been transported within the venous bloodstream to reach the heart and then the pulmonary arteries [5]. He then devised experiments to show that foreign bodies placed within the veins of animals moved proximally toward the heart. At necropsies, Virchow found clots obstructing brain, splenic, renal, and limb arteries in patients with cardiac valvular disease and left atrial thrombi. These observations showed him that clots formed locally without relation to inflammation, moved within the vascular system as emboli, and caused ischemic tissue damage [2,5].

Although the cardiac pathology was defined, clinicians were not aware of the clinical features of coronary thrombosis until the early part of the 20th century, when James Herrick described the symptoms of myocardial infarction [6]. In the 1940s cardiologists clarified the relationship between angina pectoris, coronary thrombosis, and myocardial infarction [7]. Within the brain, pathologists customarily described softenings, ramolissements, and encephalomalacia. By the turn of the century Chiari had described a single case of an intra-arterial embolus that had arisen from a thrombus in the internal carotid artery in the neck [8]. William Osler's textbook of medicine, which appeared in many editions at the beginning of the 20th century, described embolism to the brain as a cause of cerebral softenings [9]. Osler mentioned only rheumatic mitral stenosis and bacterial endocarditis as cardiac sources of embolism [9]. Osler did note that portions of clots from aneurysms, thrombi from aortic atheromas, and clots that formed in the pulmonary veins were also potential sources of brain embolism [9]. It was not until the early 1950s, when Miller Fisher described the clinical and pathological features of carotid artery thrombosis and coined the term transient ischemic attacks (TIAs) [10], that the clinical aspects of occlusive cerebrovascular disease became well known.

Although emboli were known to arise from the heart and the arterial system, early classifications of stroke equated brain embolism with cardiac-origin embolism [11]. Only two main cardiac sources were accepted—mitral stenosis with atrial fibrillation, and recent myocardial infarction complicated by a mural thrombus. Required for a stroke to be classified as embolic were the known presence of one of these two accepted cardiac sources, systemic embolism, and a sudden, maximal-at-onset, focal neurological deficit. Using these criteria very few strokes were considered embolic. Table 1 shows the frequency of strokes diagnosed as embolic in large series of stroke patients collected before 1970 [12–14].

The Harvard Cooperative Stroke Registry (HSR) [15], published in 1978, was the first study to note a high rate of embolism as a cause of stroke. This registry, unlike its predecessors, was a prospective study. All 694 stroke patients were thoroughly investigated using the technology available at that time. Embolism was diagnosed when there was a sudden obstruction of a large intracranial artery or one of its branches. The embolus could arise from any source, but predominantly the heart or one of the cervicocranial arteries that supply the brain. A sudden-onset neurologic deficit and an arteriogram that showed blockage of

Table 1 Incidence of Embolism and Other Types of Strokes (%) in Early Series

Series	n	Thrombosis	Embolism	ICH	SAH	Unknown
Aring, Merritt [12]	407	82	3	15	—	—
Whisnant et al. [13]	548	75	3	10	5	7
Matsumoto et al. [14]	993	71	8	10	6	5

ICH, intracerebral hemorrhage; SAH, subarachnoid hemorrhage.

an intracranial artery not due to local atherosclerosis were the most common evidence for embolism. Echocardiography was not available at that time, and only about half the patients had cranial computed tomography (CT), which only became available in the mid-1970s. In the Harvard Stroke Registry, 31% of strokes were classified as embolic, 53% thrombotic, and 16% hemorrhagic [15]. Note that the ratio of ischemic to hemorrhagic strokes was about the same as that in the registries listed in Table 1; only the proportion of ischemic strokes considered embolic differed dramatically. In the Harvard Stroke Registry, 215 of the 694 (31%) strokes were considered embolic. Fully 112 of the 215 (52%) embolic stroke patients had known cardiac disease. Seventy-three had atrial fibrillation and the others had recent myocardial infarction or valvular heart disease. Note that one-third of the patients with embolism had atrial fibrillation, a disorder that at that time was not considered to be an important cardiac source of embolism unless the patient also had rheumatic valvular disease [15].

Embolism requires a donor source and a recipient artery. During the last two decades, there has been a dramatic revolution in technology able to define the brain and cardiovascular abnormalities in stroke patients. This technology is now able to characterize both recipient and donor sites. Newer-generation CT scans and magnetic resonance imaging (MRI), especially with newer fluid-attenuated inversion recovery (FLAIR) techniques, are able to show brain infarcts and hemorrhages soon after the onset of neurological symptoms. Vascular imaging has also developed dramatically. Extracranial and transcranial ultrasound can now provide information rapidly about blood flow and lesions within the major extracranial and large basal intracranial arteries. CT angiography can be performed at the same time as CT by using intravenous contrast and filming with a spiral CT scanner. MR angiography can be performed at the same time as MRI, does not require contrast media, and can give accurate information about large artery lesions. Cardiac diagnostic testing, using transesophageal echocardiography (TEE), radionuclide studies, and rhythm monitoring, is also much more effective now than in the past at defining cardiac abnormalities and potential sources of embolism. TEE and Duplex ultrasound studies can also detect large aortic atheromas that might be potential sources of embolism to the brain. The available testing is rapid and relatively noninvasive when compared to angiography using contrast media.

During the past 5 years, a new capability has entered the diagnostic arsenal of clinicians—emboli monitoring using transcranial Doppler ultrasound (TCD) [16–21]. In this technique transcranial Doppler probes are positioned over brain arteries, most often the middle and posterior cerebral arteries on each side. When particles pass through the arteries being monitored, they produce an audible chirping noise and high-intensity transient signals (HITS) visible on an oscilloscope. The signal character depends on the nature of the particles (gas, thrombus, calcium, cholesterol crystal, etc.), particle size, and particle transit time. Monitoring probes can be placed on the neck and brain arteries. Emboli that arise from the heart or aorta should go equally to each side, proportionately to the anterior and posterior circulation arteries, and the signals should appear in the neck before appearing intracranially. In contrast, emboli that originate in a neck artery should go only to the intracranial arterial branches on the side of the donor artery, and embolic signals do not appear in the neck. For example, emboli from the left internal carotid artery (ICA) generate embolic signals detectable in the left middle cerebral artery and not in the neck, posterior cerebral, or right-sided arteries. This technique now allows better identification of the nature of embolic materials and their sources, and also allows some quantification of the emboli load and a means of monitoring the effect of various therapies on lessening that load.

Newer diagnostic testing has now shown that embolism is a much more common cause of stroke than it was thought to be in the past [22]. Physicians in prior decades thought that release of embolic materials was an unusual event with a high hit rate—that is, that emboli reaching intracranial arteries had a high likelihood of causing stroke and brain infarction. Recent data show that embolic particles are often found in the circulation but the hit rate is low [16–22]. These particles can arise from a variety of donor sources including the heart, the aorta, and neck and proximal intracranial arteries.

In this chapter we will first consider the pathology and pathophysiology of brain embolism and then comment on the clinical and imaging findings of patients with embolic strokes (from any donor source). Then we will turn to discussions of the various donor sources—cardiac, aortic, and arterial—and their recognition, clinical features, diagnosis, and treatment.

PATHOLOGY, PATHOPHYSIOLOGY AND LOCATIONS OF BRAIN EMBOLISM

Lodging and Movement of Emboli

When emboli are released into the circulation, they travel distally until they lodge in an extracranial or intracranial brain artery. Unlike thrombi, which are formed locally in areas of atherosclerosis or other endothelial damage, emboli are loosely adherent to the vascular walls in the region where they first land. An embolus might precipitate a vasoconstrictive response in the recipient artery. Blockage of the recipient artery causes a sudden decrease in blood flow and pressure in the artery distal to the blockage. The brain tissue supplied by the artery becomes ischemic. These changes in the supply zone of the recipient artery quickly induce collateral blood flow. One of the authors (L.R.C.) recalls vividly being present for animal experiments performed by his neurology chairman, Dr. Derrick Denny-Brown. After the dura mater had been opened, exposing the pial arteries, Denny-Brown tied the carotid artery in the neck on the side of the surgical exposure. After a very brief period of pallor of the brain and decreased blood flow through the pial arteries, there was rapid reperfusion through collateral vascular channels. Surgeons sometimes tie neck arteries that feed aneurysms, most often without causing persistent brain ischemia. Collateral blood flow develops very rapidly and is often sufficient to maintain adequate perfusion of the brain.

The sudden blockage of a brain-feeding artery often leads to symptoms of dysfunction of the area of brain supplied. When collateral blood flow develops, the symptoms may stabilize or even improve. The nonadherent embolic particles often do not remain at their initial recipient site but fragment and move distally. Sequential arteriograms, or even sequential injections during the same arteriogram, can show passage of emboli from their initial resting place [23–25]. This distal passage of emboli often occurs without causing new symptoms since the fragments may pass through the system without causing further ischemic damage. Alternatively, the embolus might block a distal branch. If collateral circulation to the supply area of that branch is not adequate, then further brain ischemic symptoms and brain infarction may develop.

Hemorrhagic Infarction

When embolism causes brain infarction, the infarcts are often hemorrhagic. Miller Fisher and Raymond Adams extensively studied their necropsy material to define the mechanism of hemorrhagic infarction in the brain [26,27]. Obstruction of a brain-supplying artery causes ischemia to neurons and also causes ischemic damage to the blood vessels within the area of ischemia. When the obstructing embolus moves distally, the previously ischemic region is reperfused with blood. The damaged capillaries and arterioles within that region are no longer competent and blood leaks into the surrounding infarcted tissue. An example of this mechanism is shown in Figure 1, from the Fisher and Adams study [27]. In this patient an embolus had initially blocked the mainstem middle cerebral artery (MCA) before its lenticulostriate branches, causing ischemia to the basal ganglia, internal capsule, and the superficial cortical territories supplied by the MCA. The embolus then moved and at necropsy had passed beyond the lenticulostriate branches but continued to obstruct the MCA more distally. The reperfused deep basal ganglionic region was very hemorrhagic at necropsy while the superficial territory of the MCA which was never reperfused showed a bland infarct.

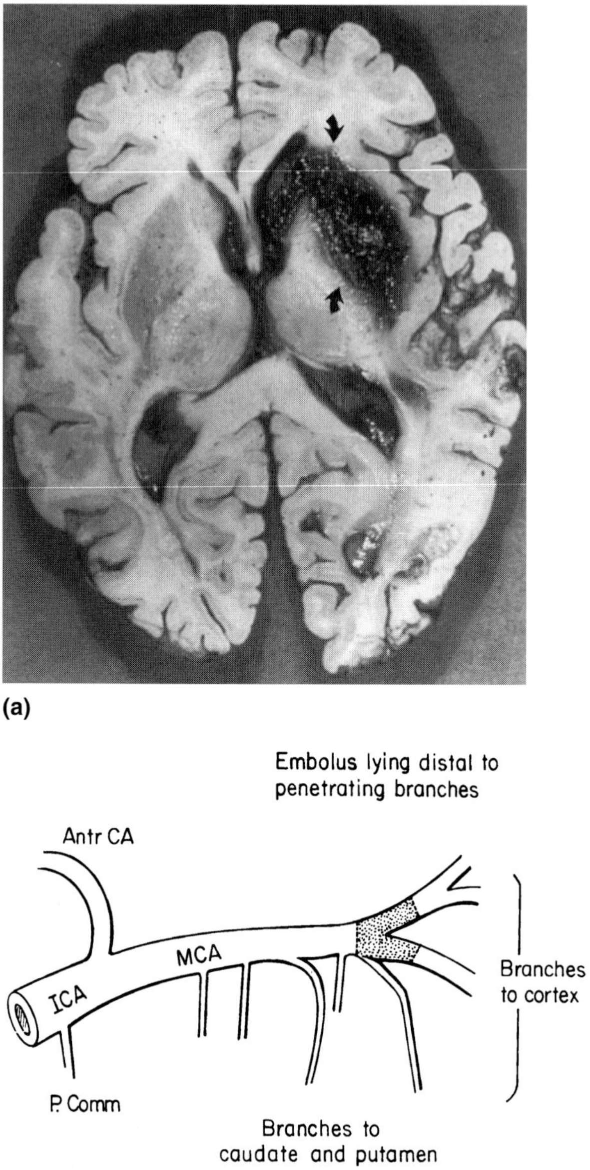

(a)

(b)

FIG. 1 (a) Coronal section of the brain at necropsy showing a hemorrhagic infarction on the right involving the caudate nucleus and putamen, regions supplied by the lenticulostriate branches of the right middle cerebral artery. (b) Cartoon of the intracranial internal carotid artery and its branches at necropsy. An embolus (hatched region) was found in the distal portion of the mainstem middle cerebral artery beyond the lenticulostriate branches that supply the caudate nucleus and putamen. This embolus, at one time, must have blocked these penetrating branches and then moved more distally in the artery. (From Ref. 27.)

The essential cause of hemorrhagic infarction is reperfusion of previously ischemic tissue. The other mechanism that causes hemorrhagic infarction besides embolism is systemic hypoperfusion. After cardiac arrest or shock, the reinstitution of effective circulation after a prolonged period of brain hypoperfusion can lead to hemorrhage within border zone infarcts. Hemorrhagic changes are extremely common in patients with brain embolism. In two series, the investigators prospectively studied the frequency of hemorrhagic infarction on sequential brain-imaging scans. Yamaguchi et al. compared the findings on CT scans performed 3 to 10 days after stroke in 120 patients with embolic brain infarcts with 109 patients whose infarcts were considered due to local thrombotic occlusive disease [28]. Hemorrhagic infarcts were found in 45 patients (40%) with embolic infarcts, compared to two (1.8%) patients with local thrombosis-related infarcts [28]. Okada and colleagues studied 160 patients who had presumed embolic brain infarcts by performing CT scans every 10 days during hospitalization [29]. Hemorrhagic infarction was found on CT at some time during the course in 65 (40.6%) patients. Hemorrhagic changes were found on the initial CT scan performed during the first 4 days in only 10 patients (6%), while the remainder of the hemorrhagic infarcts were found on follow-up CT scans. Studies at the New England Medical Center in Boston showed that all of the patients with cerebral [30] and cerebellar [31] hemorrhagic infarcts that were studied and reported had embolic causes. MRI is more sensitive than CT at detecting hemorrhagic changes, so sequential MRI probably would show a frequency of >50% for hemorrhagic changes in patients with embolic brain infarcts.

In the great majority of patients, hemorrhagic infarction consists of diapedesis of red blood cells into infarcted tissue. Often the appearance is that of scatterred petechial hemorrhages, or a confluent purpuric pattern scattered throughout the infarct [32]. Figure 2 shows a well-circumscribed hemorrhagic infarct caused by an embolus to a small branch of the middle cerebral artery. As in Figure 1a, this infarct is very hemorrhagic because of confluent bleeding into ischemic brain tissue. Figure 3 shows hemorrhagic stippling within bilateral posterior cerebral artery territory infarcts caused by an embolus to the rostral basilar artery bifurcation. In some brain infarcts, especially large ones involving more than one lobe, localized homogeneous collections of blood (hematomas) can develop within the region of hemorrhagic infarction. In the great majority of patients with hemorrhagic infarcts, the hemorrhagic transformation does not cause any alteration in the clinical symptoms and signs. The hemorrhagic changes are usually found on routine follow-up scans. Bleeding into dead tissue does not alter clinical findings unless a large space-taking hematoma develops.

When studied, anticoagulation of patients with hemorrhagic infarction due to brain embolism did not cause an increase in bleeding [30]. Internists and cardiologists are accustomed to treating patients with hemoptysis caused by pulmonary embolism with heparin followed by coumadin. These patients with pul-

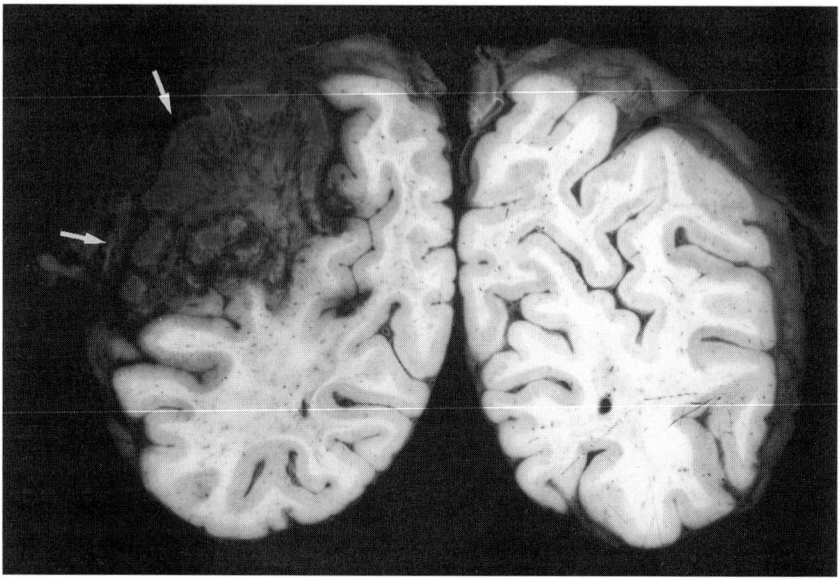

FIG. 2 Cut section of the posterior portion of the brain at necropsy. A very well circumscribed, triangular-shaped, very hemorrhagic infarct is seen within the parietal lobe on the left (white arrows). This infarct was the result of an embolus to a branch of the middle cerebral artery.

monary embolism-related hemoptysis have beefy hemorrhagic lung infarcts, and yet heparin does not seem to create a major risk for further symptomatic lung bleeding. The situation is similar within the brain. Recent studies have shown that anticoagulation of patients with hemorrhagic infarcts in the brain due to dural venous sinus occlusion have better outcomes if treated with anticoagulants [33,34]. However, anticoagulation, especially using an intravenous bolus dose of heparin, does carry a risk of hematoma formation in patients with large brain infarcts even when no hemorrhagic changes are initially present.

Location and Size of Embolic Occlusions and Brain Infarcts

About 80% of emboli that arise from the heart go into the anterior (carotid artery) circulation, equally divided between the two sides. The remaining 20% of emboli go into the posterior (vertebral and basilar arteries) circulation, a rate roughly equal to the proportion of the blood supply that goes into the vertebrobasilar

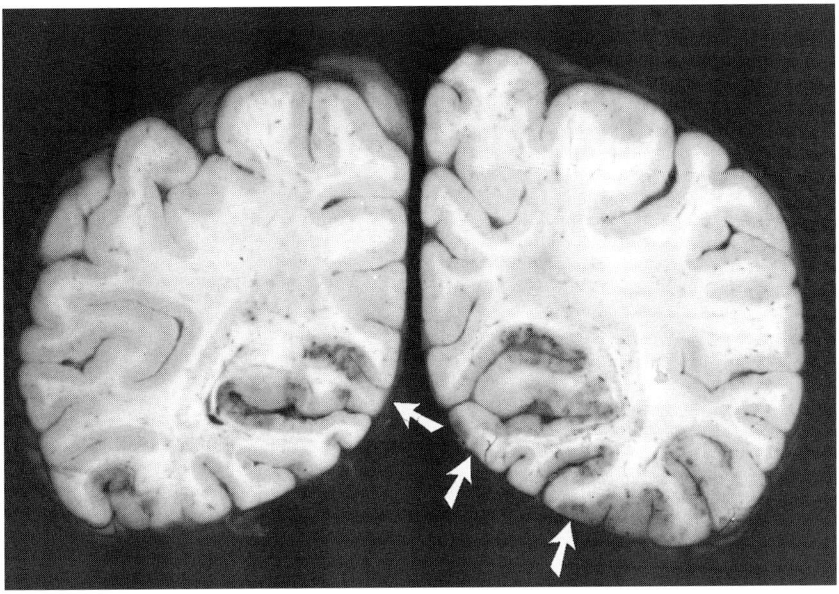

FIG. 3 Cut section of the posterior portion of the brain at necropsy showing a bilateral hemorrhagic infarct within the territories of the posterior cerebral arteries (white arrows). The black stippled areas within the infarct represent small hemorrhages. These infarcts are a result of a single embolus temporarily blocking the distal bifurcation of the basilar artery, impeding flow to the left and right posterior cerebral arteries.

arteries. In the Harvard Stroke Registry [15] 78% of emboli caused clinical anterior circulation ischemia while the frequency of anterior circulation embolism was 85% in the Michael Reese Stroke Registry [35] and 70% in the Lausanne Stroke Registry [36]. The recipient artery destination depends on the size and nature of the particles. Calcific particles from heart valves or mitral annular calcifications are less mobile and adapt less well to the shape of their recipient artery resting place than red (erythrocyte-fibrin) and white (platelet-fibrin) thrombi. The circulating bloodstream seems to be able somehow to bypass obstructing cholesterol crystal emboli, especially in the retinal arteries.

Within the anterior and posterior circulations there are predilection sites for the destination of embolic particles. Large emboli entering a common carotid artery could become lodged in the common or internal carotid artery, especially if atheromatous plaques had already narrowed the lumens of these vessels. If the emboli were able to pass through the carotid arteries in the neck, the next common lodging place is the intracranial bifurcation of the internal carotid arteries (ICAs)

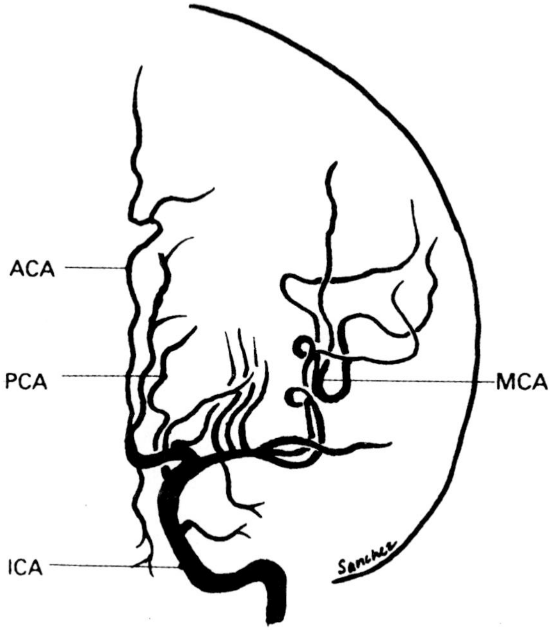

FIG. 4 Drawing of the internal carotid artery and its intracranial branches as they appear on carotid angiography, anteroposterior view. ACA, anterior cerebral artery; PCA, posterior cerebral artery; MCA, middle cerebral artery; ICA, internal carotid artery. Drawn by Dr. Juan Sanchez Ramos. (From Ref. 75.)

into the anterior cerebral (ACA) and middle cerebral (MCA) arteries. Figure 4 is a drawing of the intracranial carotid artery showing the major intracranial branches. Bifurcations are common resting places for emboli.

Emboli that pass through the carotid intracranial bifurcations most often go into the MCAs and their branches. Gacs et al. showed that balloon emboli placed in the circulation nearly always followed the same pathway and ended up in the MCAs and their branches [37]. Embolism in experimental animals produced by the introduction of silicone cylinders or spheres, elastic cylinders, and autologous blood clots, also showed a very high incidence of MCA territory localization [38]. Emboli often pass into the superior and inferior divisions of the MCA and the cortical branches of these divisions. The superior division supplies the cortex and white matter above the Sylvian fissure including the frontal and superior parietal lobes. The inferior division supplies the area below the sylvian fissure including the temporal and inferior parietal lobes. Figure 5 is a

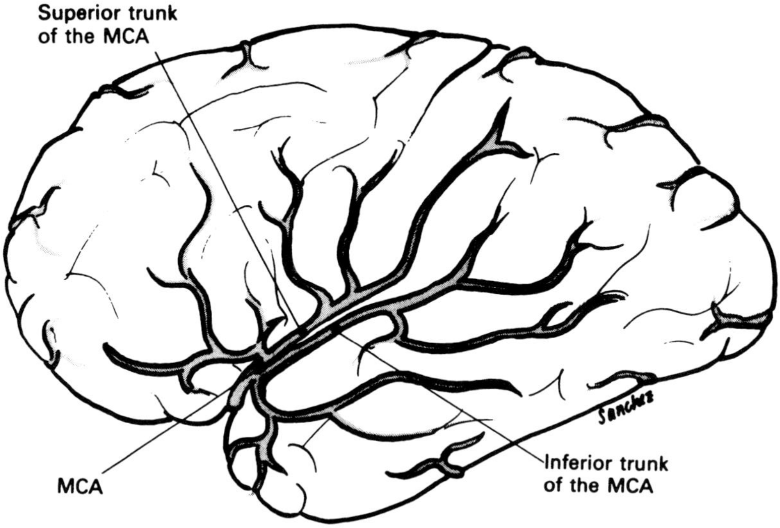

FIG. 5 Drawing of the lateral surface of the brain showing inferior trunk divisions of the middle cerebral artery and their branches. MCA, middle cerebral artery. Drawn by Dr. Juan Sanchez Ramos. (From Ref. 75.)

drawing of the convexal surface of the brain that shows the divisions of the MCA and their main branches. Figure 6 is a drawing of a cut section of the brain showing the supply zones of the different cerebral arteries. The middle cerebral artery supplies most of the convexal surface of the brain and the basal ganglia. The ACA supplies the paramedian frontal lobe. Emboli seldom go into the penetrating artery (lenticulostriate arteries) branches of the MCAs or the penetrators from the ACAs because these vessels originate at about a 90° angle from the parent arteries.

Embolism into the MCAs can cause a variety of different patterns of infarction. Figure 7 shows drawings of CT scans of nine patients with MCA embolic infarcts, and Figures 8 to 14 are imaging scans of patients with embolism involving the MCA territory. It is essential for clinicians to be able to recognize the various patterns of infarction. Blockage of the mainstem MCA before the lenticulostriate branches can cause a large infarct that encompasses the entire MCA territory including the deep basal ganglia and internal capsule as well as the cerebral cortex and subcortical white matter of both the suprasylvian and infrasylvian MCA territories (Fig. 7D, 7I).

In some patients an embolus has blocked the intracranial carotid artery,

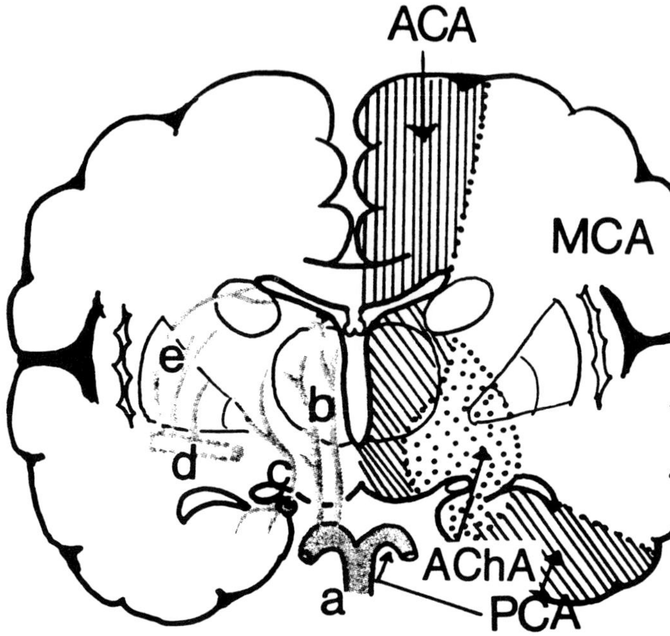

FIG. 6 Drawing of a coronal section of the brain through the cerebral hemispheres and the thalamus showing the distribution of supply of the major cerebral arteries. (a) Basilar artery. (b) Thalamoperforating artery branches of the proximal posterior cerebral artery. (c) Anterior choroidal artery. (d) Horizontal segment of middle cerebral artery. (e) Lenticulostriate arteries to the putamen and caudate nucleus. ACA, anterior cerebral artery; MCA, middle cerebral artery; AChA, anterior choroidal artery; PCA, posterior cerebral artery. Drawn by Dr Juan Sanchez Ramos. (From Ref. 75.)

causing infarction of the ACA territory as well as the entire MCA territory (Fig. 8). In young patients, when the mainstem MCA is blocked, the rapid development of collateral circulation over the convexity of the brain often leads to sparing of the superficial territory of the MCA. The lenticulostriate branches are blocked by the clot in the mainstem MCA, and collateral circulation to the deep MCA territory is poor. The resultant infarct is limited to the basal ganglia and surrounding cerebral white matter and is usually referred to as a striatocapsular infarct (Figs. 7A, 9).

Passage of an embolus into the superior division of the MCA leads to a cortical/subcortical infarct in the region of the suprasylvian convexity (Figs. 7E–G [right side], 10, 11), and embolism to the inferior division leads to an

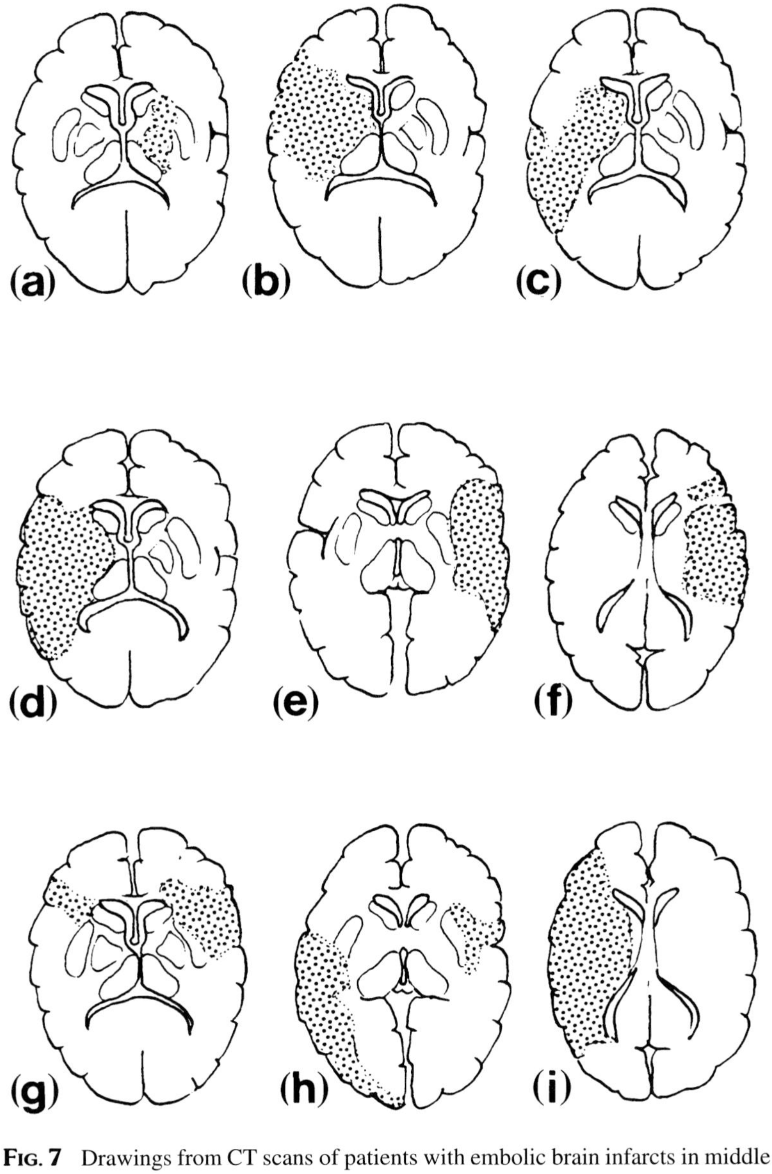

FIG. 7 Drawings from CT scans of patients with embolic brain infarcts in middle cerebral artery distribution. (a) Striatocapsular infarct. (b,c) Deep basal ganglionic-capsular and superficial territory infarcts. (d,i) Entire middle cerebral artery territory infarcts. (e–g) Superior division infarcts; (h) inferior division infarct. (g,h) Small cortical branch territory infarcts (right side). From Ref. 75. with permission.

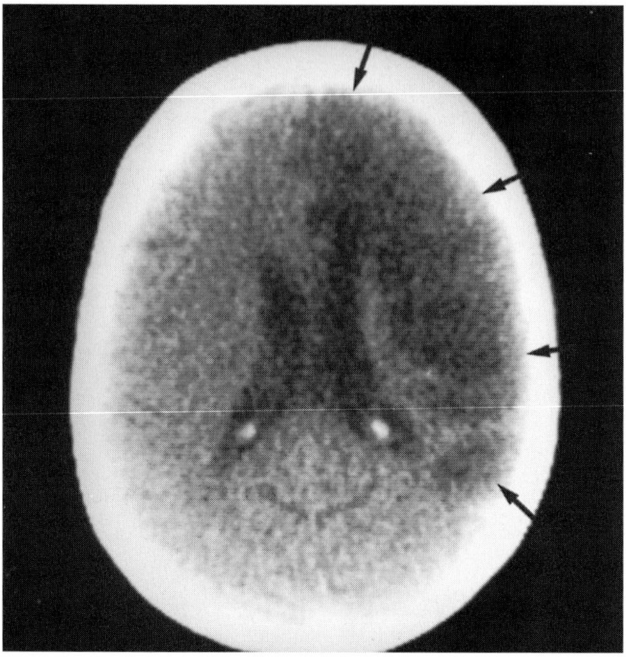

FIG. 8 CT scan showing a large infarct (black arrows) involving anterior cerebral artery territory (double arrows) and entire middle cerebral artery territory on the right.

infarct limited to the temporal and inferior parietal lobes below the sylvian fissure (Figs. 7H [left side], 12, 13). When an embolus rests first in the mainstem MCA and then travels to one of the divisional branches, infarction involves the deep territory and cortex above or below the sylvian fissure (Fig. 7B, 7C). Small emboli block cortical branches and cause small cortical/subcortical infarcts involving one or several gyri (Figs. 7G [left side], 14).

Occasionally emboli block the anterior cerebral artery or its distal branches. This causes an infarct in the paramedian area of one frontal lobe. Figure 15 is a CT scan showing a typical anterior cerebral artery territory infarct due to embolism.

Emboli that enter the posterior circulation can block the vertebral arteries in the neck or intracranially. Emboli that are able to pass through the intracranial vertebral arteries (ICVAs) will usually be able to pass through the proximal and middle portions of the basilar artery, which are wider than the ICVAs. The basilar artery becomes narrower as it courses craniad. Emboli often block the distal basi-

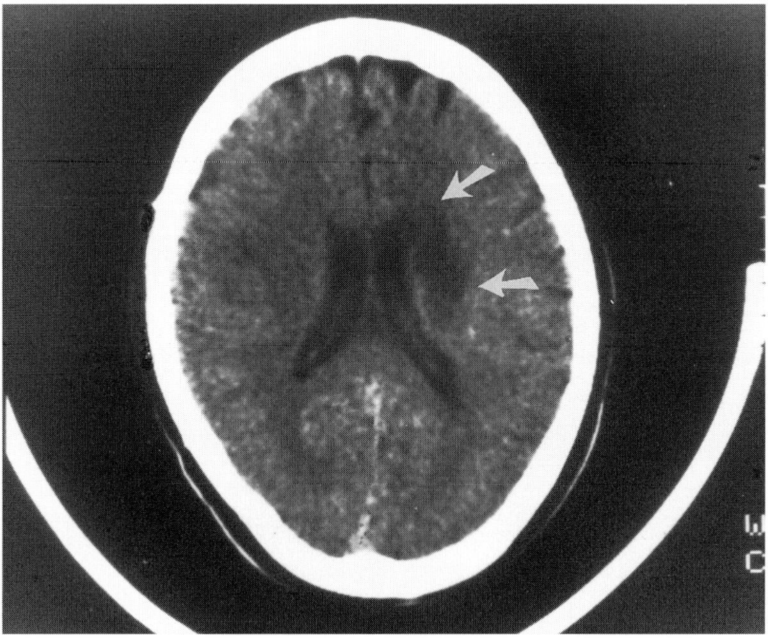

FIG. 9 CT scan showing an elliptical-shaped infarct within the basal ganglia and internal capsule on the right of the picture (white arrows).

lar artery bifurcation (''top of the basilar'') or one of its branches. The main branches of the basilar artery bifurcation are penetrating arteries to the medial portions of the thalami and midbrain, the superior cerebellar artery, which supplies the upper surface of the cerebellum, and the posterior cerebral arteries (PCAs), which supply the lateral portions of the thalami and the temporal and occipital lobe territories of the posterior cerebral arteries (PCAs). Figure 3 shows a hemorrhagic infarct in the territory of the bilateral PCAs that resulted from an embolus to the rostral basilar artery bifurcation. Figure 15 is a cartoon showing the usual loci of posterior circulation embolism. The most frequent brain areas infarcted are the posterior inferior portion of the cerebellum in the territory of the posterior inferior cerebellar artery (PICA) branch of the ICVA; the superior surface of the cerebellum in the territory of the superior cerebellar artery; and the thalamic and hemispheral territories of the PCAs. The clinical and imaging findings in patients with these lesions are described in detail elsewhere [39–41].

In the Harvard Stroke Registry, angiography was commonly used for diag-

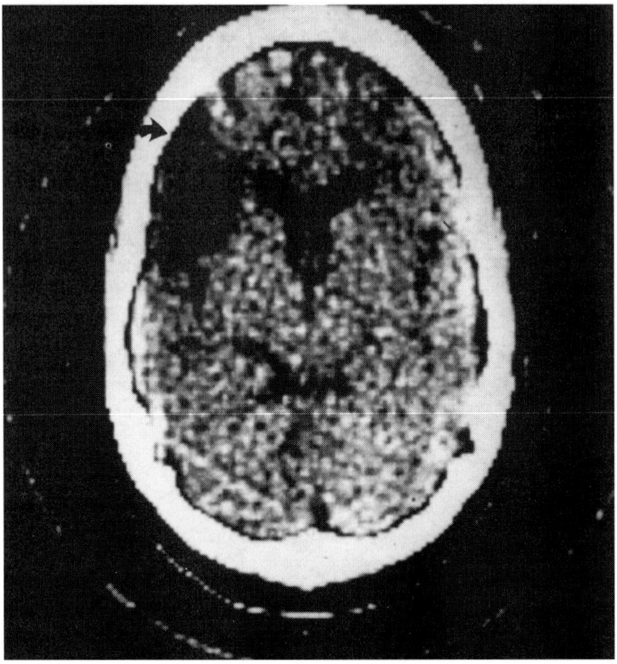

FIG. 10 CT scan showing a superior division middle cerebral artery territory infarct (single black arrow).

nosis since many patients were seen before CT scans were available. Table 2 shows the frequency of embolic occlusions in the various intracranial arteries based on angiography. The MCAs were involved in 80% of patients; the mainstem MCA and superior division branches were the regions within the MCAs that were most often occluded [15]. In the Lausanne Stroke Registry, the distribution of infarcts in patients with potential cardiac sources of emboli was based on neuroimaging using either CT or MRI [42]. Among 1311 patients in the Lausanne Registry that were tabulated, 305 (23%) had potential cardiac sources of emboli [42]. Table 3 shows the distribution of brain infarcts among these 305 patients.

Emboli of cardiac origin are often larger than those arising in the proximal arteries, so the infarcts are, on average, larger than artery-to-artery infarcts [43–45]. In the Stroke Data Bank, the medium volume of infarction on CT in patients with cardiac origin embolism was 2.4 times that found in patients with intra-arterial embolism, a highly significant difference ($P < .01$) [45]. In a study of over 2000 stroke patients, the average size of brain infarcts due to cardiac-

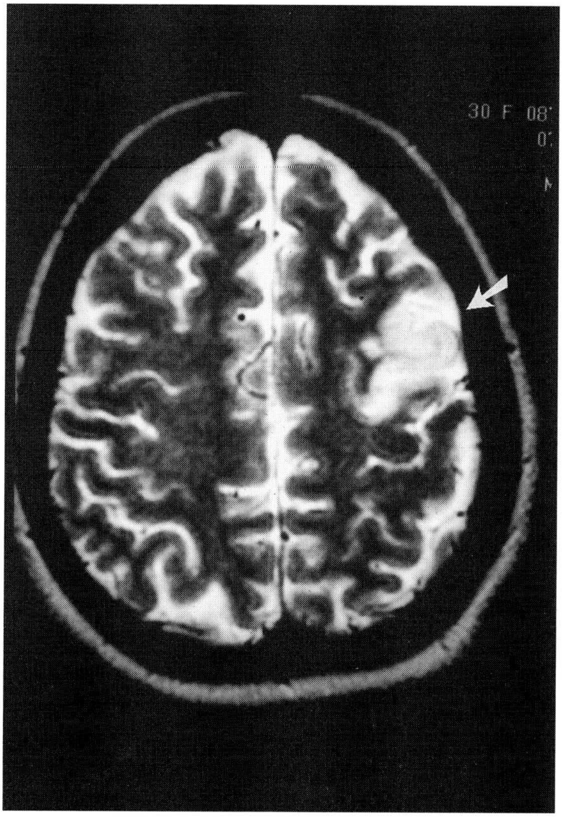

FIG. 11 MRI scan, T_2-weighted, showing a small superior division infarct on the right (white arrow).

source embolism was 73.7 cm^3, vs. 48.9 cm^3 for nonembolic infarcts [46]. A decreased level of consciousness early during the course of the stroke, a finding probably related to the size of infarction, among other factors, was also significantly more common in Stroke Data Bank patients with cardiogenic embolism compared to those with intra-arterial embolism (29.8% vs. 6.1%; $P < .01$) [45].

Another important feature of cardiac origin embolism is development of multiple cortical/subcortical infarcts in multiple vascular territories within both carotid circulations and the posterior circulation, especially in the absence of severe proximal arterial occlusive lesions. Emboli arising from the aorta probably share the same patterns as that found in cardiac-origin embolism, although recipient sites of aortic-origin emboli have not been extensively studied.

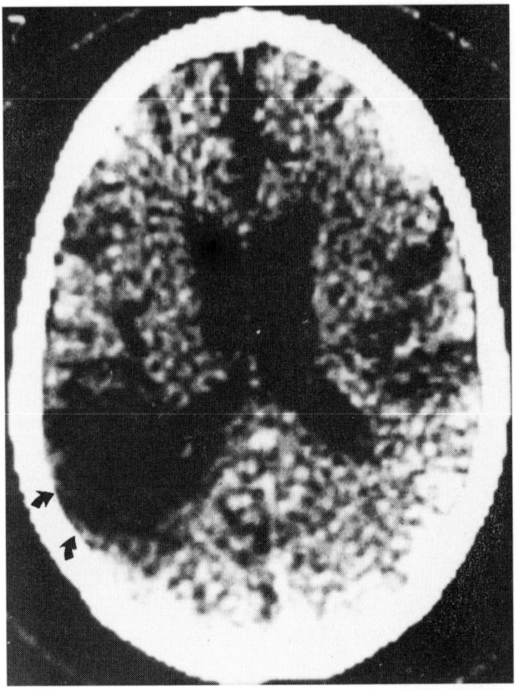

Fig. 12 CT scan showing an inferior division middle cerebral artery teritory infarct on the left (curved black arrows).

Emboli that arise from proximal arteries go only into branches of that artery. Repeated embolism into one MCA suggests an intrinsic lesion of the carotid artery on that side. The distal termination sites within the anterior and posterior circulations are the same as that described above in cardiac-origin embolism. Proximal arterial disease often induces circulatory changes with increased collateral circulation. The preexistence of collateral circulation might limit the size of intra-arterial embolic infarcts when compared to cardiac and aortic-origin embolism in which there is no such preevent adaptation. The distribution of infarcts according to superficial and deep intracranial territories also probably differs between patients with cardiac and intra-arterial sources of embolism. Table 4 shows the distribution of infarcts in the Stroke Data Bank [45]. Superficial and deep infarcts were much more common in patients with cardiac sources of embolism [45]. Large emboli more often block the mainstem MCAs and PCAs before their penetrating artery branches, leading to infarcts that are both deep and superficial.

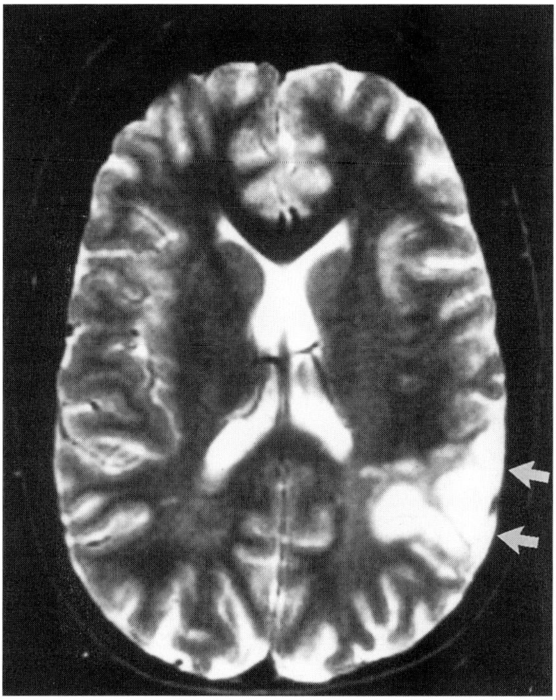

FIG. 13 MRI, T_2-weighted image, showing a small inferior division infarct on the right (white arrows).

In contrast, purely superficial infarcts were more common in patients with intra-arterial embolism [45].

CLINICAL FEATURES AND DIAGNOSIS

Early Clinical Course

The most common and most characteristic time course in patients with embolism to a brain artery is the very sudden onset of neurologic symptoms and signs that are maximal at onset. After the embolus blocks the recipient artery, collateral circulation begins to develop and some improvement occurs. The breakup and distal movement of the embolus strongly affects the subsequent clinical course. Movement of emboli is most common during the first 48 hours after symptom onset. In the Harvard Stroke Registry, angiography performed after 48 hours in

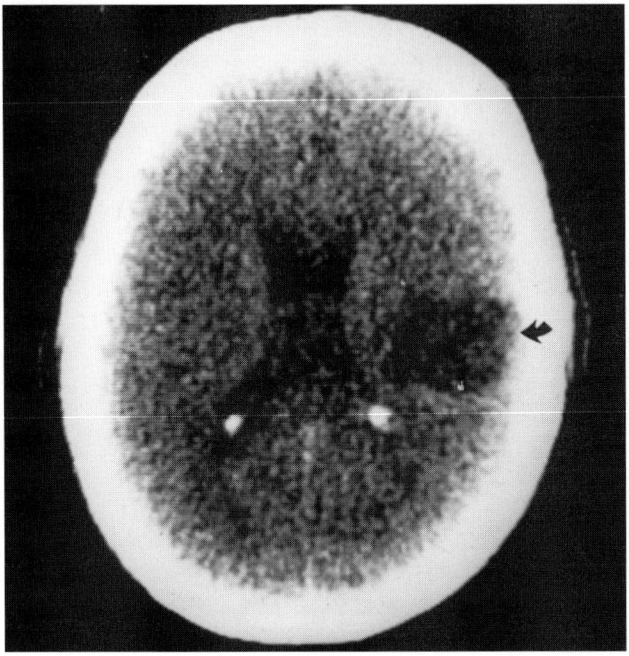

FIG. 14 CT scan showing a cortical branch middle cerebral artery territory infarct on the right (black arrow).

patients with clinical brain embolism was often normal, but immediate angiography performed within hours after symptom onset nearly always showed embolic intracranial occlusions [15]. Others have also shown a very high rate of angiographic detection of emboli when studies are performed within 8 hours after stroke onset [47,48]. Transcranial Doppler monitoring of intracranial arteries after onset of embolic strokes also shows a high frequency of emboli passage [49].

Movement of emboli before the development of irreversible brain damage allows reperfusion of previously ischemic brain tissue and is usually accompanied by clinical improvement in symptoms and signs. However, in some patients the embolus or its fragments block an important distal branch, leading to further ischemia and worsening of symptoms. For example, a patient with an embolus to the left mainstem MCA might have the sudden onset of right hemiplegia and hemisensory loss and aphasia. When the embolus passes and the lenticulostriate arteries supplying the internal capsule and basal ganglia regions are reperfused, the hemiparesis might improve. Improved cortical blood flow might be accompanied by improvement in speech. If the embolus passed into the inferior division

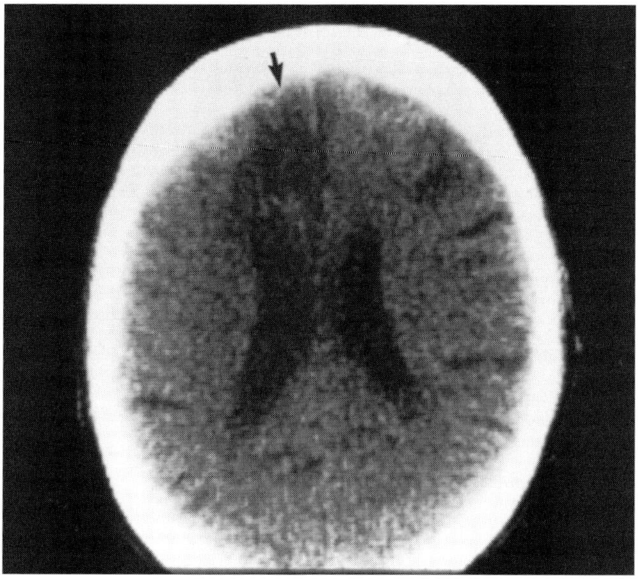

FIG. 15 CT scan showing an anterior cerebral artery teritory infarct on the left (black arrow).

of the MCA supplying the temporal lobe and occluded the artery, the patient might then have the further onset of a fluent Wernicke-type aphasia. When there is further worsening after initial improvement in patients with embolism, the worsening usually occurs in a single step and nearly always occurs during the first 48 hours. Multiple stepwise worsenings, gradual smooth worsening, and delayed worsenings are unusual. Late worsening, after 48 hours, should raise suspicion of hemorrhage into the area of infarction since hemorrhagic transformation often occurs between days 2 and 7 after stroke onset. Table 5 shows the course of deficit in various stroke registries comparing patients with embolism and in situ thrombosis [15,35,36].

Another pattern quite characteristic of brain embolism has been called ''spectacular shrinking deficit'' by Mohr [50]. This term describes sudden, complete or nearly complete clearing of a sudden-onset severe neurologic deficit. Most often the patient has had a mainstem MCA or basilar artery embolus which rapidly passed. An example of each situation will illustrate this syndrome, which is diagnostic of embolism.

A 65-year-old woman, while eating lunch, suddenly collapses and is brought to the hospital. Examination shows: her eyes are conjugately

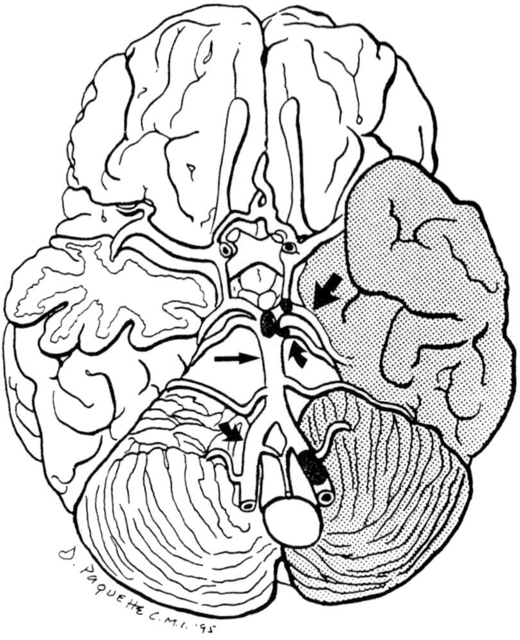

FIG. 16 Cartoon drawing showing the base of the brain and the major arteries of the posterior circulation. The left lower curved arrow is the left intracranial vertebral artery. The upper left straight arrow points to the basilar artery. The right curved artery shows the right superior cerebellar artery, and the upper right straight arrow shows the right posterior cerebral artery. The right intracranial vertebral artery, basilar artery, right superior cerebellar artery, and right posterior cerebral arteries are shown to be blocked by emboli. The resultant cerebellar and posterior cerebral artery territory infarcts are shaded gray. Drawn by Dari Paquette. (From Ref. 41.)

deviated to the left, she does not speak, her right limbs are paralyzed, she does not respond to pin or pinch on her right limbs and body, and she does not heed or look at stimuli on her right side. CT scan is negative but TCD shows no blood flow signal in the left MCA. The family sees her poor condition and is told that the outlook is quite grim. Suddenly, within an hour, the patient begins to speak and move the right limbs and quickly returns virtually to normal. Subsequent TEE evaluation shows a large protruding mobile aortic atheroma.

One evening, a 75-year-old woman coughs and becomes unresponsive. She is brought to the hospital comatose. Her pupils are small and not

TABLE 2 Vascular Recipient Arteries in the Harvard Stroke Registry Based on Cerebral Angiography

Anterior cerebral artery	3 (3%)
Middle cerebral artery	75 (80%)
Mainstem	26
Superior division	9
Superior division branch	22
Inferior division	8
Inferior division branch	1
Multiple branches	9
Posterior cerebral artery	11 (12%)
Basilar artery	5 (5%)

Source: Ref. 15.

reactive to light. Her eyes are deviated downward and inward. She does not respond to stimuli. EKG shows atrial fibrillation. The family is informed that she may be in a terminal coma and to prepare for the worst. The family members go home. CT scan is performed and is normal, as is TCD. The next morning the patient calls home and asks for her clothes and her toothbrush and berates the family for not bringing these things with them.

TABLE 3 Topography of Infarcts in the Lausanne Stroke Registry in Patients with Potential Cardiac Sources of Embolism

Anterior circulation	213 (70%)
Global MCA	33 (11%)
Superior division MCA	60 (20%)
Inferior division MCA	54 (18%)
Deep subcortical	56 (18%)
Anterior cerebral artery (ACA)	9 (3%)
ACA and MCA together	1 (0.3%)
Posterior circulation	69 (23%)
Brainstem	18 (6%)
Thalamus (deep PCA)	12 (4%)
Superficial PCA	21 (7%)
Superficial and deep PCA	3 (1%)
Cerebellum	10 (3%)

Source: Ref. 42.

TABLE 4 Distribution of Infarcts in the Stroke Data Bank

Infarct type	Cardiac-origin embolism	Intra-arterial embolism
Superficial infarcts	24%	61%
Deep small infarct	13%	10%
Deep large infarcts	9%	16%
Superficial and deep infarcts	53%	13%

Source: Ref. 45.

These two patients were cared for by one of the authors (L.R.C.). The first patient had a mainstem left MCA embolus which caused severe but transient dysfunction of the supply zone of that artery. The TCD confirmed blockage of the MCA, but CT showed no infarction. The left hemisphere was temporarily stunned, that is, not receiving enough blood containing oxygen and sugar to function, but not sufficiently deprived to develop irreversible damage. Passage of the embolus allowed rapid recovery of hemispheral function. The second patient had a top-of-the-basilar-artery embolus [39] with temporary midbrain and thalamic stunning. CT confirmed that this dysfunction was not caused by pressure from a large hemispheric lesion with herniation, and that there was no infarction in the upper brainstem. The embolus passed sometime during the night.

In one study, among 118 patients who had the abrupt onset of neurologic deficits, 14 had rapid clearing of their neurologic signs within 24 hours, and in 10, the deficit cleared within 4 hours [51]. All 14 of the patients with spectacular

TABLE 5 Early Course of Deficit in Patients with In Situ Thrombosis vs. Embolism in Various Stroke Registries

	Thrombosis			Embolism		
Course	HSR	MRSR	LSR	HSR	MRSR	LSR
Maximal at onset	40%	45%	66%	79%	89%	82%
Stepwise/stuttering	34%	30%		11%	10%	
Progressive			27%			13%
Gradual smooth	13%	14%		5%	1%	
Fluctuating	13%	11%	7%	5%		5%

HSR, Harvard Stroke Registry [15]; MRSR, Michael Reese Stroke Registry [35]; LSR, Lausanne Stroke Registry [36]. In the LSR, gradual smooth and stepwise/stuttering are considered as progressive.

shrinking deficits had cardiogenic embolism. Angiography in this series showed migration of emboli in the patients with these shrinking deficits [51].

Transient Ischemic Attacks

Temporary deficits that qualify as TIAs do occur in some patients with brain embolism. In patients with arterial sources of emboli, the attacks are always in the supply territory of the affected artery. For example, a patient with atherosclerotic stenosis of the right ICA might have attacks of right monocular visual loss and/or spells of numbness or weakness of the left arm, hand, face, or leg. A patient with right vertebral artery stenosis might have attacks of double vision, dizziness, and staggering. In patients with cardiogenic- or aortic-origin embolism, when attacks occur they are usually random and in different vascular territories.

> A patient of one of the authors (L.R.C.) awakened one night to urinate, and suddenly noted weakness and numbness of the left limbs. By morning the deficit had cleared and he did not tell his wife or a doctor. He had been feeling poorly for weeks with night sweats and fever, symptoms which he also concealed from others. The very next night, he again arose to urinate and now found that his right hand was weak. His wife heard him return to bed and noted that his voice was slurred and his speech did not make good sense. By the morning when she brought him to the doctor, he had almost returned to normal.
>
> CT showed a small left precentral gyrus infarct. The doctor was unsure whether the patient might have been confused about the side involved in the first occurrence and ordered noninvasive vascular studies of the extracranial and intracranial carotid and vertebral artery circulations, which were normal. Subsequent testing showed that the patient had bacterial endocarditis and probably had two emboli, one to the right and the other to the left cerebral hemispheres.

The definition of a TIA usually cited is that of a transient focal deficit that clears within 24 hours. This definition is quite arbitrary, and, in fact, most TIAs clear within 1 hour [52]. Despite the fact that the symptoms are transient, CT and MRI often show infarcts in regions of the brain appropriate to the symptoms [52–54]. Patients with transient focal symptoms and patients with symptoms that persist have potentially serious cerebrovascular, cardiac, or hematological conditions and are at risk for further strokes. Brain ischemia deserves thorough evaluation irrespective of the timing of clinical symptoms.

Activity at Onset

Standard clinical teaching is that strokes due to in situ thrombosis usually develop upon arising from sleep or after a nap, thrombosis having occurred while the circulation is most sluggish. In contrast, strokes related to hemorrhage and embolism are posited to occur during vigorous activity. Activity is thought to provoke leakage of blood from fragile vessels and those damaged by hypertension, and to ''shake loose'' potential emboli from their nests. Recent studies show that most strokes develop during the morning hours, between 10 AM and noon, after awakening and after daily activities have begun and not during sleep [55]. In stroke registries, activity at onset was not particularly helpful in differentiating among the various stroke mechanisms [15,35]. The great majority of strokes occurred during daily activities. In the Michael Reese Stroke Registry, only 5% of emboli and 1% of thrombotic and lacunar strokes began during vigorous physical activity or stress [35]. Occasionally, a cough, sneeze, or sudden vigorous body motion precipitates embolism although the frequency of this occurrence is relatively low. Emboli also seem to occur more often than chance after awakening at night to urinate, a so-called matudinal (morning) embolus.

Systemic Embolism

Necropsy studies of patients with brain embolism of cardiac origin nearly always show embolic infarcts in other organs, especially the spleen and kidneys. In contrast, the frequency of clinical recognition of systemic embolism is quite low. In various stroke registries, the frequencies of diagnosis of systemic embolism were: 2%, Harvard Stroke Registry [15]; 2.3%, Michael Reese Stroke Registry [35]; 3.6%, Stroke Data Bank [56]; 3%, Lausanne Stroke Registry [36]. The highest frequency of systemic embolism, 8%, was found in a study of 60 patients with cardiogenic brain embolism in whom two patients had kidney and three had peripheral limb embolism [57].

Embolism to the brain that causes ischemia usually causes transient or persistent symptoms. The brain is a bit like litmus paper, very sensitive to perturbations. Systemic embolism also causes ischemia, but the symptoms are much less specific. Embolism to a limb might cause arm pain, leg cramp, or other transient discomfort, symptoms that are very common and usually due to activity, positioning of the limb, or some other banal, everyday occurrence. Similarly, embolism to the intestinal tract might cause stomach cramps, bowel irregularity, a belly ache—rather common and nonspecific symptoms. Embolism to the kidneys or spleen causes flank or abdominal discomfort rarely diagnosed as due to systemic embolism. Hematuria and sudden-onset severe limb ischemia are probably the only two occurrences that usually lead to recognition of systemic embolism, especially in patients with known heart disease.

Headache

Headache is an extremely common symptom among stroke patients. Although brain tissue contains no pain-sensitive afferent nerve fibers, the meninges and vessel walls contain many pain-sensitive nerve endings. Stretching and dilatation of arteries on the brain surface and in the neck often produce head and neck discomfort and headache. The frequency and causes of headache vary depending on the mechanism of stroke. Some headaches are caused by mass effect in relation to brain swelling or hemorrhage within the brain. Irritation of the meninges by blood causes headache in patients with subarachnoid hemorrhage. In ischemic stroke patients, headache may also be due to distension of occluded arteries by clot, dilatation of collateral arteries, and by tears within arterial walls.

Table 6 lists frequencies of headache at or near onset of stroke in various stroke registries and series [15,36,58,59]. Headache is most common in patients with intracerebral hemorrhage. Patients with brain embolism have headache more often than patients with lacunar infarcts caused by penetrating artery disease, but less often than patients with occlusive disease of large extracranial and intracranial arteries. Headaches unusual for the individual patient may also occur before strokes. Patients with subarachnoid hemorrhage may have episodes in which a small amount of blood leaks, causing what has been referred to as a "sentinel" headache. Frequent dull or throbbing headaches often are present in the days or weeks before ischemic stroke in patients with large-artery thrombosis. These are due to distension of occluded arteries as well as dilated collateral arteries. Headaches are rarely noted before brain embolism.

Seizures

Seizures at or near stroke onset are very uncommon in patients with ischemic strokes irrespective of cause. Seizures are more common in patients with intracerebral and subarachnoid hemorrhages than in patients with ischemic strokes irrespective of the mechanism of the ischemia. In the Harvard Stroke Registry, 4% of patients with brain embolism had seizures early in their clinical course as compared to 0.3% of patients with large-artery in situ occlusions [15]. No patient with lacunar infarction in the Harvard Stroke Registry had an early seizure, an expected finding because lacunae are, by definition, small and deep and not likely

TABLE 6 Headache at or Near Time of Onset Among Various Stroke Types in Various Stroke Registries (% of Patients)

Registry	Large-artery thrombosis	Embolism	Lacunar infarction	Intracerebral hemorrhage
Harvard [15]	12%	9%	3%	33%
Lausanne [36]	17%	18%	7%	40%
Stroke Data Bank [58]	11%	10%	5%	41%
Michael Reese, Illinois [59]	26%	14%	6%	55%

to cause cortical irritation [15]. In the Stroke Data Bank only 3.1% of patients with cardiac-origin embolism had seizures [60], and no patient with presumed brain embolism in the Lausanne Stroke Registry had seizures [36]. In a thesis that analyzed the development of seizures among 770 patients with first-ever symptomatic supratentorial brain infarcts in the Maastricht stroke registry, the presence of cardiac-origin embolism meant that the patient had a relative risk of 5.14 of developing an early-onset seizure compared to patients without cardiogenic embolism [61]. Among 2000 stroke patients in another series, patients with hemorrhagic infarcts and large infarcts were most likely to have seizures [46]. The average size of infarcts in patients with seizures was 76.7 cm^3, vs. 45.6 cm^3 in patients who did not have seizures [46]. In this series 40% of the seizures in stroke patients occurred during the first day and 51% during the first week; 96% of poststroke seizures occurred during the first year after stroke [46]. Although seizures near the onset of stroke symptoms are probably more common in patients with embolism than in nonembolic causes of ischemic stroke, seizures are too infrequent to be of much diagnostic help.

Decrease in Level of Consciousness

Early decrease in the level of consciousness in stroke patients is most often due to acute brainstem tegmental ischemia related to embolism to the basilar artery. Decreased consciousness can also be related to major hemispheral ischemia caused by sudden occlusion of the major blood supply of either hemisphere. Later in the course, during days 3 to 7, persistent loss of consciousness is usually explained by brain edema and the mass effect of large cerebellar and cerebral infarcts. Transient loss of consciousness is most often seizure related, or due to a cardiac arrythmia.

Few studies have analyzed the frequency of loss of consciousness at or near the time of stroke onset. In the Stroke Data Bank, decreased consciousness early in the stroke was present in 29.8% of patients with embolism of cardiac origin, compared to a 6.1% frequency in patients with intra-arterial embolism [45]. Decreased consciousness at or near stroke onset is more common in patients with embolic occlusions than in other causes of ischemic stroke and is more common in patients with cardiac-origin embolism than in those with proximal arterial sources. The larger size of emboli of cardiac origin as compared with emboli of arterial origin is the probable explanation for the difference.

Clinical Patterns of Neurologic Symptoms

Neurological diagnoses are often made by pattern matching. Clinicians match the findings in any given patient with those usually found in patients with lesions affecting certain anatomical regions. Lesions in specific anatomical loci, in turn, are associated with occlusions of the various feeding arteries. Tables 2 through 4 show the usual common brain and vascular locations of embolic infarcts. Each location has characteristic clinical findings.

Anterior (Carotid Artery) Circulation Embolism

Among all series, the great majority of emboli are found within the MCAs and their branches. Large emboli may block the mainstem MCA near its origin, leading to infarction of the entire territory of the cerebral hemisphere supplied by the MCA (Fig. 7D, 7I). The clinical deficits in these patients are very severe and most patients die. Rare patients survive but remain severely and permanently disabled. Consciousness is reduced. The eyes usually rest conjugately toward the side of the infarct. The contralateral limbs are paralyzed and insensitive to pin stimulation or pinch. Although the patient may attend to voices, visual objects, and people situated on the same side of space as the brain infarct, they often will ignore identical stimuli on the contralateral side of space. When the left MCA is occluded, patients do not speak or heed directions or queries. Within the first 24 to 48 hours stupor deepens, then coma develops, and the patient dies. Recently some patients have been saved by removing the overlying skull plate to give the brain room to expand [62,63]. Later, the cranial bone plate can be placed back in its former position. Unfortunately, many survivors are left badly damaged and disabled. In some young patients much of the brain swelling is due to edema, and survival after craniectomy is reasonably good.

Occasionally, patients with mainstem MCA emboli who have very severe clinical signs rapidly, almost miraculously, recover. This so-called spectacular shrinking deficit is due to reperfusion of brain that was reversibly ischemic (''stunned'') [50,51]. CT scan and other neuroimaging tests can be helpful in predicting the prognosis for recovery. The presence of early signs of infarction bodes poorly for recovery. When the CT scan is normal initially, the prognosis is more hopeful.

Occlusion of the MCA proximal to the lenticulostriate branches sometimes produces an infarct that includes the deep basal ganglionic and capsular territory as well as superficial MCA territory. (Fig. 7B, 7C) This pattern of infarction, involvement of superficial and deep MCA territory, was found in over half of the patients in the Stroke Data Bank series with cardiac-origin embolism (Table 4) [45]. These patients invariably have a hemiparesis involving the face, arm, and leg on the side contralateral to the lesion. They usually also have some degree of hemisensory loss. Conjugate eye deviation and inattention to the contralateral side of visual space are variable findings that depend on the size of the infarct and its distribution in the white matter and cerebral cortex. Cortical function abnormalities such as aphasia, abnormal drawing and copying, visual neglect, and lack of awareness of the neurological deficit depend on the location and extent of cortical infarction and whether the left or right cerebral hemisphere is involved.

Occlusion of the superior division of the MCA causes ischemia in the territory of the artery that lies above the sylvian fissure. (Figs. 7E–7G, 10, 11) This includes the frontal and superior parietal lobes. The temporal lobe is spared. Patients with left superior division infarcts have a right hemiparesis more severe in the hand, arm, and face than in the lower extremity. They also have diminished touch and position sensation in the right hand and face. Patients usually fail to identify objects placed in their right hands. Aphasia is invariably present and is usually of the nonfluent type characterized by decreased amount of speech and effortful, poorly pronounced words. Comprehension of spoken language is usually relatively preserved. Patients with right superior division MCA territory infarcts have left hemiparesis more severe in the hand and face, left hemisensory loss, inattention to the left side of visual space, and diminished awareness of their left limb dysfunction.

Inferior division MCA territory infarcts involve the posterior temporal and parietal lobes (Figs. 7H [left side], 12, 13). Patients with left cerebral hemisphere infarcts have a fluent aphasia characterized by effortless speech that contains many wrong and nonexistent words, and jargon. There may also be a right upper quadrant visual field defect. Some patients become agitated and paranoid. Patients with right inferior division MCA territory infarcts have a left upper quadrant visual field defect and a hyperactive state with agitation [64]. They draw and copy drawings poorly.

Occasionally the recipient artery is the anterior cerebral artery (ACA). Infarction involves the medial frontal and parietal lobes above the corpus callosum near the midline (Fig. 15). The limbs contralateral to the infarct may show a distinct pattern of weakness with paralysis most severe in the foot, leg, and thigh and some weakness of shoulder shrug and shoulder abduction. Some patients have difficulty controlling urination. Decreased spontaneity, apathy, and decreased amount of speech also may occur due to frontal lobe infarction.

Posterior Circulation (Vertebrobasilar Arteries) Embolism

About one-fifth of emboli go to one of the vertebral arteries and enter the intracranial posterior circulation arteries. The most common clinical patterns of symptoms occur in patients with cerebellar, PCA, and ''top-of-the-basilar'' territory infarctions [41].

Emboli that block one of the ICVAs often cause infarction in the posterior undersurface of the cerebellum in the territory of the posterior inferior cerebellar artery (PICA) branch of the ICVA. Dizziness, headache in the back of the head and sometimes the neck, vomiting, and gait ataxia are the most common symptoms [41,65,66]. Examination shows severe gait ataxia. Many patients lean to the side of the infarct and have difficulty standing or even sitting without support. There may be decreased tone in the ipsilateral arm and nystagmus. Some patients with large PICA territory cerebellar infarcts develop compression of the ventricular system and brainstem, and can become stuporous and die. Removal of the soft, edematous, necrotic cerebellum can be life-saving in these patients with so-called pseudotumoral cerebellar infarcts [41].

Embolism to one of the posterior cerebral arteries (PCAs) causes infarction in the temporal and occipital lobes [41,67,68]. When the proximal PCA is blocked, the infarct often includes the thalamus. The most common symptoms and signs are visual and sensory. Patients with right PCA territory infarcts have a left visual field defect (entire left field or upper or lower quadrant), and may also report numbness and tingling and loss of sensation in their left limbs and trunk. Patients with left PCA territory infarcts have right visual field and hemisensory abnormalities. They may also be unable to read despite retaining the ability to write and may also have difficulty making new memories. Bilateral PCA territory infarcts cause cortical blindness or less severe bilateral visual field defects, severe amnesia, and an agitated delirium [39,41].

When emboli block the very distal end of the basilar artery, infarction often involves the paramedian thalamus, rostral midbrain, and both PCA territories [39–41]. Infarction can be limited to the posterior portions of the cerebral hemispheres (Fig. 3) or to the midbrain and thalamic portions of the brainstem. Bilateral infarction in the paramedian posterior thalamus usually causes reduced alertness, with hypersomnolence, loss of upgaze, and amnesia. Sometimes patients also cannot look down. When the upper midbrain is involved, patients have unilateral or bilateral third-nerve palsies (ptosis with eyes down and out) and may also have bilateral limb weakness. Cortical blindness, amnesia, and agitated delirium are added when bilateral PCA territory infarcts are also present.

IMAGING AND LABORATORY EVALUATION OF POTENTIAL RECIPIENT ARTERY SITES

Neuroimaging of the Brain

CT and MRI are indispensable in the diagnosis of brain embolism. These brain neuroimaging tests are able to separate brain infarcts from hemorrhages. CT scans have been used traditionally to exclude hemorrhage since hematomas are visible immediately after stroke onset and are easily seen as hyperdense, well-circumscribed lesions. Susceptibility-weighted MRI scans also can detect hemorrhages early in their course. Brain infarcts are usually not visible on very early, acute CT scans, while MRI is probably more sensitive in detecting early infarction.

MRI is clearly superior to CT in detecting and showing infarcts in the cerebellum, brainstem, and inferior temporal lobes. When infarcts are present, their location, size, and multiplicity can help predict the mechanism of infarction.

Careful inspection of CT scans performed within 6 hours of stroke onset sometimes shows subtle signs of early infarction. Loss of definition of the gray-white matter junction in ischemic regions, edema which causes effacement of sulci in one cerebral hemisphere or one vascular territory, loss of definition of the basal ganglia and the insular region, are all early signs of infarction. Another common finding on noncontrast CT scans is opacification of the middle cerebral or other arteries—the so-called hyperdense middle cerebral artery sign. The hyperdensity is caused by a thrombus within the artery. Sometimes hyperdense basilar and posterior cerebral arteries are evident in patients with ischemia in those vascular territories. Hyperdense arteries on noncontrast scans were found in 10% of acute strokes in one study [69], in 21% [70] and 22% [71] of acute thromboembolic MCA occlusions in other studies, and in 31% of acute anterior circulation brain infarcts in another study [72]. The hyperdense MCA sign has a relatively low sensitivity (about 50%) but a high specificity (about 90%).

CT and MRI can also be useful in deciding on treatment and rendering a prognosis. Patients who have embolic brain ischemia are candidates for thrombolytic treatment if seen early enough in their course. If a patient with a suspected MCA territory embolus had a large infarct already visible on CT or MRI at the time that thrombolytic treatment was contemplated, the likelihood of a good outcome would be small, since much brain was likely already infarcted and would be unlikely to recover after reperfusion. The risk of hemorrhage after thrombolytic treatment is also considerably higher when sizable infarction is present before treatment [73]. Decisions on the timing of anticoagulation also depend on the imaging results. When large infarcts are present, the risk of hemorrhage after heparin anticoagulation is higher.

CT and MRI are useful even when the neurological symptoms are transient. Scans in that circumstance may show unexpected infarcts despite the negativity of the history and neurological examinations. Such so-called silent infarcts are common. Neurological symptoms may have been present but forgotten by the patient. In other instances, the symptoms may have been trivial; for example, the patient may ignore a temporary limp, a short period of less precise articulation or word finding difficulty, transient numbness in a limb. Often the neurological symptoms are misinterpreted as representing transient compression of a nerve in a limb or other banal nonstroke causes. When there are multiple unsuspected brain infarcts in different vascular territories, cardiogenic or aortogenic embolism is likely. The presence of multiple infarcts in one vascular territory, such as the right ICA territory, should lead to the conclusion that there is most likely disease in that artery, in this case the right ICA or MCA.

Vascular Imaging

Vascular studies have a dual purpose: to define the lesion within recipient arteries and to image any possible arterial sources of embolism. Since angiography was the first vascular imaging test used to detect emboli and to define vascular lesions, knowledge of the diagnostic angiographic findings will help physicians interpret the results of less invasive vascular tests. Angiographic findings that suggest embolism are the following.

Blockage of Superficial Branches of Intracranial Arteries

Atherosclerosis rarely affects branch arteries but is much more common in the major extracranial and basal intracranial arteries.

Absence of Any Vascular Occlusive Lesion in the Artery Supplying an Infarcted Zone

For example, if a patient has a sizable acute right MCA territory infarct and the right ICA and MCA are normal angiographically, then one can conclude that there must have been temporary blockage of the right MCA by an embolus that remained long enough to cause infarction and later passed.

Movement or Disappearance of a Vascular Obstructing Lesion on Sequential Angiographic Films

Movement of occlusive particles is diagnostic of emboli.

Sudden, Sharply Demarcated Occlusion of Major Intracranial Arteries

Especially, the MCAs, PCAs, and cerebellar arteries in the absence of atherosclerosis in those vessels are occluded. Patients who have in situ thrombi form at sites of previous atherosclerosis usually have had promonontory TIAs, and the occlusion is tapered. The occluded artery shows some signs of prior atherosclerotic stenosis.

A Filling Defect Within a Symptomatic Intracranial Artery

This is highly suggestive of embolism.

Angiography also gives information about possible proximal arterial sources of embolism. In a patient with a right MCA territory infarct, severe stenosis of the right ICA in the neck is highly suggestive of intra-arterial embolism arising from the right ICA.

Newer, less invasive vascular imaging tests are now used instead of angiography in most patients. We recommend that noninvasive imaging always precede angiography even when it has already been decided that angiography is needed [74]. The results of noninvasive vascular tests can help better target angiography and limit the number of arteries that require study and so reduce the amount of contrast media needed and the length of the procedure. CT angiography (CTA) can be performed at the same time that CT brain images are acquired. Intravenous dye is injected, and spiral CT scanners are able to generate images of the major extracranial and intracranial arteries. MR angiography (MRA) can be performed at the same time that MRI brain images are generated. MRA does not require injection of any substance. CTA and MRA can generate accurate images of the major extracranial and intracranial arteries but do not show branches very well. Clinicians should view the films using the same criteria for embolism that were discussed for angiography.

Ultrasound is another very important diagnostic modality that has a number of advantages. Machines are portable. Testing is safe and without risks. Ultrasound testing is much less expensive than angiography, MRA, or CTA. Ultrasound testing can be repeated in order to document changes in blocked recipient arteries. In some European centers, ultrasound equipment is available at the bedside and is used by physicians to extend the vascular physical examination much as ultrasound is now used by nurses and physicians in intensive-care units to monitor peripheral vessels.

Intracranial arteries are insonated using a small probe placed at regions of the skull where there are foramina or natural soft spots. The usual windows are the orbit, foramen magnum, and temporal bone (Fig. 17). Transcranial Doppler (TCD) probes are placed perpendicular to arteries, for example, the MCAs, while the technician or physician performing the test listens for the characteristic pulsatile swooshing sound that indicates that the probe is in the correct position. The computer allows the person performing the TCD examination to view the Doppler spectrum at successive 5-mm depths along the insonated artery. Figure 18a shows a probe insonating the MCA on one side, and Figure 18b shows a characteristic spectrum from that MCA. TCD measures blood flow velocities along insonated arteries.

Most people have had the experience of trying to wash a pavement or paved patio with a garden hose. Figure 19 illustrates the water flow when the spigot is turned fully on and the nozzle is not turned. When the nozzle of the hose is turned, a stronger, more targeted water spray is generated (Fig. 20). Turning the nozzle reduces the size of the lumen at the end of the hose. The velocity of flow in the water jet is inversely proportional to the luminal size until a critical luminal size is reached, at which time flow is reduced. If the nozzle is turned fully, then water stops flowing or dribbles out the end of the hose (Fig. 21). Similarly, if an insonated artery is stenotic, then the blood flow velocities are increased at the

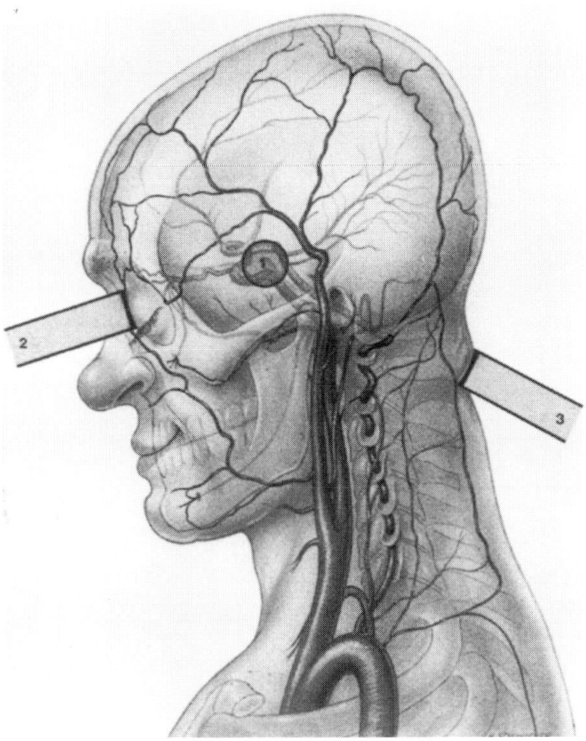

FIG. 17 Anatomical drawing of the neck and head of a man, lateral view, showing the insonation sites for transcranial Doppler ultrasound. (1) Temporal window. (2) Orbital window. (3) Suboccipital, foramen magnum window. (From Ref. 76.)

site of narrowing. If the artery is blocked by an embolus or in situ thrombus, then no or very low signals are obtained.

In a patient with a right MCA territory stroke, the absence of Doppler signals over the right MCA, when left MCA signals are normal, is strongly suggestive of right MCA occlusion. Subsequent appearance of signals in the right MCA shows that the obstruction has moved along or passed. Unfortunately, in some patients, especially older women, it is not possible to obtain signals from the MCAs because of the lack of a suitable temporal window. The ICVAs can be insonated through the foramen magnum. Figure 22 shows the vertebral arteries in the upper neck, foramen magnum, and intracranially.

Extracranial ultrasound using Duplex equipment (combined B-mode ultrasound and pulsed Doppler) can detect significant occlusive and stenotic lesions

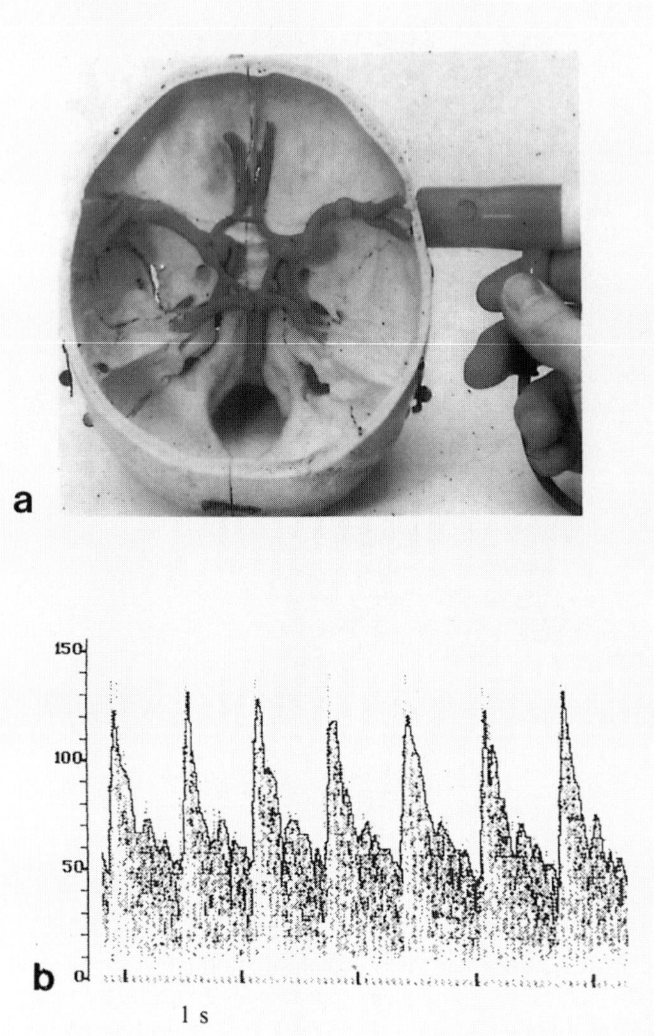

FIG. 18 (a) Base of the skull with the arteries shown as they would appear in situ. The transcranial Doppler probe is placed on the right of the figure perpendicular to the middle cerebral artery. (b) Doppler spectra from the middle cerebral artery. (Courtesy of Durchblutsstorungen des Gehirns—neue diagnostiche Moglichkeiten. Verlag Bertelsman Stiftung, Gutersloh, 1987.)

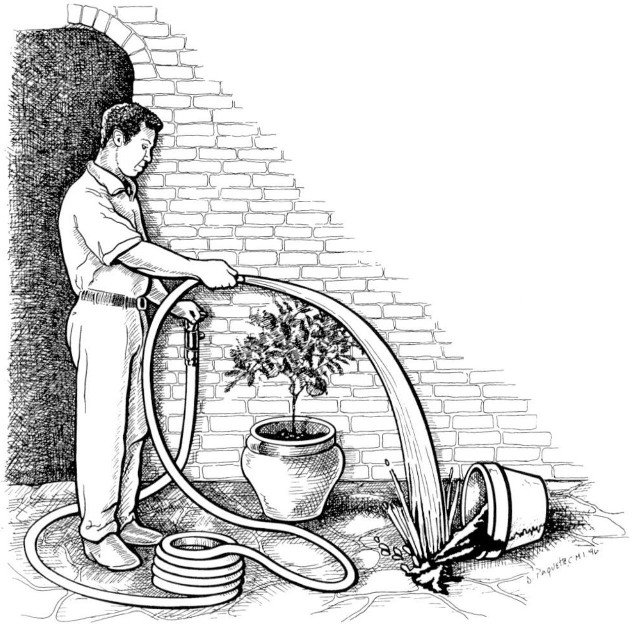

Fig. 19 Drawing of a man cleaning a patio with a hose. The water spigot is opened fully and the nozzle is wide open. Drawn by Dari Paquette.

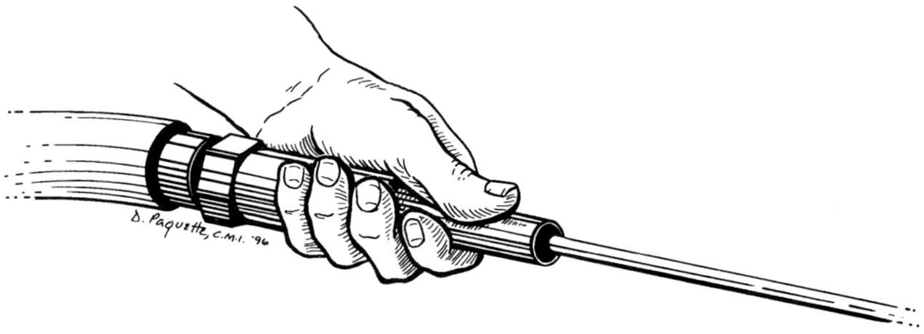

Fig. 20 The nozzle is turned making the lumen of the hose smaller and narrowing the jet of water. Drawn by Dari Paquette.

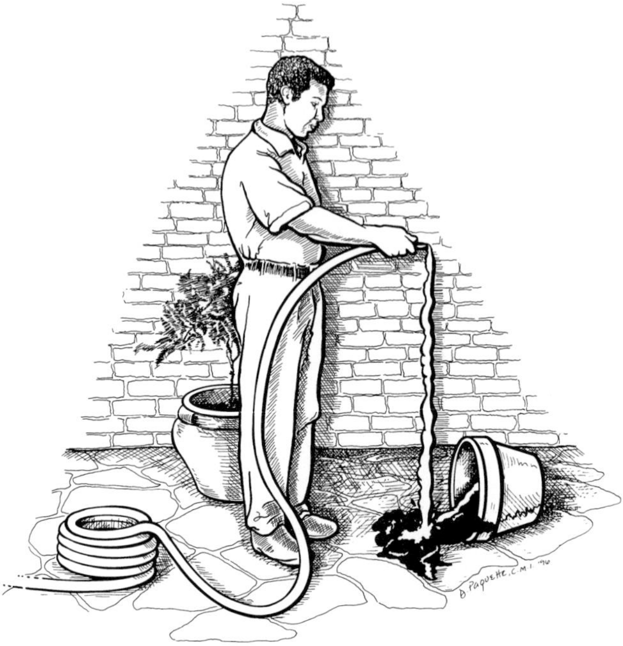

Fig. 21 The nozzle has been turned nearly fully, obliterating the lumen of the hose. Only a dribble of water escapes from the hose. Drawn by Dari Paquette.

of the extracranial carotid and vertebral arteries [75,76]. Newer technology such as color-flow and power Doppler improve diagnostic accuracy of the vascular images. A continuous-wave (CW) Doppler probe can be moved along the neck arteries to show whether flow is antegrade, retrograde, or mixed. Extracranial ultrasound helps identify potential arterial sources of embolism. Occasionally, emboli can block the carotid or vertebral arteries in the neck. Sequential ultrasound tests can show disappearing embolic occlusions [77].

Monitoring of Emboli

TCD can also be used to monitor for embolism [16–21]. Monitoring is performed in patients who are being evaluated for TIAs or acute strokes, and during procedures such as carotid and vertebral artery angioplasty, carotid endarterectomy, and cardiac surgery. Monitoring can show that microembolism is occurring and can suggest the source. Monitoring can also quantitate the frequency of microembolic signals and can be performed sequentially to monitor the effects of treat-

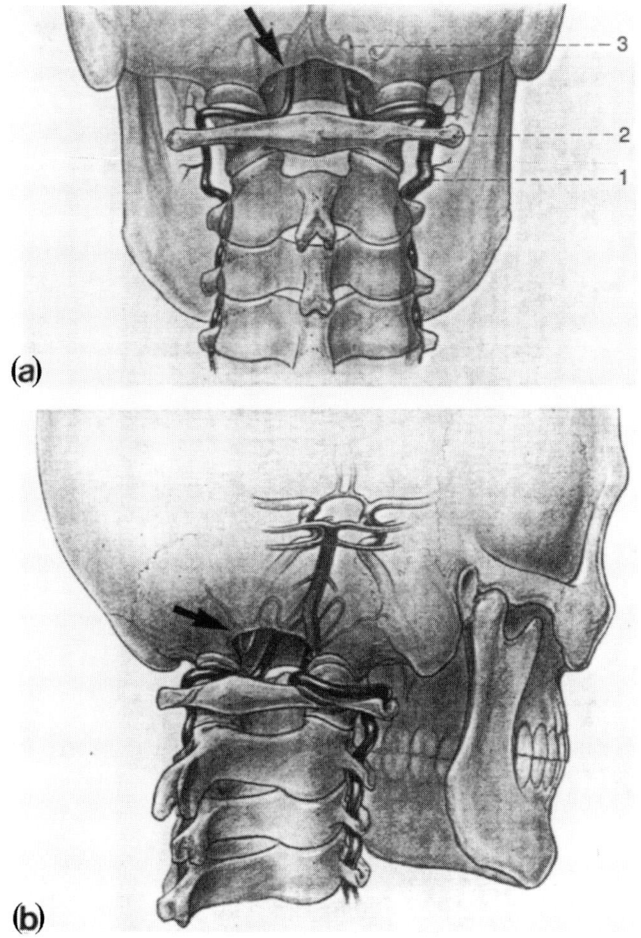

FIG. 22 Posterior views of the upper neck vertebrae and the skull, showing the vertebral arteries and the foramen magnum (black arrows). (a) Direct anteroposterior view: 1, vertebral artery; 2, transverse process of the atlas; 3, posterior inferior cerebellar artery (PICA) branch of the intracranial vertebral artery (ICVA). (b) An oblique view of the same structures.

ment. Figures 23 and 24 show some examples of embolic signals that were detected after a small quantity of air was injected into a peripheral vein in a patient with a patent foramen ovale.

In one study, Daffertshofer and colleagues monitored 280 patients with acute ischemic events in MCA territorry as well as 118 asymptomatic controls

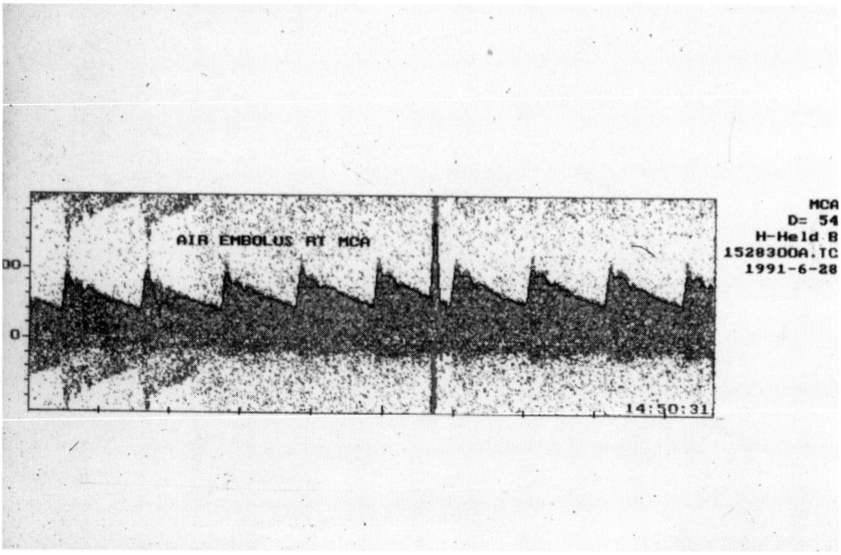

FIG. 23 Doppler spectrum from monitoring of the right MCA in a patient with a patent foramen ovale. An embolic signal is seen after introduction of a small quantity of air into a peripheral arm vein.

for periods of 30 to 60 minutes [20]. Only two controls (1.7%) had microembolic signals. No microembolic signals were detected among 78 patients who had no identified sources of embolism, while 12.9% of patients with sources of emboli had microembolic signals [20]. In this study, microembolism was more common in patients with vascular sources of embolism such as ICA stenosis (17.1%), compared to 6.2% in patients with cardiac sources of embolism. One-fifth of patients with ICA stenosis >70% had microembolic signals, compared to 13% in patients with <70% ICA stenosis.

Sliwka et al., during a 6-month period, attempted to monitor 109 consecutive patients with atrial fibrillation or other potential cardiac sources of embolism [19]. Nine of the patients had insufficient temporal windows, so they could not be monitored with TCD. Microembolic signals were detected in 36 of the 100 patients successfully monitored. The average number of microembolic signals was 2.69 ± 2.7 per 30 minutes (range 1 to 12) [19]. Patients with atrial fibrillation who had coronary atherosclerotic heart disease with ejection fractions of <30%, dilated cardiomyopathy, or mitral stenosis had the highest percentage of microemboli detection [19]. In another study, 38 patients with acute strokes were monitored with TCD. Only four had microembolic signals [18]. Two of the emboli-positive patients had mechanical prosthetic valves; one had severe ICA ste-

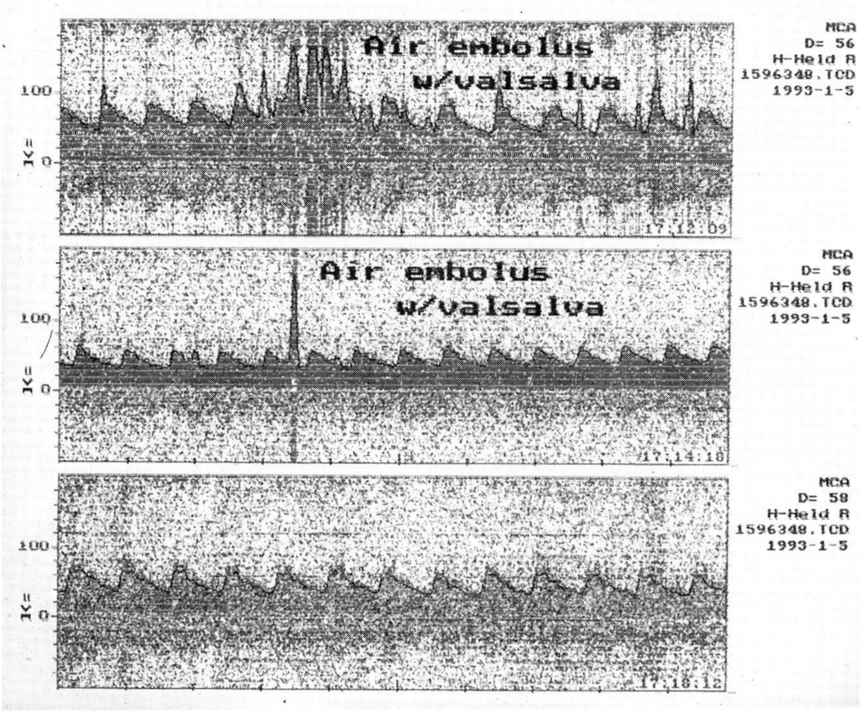

FIG. 24 Doppler spectra from same patient studied in Figure 23. More emboli are seen after Valsalva maneuver.

nosis; and one had a patent foramen ovale, and echocardiography showed mitral valve strands [18].

Georgiadis and colleagues monitored 300 patients with potential cardiac sources of emboli and 100 patients with severe ICA disease using TCD [78]. They found the following frequencies of microembolic signals among their monitored patients: infective endocarditis, 43%; left ventricular aneurysm, 34%; intracardiac thrombus, 26%; dilated cardiomyopathy, 26%; nonvalvular atrial fibrillation, 21%; native valvular disease, 15%; prosthetic valves, 55%; ICA disease, 28% (symptomatic ICA disease 52%, asymptomatic disease 7%); and 5% among controls [78].

Monitoring during cardiac and angiographic procedures and cardiac and vascular surgery can help the teams performing the procedures modify their techniques according to the frequency of microembolic signals. The results of TCD monitoring have varied considerably in different studies. Undoubtedly the technology available will improve. Standardization and interpretation of results are necessary. The technology promises to be important both in diagnosis and in monitoring the results of treatments and procedures.

SOURCES OF EMBOLI

The great majority of emboli to the brain arise from the heart, aorta, or the cervicocranial arteries. Figure 25 is a cartoon which illustrates these major sources.

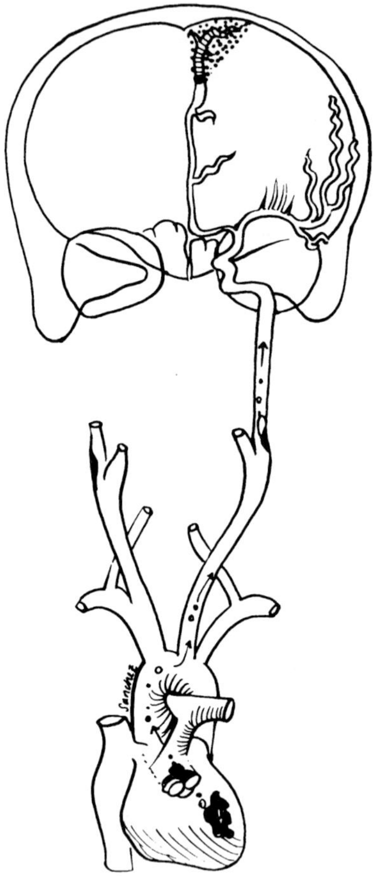

FIG. 25 Cartoon showing at the top of the figure blockage of an anterior cerebral artery by an embolus. Black regions within the heart, aorta, and carotid arteries represent potential donor sources of the embolus. Drawn by Dr. Juan Sanchez Ramos. (From Ref. 75.)

Occasionally foreign materials such as air, fat, or cancer cells enter the circulation and embolize to various systemic organs.

Cardiac Sources

In the 1950s the only two cardiac disorders that were accepted as having an important risk of causing embolism were rheumatic mitral stenosis with atrial fibrillation, and recent myocardial infarction. We now know that many cardiac lesions and disorders carry some risk of cardiac thrombosis and embolism. Data from stroke registries and more modern cardiac diagnostic testing have made it possible during the past two decades to diagnose cardiac disorders more definitively and to attempt to quantify the risk of embolism. Cardiac disorders that carry a risk of brain embolism can be divided into six groups: (1) *arrythmias*, especially atrial fibrillation and sick-sinus syndrome; (2) *valvular heart diseases*, especially mitral stenosis, prosthetic heart valves, infective endocarditis, and marantic endocarditis; (3) *ventricular myocardial abnormalities*, especially related to coronary artery disease, myocarditis, and other dilated cardiomyopathies; (4) *lesions within the cavity of the ventricles*, especially tumors such as myxomas and thrombi; (5) *shunts*, especially intra-atrial septal defects and patent foramen ovale which allow passage of emboli forming in the peripheral veins to enter the systemic circulation causing so-called *paradoxical embolism*; and (6) *atrial lesions* such as dilated atria, atrial infarcts and thrombi, and atrial septal aneurysms.

Virchow, in 1856, described three antecedent conditions for the development of thrombi within the chambers of the heart: a region of circulatory stasis, injury to the endothelial surfaces of the heart, and increased blood coagulability [79,80]. In areas of stasis a low shear rate and other factors activate the classical coagulation cascade, leading to the formation of erythrocyte-fibrin thrombi. Stasis occurs most often in the atria and atrial appendages in patients with atrial fibrillation, and in the ventricular chambers in patients with global and focal regions of decreased myocardial contractility. Altered myocardial endothelium occurs in patients with myocardial infarcts, ventricular aneurysms, and inflammatory and other myocardiopathies and endocardial disorders. Valvular endothelium can be damaged by many different conditions. Loss of a protective endothelial surface exposes circulating blood to the underlying tissues and causes platelet activation, adhesion, and secretion, as well as activating the coagulation cascade [80,81]. Recent studies have begun to show increased platelet activation and blood coagulability in patients with cardiac-source embolism [82,83].

In this section, we will first comment on the cardiac disorders known to predispose to brain embolism and discuss specific treatment studies when available. We will then note the frequency of these sources in various stroke registries, and then discuss general diagnostic and treatment issues. Embolism during and after surgery and after diagnostic procedures will be discussed in Chapters 4 and 5.

Arrythmias

Atrial fibrillation

Atrial fibrillation is one of the most common cardiac disorders. About 0.4% of the population have atrial fibrillation, and the disorder becomes much more common as patients age. Perhaps as many as 5% of individuals over age 60 have atrial fibrillation [84,85]. Epidemiological studies during the past two decades have firmly established that atrial fibrillation is a very important risk factor for stroke, that stroke is most often due to cardiogenic embolism, and that standard antithrombotic treatment substantially reduces the frequency of brain embolism in patients with atrial fibrillation. In four large studies the relative risk of stroke was 5.6 (Framingham, U.S.) [86], 5.6 (Shibata, Japan) [87], 7.1 (Reykjavik, Iceland) [88], and 6.9 (Whitehall, U.K.) [89] times that of patients without atrial fibrillation.

Clearly, the etiology of atrial fibrillation and associated cardiac and other medical factors affect the risk of stroke in patients with atrial fibrillation. In the Framingham study, the presence of rheumatic heart disease and atrial fibrillation conveyed a 17.6 × risk of stroke, compared to the lone atrial fibrillation rate of 5.6 × [86]. Advanced age, congestive heart failure, a history of hypertension, previous myocardial infarction, and prior thromboembolism all increase the risk of stroke in patients with atrial fibrillation [90,91]. These features should be known from the medical history.

A collaborative analysis of five atrial fibrillation stroke prevention studies analyzed the contribution of various historical risk factors on the development of stroke during follow-up [92]. The relative risks (RRs) as determined by multivariate analysis of all the data were: history of previous stroke or TIA (RR 2.5); diabetes mellitus (RR 1.7); history of hypertension (RR 1.6); and increasing age (RR 1.4 for each decade) [92]. These calculated relative risks were for the occurrence of any stroke and were not limited to those attributable to cardiogenic embolism.

Information derived from echocardiography is also very helpful in assessing the risk of brain embolism in individual patients with atrial fibrillation [93–95]. Transesophageal echocardiography (TEE) can detect *left atrial and left atrial appendage thrombi*. In patients with atrial fibrillation who do not have valvular disease, thrombi often form in and dislodge from the left atrial appendage, while patients with atrial fibrillation and valvular disease have more left atrial thrombi [95,96]. In patients with valvular disease and atrial fibrillation, thrombi have been detected in 9% to 29% of patients, compared to 10% prevalence in patients without valvular disease [95]. Small thrombi, < 2 mm, and those that have already dislodged are not readily detected. The sensitivity of TEE in detecting left atrial and left atrial appendage thrombi has been estimated at between 83% and 100% [94]. *Left atrial enlargement* [93–95] and *abnormal left atrial appendage function* as determined by Doppler TEE [95,97–100] also convey an increased risk for cardioembolic stroke. The presence of *mitral annulus calcification* [100] and *left ventricular dysfunction* [94,95] also increase the risk of stroke in patients with atrial fibrillation.

Spontaneous echo contrast (also called ''smoke'') is probably one of the most important factors that predict the future likelihood of cardiogenic embolism in patients with atrial fibrillation. First described in patients with mitral valve disease [101], spontaneous echo contrast refers to swirling hazes of echogenicity within the cardiac chambers. The echogenic swirls can move repeatedly within the cavity and may disappear when blood flow increases or when local stasis resolves. The intensity can vary from a faint, cloudlike appearance to bright echo contrast. Spontaneous echo contrast is probably due to the interaction between plasma proteins and erythrocytes at low shear rates [95,102]. The major determinants of spontaneous echogenicity are the hematocrit, fibrinogen levels, and slow intracardiac flow [103]. The frequency of spontaneous echo contrast has been evaluated in several studies of patients with atrial fibrillation [96,104–106]. In one study, among 33 nonanticoagulated patients with atrial fibrillation without valvular disease, 11 had spontaneous echo contrast [96]. Tsai et al. found spontaneous echo contrast using TEE in 25 of 103 atrial fibrillation patients (24%) who did not have valvular disease [106]. In this study 21 of 35 patients (84%) who had thromboembolism had spontaneous echo contrast [106].

The presence and nature of valvular disease is an important factor in predicting the presence of echo contrast. DeBelder et al., in a study of atrial fibrillation patients, reported echo contrast in 67% (10/15) patients with mitral stenosis, in 50% (4/8) patients with prosthetic mitral valves, and in 21% (12/57) of patients without these conditions [104]. Echo contrast was found in 65% of patients who had a history of thromboembolism. Leong and colleagues prospectively followed a series of 272 patients with atrial fibrillation who had no valvular disease [107]. Twenty of the 161 (12.4%) patients with spontaneous echo contrast had cerebrovascular events, and two had systemic embolism (total event rate 12% per year); only five of 111 (4.5%) patients who did not have echo contrast had cerebrovascular events (event rate of 3% per year) [107]. Chimowitz and colleagues showed that the presence of spontaneous echo contrast was highly associated with prior strokes in patients who had either atrial fibrillation or mitral valve stenosis [108].

Atrial fibrillation is a common finding in the elderly. Many patients with atrial fibrillation have other conditions, such as hypertension, diabetes, duplicated extracranial and intracranial occlusive disease, and aortic atheromas, which explain their strokes; also, many strokes that occur in patients with atrial fibrillation are not cardioembolic. The Stroke Prevention in Atrial Fibrillation investigators

(SPAF) analyzed the most likely mechanisms of stroke among 63 patients with atrial fibrillation studied in their trial [109]. Twenty-two of the 63 strokes were deemed most likely cardioembolic; four were atherothrombotic; seven due to the penetrating artery disease underlying lacunar infarction; three to other specific causes; and 27 were of uncertain cause [109]. In the European Atrial Fibrillation Trial (EAFT), investigators analyzed the presence of infarcts on CT scans in patients in their atrial fibrillation trial [110]. Among 985 patients, 14% had so-called silent infarcts on CT scans, i.e., infarcts for which there was no relevant history. The most common type of silent infarcts (43%) were small, deep, lacunar infarcts most likely related to associated penetrating artery disease, and were probably not cardioembolic [110]. In the Lausanne Stroke Registry, only 18% of patients with atrial fibrillation and stroke had atrial fibrillation as the only potential cause of stroke [111]. Coexisting large and penetrating artery disease and other cardiac sources of embolism were common. Using extracranial ultrasound, among 159 patients with atrial fibrillation and brain infarcts, abnormal findings in the ipsilateral ICA (107; 67%) and the contralateral ICA (92; 58%) were very common [111].

During the last decade there have been major advances in our knowledge about stroke prophylaxis in patients with atrial fibrillation who do not have valvular heart disease. Table 7 reviews the six major randomized trials that studied this issue [100,111–117]. Another trial, the Canadian Atrial Fibrillation Anticoagulation Study (CAFA), was prematurely stopped after randomization of 383 patients to receive warfarin (INR 2–3) or placebo after the results of other studies were published [118]. Warfarin-treated patients had fewer primary outcome events (nonlacunar brain infarcts, systemic embolism, and fatal intracranial bleeding episodes) 3.5%/year compared to 5.2%/year in the placebo-treated group, but the results lacked statistical power because of premature termination of the study [118]. All trials showed a consistent and considerable risk reduction for stroke in patients treated with warfarin.

The European Atrial Fibrillation Trial (EAFT) study group addressed specifically the question of the optimal level of anticoagulation by reviewing the results of their own trial [119]. No treatment effect was found with anticoagulation responses below INRs of 2.0. The rate of thromboembolic events was lowest at INRs from 2 to 3.9; most major hemorrhages occurred at INRs of 5.0 and above. The EAFT group recommended a target of 3.0 with a range from 2 to 5.0 [119]. Fixed-dose warfarin with a target of 1.3 to 1.5 was not as effective as standard adjusted-dose warfarin at an average INR of 2.4, even when aspirin 325 mg/day was added to the low fixed-dose warfarin in another study [116]. Warfarin is about 50% more effective than aspirin in reducing the rate of stroke in patients with atrial fibrillation without valvular disease [120]. The rates of intracranial hemorrhages and major bleeding episodes were low in all groups in all trials except in warfarin-treated patients over 75 in the SPAF II study. In that

Table 7 Trials of Prophylactic Therapy in Patients with Atrial Fibrillation Without Valvular Disease

Trial	Design	Results
Copenhagen AFASKA [112]	1007 patients; mean age 73; coumadin (INR 2.8–4.2) vs. aspirin (75 mg/day) vs. placebo.	Thromboemboli (stroke, TIA, systemic embolism). Coumadin 2%/year; aspirin 5.5%/year; placebo 5.5%/year.
BAATAF [100]	628 patients; mean age 68; coumadin (INR 1.5–2.7) vs. other medical Rx (could include aspirin).	Coumadin 2 strokes (0.4%/year); control 13 (3%/year). No benefit of aspirin (8 of 13 strokes in controls or aspirin); 2 hemorrhages—1 each group.
SPAF [113]	1330 patients; mean age 67; Warfarin-eligible patients randomized to warfarin (INR 2–3.5), aspirin (325 mg/day), or placebo. Warfarin-ineligible patients randomized to aspirin or placebo.	Warfarin 2.3%/year vs. 7.4%/year placebo; stroke in warfarin-ineligible aspirin group 3.6%/year vs. 6.3% in placebo group. Major bleeding 1.5%, 1.4%, 1.6% in warfarin, aspirin, placebo groups.
EAFT [114]	1007 patients; mean age 73; Warfarin-eligible patients randomized to warfarin (INR 2.5–4), aspirin (300 mg), or placebo. Warfarin-ineligible to aspirin or placebo.	Strokes in 8% of 225 in warfarin group, 15% of 404 in aspirin group, 19% of 378 in placebo group. Major bleeding 2.8%/year warfarin group, 0.9%/year aspirin group.
SPAF II [115]	1100 patients; mean age 69.6; warfarin (INR 2–4.5) vs. aspirin (325 mg/day compared in patients <75 and patients >75	715 patients <75; ischemic stroke, systemic embolism 1.3%/year. Warfarin vs. 1.9%/year aspirin; major hemorrhage 0.9%/year aspirin, 1.7%/year warfarin. 385 >75; ischemic stroke, systemic embolism 3.6%/year warfarin; 4.8%/year aspirin; major bleeds 4.2% warfarin,[a] 1.6% aspirin
SPAF III [116]	1044 patients with 1 or more risk factors; mean age 72; low-intensity fixed-dose warfarin (INR 1.2–1.5) plus aspirin (325 mg/day vs. adjusted-dose warfarin (INR 2–3)	INR 1.3 fixed-dose warfarin vs. INR target 2.4 adjusted group. Ischemic stroke, systemic embolism in 7.9% of fixed-dose aspirin vs. 1.9% in adjusted-dose group
SPAF III [117]	892 patients with posited low risk were given 325 mg aspirin	Rate of ischemic stroke was low (2%/year) and disabling ischemic stroke only 0.8%/year. Rate of major bleeding was 0.5%/year.

AFASAK, Copenhagen Atrial Fibrillation Aspirin Anticoagulation Study; BAATAF, Boston Area Anticoagulation Trial for Atrial Fibrillation; SPAF, Stroke Prevention in Atrial Fibrillation Study; EAFT, European Atrial Fibrillation Trial.

[a] 71% of intracranial hemorrhages fatal; 29% had residual deficit.

study seven of 197 warfarin-treated older patients had intracranial hemorrhages which were most often fatal [116]. Aspirin is also an effective treatment; in aggregate, aspirin conveys a stroke risk reduction of 20% to 25% with no clear relationship to aspirin dose [120].

A collaborative analysis showed that the annual stroke rate in patients with atrial fibrillation without clinical risk factors (prior stroke or TIA, diabetes, hypertension, older age) was very low, especially in patients <60 years old [92]. The rates of stroke in those without risk factors were 0 in 112 patients <60, 1.6% in 132 patients 60 to 69 years old, and 2.1% in 138 patients 70 to 79 years old [92,120]. The SPAF II [113] and SPAF III investigators [114a] and others [117] recommend that young patients with atrial fibrillation who have no additional risk factors are probably adequately protected by aspirin therapy. The SPAF III investigators enrolled 892 patients with atrial fibrillation who had none of the four prespecified risk factors: (1) recent congestive heart failure or left ventricular fractional shortening <25%; (2) previous thromboembolism; (3) systolic blood pressure >160 mm Hg; and (4) women >75 years of age [117]. The rates of ischemic stroke (2%/year) and disabling ischemic stroke (0.8%/year) were low and were just above the rate of major bleeding with aspirin therapy (0.5%/year) in this study [117].

Individuals with clinical and/or echocardiographic risk factors should be treated with warfarin with an INR maintained between 2 and 4 (target 2.6 to 3.0). In older patients (>75 years) the risk of serious hemorrhage is higher. Koudstaal, in discussing treatment of patients >80 years, said it well: ‘‘Very elderly atrial fibrillation patients have most to win but also most to lose from anticoagulation treatment’’ [121]. Treatment should be decided on an individual basis, with the clinician weighing the risk of stroke without warfarin versus the risk of important hemorrhage on warfarin treatment. Koudstaal emphasized that there was no good reason to deny anticoagulant treatment to an 85-year-old patient with a recent stroke due to atrial fibrillation if that patient had no major risk factors for hemorrhage and was expected to be compliant with testing and treatment [121].

The use of anticoagulants to manage patients having cardioversion is more controversial. There is general agreement that anticoagulation for 3 weeks before cardioversion greatly reduces the risk of cardiac-origin embolism at the time of cardioversion [122–124]. The main issues are whether anticoagulation is needed when the duration of atrial fibrillation is short (<72 hours), and whether anticoagulants are needed when TEE prior to cardioversion does not show atrial or atrial appendage thrombi [124]. Stoddard and colleagues showed that left atrial appendage thrombi are sometimes found in patients with short-duration atrial fibrillation (<48 hours) who have had recent embolic events [125]. Emboli can occur in patients in whom no thrombus is found before cardioversion [124,126].

Fatkin and colleagues showed that thrombi can develop after cardioversion [126]. They attributed the development of thrombosis after restoration of sinus rhythm to atrial stunning. They posited a delay between the restoration of electrical sinus rhythm and the return of effective atrial contractions. This can be viewed as atrial electrical-mechanical disassociation. Thrombi can form in the stunned atrium and embolize after atrial contractions are restored [124,126]. When there are no contraindications, it is probably wise to anticoagulate all patients before cardioversion. In patients with important risks for anticoagulation, it is probably relatively safe to cardiovert patients without prior anticoagulation in whom left atrial and left atrial appendage thrombi are not visible by technically adequate TEE performed by very experienced physicians.

Sick Sinus Syndrome

Although sinus node dysfunction has been recognized clinically since the very early years of the 20th century, identification of the malfunctioning atrium as a source of embolism was first recognized during the 1970s [127,128]. A variety of names are used for this condition including sick sinus syndrome, sinoatrial disorder, and bradycardia-tachycardia syndrome. Essential for the diagnosis is demonstration of sinus node dysfunctioning. Patients often present with slow and/or fast cardiac rhythms. Diagnosis depends on showing sinoatrial block, sinus arrest, sinus pauses >3 seconds, and sinus bradycardia with a ventricular rate of <50 [129]. Lown characterized the disorder as consisting of chaotic atrial activity, changing p-wave contour, and bradycardia admixed with multiple and recurrent ectopic beats and runs of atrial and nodal tachycardia [130]. Many patients also have atrial fibrillation or flutter with a relatively slow ventricular response (<70 beats per minute) [129].

Sinus node dysfunction can be caused by failure of impulse formation within the sinus node or by blocking transmission of the sinus impulse to the perinodal tissue in the atrium, so-called exit block. The condition becomes more common as patients age. In adults, sinus node dysfunction is most often due to degenerative changes in the sinus node and replacement with collagen. Apoptosis of the cells in the sinus node that are responsible for spontaneous depolarization occurs with increasing frequency as patients grow older. Damage to the sinus node can also be caused by coronary artery diseases of varying etiologies. Sinus node dysfunction can also follow cardiac surgery. In young patients a variety of different disorders that affect the myocardium and pericardium cause sinus node dysfunction [129]. An analysis of cardiovascular disease in Rochester, Minn., showed that 2.9% of men and 1.5% of women aged 75 or older had the sick sinus syndrome [131].

The first major study of embolism in patients with sinoatrial disorders was that of Fairfax, Lambert, and Leatham [127]. These authors studied 100 patients with chronic sinoatrial disorders whose mean age was 64.7. In 15 the cause was considered to be coronary artery disease; in 75 the cause was unknown. Sixteen patients (16%) had 27 episodes of embolism, compared with a 1.3% incidence

that idiopathic calcific aortic valve disease of the elderly is due to the atherosclerotic process, but definite proof of this hypothesis is not available. Microthrombi with evidence of organization have been found at necropsy in 53% of stenotic aortic valves [142]. Changes in the aortic valve are progressive. Thickening of previously diseased valves is thought to result from the deposition of fibrin. Fibrin deposits become organized and calcified with resultant distortion of the normal valve architecture. Bicuspid and calcific aortic valves are not able to open freely. Narrowing and irregularity of the valve orifice contribute to turbulent blood flow. Eddies form in the region of the sinus of Valsalva and also adjacent to any regurgeant jetstream, which flows into the left ventricle [155]. Abnormal flow and abnormal valve surfaces activate platelets and induce fibrin deposition, accounting for the prevalence of microthrombi along valve surfaces.

Embolism has been considered a much less common occurrence in patients with aortic valve disease when compared with mitral valve disease. Pleet et al. in 1981 reported four patients who had bicuspid aortic valves and cerebrovascular events [156]; three had sudden-onset strokes and the other had recurrent stereotyped TIAs. Full evaluation showed no cause for the brain infarcts in the three patients with strokes except for the bicuspid valve, and the authors attributed the strokes to brain embolism from the congenitally abnormal valves. The fourth patient, who had repeated TIAs, had a chronic hematological disorder and may not have had brain embolism. Others have reported instances of spontaneous brain embolism from calcific aortic valves [157–159]. In each patient the calcific embolus was seen on noncontrast CT as a dense, calcified region, and vascular studies (MRA, spiral CTA, and contrast angiography, each performed in individual patients) showed that the calcific density was within intracranial arteries (the supraclinoid carotid artery [157], the M1 segment of the MCA [158], and the M2 MCA segment [156] and was occlusive. The two young patients, men aged 36 [157] and 40 [158], had calcified bicuspid valves, while the 73-year-old patient [159] had calcific aortic stenosis without known underlying cause. Kapila and Hart described a patient with calcific aortic stenosis who developed a left hemiparesis 2 days after cardiac catheterization, and a calcific embolus was seen on CT scan occluding the right MCA [160].

Some clinical and necropsy studies show that embolism from calcific aortic valves is probably not rare. Soulie et al. found emboli in 33% of 81 patients with calcific aortic stenosis [161]. Holley et al., in another autopsy study, found calcific emboli in 37 of 165 (22%) patients with calcific aortic stenosis [162]. Thirty-two emboli were found in the coronary arteries, 11 in the renal vessels, one in the central retinal artery, and one in the MCA [162]. Although the MCA was occluded by a calcific embolus in one patient, no neurologic signs were recorded and no infarct was found [162]. During life, calcific emboli have often been identified in the eye because of their typical morphology on fundoscopic examination of the retina [163,164]. Calcific retinal emboli appear as white, irregular, immovable densities and are usually distinguishable from bright cholesterol crystals, and fibrin-platelet plugs. Among 103 patients with retinal artery occlusions and cardiovascular disease, aortic stenosis was present in 11 patients and was the most common cardiac lesion [164]. In all clinical studies, symptoms that reflect embolization occur more commonly after cardiac procedures (catheterization and surgery) than occur spontaneously. Aortic valve surgery is especially associated with a high frequency of embolism. Holley and colleagues found 82 instances of embolization among 38 of the 62 patients (61%) who had closed valvulotomy or aortic valve replacement and who died at various intervals after surgery [165]. Embolization is also more common in patients with bacterial endocarditis superimposed upon bicuspid or calcific aortic valves than it is in noninfected valves. The discrepancy between (1) the relatively high frequency of calcific emboli found at necropsy and in the eye and (2) the low frequency of clinically symptomatic brain and visceral organ ischemic events, is probably explained by the small size of the embolic particles and the fact that visceral emboli are much harder to diagnose than brain emboli.

Hypertrophic cardiomyopathy, also called idiopathic hypertrophic subaortic stenosis (IHSS), has become more frequently recognized since the advent of echocardiography. This disorder is characterized more by disproportionate and asymmetric hypertrophy of the left ventricular myocardium in the region of the ventricular septum than in the left ventricular free wall. Septal hypertrophy is associated with systolic anterior motion of the mitral valve and variable left ventricular outflow obstruction, depending on myocardial contractility. Structural abnormalities of the mitral valve often accompany the hypertrophic cardiomyopathy [166].

The rate of stroke in patients with hypertrophic cardiomyopathy is low, and stroke rarely occurs early in the course of the disease. When stroke occurs it is usually due to embolism in relation to atrial fibrillation, bacterial endocarditis, mitral valve dysfunction, or mitral annular calcification. Atrial fibrillation tends to develop late in patients with hypertrophic cardiomyopathy and is often accompanied by left atrial enlargement [167,168]. Mitral annulus calcification is also associated with IHSS [169]. In one study, among 150 patients with subaortic stenosis followed for an average of 5.5 years, only 11 patients (7%) had cerebrovascular events: five (3%) had a stroke, and six (4%) had TIAs [170]. Among those with stroke, atrial fibrillation, left atrial enlargement, and mitral regurgitation were common. Four patients were hypertensive and three had coronary artery disease, so some of the strokes were likely attributable to coexistent occlusive vascular disease [170].

Little has been written about embolism in patients with aortic insufficiency. Aortic regurgitation is caused by dysfunction of the aortic valve leaflets or the aortic root. Rheumatic valvulitis and infective endocarditis are probably the most common cause of aortic leaflet disease, causing aortic insufficiency, while Marfans, aortic dissection, and annuloaortic ectasia due to aging and hypertension are the usual causes of aortic root disease [153]. Syphillis was formerly a common cause of aortic valve insufficiency but is now rare. Rheumatic aortic valvulitis and vegetations on the aortic valve are likely potential sources of brain and systemic embolism in patients with aortic regurgitation, but there is little information on this topic. Cerebral emboli monitoring of patients with aortic insufficiency using TCD may prove interesting in the future.

Mitral Valve Prolapse

The topic of embolism in patients with mitral valve prolapse (MVP) has always been controversial. Barlow and Bosman in an early report of the midsystolic click-mitral valve prolapse syndrome described a 23-year-old woman who had transient left arm weakness, and evaluation showed mitral valve prolapse. No details of the neurological symptoms or signs were included and the relationship of the neurological event to her heart condition was not considered [171,172]. Since then a number of case control and necropsy studies have shown that patients with MVP do have cardiogenic embolism but not very often. For unclear reasons, cerebrovascular events in patients with MVP have a relatively low recurrence rate even without treatment. MVP is now the single most frequently diagnosed cardiac valvular abnormality. Estimates of prevalence range from 5% to 21%, with the rate being slightly higher in girls and women [172,173]. The basic pathological process is disruption of collagen and infiltration by a myxomatous substance rich in mucopolysaccharide. The mitral valve is often thickened, and the chordae tendinae and the mitral annulus may also contain myxomatous deposits which can cause elongation of the chordae, sometimes with rupture and dilatation of the mitral valve annulus [174]. Abnormal mitral valve leaflet motion can cause fibrosis and thickening of the endocardial surface of the valve leaflets. The tricuspid and aortic valves sometimes also have a myxomatous degeneration. When there is enough slippage that a portion of the mitral valve fails to coapt against the rest of the leaflet, then mitral regurgitation develops. Patients with MVP sometimes have abnormal left ventricular contraction, most often characterized as a vigorous contraction ring of the basal inferior wall of the ventricle [175]. At necropsy, thrombi have been found especially in the angle between the posterior leaflet of the mitral valve and the left atrial wall [176,177]. The development of an adherent thrombus in the cul-de-sac created between the ballooning posterior mitral valve leaflet and the atrial wall is usually attributed to a mitral regurgitant jetstream [172]. Transformation of the normally rigid valve into loose myxomatous tissue results in stretching of the valve leaflets, loss of endothelial continuity, and rupture of subendothelial connective tissue fibers. These changes could promote the formation of platelet-fibrin thrombi on the valve surface. A friable granular yellow thrombus composed of fibrin and platelets was found at necropsy in a 21-year-old patient who died after the sudden onset of a left hemiplegia [178]. Fibrin emboli were found in the coronary and renal arteries as well as frontal MCA branches in the brain [178].

MVP is diagnosed now by echocardiography when there is abnormal posterior movement of the coapted anterior and/or posterior leaflets of 2 mm or more; a midsystolic ''buckling'' or pansystolic ''hammocking'' of the valve leaflets is also described [172]. One or both of the mitral valve leaflets are displaced during systole into the left atrium above the plane of the mitral annulus using the parasternal long-axis view during echocardiography [179,180]. Mitral valve thickening and redundancy and the presence of mitral regurgitation are important additional criteria for the presence of important myxomatous mitral valve changes [180–182]. About 8% of patients with MVP develop severe mitral regurgitation leading to congestive heart failure and necessitating mitral valve replacement. Atrial fibrillation can occur at any time but is more common in older patients, especially those with mitral regurgitation and large left atria. Myxomatous valves can become infected during bacteremia, but the frequency of infective endocarditis is quite low. MVP occurs in patients with inherited connective tissue disorders such as Marfans, Ehlers-Danlos, and osteogenesis imperfecta [172].

The first report of a possible relation between MVP and brain ischemia was by Barnett in 1974 [183]. The initial report was of four patients, but Barnett and his colleagues later expanded the number of cases to 14 patients [176,184]. All patients were relatively young (10 to 48 years old), and none had cardiovascular risk factors or occlusive vascular lesions. Barnett and colleagues published a case control series in 1980 that provided further evidence of a relationship between MVP and brain ischemia in young patients [185]. The frequency of MVP among 141 patients >45 years old who had brain ischemic events was 5.7%, compared to a frequency of 7.1% among age-matched controls who had no history of cerebral or cardiac disease [185]. A second group of 60 patients <45 (mean age 33.9 years) with brain ischemic events was also studied. MVP was detected in 24 (40%) of the younger patients, compared to five (6.8%) of 60 age-matched controls (odds ratio of 9.3) [185]. Six of the 24 patients had other potential causes of stroke, but 18 had no other recognized cause of brain ischemia. Barletta and colleagues later compared echocardiographic findings among 39 patients with MVP who had brain ischemic events with the findings among 111 patients with mitral valve prolapse who had no history of brain ischemia [186]. Aortic valve prolapse (62% vs. 34%; $P < .01$) and multiple valve prolapse with diffuse valvular thickening (26% vs. 7%; $P < .01$) were more frequent in patients with brain ischemia [186]. Among two series of patients with MVP and brain ischemia [176,181], the frequency of atrial fibrillation was high. In the series of Nishimura et al. 60% of the patients with brain ischemia had atrial fibrillation [181].

Among six series of patients [176,177,187–190] with MVP and brain ischemic events reviewed by Lauzier and Barnett [172], there were 114 patients—

46 men and 68 women. Among those in whom the information was recorded, 39 (53%) had a single attack and 23 (31%) had multiple attacks. Two-thirds of the events were strokes and the remainder were TIAs. The great majority of events were within the carotid artery territory (84%); 16 of the patients had an arrhythmia detected by rhythm monitoring including eight with atrial fibrillation.

Abnormalities of platelet function have been shown in patients with MVP and thromboembolism. Shortened platelet survival time, an increase in circulating platelet aggregates, and increased levels of beta-thromboglobulin and platelet factor 4 were found in patients with mitral valve prolapse [172]. Interaction of circulating platelets with abnormal endocardial and valve structures found in patients with myxomatous valve degeneration causes increased platelet aggregation, adhesion, and secretion. Platelet fibrin aggregates adhere to abnormal valve surfaces and later embolize or promote formation of erythrocyte-fibrin clots.

The recurrence rate of stroke in patients with MVP is relatively low. In patients with mitral regurgitation and large left atria, and in those with atrial fibrillation and atrial or valvular thrombi shown by echocardiography, warfarin anticoagulation is probably indicated. In the great majority of patients who do not have atrial fibrillation, endocarditis, or severe mitral insufficiency, the treatment of choice is probably aspirin or another antiplatelet aggregant such as ticlopidine or clopidogrel. We prefer the dose of two 5-grain tablets (325 mg) of aspirin a day, but others favor larger or smaller doses.

Mitral Annulus Calcification

Mitral annulus calcification (MAC) is a degenerative disorder of the fibrous support structure of the mitral valve that occurs rather commonly in the elderly, especially in women. McKeown found MAC at necropsy in 27% of 100 elderly patients [172,191]. Among 5694 individuals in the Framingham project who had M-mode echocardiography, 2.8% had posterior submitral calcification; 95% of those patients who had MAC came from the 40% of subjects that were over 59 years of age, and twice as many women as men had mitral annulus calcification [192]. In the original description of MAC published in 1962, four of the 14 patients described by Korn and colleagues had brain infarcts, multiple in three [193]. The occurrence of brain infarction was noted in a table in the paper but was not commented on in the text [193]. The first important description of MAC as a potential cause of stroke was by DeBono and Warlow [194]. These authors in 1979 studied 151 consecutive patients with retinal or brain ischemia and found MAC in eight patients compared to no instances of MAC in age- and sex-matched controls who did not have brain or eye ischemia [194].

Among 127 patients in the Michael Reese Stroke Registry with brain embolism, seven had MAC [35]. Perhaps the most definitive epidemiological study of the relationship of MAC with stroke was the Framingham study [195]. Between 1979 and 1981, 426 men and 733 women in the Framingham study cohort (average age 70 years) who had not had strokes had M-mode echocardiograms. Among these 1159 patients, 44 men (10.3%) and 116 women (15.8%) had MAC. During 8 years of follow-up, 51 patients with MAC (5.1%) had strokes, compared to 22 patients without MAC (13.8%); MAC was associated with a 2.10 relative risk of stroke (95% confidence interval 1.24 to 3.57; $P = .006$) [195]. There was a continuous relation in this study between frequency of stroke and severity of MAC; each millimeter of thickening on the echocardiogram represented a relative risk of stroke of 1.24. Even when patients with atherosclerotic heart disease and congestive heart failure were excluded, patients with MAC still had twice the stroke risk of those without MAC [195].

Pathological data are more convincing, in my opinion, in linking MAC to brain embolism. Korn et al. reported the clinical and necropsy data on 14 patients with MAC [193]. They noted that calcification has a predilection for the posterior portion of the mitral annulus ring. Calcific masses often extended as far as 3.5 cm into the adjacent myocardium, and often projected superiorly toward the atrium and centrally into the cavity of the left ventricle [193]. Pomerance later noted ulceration and extrusion of the calcium through the overlying cusp into the ventricular cavity in some patients with MAC studied at necropsy, and thrombi were attached to the ulcerated regions in four patients [196]. Fulkerson reported 80 patients with MAC among whom five had episodes of arterial embolization; four had peripheral arterial embolectomies, and one had calcific retinal emboli [197]. Ridolfi and colleagues reported a 53-year-old patient with MAC studied clinically and at necropsy who had multiple calcific coronary and anterior and posterior circulation emboli originating from a calcified mitral annulus [198]. The embolic material can be either calcium (as has also been shown in calcific aortic stenosis) or thrombus. Mouton et al. reported an elderly woman with MAC who, on cranial CT scans, had multiple flecks of calcium that were blocking arteries that supplied infarcted regions [199].

Thrombi attached to calcified mitral annuli have also been shown by echocardiography. Stein and Soble reported two such patients [200]. Multiplane TEE showed a 2-mm mobile thrombus attached to the atrial surface of the calcified posterior portion of the mitral annulus in a 74-year-old woman who had developed a sudden-onset right hemiparesis and aphasia. There were no other cardiac sources of emboli. After 8 weeks of warfarin, a repeat echocardiogram showed that the thrombus was no longer present [200]. In a second patient, who had a parietal lobe brain infarct, TEE showed a 5-mm mobile thrombus attached to an 8-mm calcified nodule on the posterior mitral valve leaflet. Subsequent echocardiograms revealed that the thrombus was first smaller and later gone after warfarin anticoagulation [200].

MAC is a very common finding, especially in older women, and is often accompanied by mitral regurgitation and atrial fibrillation. Bacterial endocarditis can be superimposed. Hypertension, coronary atherosclerotic heart disease, and occlusive cerebrovascular disease are also often present in the population of patients that have MAC. There are no data on the utility of any prophylactic treatment on the prevention of brain or arterial embolism in patients with MAC.

Prosthetic Cardiac Valves

Advances in cardiac diagnosis and cardiac surgery have led to increasingly frequent replacement of heart valves. There are now more than 80 different models of prosthetic valves, and >60,000 valve replacements are performed annually in the United States alone [201]. Mechanical valves are made primarily with metal and carbon alloys and are quite thrombogenic. Thrombogenic potential is highest with caged-ball prostheses (e.g., Starr-Edwards valve), lowest in individuals with bileaflet-tilting-disk prostheses (e.g., St. Jude Medical), and intermediate with single-tilting-disk valves (e.g., Bjork-Shiley) [201]. Bioprosthetic valves are most commonly heterografts derived from pig or cow pericardial or valve tissues mounted on metal supports. Homografts in the form of preserved human valves are occasionally used for valve replacements. Bioprosthetic valves have low thrombogenic tendencies (but still higher than native valves), so long-term anticoagulation is ordinarily not prescribed. Unfortunately bioprosthetic valves are less durable than mechanical valves [201].

Valve thrombosis is an important complication in patients with both mechanical and bioprosthetic valve prostheses. Important valve thrombosis causes pulmonary congestion, reduced cardiac output, and brain and systemic embolism. The frequency of prosthetic valve thrombosis is estimated to be between 0.1% and 5.7% per year [202,203]. Alteration of blood flow related to mechanical valves, as well as the inherent thrombogenicity of the materials used, promotes thrombosis and thromboembolism. Flow velocity studies show turbulent flow patterns that contribute to vascular stasis and thrombus formation around mechanical valve prostheses [204]. Hematological studies in patients with mechanical valves show elevation of platelet-specific proteins that indicate platelet activation and decreased platelet survival in patients with artificial heart valves [205–207].

The pathophysiological events that promote thromboembolism begin during heart surgery. Prosthetic materials and injured perivalvular tissues cause platelet activation as soon as circulation is restored. Dacron sewing rings, common to all prosthetic valves, form a fertile nidus for platelet activation and adhesion [80]. Prosthetic material also activates the intrinsic pathway of the coagulation cascade [208]. Both platelet activation and activation of the coagulation cascade promote the formation of red erythrocyte-fibrin thrombi. Degenerative changes in bioprosthetic valves also can lead to the deposition of white platelet-fibrin thrombi [209]. Late thrombosis has also been shown in the cusp sinuses of bioprosthetic mitral valves that have undergone fibrosis and calcification [210,211].

Embolism is an important complication in patients with both mechanical and bioprosthetic valves. The frequency of major embolism in patients with mechanical valves is estimated to be about 4% per year if no antithrombotic therapy is used [212]. This figure is reduced to about 2% per year by medications that decrease platelet aggregation and to 1% per year with warfarin anticoagulation [212]. Most symptomatic emboli go to the brain. Patients with mitral mechanical valves have a slightly higher frequency of embolization than those with aortic valves, probably related to the higher frequency of associated atrial fibrillation and large left atria in patients with mitral valve prostheses. Patients with bioprosthetic valves also have a risk of embolism. In one series of 128 patients with porcine bioprosthetic valves inserted, during 5 to 8 years of follow-up, two of 43 patients with aortic valve replacement, nine of 62 with porcine mitral valves, and four of 18 with both mitral and aortic prosthetic valves had clinical thromboemboli [213]. Among the 15 patients with thromboemboli in this series, 13 had atrial fibrillation and the other two had heart block [213]. Large left atria, atrial fibrillation, left ventricular dysfunction, and infective endocarditis are important associated conditions in patients with prosthetic valves that can cause thromboembolism.

Monitoring of patients with prosthetic heart valves using TCD has shown a high frequency of microembolic signals [214–217]; the rate is higher in children than adults [213]. Studies using hyperbaric oxygen and varying partial pressures of oxygen in the blood show that the great majority of microemboli are gaseous and are about 3 to 4 μm in size [218]. The gas represents cavitation bubbles produced by valve contact with the blood. The small size of particles allows passage through the capillary bed without blocking the microcirculation. Occasionally, embolic metallic fragment artifacts are found on cranial MRI scans of patients with mechanical prosthetic heart valves, even in the absence of neurological symptoms indicating brain embolism [219].

Anticoagulation is recommended for all patients with prosthetic heart valves. Patients with bioprosthetic valves are usually treated for the first 3 months after surgery using a target INR of 2.0 to 3.0 [201,220,221]. Oral anticoagulant therapy reduces the incidence of embolism in patients with mechanical valve prostheses, and the intensity of anticoagulation has been recommended to be higher than that used with bioprosthetic valves (INR of 2.5 to 4.9). Patients with caged-ball prostheses may require a higher intensity of anticoagulation than those with bileaflet disk valves and those with single-tilting disk valves [201]. Adding antiplatelet medications such as dipyridamole or aspirin can further reduce the frequency of embolism. Aspirin (100 mg/day) added to warfarin (INR target 3.0 to 4.5) in patients with mechanical prosthetic valves or tissue valves and atrial fibrillation, reduces mortality and the frequency of embolization [222]. Bleeding is increased during high-intensity anticoagulation with aspirin therapy. Aspirin and lower-intensity anticoagulation (INR 2.0 to 3.0) is probably as effective as high-intensity anticoagulation and has less risk of serious bleeding. Since prosthetic valves induce formation of both white platelet-fibrin and red erythrocyte-fibrin clots, the use of combined antiplatelet aggregant and anticoagulant therapy makes sense. Ticlopidine or clopidogrel could also be used with warfarin but the effects of these combinations have not been reported. Pregnant women with prosthetic valves should be treated with heparin or low-molecular-weight heparin during pregnancy since the incidence of thromboemboli is increased while pregnant and also in the puerperium [201,223,224].

The optimal intensity of anticoagulant therapy has been examined in several studies. Turpie et al. compared two levels of anticoagulation (INR 2.0 to 2.5 among 106 patients vs. INR 2.5 to 4 among 108 patients) that were given for 3 months after bioprosthetic valve implantation [221]. The rate of embolic events was the same but there was significantly more bleeding in patients with higher-intensity anticoagulation [221]. Altman et al. compared the outcomes of patients who had received tilting-disk valves according to anticoagulant intensity [224a]. In this study 51 patients had INRs between 2.0 and 3.0, while 48 patients had INRs between 3.0 and 4.5; all patients also received aspirin 330 mg and dipyridamole 75 mg twice daily. No difference was found in the embolic rate, but bleeding events were more common in the higher-intensity anticoagulation group [224a]. Butchart and colleagues compared two levels of anticoagulation—INRs of 2.5, and INRs of 3.0, among patients with tilting-disk mitral or aortic prosthetic valves [224b]. Among mitral prostheses the 103 patients with INRs of 2.5 had significantly more events (23 vs. 4) than the group with INRs of 3.0 without more bleeding events. However in the group with aortic prostheses, the group with moderate-intensity anticoagulation (INR of 3.0) had more bleeding without a difference in thromboembolic events [224b]. Horstkotte et al. compared three intensities of anticoagulation (INRs of 1.8 to 2.7, 2.5 to 3.2, and 3.0 to 4.5) in patients with St. Jude mechanical valves in both the mitral and aortic positions, and found equivalent protection from thromboembolism in all groups but less bleeding in the lowest-intensity anticoagulation group [224c]. In the large French AREVA trial, low-intensity (INR 2.0 to 3.0) and higher-intensity (INR 3.0 to 4.5) anticoagulation was compared among 354 patients with St. Jude bileaflet valves and 80 tilting-disk valves; 414 prosthetic valves were aortic and only 19 were mitral [224d]. No significant differences were noted in the frequency of thromboembolism, but there were fewer hemorrhagic complications in the lower-intensity anticoagulation group [224d]. A group of physicians at the Mayo Clinic recently reviewed the literature concerning the intensity of anticoagulation in patients with prosthetic heart valves and made recommendations about treatment [224e]. Their recommendations are listed in Table 8.

Infective Endocarditis

Although neurological complications of infective endocarditis have been well known since the time of Osler [225], the clinical spectrum of endocarditis has changed dramatically during the past decades. Compared with endocarditis pa-

TABLE 8 Anticoagulant Guidelines for Patients with Prosthetic Cardiac Valves

Factor	Target INR	Aspirin (mg/day)
Aortic valves		
Newer-generation bileaflet mechanical valves	2.5	81
All other mechanical valves	3.0	81
Bioprosthetic valves	2.5, 3 months	325[a]
with thromboembolic risk factors	2.5, indefinitely	81
Mitral valves		
First-generation tilting disk valves	3.5	81
All other mechanical valves	3.0	81
Bioprosthetic valves	2.5, indefinitely	81
Low thromboembolic or high bleeding risk	2.5, 3–6 months	325[a]
Mitral valve repair	2.5, 3 months	325[a]
Thromboembolic risk factors	2.5, indefinitely	81

[a] Treatment continued indefinitely even after coumadin was stopped.
Source: Ref. 224e.

tients three decades ago, present-day series of patients with infective endocarditis are on average older, contain more drug addicts, have more examples of tricuspid valve involvement, usually in intravenous drug addicts, and have more patients with infection of prosthetic valves. Diagnostic capabilities have also changed. Echocardiography and newer brain and cerebrovascular imaging techniques allow better clarification of the cardiac and brain pathology and pathophysiology.

In 1969, Mayo Clinic neurologists reviewed their experience accumulated during the period 1950 to 1964 [226]. Among 385 patients with endocarditis, 110 (29%) had neurologic complications including 55 with cerebrovascular disease. The neurological complications described by Jones et al. remain the major syndromes still seen today [226]. Forty-four of the 55 individuals (80%) with cerebrovascular complications had brain infarcts (38 carotid system; six vertebrobasilar). Among the 11 patients with brain hemorrhage, eight were into the brain substance (intracerebral) and three were subarachnoid [226]. Twenty-one patients in the Mayo Clinic series had acute encephalopathy and seven had meningitis. These syndromes—brain ischemia, intracerebral hemorrhage, subarachnoid hemorrhage, encephalopathy, and meningitis—remain the major neurological complications found in recent series of patients with both native valve and prosthetic valve endocarditis [227–231].

Brain ischemia is invariably due to embolism. About one-fifth of patients with endocarditis develop brain infarcts. At necropsy, small cortical or subcortical bland infarcts are found—usually multiple. In one series, 19/33 (58%) infarcts were small, 11/33 (33%) were moderate in size, and 3/33 (9%) were large [228]. The larger infarcts were found in patients with *Staphylococcus aureus* endocarditis. Ischemia can take the form of transient ischemic attacks that involve the brain or the retina. In one series, among 133 episodes of endocarditis, three patients had transient monocular visual loss and one patient had a retinal infarct [228]. Brain ischemia may be the presenting sign of endocarditis and is most common early in the course of the disease. Ischemic strokes can also occur in the days after antibiotic treatment is begun. Monitoring of patients with endocarditis using TCD shows that microemboli continue to occur even after antibiotic treatment, although more emboli are detected before and shortly after antibiotics are given. Brain ischemia was described in 17% [227], 19% [228], and 15% [231] of patients in various recent infective endocarditis series.

Brain hemorrhage is much less frequent than ischemia, but the effects of hemorrhage can be devastating or mortal. Intracerebral hemorrhage was found in 6% [227], 7% [228], 2.8% [230], and 5.6% [231] of patients in various endocarditis series. Recent series that included modern brain imaging and necropsy studies have clarified the mechanisms of intracerebral hemorrhage in endocarditis [229,232,233]. Some patients have bleeding into bland infarcts. This usually takes the form of hemorrhagic infarction—petechial and larger hemorrhagic mottling within the infarct without formation of a frank discrete hematoma. In some patients, large hematomas develop. Hematomas are often found in patients treated with anticoagulants. In other patients intracerebral hemorrhage results from rupture of a septic arteritis caused by embolization of infective material to the artery with necrosis of the arterial wall [232,233]. In a small minority of cases, intracerebral hemorrhage is due to rupture of a mycotic aneurysm into the brain substance. Brain hemorrhage, similar to the situation in patients with brain ischemia, is most common at or near presentation of the patient and is less common after effective antibiotic treatment. Many patients who develop brain hemorrhage have had an attack of transient or persistent brain ischemia in the hours or days before the hemorrhage. This prodromal ischemia is explained by an arterial embolus causing brain infarction. Hemorrhage into an infarct or rupture of the artery that received the infected embolus causes the hemorrhage, which often proves fatal [232,233].

The need for angiography to detect mycotic aneurysms and the indications for surgical treatment of aneurysms found by angiography are controversial topics. In a review by Hart et al., among 2119 patients with endocarditis, only 5% of patients with brain hemorrhages had identified mycotic aneurysms [232]. Mycotic aneurysms are caused by embolization of infected material into the wall and adventitia of brain arteries. The aneurysms usually occur distally along arteries and tend to be multiple. The location of aneurysms in patients with infective endocarditis is similar to those found in patients with atrial myxomas, probably because of similar embolic etiologies. In contrast, ordinary saccular "berry" aneurysms occur proximally along the basal arteries of the circle of Willis. Angiography of patients without brain hemorrhage seldom shows mycotic aneurysms. Mycotic aneurysms have been shown to disappear in some patients on sequential angiography performed after bacteriological cure [234–236]. This information suggests a nonaggressive approach to the diagnosis and treatment of mycotic aneurysms [232]. However, mycotic aneurysms can rupture, sometimes after bacteriological cure, and rerupture can prove fatal. Some neurologists and neurosurgeons recommend that angiography be performed in all patients suspected of harboring aneurysms [234,237]. At present the decision on angiography, and on surgical treatment if an aneurysm is found, must rest on the total clinical picture in individual patients.

Diffuse brain-related symptoms, usually referred to as *encephalopathy*, are very common in patients with endocarditis. Symptoms include lethargy, decreased level of consciousness, confusion, agitation, and poor concentration and memory. Encephalopathy has different explanations. Often the encephalopathy is toximetabolic and is explained by systemic factors such as azotemia, pulmonary dysfunction, hyponatremia, etc. In many patients encephalopathy is a toxic effect related to fever and to the acute infection. Patients with *Staph. aureus* acute endocarditis are more often toxic than in endocarditis caused by other organisms. Necropsy and CT/MRI studies of patients with encephalopathy often reveal multiple small, scattered brain infarcts and/or microabscesses [229,238]. Encephalopathy usually develops during uncontrolled infection with more virulent organisms, supporting the role of microscopic-size septic emboli as the cause [229,239].

Meningitis also occurs in patients with endocarditis. The presentation is often headache with fever. Since the usual infecting organism is not very virulent, the patient is not as ill as in other acute forms of bacterial meningitis. Meningitis occurred in 6.4% [226] and 1.1% [227] in two series of patients with endocarditis. Meningeal infection is due to embolization of infected vegetations to meningeal arteries.

Valvular vegetations in patients with infective endocarditis are composed of platelets, fibrin, erythrocytes, and inflammatory cells attached to damaged endothelium of native and prosthetic valves. Organisms are enmeshed within the fibrinous material, often deep within the vegetations, explaining why antibiotics have difficulty sterilizing the lesions. Vegetations range in size from several millimeters to several centimeters, and their potential for embolization relate to their size and friability. The mitral valve is most often involved. However, mitral valve disease is also more frequent than other valve disease. Salgado et al. compared valve involvement in patients with and without neurologic complications of endocarditis [227]. Aortic valve disease was present in 38/64 (59.4%) patients with neurologic complications, vs. 65/111 (59.6%) endocarditis patients without neurologic complications. Mitral involvement occurred in 22/64 (34.4%) patients

TABLE 10 Infecting Organism in Various Series of Patients with Neurological Complications of Infective Endocarditis

Bacteria	Kanter [229]	Matsushita [231]	Salgado [227]	Jones [226]
Staph. aureus	36 (27%)	3 (12.5%)	13 (20%)	26 (24%)
Staph. epidermis	7 (5%)	1 (4%)	5 (8%)	
Strep. viridans	69 (51%)[a]	20 (83%)	20 (31%)	60 (55%)
Strep group D			15 (23%)	12 (11%)
Beta strep	6 (4%)			
Others	16 (12%)		13 (20%)	12 (11%)

[a] Group D strep included in this group.

normal or may contain slightly increased protein levels and increased numbers of erythrocytes and leukocytes. Usually the pleocytosis is moderate (<300 cells/cc) and may be predominantly lymphocytic or polymorphonuclear, unless a clinical picture of meningitis is present, in which case there may be more white blood cells. The frequency of detection of vegetations on echocardiography depends on the technique used and the frequency of examinations. Infective vegetations appear as bright, usually mobile echo-dense lesions attached to valve leaflets. Lesions <2 mm in size are probably not reliably identified by echocardiography. In the series of Hart et al. (M-mode and 2D TTEs), vegetations were found on 41% of initial echocardiograms in patients with *Staph. aureus* endocarditis, compared with 57% of initial studies in patients with streptococcal species endocarditis [228], TEE is likely to show vegetations more often than TTE. An echocardiogram that fails to show a vegetation clearly does not exclude the diagnosis of endocarditis. Angiography can show occluded arteries or mycotic aneurysms [231] but has seldom been performed routinely in series of patients with neurologic complications of endocarditis.

The most important treatment is the rapid introduction of specific antimicrobial drugs. Most neurologic complications occur before or near the time of diagnosis and initial antibiotic treatment. Recurrent strokes do occur after bacteriologic cure, but rarely. In one series, among 147 patients discharged from the hospital after treatment of infective endocarditis, 15 developed strokes after discharge; all except one of the stroke patients had prosthetic valve endocarditis [227]. Strokes in this series occurred long after discharge (median 22 months) and were better explained by recurrence of endocarditis, complications of anticoagulants, or noninfective disease of the prosthetic valves than cerebrovascular complications of the original endocarditic episode [227]. There is general agreement that native valve endocarditis is not an indication for anticoagulation even when brain or systemic embolism has occurred. Controversy surrounds the issue of maintenance of anticoagulation in patients who have mechanical valve endocarditis, but most clinicians favor cautious continuation of anticoagulants unless a brain hemorrhage develops. When a hemorrhagic infarct or brain hemorrhage develops, anticoagulation with warfarin is usually stopped for 1 to 2 weeks. In patients with a major risk of recurrent embolization it may be safe to use heparin beginning soon after the hemorrhage is discovered, and later switch back to warfarin. Cardiac surgery to debride or replace infected valves is performed for cardiac indications—mostly heart failure related to valve dysfunction, lack of control of infection, valve infection with fungal or other virulent organism not controllable by antimicrobial drugs, and valve or chordae tendinae rupture.

Noninfective Fibrous and Fibrinous Endocardial Lesions (Including Valve Strands)

In a variety of other circumstances, fibrous valve thickening, often with grossly visible vegetations that contain mixtures of blood platelets and fibrin, are found on the heart valves and adjacent endocardium in patients who have no evidence of either rheumatic fever or bacterial endocarditis. The first detailed description of such lesions was in 1924 by Emanuel Libman and Benjamin Sacks, who reported four patients studied clinically and pathologically of an ''atypical verrucous endocarditis'' [241]. The patients included three women, aged 24, 37, and 10, and a 19-year-old man. Necropsy showed fibrous thickening of valves with vegetations especially along the closure lines of the valves and on the valve leaflets. The vegetations spread to the papillary muscles and ventricular endocardium. The histopathology was thought to be unique by the authors. In one patient:

> In the mitral valve, there was a deposit of agglutinated blood platelets over large flat areas, beneath which the endocardial tissues were densely infiltrated with polymorphonuclear leukocytes and round cells. . . . The valve itself was enormously thickened owing to an old chronic inflammatory process. . . . The blood platelet masses showed a tendency in places to fibroblastic invasion. The inflammatory process extended throughout the entire thickness of the valve, and the vegetative deposit was therefore present on both the auricular and the ventricular aspects of the valve [241].

Fibrinous pericarditis was present in three of the patients, and rash, bleeding, arthritis, anemia, and glomerulonephritis were common clinical features. The fourth patient was the only one with prominent clinical neurologic abnormalities, a unilateral paralysis, and seizures which developed shortly before death in this patient; the authors speculated that these findings might have been caused by emboli from the valvular vegetations (the brain was not available for examination in this patient). Libman and Sacks were uncertain of the diagnosis but noted that the clinical picture resembled some of the erythematous diseases that Osler had

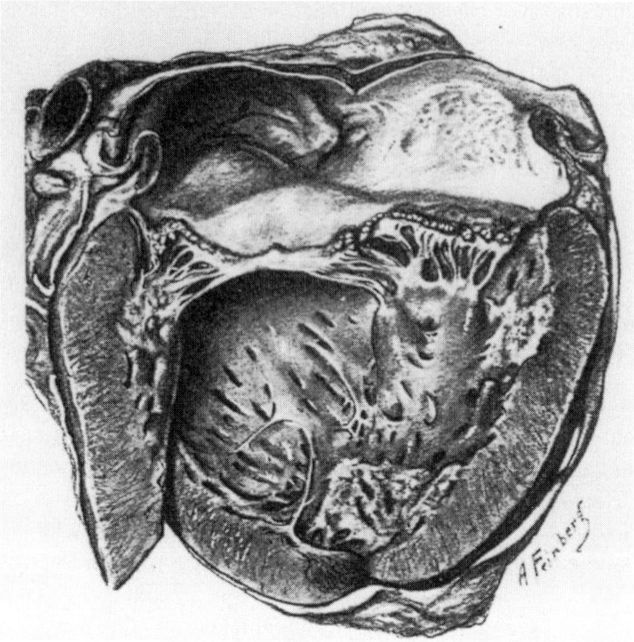

FIG. 27 Drawing of a heart at necropsy. The left side of the heart shows verrucous vegetations along the line of closure of the mitral valve extending in places to the free edge. There are areas of endocarditis on the papillary endocardium and adjacent mural endocardium, and an isolated patch of mural endocarditis in the region of the apex of the ventricle. A healing fibrinous pericarditis is also present. (From Ref. 241.)

mentioned in his textbook of medicine [241]. Figure 27, from the original report by Libman and Sacks, is a drawing of the cardiac vegetations found in one patient at necropsy. Klemperer, Pollack, and Baehr, the very next year, published the pathological findings in disseminated lupus erythematosis [242], and Baehr and colleagues, in 1935, published a series of 23 patients who had acute disseminated lupus erythematosis among whom 13 had a nonrheumatic verrucous endocarditis similar to that described by Libman and Sacks [243]. These clinical and pathological reports brought the disease lupus erythematosis, known previously as predominantly a skin disorder, to the attention of the medical community as an acute disseminated systemic disease. Gross, a younger colleague of Libman and Sacks at Mount Sinai Hospital in New York, in 1940, reported a detailed study of 27 hearts, 23 of whom were fatal cases of acute lupus erythematosis [244]. It was Gross who pointed out that the patients in the original report from the Mount Sinai Hospital had the typical clinical findings of lupus erythematosis, and Gross suggested that the endocarditic lesions be named after Libman-Sacks, and that the verrucous endocardial lesions were diagnostic of lupus erythematosis [244]. Libman and Sacks [241] and Gross [244] were aware that similar endocarditic lesions also occurred in terminal or cachectic diseases such as carcinoma, tuberculosis, and leukemia and had usually been called nonbacterial thrombotic endocarditis. Since these early reports, we now know that similar lesions of the cardiac valves and endocardium occur in patients with systemic lupus erythematosis (SLE), the antiphospholipid antibody (APlA) syndrome, and marantic nonbacterial thrombotic endocarditis (NBTE). Presumably all have a similar pathogenesis.

Fox et al., in 1980, described a patient with clinical and serological evidence of SLE who developed systemic and brain emboli [245]. The mitral valve ''was covered on both surfaces with several granular, friable hemorrhagic vegetations that measured up to 1 cm in diameter'' (Fig. 13). The brain, spleen, kidneys, and skin contained multiple infarcts, and many arteries were blocked by fibrin-platelet emboli and particles arising from the vegetations on the mitral valve [245]. This was probably one of the first cases in which brain embolism from Libman-Sacks lesions was well documented.

Most observers had concluded that endocarditic lesions in patients with SLE were of interest but rarely caused important heart dysfunction or embolism. Harvey et al. in their review of 138 patients with SLE found cardiac valvular vegetations in one-third of patients but concluded, ''The presence of endocarditis had no effect on the heart or circulation'' [246]. There were frequent neurologic findings among the 138 patients reviewed including, hemiparesis, seizures, and aphasia, which were attributed to ''lupus vasculitis'' by the authors [246]. However, in a review of the neurological and neuropathological manifestations of SLE, Johnson and Richardson found true vasculitis to be quite rare in the nervous system although their study did include patients with brain infarcts [247]. Devinsky and colleagues were unable to find a single case of vasculitis causing stroke or brain infarction among 50 SLE patients who had detailed neuropathological examinations [248]. They attributed cerebrovascular lesions to emboli from Libman-Sacks endocarditis and coagulopathies [248].

More recently, a number of echocardiographic studies have attempted to define the frequency and importance of endocarditic lesions in series of patients with SLE [249–251]. Galve et al. performed echocardiography (M-mode and 2D) on 74 patients with SLE on two occasions approximately 5 years apart [249]. Clinically important valve disease was found in 18% of patients including seven with vegetations mostly on the mitral and aortic valves. Nine patients had thickening and stiffness of valves, causing stenosis or regurgitation in six and causing calcification in two. Six of the 74 patients required valve surgery during 5 years' follow-up, and one developed vegetations not present 5 years previously [249]. Roldan et al. performed TEE on 69 SLE patients on two occasions averaging 29 months apart [245]. Valvular abnormalities were found in 61% of patients on the initial TEE and in 53% on the second echocardiographic study. Valve thickening (61%), vegetations (43%), valve regurgitation (25%), and stenosis (4%) were found on the initial echocardiograms. Involvement of the mitral valve was often followed closely by involvement of the aortic valve; tricuspid valve disease occurred occasionally but pulmonic valve involvement was rare. The combined incidence of stroke, peripheral embolism, heart failure, and superimposed infective endocarditis was 22% in those with valvular disease on TEE [250]. Crozier et al. found a high frequency of mitral regurgitation (46%) among 50 female Chinese patients with SLE [251]. Our own experience is similar to that of Devinsky et al. that stroke and microinfarcts in patients with SLE are most often attributable to brain embolism from valvular lesions or coagulopathy. The presence of coagulopathy and thrombocytopenia in SLE probably correlates with the presence of valvular disease, although this relationship has not been well studied.

The antiphospholipid antibody (APlA) syndrome has become recognized within the past two decades as a prothrombotic syndrome separate from SLE. The APlA syndrome is characterized by frequent fetal loss, strokes, myocardial infarcts, phlebothrombosis, pulmonary emboli, and thrombocytopenia. Serological testing reveals positive assays for the lupus anticoagulant and/or anticardiolipin antibodies. Recently, echocardiographic studies have shown that there is a relatively high frequency of valvular cardiac lesions in patients with this syndrome and that the valve lesions are indistinguishable from those found in patients with SLE. Brenner et al. studied 34 patients with the APlA syndrome using 2D and Doppler echocardiography [252]. Fourteen patients had arterial thromboembolism, six had venous thrombosis, and 14 had recurrent fetal loss. Valvular lesions (mostly mitral and aortic thickening and vegetations) were found in 11 patients (32%) including 9/14 (64%) of those with arterial thromboembolism [252]. Barbut et al. studied the prevalence of antiphospholipid antibodies among patients in whom echocardiography showed mitral and/or aortic regurgitation [253]. Among 87 consecutive patients with these valve dysfunctions, 26 (30%) had immunoglobulin G or M anticardiolipin antibodies. Focal cerebral ischemic events occurred in eight of these patients (seven judged embolic), including seven of the IgG anticardiolipin-positive patients [253].

Barbut and colleagues studied 21 patients with APlA antibodies who had focal cerebral ischemic events [254]. Twelve of 14 (86%) stroke patients and three of seven (42%) nonstroke lesion patients had echocardiographic evidence of mitral or aortic valve abnormalities. Eight of the 21 patients with APlAs had SLE in this study [254]. In a large cooperative study performed by the Antiphospholid Antibodies in Stroke Study Group, among 128 patients who had brain or ocular ischemia and were APlA-positive, 16 (22.2%) had mitral valve abnormalities on echocardiograms and two had aortic valve abnormalities [255]. Figure 28 shows the CT scan findings in a patient with multiple embolic brain infarcts and high titers of APlAs. Figure 29 shows the echocardiographic findings in this

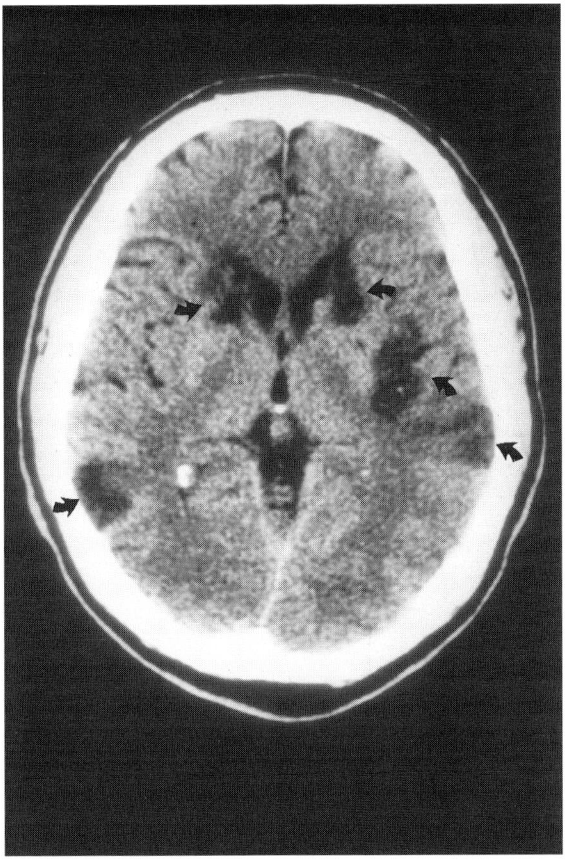

FIG. 28 CT scan showing five brain infarcts (curved black arrows) located in the basal ganglia and temporal lobes bilaterally.

patient, and Figure 30 is a photograph of the mitral valve removed at surgery showing the vegetations. Phospholipids are important constituents of cardiac valve endothelium, blood platelets, vascular endothelium, and coagulation proteins. At present, assays for antiphospholipid antibodies only include testing for lupus anticoagulant and anticardiolipin antibodies. We and others have cared for patients with the clinical features of the APlA syndrome who have negative antibody assays. Some of these patients also have prominent valve vegetations and cardiogenic brain embolism.

Both hypercoagulability and nonbacterial thrombotic endocarditis (NBTE) have long been known to occur in patients with cancer and other debilitating

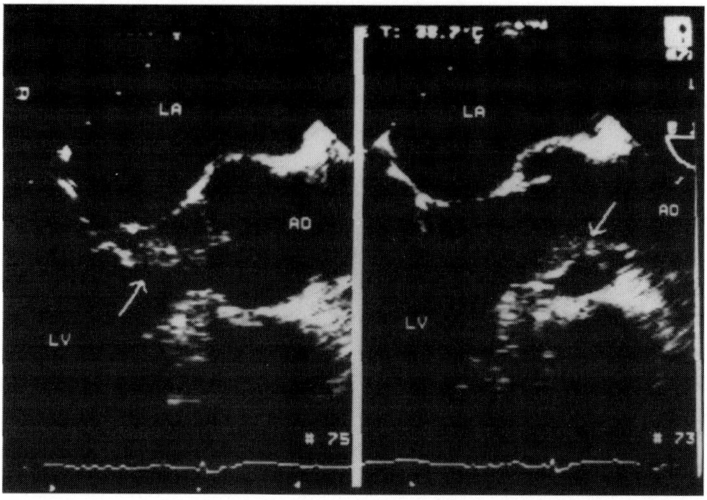

Fig. 29 Echocardiography showing a pedunculated, mobile lesion on the mitral valve (white arrows). LA, left atrium; LV, left ventricle; AO, aorta.

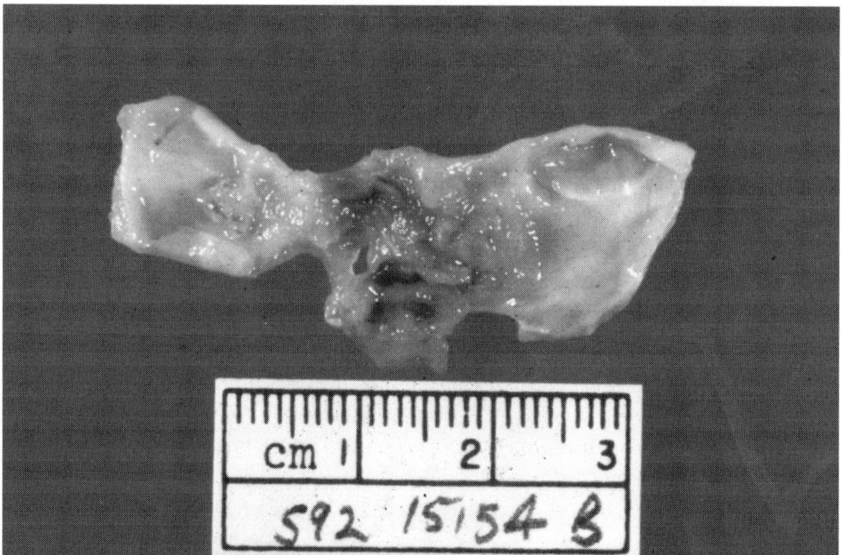

Fig. 30 Mitral valve removed surgically showing vegetations.

chronic diseases. Most often the cancers are mucinous adenocarcinomas [256]. In one study, among 20 cancer patients who had thromboembolic disease of the brain and other organs, 16 (80%) had NBTE at necropsy [257]. Valvular involvement was mitral in eight patients, aortic in four, mitral and aortic in three, and tricuspid in one. Large-vessel occlusive emboli and multiple infarcts and microvascular occlusions were found in the brains of these patients. In another study, among 18 patients with cancer and NBTE, eight developed a stroke, and in five stroke was the initial clinical manifestation of cancer [258]. Edoute et al. performed prospective echocardiograms on 200 cancer patients and found a 19% frequency of NBTE [258a]. The valve lesions equally involved the mitral and aortic valves, and an elevated plasma D-dimer level, a marker for hypercoagulability, was also often found in the cancer patients with clinical thromboembolism [258a]. NBTE is characterized by friable white or tan vegetations, usually along lines of valve closure. The vegetations can be large. Microscopy usually shows degenerating platelets interwoven with strands of fibrin and some leukocytes forming eosinophilic masses of tissue. All three conditions—SLE, APlA syndrome, and NBTE—are associated with hypercoagulability, strokes, and platelet abnormalities. The cardiac valve and endothelial lesions in these three conditions are very similar and probably indistinguishable grossly and microscopically. Platelet deposition, incorporation of fibrin, and the formation of platelet thrombi on valve and endocardial surfaces are common to all three conditions. Treatment of these conditions has not been formally studied. In theory drugs that alter platelet aggregation, secretion, and adhesion might be effective. In patients with SLE and APlA, antibodies that are associated with hypercoagulability, heparin, and warfarin compounds are usually prescribed to treat the hypercoagulability and prevent venous and arterial occlusions.

Noninfective valve lesions are also found in patients with carcinoid tumors (probably causally related to elevated serotonin levels in the blood), and after the use of some drugs (ergotamine, methysergide, dexfenfluramine, and fenfluramine and phentermine) [259]. The valve and endocardial lesions that result are similar to each other morphologically and consist of fibrotic thickening of the valves with reduced pliability. To date embolism has not been reported as a consequence of this type of valve disease.

Echocardiographic examinations often show *strands of mobile tissue* attached to valve surfaces. The cause and significance of these strands remain uncertain. Lambl in 1856 had originally described such filamentous outgrowths from the ventricular surfaces of the aortic valves sometimes found at necropsy [260] so these fibrous strandlike lesions have often been called Lambl excrescences. Later Magarey found similar filiform strands on the atrial surface of mitral valves [261]. The strands, which were composed of a cellular connective tissue core covered by endothelium, were usually <1 mm thick and ranged in length from 1 to 10 mm [261]. Magarey related the strands to mitral valve thickening and posited that they originated from fibrinous deposits on the valve surface [261]. Freedberg et al. reviewed retrospectively a series of 1559 patients having TEEs during a 2-year period and found mitral valve strands in 63 (4%) [262]. Aortic valve strands were found in 26 (1.7%) patients. Strands were found in 10.6% of patients referred because of suspected recent embolic events, compared to 2.3% of those referred for other indications [262]. Tice and colleagues specifically prospectively looked for mitral valve strands among all patients with native mitral valves studied by transesophageal echocardiography during a 2-year period at their hospital [263]. Among 968 patients, 22 (2.3%) had mitral valve strands. Twenty of these 22 patients were studied because of brain ischemic events. In total, 6.3% of 318 patients having TEE because of brain ischemia had strands, compared to 0.3% of 650 patients having TEE for other indications [263].

Nighoghossian et al. reported three patients who had brain ischemic events presumably related to mitral valve strands and who had had cardiac surgery [264]. Extensive evaluation including cerebral angiography and serological testing showed no cause for stroke other than the valve lesions. The valve lesions were described as a floating mass 6 mm thick on the ventricular surface of the mitral valve, a 6-mm lesion on the anterior mitral valve leaflet, and a sessile 5-mm lesion on the anterior mitral valve leaflet [264]. One patient had immediate cardiac surgery when the valve lesion was found; the other two patients had surgery when they had subsequent strokes despite anticoagulant therapy. Histopathological examinations showed that the lesions were composed of an acellular fibrous core with rings of granular material and endothelial cells. In two patients thrombi were attached to the lesions [264].

Roberts and colleagues compared the frequency of strands among patients referred for TEE because of brain ischemia and those referred for other indications [260]. An association between brain ischemia and strands was found (odds ratio 4.4; 95% confidence interval 2.0 to 9.6). The association was true for men and women and all racial groups. The association was strongest for younger patients and those with both mitral and aortic valve strands. The effect of strands did not depend on valve thickness [265]. Cohen et al. studied 338 patients referred to their echocardiographic laboratory in Paris because of brain ischemia and compared the findings to 276 patients who had no history of brain ischemia [266]. Strands were found in 22.5% of brain ischemia patients, vs. 12.1% of controls (crude odds ratio of 2.1; 95% confidence interval 1.3 to 3.4; $P < .005$).

Strands were found equally in patients with other likely sources of brain infarction as in those with no other sources. The risk of recurrent stroke in patients with strands was low. In this study, and in another echocardiographic study [267], strands were often found in patients with mitral valve thickening [266]. These data and the pathological studies of Magarey [261] suggest that strands are probably most often formed because of a degenerative process that causes fibrinous deposits on valve surfaces. Emboli can arise from the abnormal valves, or on occasion from the strands, or from thrombi formed on the surface of the valve or on the strands. Strands may, in some patients, share a pathogenesis with valve lesions found in patients with SLE, APlAs, and cancer. Some patients with strands have APlAs [268]. Treatment of patients with strands has not been formally studied, but anticoagulants were unsuccessful in preventing brain emboli in two reported patients [264] and are probably also not effective in patients with NBTE. Antiplatelet aggregants or a combination of antiplatelet aggregants and anticoagulants might be more effective in preventing thrombus formation and embolism than either agent alone.

Myocardial and Cardiac Chamber Lesions

Myocardial Infarction and Coronary Artery Disease

Systemic embolism is apparent clinically in about 3% (range 0.6% to 6.4%) of patients with acute myocardial infarction [269–274]. Most clinically detected emboli are those that involve the brain and present as acute strokes. Most strokes that occur in patients with acute myocardial infarcts are caused by embolization of thrombi formed in the left ventricle, but some strokes are related to left atrial thrombi, hypotension, and extracranial occlusive vascular disease. Vascular occlusions, including coronary artery thrombosis, are followed by an increase in acute-phase reactants including serine protease coagulation proteins. Venous thromboses and occlusion of atherostenotic craniocervical arteries may occur in the days and weeks after myocardial infarction because of this hypercoagulability. The stroke occurrence with and without anticoagulation from three trials of large numbers of patients with myocardial infarcts is shown in Table 11 [272–275]. These trials were carried out in the period 1969 to 1973, when the intensity of anticoagulation was much higher than that recommended now. Despite the high intensity of anticoagulation, the complication rates attributable to anticoagulants were low. Minor bleeding occurred in 7%, major bleeds in 1.5%, and intracranial hemorrhages in 0.05%; there were no fatal hemorrhages [272–275].

TABLE 11 Acute Myocardial Infarction, Stroke Occurrence, and Anticoagulation

Trials	No. patients	Strokes (no anticoagulants)	Strokes (anticoagulated)
Veterans [273]	999	3.8%	0.8%
MRC (U.K.) [274]	1427	2.5%	1.1%
Bronx Hospital [275]	1136	2.3%	1.7%
Totals	3562	2.9%	1.2%

Source: Ref. 272.

Left ventricular thrombi can be detected in 20% to 40% of patients with acute anterior myocardial infarcts but are unusual in patients with inferior infarction [271,276,277]. Most thrombi form on the apical wall of the left ventricle, probably in relation to regions of reduced ventricular contractility. Mural thrombi are more likely to form in patients with transmural and large anterior myocardial infarcts than in those with small infarcts. Areas of decreased ventricular contractility, low ejection fraction, and development of a left ventricular aneurysm predispose to thrombus formation. Large thrombi most often occur within the first 3 days after myocardial infarction, especially in patients with large infarcts that carry a poor prognosis [278,279]. Systemic embolization occurs on average 14 days after myocardial infarction and is unusual after 4 to 6 weeks [280]. Pedunculated, mobile thrombi that project into the left ventricular cavity pose the greatest risk for embolization. Anticoagulants clearly reduce the rate of stroke in patients with acute myocardial infarcts. In a study of 999 patients with acute myocardial infarction, short-term warfarin treatment for 28 days reduced the rate of stroke (0.8% vs. 3.8% in nonanticoagulated controls; $P < .001$) [281]. Anticoagulation is indicated in patients with infarcts and echocardiographic findings that predict a high rate of mural thrombus formation and systemic embolism.

Regions of akinesis and dyskinesis, and frank ventricular aneurysms often persist after acute myocardial infarction. In the Coronary Artery Surgery Study (CASS), 7.6% of patients had angiographically defined left ventricular aneurysms [282]. Aneurysms are usually anterior, apical, or anteroapical; posterior aneurysms involving the diaphragmatic wall occur but are rare. Although aneurysms are relatively common and mural thrombi often form within aneurysms, the risk of stroke is relatively low—about 5% [211,283]. Posited reasons for a rather low rate of embolization despite aneurysm formation include: mural thrombi become organized and adherent to the aneurysm walls; thrombi often have a relatively small area of contact with blood flow in the ventricle; and there is a loss of projectile force generated by the underlying adjacent myocardium [211,284]. Considering all patients who have recovered after myocardial infarction, the risk of stroke in patients with impaired left ventricular function after myocardial infarction is substantial. Among 2231 patients with left ventricular dysfunction after acute myocardial infarction who were followed for an average of 42 months, 103 (4.6%) developed strokes [285]. The estimated 5-year stroke rate was 8.1% and the actual stroke rate was 1.5% per year of follow-up [285]. Large size of myocardial infarcts and reduced left ventricular ejection fraction were the two most important predictors of the development of stroke in this study. Patients with ejection fractions of <28% were at highest risk, and for every absolute decrease of 5% in the left ventricular ejection fraction the risk of stroke increased by 18% [285]. In this study (Survival and Ventricular Enlargement [SAVE] trial), beneficial effects of anticoagulation in preventing stroke were found in patients with moderate to severe decreases in left ventricular ejection fraction and also in patients with better preserved function (ejection fractions >35%) [285]. The benefit of anticoagulation for stroke prevention after myocardial infarction was also shown in two other trials [286,287].

Some patients with brain embolism are unexpectedly found to have thrombi within their left ventricles [288,289]. Many such patients do not have a history of acute myocardial infarction, and the cardiac cavity lesions are often first thought to represent myxomas or other cardiac tumors. Sequential echocardiography shows that these thrombi can gradually regress, or suddenly disappear [289–291], often without development of neurologic or other symptoms of embolism. Thrombus formation, and spontaneous endogenous fibrinolysis and fragmentation of thrombi, are dynamic processes. Thrombolytic treatment of patients with cardiac thrombi poses the theoretical risk of breakup of large thrombi into portions which could embolize and cause stroke and systemic embolism. Thrombi often disappear during anticoagulation without apparent symptoms or signs of embolism.

Myocardiopathies

Conditions that affect the endocardium and myocardium promote the formation of cardiac mural thrombi and systemic and brain embolism. Probably the three most important factors that determine thrombus formation are involvement of the endocardial surface, ventricular contractility and blood flow and ejection patterns within the ventricles, and activation of platelets and the coagulation system. Among the three categories of cardiomyopathies—dilated, restrictive, and hypertrophic—mural thrombus formation and embolism are most common among the disorders that cause a dilated cardiomyopathy. Intraventricular thrombus formation is enhanced by stasis of blood and by the loss of normal subendocardial trabeculation. The network of subendocardial trabeculae can act as many small compartments that produce high levels of force within the ventricle propelling blood away from the endocardial surface [291a]. As left ventricular function deteriorates and the left ventricular ejection fraction becomes <40%, thrombi are more likely to form and patients have an increased risk of thromboembolism [291a].

In one study of patients with idiopathic dilated cardiomyopathy, 60% had mural thrombi defined by echocardiography, and even more had clinical or necropsy evidence of systemic embolism [292]. Conditions as diverse as muscular dystrophies [293,294], cardiac amyloidosis [295], peripartum cardiomyopathy [296,297], cocaine-related cardiomyopathy [298], noncompaction of the myocardium [299], and cardiac sarcoidosis [300] have been associated with thromboembolism arising from the heart disease. Mural thrombi form mostly within the trabeculae carnae near the cardiac apex. Atrial fibrillation develops in some patients with cardiomyopathies and further increases the frequency of embolism. Embolism is unusual in patients with hypertrophic cardiomyopathies unless they develop atrial fibrillation.

Some reports conclude that anticoagulation in patients with dilated cardiomyopathies is effective, but other studies have shown poor effectiveness in preventing thromboembolism [299a]. In one study reported by Fuster and colleagues, among 103 patients who were not anticoagulated there were 19 embolic events that occurred during 624 patient-years compared to no embolic events among 32 patients who were anticoagulated during 101 patient-years [299b]. However, in the Vasodilators in Heart Failure trials, there seemed to be no important protective effect of anticoagulation [299a].

Cardiac Myxomas and Other Tumors

Although cardiac tumors are rare, they are an important cause of embolism and are very important to diagnose. *Myxomas* are the most common heart tumors and were found in 0.025% of patients in an unselected autopsy study [301]. The cells of origin are endocardial and arise from multipotential mesenchymal cells that persist as embryonal remnants during septation of the heart [302]. About 75% originate in the left atrium, and 15% to 20% in the right atrium [302,303]. Most myxomas originate from the interatrial septum at the edge of the fossa ovalis, but some originate from the posterior or anterior atrial walls or the auricular appendage [302,303]. About 6% to 8% of myxomas are found in the ventricles, equally divided between the left and right ventricles [302,303]. Rarely, myxomas can arise from the region of the heart valves. Biatrial myxomas have been described in which the tumor usually projects into the contralateral atrium through a patent foramen ovale [302]. Myxomas project from their endocardial attachments into cardiac chambers. Myxomas are most often found in patients between the ages of 30 and 60; women are slightly more often affected than men, and there are instances of familial occurrence of myxomas.

Embolism is estimated to occur in 30% to 50% of patients with cardiac myxomas [302,304–306]. Most emboli arise from the left atrium and go to the brain or systemic organs. Occasional cases of right atrial myxomas with systemic embolism have been reported in the presence of a patent foramen ovale [307–309]. The most common recognized site of embolism is to the brain, but embolism to the eye can cause transient or persistent visual loss, and embolism to the spinal cord has also been reported [302,310,311]. Most often, patients with brain embolism present with a sudden-onset focal neurologic deficit. Transient deficits sometimes occur. Often there has been more than one brain embolism before atrial myxomas are diagnosed. Usually the diagnosis of myxomas is made by echocardiography. Although echocardiography is very sensitive for the detection of myxomas, in one patient with recurrent brain embolism to the posterior circulation from a left atrial myxoma, the initial echocardiogram was negative [312]. Small size of tumor or embolization of the bulk of the tumor could explain the initially negative echocardiogram. Emboli can consist of tumor fragments and/or thrombus. Patients with progressive demetia caused by multiple small brain infarcts [313], and sudden coma due to a shower of tumor emboli to multiple brain arteries have been reported [314].

Occasional patients with brain emboli from myxomas have subarachnoid or intracerebral hemorrhage [315–317]. Bleeding is related to the development of hemorrhagic infarction or rupture of aneurysms. Embolism from myxoma tissue to the wall of brain arteries causes aneurysms that are identical to mycotic aneurysms found in patients with bacterial endocarditis. Usually the aneurysms are relatively small, multiple, and on peripheral branches of brain arteries [316,317]. Some aneurysms are quite large [316]. The peripheral location of aneurysms in patients with myxomas and endocarditis differs from that usually found in patients with saccular (berry) aneurysms. Delayed progressive brain ischemia and enlargement of aneurysms can develop after the initial embolic event [315]. Although delayed growth and rupture of aneurysms [315–319] and metastatic tumor growth [319–321] do occur, their frequency is probably very low. In a review of 35 patients with atrial myxomas followed at the Mayo Clinic, none had subsequent delayed neurological events attributable to their myxomas [319]. Recurrent cardiac tumors after surgery can, however, give rise to recurrent embolization.

Papillary fibroelastomas are another type of cardiac tumor that often give rise to brain embolism [322,323]. The lesions consist of multiple papillary fronds that radiate from an avascular fibrocollagenous core attached by a short pedicle to the endothelium. They most often arise from the aortic valves [324]. Angina and coronary ischemia are caused by embolism to the coronary arteries. Multiple brain infarcts usually occur before the diagnosis is made by echocardiography. *Rhabdomyomas* are often multiple, arise from the ventricular myocardium, and project into the ventricular cavity. Tuberous sclerosis is present in about 33% of patients with rhabdomyomas [325]. Other cardiac tumors include *lipomas*, which often involve the interatrial septum and can arise from the mitral or aortic valves, rhabdomyosarcomas, angiosarcomas, and metastatic tumors. These rarely have been associated with brain embolism [331]. Patients with neurofibromatosis may develop rhabdomyosarcomas, which have been reported to cause brain emboli [327].

Anticoagulants are probably not effective in preventing embolism in patients with cardiac tumors. Emboli often represent tumor fragments. Theoretically, white platelet-fibrin nidi might develop on the surface and crevices of cardiac tumors, as might red erythrocyte-fibrin thrombi. For this reason, agents that affect platelet aggregation and function and standard anticoagulants might have some therapeutic effect, but there are no studies of their utility in patients with myxomas or other cardiac neoplasms. The only definitive treatment is surgical whenever possible.

Paradoxical Embolism and Cardiac Septal Lesions

While once considered to be very rare, emboli entering the systemic circulation through right-to-left shunting of blood are becoming more frequently recognized with the advent of newer diagnostic technologies. By far the most common potential intracardiac shunt is a residual patent foramen ovale (PFO). The high frequency of PFOs in the normal adult population has made it difficult to be certain in an individual stroke patient with a PFO whether paradoxical embolism through the PFO was the cause of their stroke or the PFO was merely an incidental finding. Autopsy series have shown that about 30% of adults have a probe patent foramen ovale at necropsy [328]. Hagen et al. studied 956 patients with clinically and pathologically normal hearts and found a PFO in 27.3% [328]. The frequency of PFOs declined with age: 34.3% during the first three decades of life; 25.4% during the fourth to eighth decades; and 20.2% during the ninth and 10th decades. The average diameter of PFOs was 4.9 mm and the size tended to increase with age [328]. Echocardiographic studies have shown that PFOs are more commonly found in patients with stroke than in controls and that PFOs are more common in patients with an undetermined cause of stroke (''cryptogenic stroke'') than in those in whom another etiology has been defined. Lechat and colleagues examined 60 adults <55 years old with stroke and 100 controls using 2D echocardiography and injections of 5 to 10 mL of agitated saline containing air bubbles [329]. The frequency of PFOs was higher in the stroke group (40%) than in controls (10%). Among patients with an identifiable stroke cause, 21% had PFOs; 40% of patients with possible risk factors for stroke such as migraine, mitral valve prolapse, or use of oral contraceptives had PFOs. The frequency of PFO detection was highest (54%) in those patients with no identifiable risk factor or cause of stroke [329].

DiTullio and colleagues studied 146 patients among whom 31% had no known cause of stroke and 69% had identifiable causes other than paradoxical embolism [330]. Among the total group of patients, 26 (18%) had PFOs. Patients with cryptogenic stroke had a higher prevalence of PFOs than those with identifiable causes, both in the group <55 years old (48% compared to 4%) and those >55 years old (38% vs. 8%) [330]. Petty et al. studied the presence of PFOs among 160 patients with brain infarcts and also found that PFOs were more common among patients with infarcts of uncertain cause (40%) compared with 25% of infarcts with a known cause [331].

Review of series of patients with paradoxical embolism [332–334] through a PFO and our own experience allow us to arrive at five criteria that, when four or more are met, establish with a high degree of certainty the presence of paradoxical embolism:

1. *A situation that promotes thrombosis of leg or pelvic veins*, e.g., long sitting in one position, recent surgery, etc.
2. *Increased coagulability*, e.g., the use of oral contraceptives, presence of Leiden factor with resistance to activated protein C, dehydration
3. *Sudden onset of stroke during sexual intercourse, straining at stool, or other activity that includes a Valsalva maneuver* or that promotes right-to-left shunting of blood
4. *Pulmonary embolism* within a short time before or after the neurological ischemic event
5. Absence of other putative causes of stroke after thorough evaluation

A recent patient of one of the authors (L.R.C.) provides an example of the diagnosis of paradoxical embolism:

> A 29-year-old woman and her husband took their four children home from a trip on an 8-hour car ride. The day was very warm and she had nothing to drink during the ride. She spent much of the time acting as a policeman for the children, disciplining them while kneeling on her seat facing the children, who were cavorting in the rear of the station wagon. When they got home, they fed the children and put them to bed. She showered and immediately thereafter had sex with her husband. At the point of climax, she became unable to speak and her right arm was weak and numb. Examination showed a right hemiparesis and aphasia. CT showed a left upper division MCA territory infarct. Echocardiography revealed a PFO with increased flow during a Valsalva maneuver. The heart and aorta were otherwise normal, and an MRA examination of the cervicocranial arteries was normal. She made a good recovery but had some residual right-hand numbness and dysnomia.

Gautier and colleagues reported 29 patients with paradoxical embolism and reviewed 31 patients reported by others [334]. Situations that promoted venous occlusions among these 60 patients included surgery (seven), postpartum, lower-extremity injury, and jugular vein catheterization. Strokes occurred after sex (two), straining at stool (seven), weight-lifting (two), blowing the nose with great effort, asthmatic attack, gymnastics, decompressing the ears, and martial arts. Venous thrombosis was detected in very few patients and very few had clinical pulmonary emboli. Lung radionuclide scans, pulmonary angiography, and necropsy did show pulmonary emboli in an important number of patients [334]. Patients were not fully evaluated for hypercoagulability. The most common territory of stroke was the MCA, which was involved in 25 patients, while 15 had vertebrobasilar territory embolic infarcts [334]. The 37.5% of posterior circulation infarction is more than expected since only 20% of blood flow to the brain goes through the posterior circulation [41]. A study of the distribution of microemboli in patients with PFOs also showed that there is an unexplained predilection for embolic material to go to posterior circulation vessels [335].

Paradoxical embolism has also been described through ventricular septal defects [336], atrial septal defects [337], and pulmonary arteriovenous fistulas [338]. Venous thrombosis can be detected if studies are performed early in the course. Some venous thrombi involve the pelvic veins and might be detected by abdominal and pelvic imaging techniques. Stollberger et al. studied 49 patients with paradoxical embolism through PFOs including 41 patients with stroke and eight with acute limb embolism [339]. Venous thrombosis was suspected clinically in six patients and documented by venography in 24 of 42 (57%) patients studied. Venous diagnostic studies were more likely to be positive when patients were studied soon after systemic embolism [339].

The advent of TEE has undoubtedly facilitated recognition and quantification of PFOs and atrial septal defects. TEE was able to show a serpentine thrombus actually traversing a PFO [340] and to detect fat emboli during surgery for a femoral fracture [341]. Transcranial Doppler ultrasound (TCD) has also been used effectively to diagnose the presence of right-to-left cardiac or pulmonary shunting [342,343]. The technique involves injection of a small amount of saline which has been agitated vigorously with a small amount of air, or mixed with a polygelatine contrast agent [343] into a cubital vein. During and after the injection, the MCA is insonated using TCD. Appearance of microbubbles in the MCA within the first three to five cardiac cycles ($<$10 seconds) indicates the presence of right-to-left shunting of blood [342,343]. The test is usually done with and without a Valsalva maneuver. The technique has the advantage of being able to be used at the bedside since TCD is portable.

Investigators have compared the utility of TCD and echocardiography in detecting right-to-left shunts [343–347]. TTE was less sensitive than TEE and detected only 9/19 (47%) in one series [344]. The results depended heavily on the frequency of adequate heart visualization during TTE. The sensitivity of TCD was 91.3%, specificity 93.8%, and overall accuracy 92.8% in one study using TEE as the gold standard for recognition of a PFO [346]. In all of the series, some patients with PFOs were detected by one or the other technique (TCD or TEE) but missed by the other [343–347]. TCD can merely suggest the presence of a right-to-left shunt and is not specific for a cardiac source; patients with pulmonary shunting will also have positive TCDs. TCD can be used as a screening test. If positive, then echocardiography is indicated.

Predictors for the likelihood of paradoxical embolism through PFOs have been sought using TEE [348,349]. In one study, the presence of an atrial septal aneurysm accompanying the PFO was an important finding, favoring the presence of paradoxical embolism [348]. In another study, PFOs were significantly larger

(2.1 ± 1.7 mm vs. 0.57 ± 0.78 mm), and there were more microbubbles (13.9 ± 10.7 vs. 1.6 ± 0.8 per mm^3) in patients with cryptogenic stroke than in those with identified causes of stroke [349].

Electrocardiographic findings can also raise the suspicion of the presence of PFOs and ostium secundum atrial septal defects. Ay and colleagues recently described the finding of an M-shaped notch on the ascending branch or on the peak of the R-wave in inferior ECG leads (II, III, avF) as an indicator of the presence of PFOs or atrial septal defects [349a]. This notched pattern has been called ''crochetage'' because of its resemblance morphologically to a crochet needle [349a,349b]. Crochetage was found in 10 of 28 (36%) of patients with echocardiographically documented PFOs [349a]. Heller and colleagues had previously shown that corchetage was a useful indicator of ostium secundum atrial septal defects [349b].

Atrial septal aneurysms have recently received increased attention in relation to their possible role in contributing to brain embolism. Fusion of the septum primum closes the foramen ovale and leads to a depression on the right side of the interatrial septal wall. Bulging of the septum primum tissue of the atrial septum through the fossa ovalis into either the right or left atrial cavity is called an atrial septal aneurysm. Atrial septal aneurysms were first reported in 1934 [350]; they were found in 1% of necropsies by Silver and Dorsey [351] and are found in 3% to 4% of TEEs [352]. Belkin et al. analyzed the findings among 36 consecutive patients with echocardiographically documented atrial septal aneurysms [353]. Ten of the patients had cerebrovascular ischemic events and one had a peripheral limb embolus. The authors judged that 6 (17%) patients had definite and 8 (22%) had probable embolic events. In this study 28/31 (90%) patients also showed atrial shunting of agitated saline contrast [353]. Nater and colleagues studied 12 patients who had brain ischemic events (11 strokes and one TIA) and atrial septal aneurysms [352]. Ten patients (83%) also had a patent foramen ovale. The clinical data suggested brain embolism in each case [352].

Cabanes et al. studied the frequency of atrial septal aneurysms, patent foramen ovale, and mitral valve prolapse among 100 fully evaluated stroke patients <55 years old and among 50 controls [354]. Atrial septal aneurysms were found in 28% of stroke patients and 8% of controls. A patent foramen ovale was found in 72% of patients with atrial septal aneurysms, and 25% of patients without atrial septal aneurysms. The presence of an atrial septal aneurysm (odds ratio 4.3; 95% confidence interval 1.3 to 14.6; $P = .01$) or a PFO (odds ratio 3.9; 95% confidence interval 1.5 to 10; $P = .003$) was strongly associated with cryptogenic stroke. The stroke odds ratio of a patient with both an atrial septal aneurysm and a PFO were 33.3 (95% confidence interval 4.1 to 270) times the stroke odds of a patient who had neither. Atrial septal aneurysms with >10 mm excursion were eight times more likely to be associated with stroke than those with smaller excursions [354]. The presence of mitral valve prolapse in this study did not increase the odds of cryptogenic stroke. The data from these three echocardiographic studies [352–354] are conclusive that there is a strong association between atrial septal aneurysms and interatrial shunts, and that the presence of either atrial septal aneurysms and/or PFOs is strongly associated with the presence of cryptogenic stroke, especially among young stroke patients. The exact mechanism by which atrial septal aneurysms contribute to brain embolism has not been satisfactorily clarified but these lesions can harbor thrombi. Thrombus was seen within an atrial septal aneurysm in one patient [355] and has been found within the base of atrial septal aneurysms at necropsy [351].

The recurrence rate of stroke in patients with PFOs and the effect of various treatments on recurrence has occasionally been studied [348,356–359]. In one small study, no recurrences occurred among 15 patients taking aspirin (six), warfarin (seven), or after surgical closure (two) [348]. Bogousslavsky and his Swiss colleagues studied stroke recurrence among 140 consecutive patients who had PFOs and brain ischemic events [356]. One-fourth of the patients also had atrial septal aneurysms. During a mean follow-up period of 3 years, the stroke or death rate was 2.4% per year. Only eight patients had a recurrent brain infarct (1.9% per year) [356]. Ninety-two (66%) took aspirin 250 mg per day, while 37 (26%) were given anticoagulants and 11 (8%) had surgical closure of the PFO within 12 weeks of the stroke after being treated with anticoagulants. There was no significant difference in the effect of any of the treatments on recurrence. The relatively low rate of recurrence contrasted with the severity of the initial stroke which left disabling effects in half the patients [356]. In a French multicenter study, 132 patients with PFOs and/or atrial septal aneurysms and cryptogenic stroke were followed for an average of 22.6 months [357]. The recurrence rate was approximately 2% to 3% at 2 years and was higher in patients with both PFOs and atrial septal aneurysms. Recurrences occurred in four patients who were taking antiplatelet agents and in one who was treated with anticoagulants [357]. In another study, Lausanne investigators found no recurrence of stroke during an average follow-up of 2 years among 30 patients who had suture closure of PFOs during cardiopulmonary bypass surgery [358]. None of the patients were given antiaggregants or anticoagulants after surgery. There were no serious surgical complications. After surgery, two patients had interatrial shunting as determined by TCD and TEE, but the shunts were much smaller than before surgery [358].

PFOs have also been closed using an umbrella device placed through a catheter. Bridges and colleagues reported the results of transcatheter closure of PFOs among 36 patients with PFOs of whom half had multiple ischemic events [359]. Twelve patients had had ischemic events while taking warfarin before closure. In 28 (78%) the closure was complete and another five had nearly complete closure. No patient had a recurrent stroke during 8.4 months of follow-up, but four patients had transient ischemic events [359]. The available data regarding treatment are inconclusive but all studies have shown a very low recurrence rate (about 2% per year) among stroke patients with PFOs. The presence of both a PFO and an atrial septal aneurysm substantially increases the risk of stroke recurrence. Warfarin and surgical or transcatheter closure are posited to be more effective than drugs that affect platelet functions, but studies have not definitively shown their superiority.

Frequency of Various Cardiac Sources of Emboli in Stroke Registries

Unfortunately, there are very few analyses of the frequency of various cardiac sources of embolism among well-studied series of stroke or brain ischemia patients. The Stroke Data Bank, which included 1805 patients among whom 1290 had brain infarcts, did report the frequency of various cardiac lesions among their patients with brain infarcts [56]. Based on a literature review, the Stroke Data Bank investigators first divided cardiac lesions into those considered at high risk for cerebral embolism and those considered at lesser risk. Historical features, ECG, and 2D TTE data were used to categorize the cardiac lesions. Patients were considered to have a high-risk condition if they had past valve surgery, a history or ECG evidence of atrial fibrillation, atrial flutter or sick sinus syndrome, echocardiographic evidence of ventricular aneurysm, akinetic ventricular segment, mural thrombus, left ventricular hypokinesis, or cardiomyopathy. There were 250 patients who had one or more of these high-risk cardiac sources [56]. Patients with cardiac lesions considered to have less risk of brain embolism (called medium-risk by the investigators) had to have no high-risk conditions and a history of myocardial infarction within 6 months, aortic or mitral stenosis or regurgitation, congestive heart failure, history or echocardiographic evidence of mitral valve prolapse, echocardiographic evidence of mitral annulus calcification, a hypokinetic ventricular segment, or decreased left ventricular function. There were 166 patients who met criteria for medium-risk donor sources [56]. Some patients had more than one cardiac condition; for example, atrial fibrillation and congestive heart failure.

Table 12 shows the frequency of the various cardiac conditions in the Stroke Data Bank. The commonest cardiac problem by far was atrial arrythmia; 190 patients in the high-risk group (76%) had atrial fibrillation, atrial flutter, or sick sinus syndrome. Most patients with atrial arrythmias did not have cardiac valve disease (162/190; 85%). Congestive heart failure was the next most common abnormality and was present in 92 (37%) patients in the high-risk and 95 (57%) patients in the medium-risk categories. Akinetic regions on TTE were the next most common category in the high risk group and were found in 52 (21%) of Stroke Data bank patients [56]. The Stroke Data Bank investigators mentioned endocarditis and right-to-left cardiac shunts as potential cardiac donor sources

Table 12 Patients in the Stroke Data Bank with Selected Cardiac Characteristics[a] in High and Medium Cardiac Risk Groups

Cardiac risk categories	High risk (n = 250)	Medium risk (n = 166)
High-risk categories		
Valve surgery	15	
A fib, A flutter, sick sinus with valve disease	28	
A fib, A flutter, sick sinus but no valve disease	162	
Ventricular aneurysm[b]	5	
Mural thrombus[b]	12	
Cardiomyopathy or left ventricle hypokinesis[b]	7	
Akinetic region[b]	52	
Medium-risk categories		
Myocardial infarct within 6 months	25	18
Valve disease without A fib, A flutter, sick sinus	31	19
Congestive heart failure	92	95
Decreased left ventricle function[b]	0	3
Hypokinetic segment[b]	0	12
Mitral valve prolapse (by history or echocardiogram	5	13
Mitral annulus calcification[b]	14	46

[a] Some patients had more than one characteristic.
[b] By echocardiography.
Source: Ref. 56.

of embolism, but they did not tabulate the occurrence of these conditions in the two risk groups. Patent foramen ovale, atrial septal defects and aneurysms, spontaneous echo contrast, and lesions in the ascending aorta and aortic arch were not tabulated probably because the Stroke Data Bank patients were studied before TEE and only TTE was used [56].

The Lausanne Stroke Registry reported the frequencies of various potential cardiac sources of embolism (PCSEs) among the first 1311 patients admitted to the hospital with a first-ever stroke [42]. Among these patients, a total of 305 (23%) had PCSEs. Atrial fibrillation (141; 46%) was the commonest abnormality; atrial fibrillation was an isolated finding in 118 patients and was accompanied by myocardial abnormalities in 12 patients and by valve disease in 11 other patients. Myocardial abnormalities were the next most common PCSE in the Lausanne Stroke Registry, occurring in 84 (27.5%) of patients with cardiac donor sources. Among the 305 patients with PCSEs, 33 (11%) also had large-artery atherostenotic lesions and 125 (40%) had atherosclerotic plaques associated with lesser severity of stenosis, lesions which represented potential arterial donor sources of embolism [42]. TEE was also not available among these reported patients, and only

TABLE 13 Potential Cardiac Sources of Embolism in the Lausanne Stroke Registry

Cardiac abnormalities	No. patients (%)
Isolated myocardial abnormalities	84 (27.5%)
Focal left ventricle akinesia without thrombus	61 (20%)
Focal left ventricle akinesia with thrombus	7 (2.3%)
Global ventricular hypokinesia	7 (2.3%)
Patent foramen ovale	6 (2%)
Left atrial myxoma	2 (0.7%)
Left ventricle thrombus	1 (0.3%)
Isolated valve abnormalities	71 (23.3%)
Mitral valve prolapse	51 (16.7%)
Mitral stenosis or insufficiency	10 (3.3%)
Prosthetic mitral or aortic valve)	10 (3.3%)
Isolated arrhythmia	127 (41.6%)
Atrial fibrillation	118 (38.7%)
Sick sinus syndrome	9 (2.9%)
Arrhythmias + myocardial abnormalities	12 (3.9%)
Atrial fibrillation + Focal left ventricular akinesia without thrombus	6 (2%)
+ Focal left ventricular akinesia with thrombus	1 (0.3%)
+ Global hypokinesia	3 (1%)
+ Left ventricular thrombus	2 (0.7%)
Arrythmias + valve abnormalities	11 (3.6%)
Atrial fibrillation + mitral valve prolapse	6 (2%)
+ Mitral stenosis	2 (0.7%)
+ Prosthetic valve	3 (1%)

Source: Ref. 42.

nine patients <40 years old had microbubble injections searching for patent foramen ovale; six had PFOs detected by this method. The PCSEs in the Lausanne Stroke Registry are shown in Table 13.

The frequency of cardiac conditions among echocardiographic series of patients is heavily dependent on referral bias. Atrial fibrillation is undoubtedly the most commonly recognized cardiac donor source of embolism. Myocardial disease, most often coronary artery related, represents the next most important cardiac source followed by valve disease.

Aorta as a Source of Brain Embolism

Studies of patients with stroke and TIA have now firmly established that the thoracic aorta is an important source of brain embolism. The first report on this subject was published half a century ago. Meyer described two patients with syphilitic aortic aneurysms that developed cholesterol crystal embolism [360]. A decade later Winter also described two patients with syphilitic aneurysms of the proximal aorta [361]. The ascending aorta of Winter's first patient was ''covered by innumerable atheromata most of which were eroded and partly calcified. Soft thrombi containing cholesterol crystals were adherent to many'' [355]. Many brain arteries were blocked by cholesterol crystal-containing thrombi. In the second patient, who also had multiple brain cholesterol crystal emboli, the ''entire intimal surface of the aorta, but in particular the aneurysm, was covered by astheromatous plaques many of which were ulcerated and covered by soft thrombi'' [361]. In 1965, Miller Fisher, Paul Dudley White, and colleagues examined the aorta and extracranial and intracranial arteries among 178 patients and found that only 37 aortas were free of ulceration and that the aorta was two to four times more likely to show severe atherosclerosis than the cervical carotid and vertebral arteries [362].

Although it is well known that the aorta was an important site of atheromatous disease, there was almost no mention of aortic atherosclerotic disease as an important cause of stroke until the beginning of the last decade of the 20th century. Tunick and his colleagues at the New York University Medical Center published two reports that included four patients with unexplained brain ischemic events in whom TEE showed large protruding, often mobile atheromas [363,364]. In one patient who had brain, leg, and arm emboli, TEE showed ''a large mass with smaller mobile components, protruding into the lumen of the aortic arch'' [364]. Several aortic masses in this patient were removed surgically and showed severe atherosclerotic plaques with superimposed thrombi [364]. Shortly after publication of these case reports, Tunick and colleagues reported the TEE results among 122 patients who had stroke, TIAs, or peripheral emboli, and 122 age- and sex-matched controls [365]. Protruding atheromas were strongly related to the occurrence of embolic events (odds ratio 3.2; 95% confidence interval 1.6 to 6.5; $P < .001$), and atheromas with mobile components were only found in patients with embolic events [365]. Karalis and colleagues also reported an observational TEE study of their experience with aortic atheromas [366]. ''Intra-aortic atherosclerotic debris'' was found in 7% of 556 patients studied by TEE; 11 patients with these atheromatous aortic lesions (31%) had embolic events [366]. Embolic events were more often associated with pedunculated and mobile aortic lesions than those that were layered and immobile [366].

These observational studies and case reports alerted the medical community to the possible importance of aortic atheromas as a cause of stroke and peripheral embolism. In 1992, Pierre Amarenco and his Paris colleagues published two reports which showed definitively that aortic atheromatous disease was an important cause of stroke and could be identified clinically [367,368]. Amarenco et al. first published a necropsy study of 500 patients who had stroke or other neurologic diseases. Ulcerated aortic plaques were found in 26% of 239 patients with cerebrovascular disease, compared to only 5% of 261 patients with other neurologic diseases ($P < .001$) [367]. The prevalence of aortic atheromas was 61% among patients with brain infarcts and no demonstrated cause, and 22% among those with other defined causes ($P < .001$) [367]. The presence of ulcerated plaques in the aortic arch did not correlate with the presence of carotid artery stenosis, suggesting that aortic and carotid artery disease were independent risk factors for stroke [367].

Amarenco and Cohen and their colleagues also reported a study of 12 consecutive patients with cryptogenic stroke studied by TEE [368]. Six (50%) had intraluminal echogenic masses in the aortic arch, most often at the junction of the ascending aorta and the arch. In one patient the mass was pedunculated but in the other five the attachment was broad-based with a very irregular surface. The masses extended from 3 to 15 mm into the aortic lumens. Cholesterol emboli were found in quadriceps muscle biopsies in two patients with aortic masses [368]. Tobler et al. studied at necropsy the presence and distribution of atherosclerotic plaques in the ascending aorta [369]. Among 97 ascending aortas, 38% had atherosclerotic plaques >8 mm in diameter; the average diameter of plaques was 19 mm. Most of the 66 plaques were distributed anteriorly or posteriorly on the right side of the ascending aorta, and the upper and lower halves of the ascending aorta were equally involved [369]. Plaques were also prevalent in the aortic arch, especially at the orifice of the innominate artery (21% of 48 arch specimens) [369].

TEE studies in the United States [370,371] and Japan [372] confirm the importance of aortic lesions as a source of brain and peripheral embolism. Masuda et al. analyzed the clinical features and the distribution and pathology among 15 patients with brain atheromatous embolism studied clinically and at necropsy [373]. Cardiac surgery, cardiac catheterization, and angiography triggered embolism in six (40%) of patients in this series. Nine (60%) patients had extensive cortical, often hemorrhagic infarcts in the regions of the arterial border zones between the anterior and middle cerebral arteries and between the middle and posterior cerebral arteries. Six (40%) patients had territorial infarcts of different sizes caused by occlusion of major or branch cerebral arteries [373]. All patients had complicated atheromas in the ascending aorta and the aortic arch. Calcification, ulcerations, mural thrombi, and aneurysmal dilatations were prevalent. Cholesterol crystal emboli were often found in arteries within the border zone regions [373].

Two recent studies investigated the frequency of occurrence of vascular events in patients who had TEE-documented aortic arch atherosclerosis [374,375]. The French Study Group followed 331 patients who presented with brain infarcts for 2 to 4 years [374]. The frequency of subsequent brain infarction and other vascular events was closely correlated with the thickness of the aortic wall. The frequency of recurrent brain infarcts was 11.9 per 100 patient-years in those who had an aortic thickness of >4 mm, compared to rates of 3.5/100 patient-years for those with 1- to 3.9-mm-thick aortic walls, and 2.8/100 patient-years in those with aortic walls <1 mm thick. After controlling for other confounding factors the relative risk of brain infarction was 3.8 (95% confidence interval 1.8 to 7.8; $P = .0012$) and of all vascular events 3.5 (95% confidence interval 2.1 to 5.9; $P < .001$) in patients with aortic wall plaques >4 mm [374]. In a prospective study conducted in two German university hospitals, physicians followed 136 patients with flat plaques <5 mm in thickness, and 47 patients with either thick plaques >5 mm thick or complex plaques with mobile components for an average of 16 months [375]. Embolic events occurred in 15 patients; the incidence was 4.1/100 patient-years in patients with flat plaques, vs. 13.7/100 patient-years in those with complex, thick, or mobile plaques [375].

Atherosclerosis is not the only disease of the aorta that can give rise to embolism. Syphilitic aortitis and aneurysms have long been known to ulcerate and cause thromboembolism [360,361]. Physicians in Sri Lanka described 10 patients who had an inflammatory aortitis different from Takayasu's disease that caused brain embolism and strokes [376]. The earliest histological changes in this condition were focal fragmentation of elastic lamella and an acute inflammatory aortitis in the media of the aortic arch. The aortic intima was edematous and mural thrombi often formed on the endothelial surface of the aorta and embolized intracranially [376]. Takayasu's disease, aortic trauma, and aortic dissection are probably also occasionally complicated by embolism arising from the aorta. In the case of aortic dissection, thrombus formation within the aorta and subsequent embolism should be separated from obliteration of the orifices of the branches of the arch by the dissection, and from concurrent dissection of brachiocephalic arteries, which often accompanies aortic dissections [377–379].

Treatment of aortic atheromatous disease is controversial. Anticoagulants have been posited to aggravate cholesterol crystal embolism [380], but in several patients aortic thrombotic masses have disappeared after anticoagulant therapy [381,382]. By preventing the formation of thrombi over ulcerated areas of aortic atheromas, heparin and/or coumadin could theoretically facilitate contact of the atheromatous material with the lumen and promote cholesterol embolism. Cholesterol embolism has also been described after thrombolytic treatment of patients with acute myocardial infarction [382a]; similar to anticoagulants, thrombolytic agents could expose ulcerated areas to the circulation if thrombi were lysed. Intravenous thrombolytic treatment [383] and surgical removal of protruding atheromas [364] have also been reported to be successful in treating patients with aortic atheromas. In one patient who had a carpet of protruding atheromas that involved the orifices of several brachiocephalic arteries, the aortic arch was removed and replaced with a graft [384]. This patient had had three brain embolic events despite warfarin anticoagulation [384]. Agents that affect platelet aggregation and function, and combinations of antiplatelet drugs and anticoagulants might be effective in preventing embolism from aortic plaques but have not been systematically studied.

Arterial Sources of Embolism

The extracranial and intracranial large arteries often serve as the donor source for embolism to the brain. Arterial-source embolism is referred to as artery-to-artery, intra-arterial, or ''local'' embolism. This subject is complex and has been reviewed extensively elsewhere [41,75]. Herein, we include only a very brief review of this topic.

Disease, Pathology, and Pathophysiology

Although atherosclerosis is by far the most common condition that leads to intra-arterial embolism, other vascular diseases can also serve as donor sources. Trauma and dissections of arteries lead to local thrombus formation and embolism. Occasionally, inflammatory diseases of the brachiocephalic branches of the aortic arch such as temporal arteritis and Takayasu's disease can lead to intra-arterial embolism. Thrombi sometimes form within arterial aneurysms, both saccular [385,386] and fusiform dolicocephalic aneurysms [387], and can then break off and embolize to distal branch arteries. Fibromuscular dysplasia (FMD) is an important but relatively uncommon vascular disease which affects the pharyngeal and occasionally the intracranial portions of the carotid and vertebral arteries that can also serve as a source of distal intra-arterial embolism. Thrombi can, on occasion, form within large arteries in the absence of important arterial disease in patients with cancer and other causes of hypercoagulability [388]. These luminal thrombi then embolize to intracranial arteries, causing strokes.

Atherosclerosis is the predominant cause of intra-arterial embolism. The initial arterial lesion is a fatty streak which develops in the intima and then enlarges into a raised atherosclerotic plaque. Plaques contain a mixture of lipid, smooth muscle, fibrous and collagen tissues, and inflammatory cells [10,389,390]. Plaques can enlarge quickly when hemorrhages occur within the plaques. When a critical plaque size and reduction in the lumen are reached, the atherosclerotic process accelerates. Reduced luminal area and the bulk of the protruding plaque alter the physical and mechanical properties of blood flow and create regions of local turbulence and stasis. Platelets often adhere to the irregular surfaces of plaques. Secretion of chemical mediators within platelets and within the underlying vascular endothelium causes aggregation and further adherence of platelets to the endothelium. A ''white clot'' composed of platelets and fibrin develops and, at first, is rather loosely adherent to the vascular wall. Plaques often interrupt the endothelium and ulcerate. Breaches in the endothelium allow cracks and fissures to form, allowing contact of the constituents of the plaque with the luminal contents. The coagulation cascade is activated by this contact, and a ''red thrombus,'' composed of erythrocytes and fibrin, forms within the lumen. Platelet secretion can also activate the serine proteases that form the body's coagulation system and so also promote the formation of red clots. When thrombi first form, they are poorly organized and only loosely adherent. They often propagate and embolize. Within a period of 1 to 2 weeks, thrombi organize and become more adherent and fragments are less likely to break off and embolize. A variety of different materials— cholesterol crystals, calcified plaque fragments, white clots, and red thrombi—can form the substance of intra-arterial emboli.

Arterial dissections are probably the second most common disease that leads to artery-to-artery brain embolism. Stretching or tearing within the arterial media causes formation of an intramural hematoma. Blood within the media dissects longitudinally along the vessel wall. Expansion of the arterial wall compromises the lumen. The expanding intramural hematoma can tear through the intima and inject fresh red congealed hematoma containing thrombuslike material into the arterial lumen. This material is, at first, not adherent to the endothelium and often embolizes. The intimal tear and the underlying medial hematoma cause some irritation of the endothelium which, in turn, causes activation of platelets and the coagulation cascade promoting the formation of a thrombus in situ within the lumen. Compromise of the lumen by the expanding intramural lesion alters blood flow within the lumen, which also promotes thrombus formation. Thus thrombus can form in situ within the dissected artery or reach the lumen by introduction of the intramural contents. In either case, the acute luminal thrombus is poorly organized and nonadherent and readily embolizes distally [41,75,391,392].

Relation of Symptoms to Severity of Arterial Stenosis

Unlike the situation within the coronary arteries, there is a very close relationship between brain ischemia and the severity of arterial stenosis. Transient or persistent brain ischemia is far more likely to develop when the arterial lumen is compromised. The arterial process causes brain ischemia either by substantially reducing blood flow to a region of the brain supplied by the artery (hypoperfusion) or by providing the donor source for intra-arterial embolism. Most sizable brain infarcts in patients with arterial stenoses and occlusions are thought to be embolic. Transcranial Doppler (TCD) studies that show an increased rate of high-intensity transient microembolic signals in patients with severe ICA stenosis support this explanation [20,393–395].

Severity of stenosis is widely accepted as the most important prognostic risk factor that indicates the likelihood of future development of stroke in patients with symptomatic ICA disease in the neck [396–398]. Although less pronounced, the direct relationship between severity of arterial stenosis and subsequent stroke is also found in patients with asymptomatic carotid artery stenosis [399–402]. Norris and colleagues found increasing cumulative rates of transient ischemia and stroke in relation to increasing grades of arterial stenosis [402]. The incidence of ischemic events also correlated very closely with progression of the luminal compromise [402]. Norris estimated that the annual stroke rate in asymptomatic patients with <75% ICA stenosis in the neck was 1% to 2%, compared to a rate of 5% to 6% in patients with >75% stenosis [395]. The North American Symptomatic Carotid Endarterectomy Trial (NASCET) [396] and the European Carotid Surgery Trial (ECST) [397] each found a clear advantage of carotid endarterectomy over medical therapy in symptomatic patients with severe ICA stenosis, but patients with less severe stenosis did not benefit from carotid artery surgery. The Asymptomatic Carotid Atherosclerosis Study (ACAS) also found a benefit for carotid surgery in asymptomatic patients with severe ICA stenosis [403].

In the NASCET study, the risk of stroke correlated highly with the degree of ICA stenosis in all patients with transient monocular blindness, transient hemispheral ischemic attacks, and minor strokes [396,398]. Table 14 shows that the hazard rates for ipsilateral strokes in patients with severe ICA stenosis (>70% luminal narrowing) in patients with first-ever retinal and hemispheric TIAs treated medically increase proportionally with the severity of stenosis [398]. Nicolaides et al. analyzed patients with transient ischemic attacks and minor strokes who had good recovery for the presence of CT scan infarcts (Table 15) [404]. In all groups studied, patients with severe stenosis and occlusion had more frequent brain infarcts [403]. The presence of ''silent infarcts'' on MRI [405] and even the size of brain infarcts [406] have been shown to depend on the severity of ICA stenosis in the neck. The severity of intracranial arterial stenosis has also

TABLE 14 Hazard Rate Estimates at 24 Months for Development of Ipsilateral Strokes in Patients with First-Ever Transient Retinal and Hemispheric TIAs Studied in the NASCET Trial[a]

% ICA luminal narrowing	Retinal TIA (n = 59)	Hemispheral TIA (n = 70)
75% ICA stenosis	11.2	37.4
85% ICA stenosis	17.8	60
95% ICA stenosis	28.9	96.3

[a]Estimates made using proportional hazards regression analysis.
Source: Ref. 398.

Table 15 CT Scan Infarcts on the Symptomatic Side in Patients with TIAs and Minor Strokes

Duplex scan ICA stenosis grade	Transient monocular blindness		Transient hemispheral attacks		Minor strokes with good recovery	
	n	CT infarct	n	CT infarct	n	CT infarct
Normal	16	3 (19%)	33	8 (24%)	41	24 (59%)
1–14% stenosis	23	3 (13%)	34	10 (29%)	40	21 (52%)
15–49% stenosis	10	1 (10%)	15	5 (33%)	21	11 (52%)
50–99% stenosis	21	9 (43%)	21	10 (48%)	26	17 (65%)
Occlusion	9	5 (56%)	6	3 (50%)	7	6 (86%)

Source: Ref. 404.

been shown to correlate highly with severity of stenosis [407–409]. When stenosis is severe, the altered physical characteristics of blood flow strongly facilitate thrombus formation within the lumen, and thromboembolism develops.

Some patients with lesser degrees of arterial stenosis do develop intra-arterial embolism. Most often these emboli are white clots that cause transient ischemia or minor strokes—a phenomenon that Miller Fisher calls ACME (acceptible minor embolism). The morphological characteristics of plaques from specimens removed at endarterectomy correlate with symptoms [410]. Some features of plaques as they appear on B-mode images of the cervical arteries, their degree of surface irregularity, heterogenicity, and echogenicity are helpful in predicting the likelihood of related stroke. Echolucent plaques are rich in lipids and are associated with elevated levels of triglyceride-rich lipoproteins [411,412]. Soft, heterogeneous plaques with irregular surfaces are more often associated with symptoms than are calcified, dense plaques with regular surfaces [412,413].

Distribution of Arterial Lesions

There are important racial and sex differences in the distribution of arteriosclerotic occlusive lesions [414–417]. In white men, the predominant cerebrovascular occlusive lesions are in the carotid and vertebral arteries in the neck. Blacks, individuals of Asian origin, and women more often have occlusive lesions in the large intracranial arteries and their main branches, and less often have severe occlusive vascular lesions in the neck. White men who have carotid artery disease also have a high frequency of coexisting coronary artery and occlusive lower limb artery disease, as well as hypertension, hypercholesterolemia, and smoking. After the menopause the frequency of extracranial occlusive disease increases in

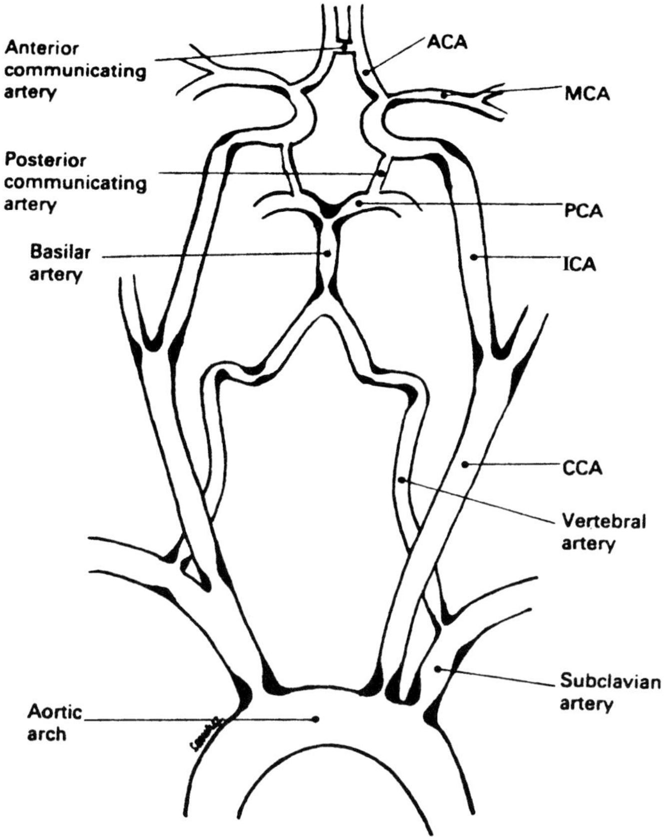

FIG. 31 Diagrammatic representation of the cervicocranial arteries showing the predilection sites for atherosclerotic narrowing in white men. The black areas represent atherosclerotic plaques. Drawn by Dr Juan Sanchez Ramos. ACA, anterior cerebral artery; MCA, middle cerebral artery; PCA, posterior cerebral artery; ICA, internal carotid artery; CCA, common carotid artery. (From Ref. 75.)

women. Figure 31 shows the predilection sites for atheromatous plaques in white men.

Within the anterior circulation, the most frequent and most important occlusive lesion in white men is within the ICA in the neck. Atherosclerotic lesions usually begin within the common carotid artery (CCA) along the posterior wall of that vessel opposite the flow divider between the ICA and the external carotid

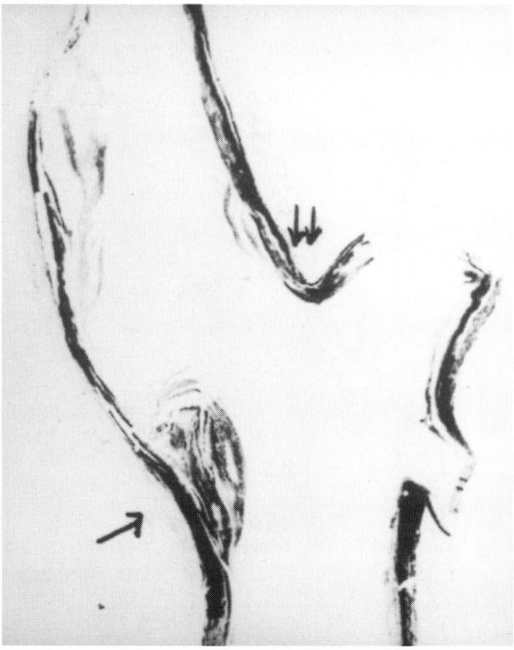

FIG. 32 Drawing of a stained specimen of the carotid arteries. The double black arrows point to the flow divider between the internal and external carotid arteries. The single arrow shows a protruding plaque in a characteristic location along the posterior wall of the internal carotid artery opposite the flow divider. (From Ref. 75.)

artery (ECA) [362,389,390]. Figure 32 illustrates this localization of plaque. Atherosclerotic plaques grow in diameter and often spread rostrally within the CCA, the proximal ICA, and ECAs. The next most common atherosclerotic lesions in white men are found within the intracranial ICA in the proximal intracranial portion of the artery, called the carotid siphon because of its S shape, and within the proximal portions of the middle cerebral arteries (MCAs). These lesions all produce symptoms by causing hypoperfusion of supplied brain territories or by embolism of fragments of clots that form upon the vascular endothelium of plaques or of particles of the plaques themselves. Women, blacks, and Asians often develop occlusive lesions within the MCAs and their branches. ICA siphon and neck lesions are less often found. Blacks, Asians, and women who develop occlusive neck lesions usually smoke and have important coexisting atherosclerotic risk factors such as hypertension and hypercholesterolemia.

Within the posterior circulation, the commonest occlusive lesion among white men is at the vertebral artery origin in the neck and within the adjacent subclavian artery. The next most common lesion is within the basilar artery. White men with occlusive extracranial vertebral artery (ECVA) disease also have a high frequency of coexisting carotid artery disease [41,362,418,419], as well as hypertension and hypercholesterolemia. Intracranial lesions are also very common both in white men and in women, blacks, and Asians. The predominant lesions are within the intracranial vertebral arteries (ICVAs). Atherosclerotic lesions within the ICVAs are often bilateral. Atherosclerotic lesions involving the posterior cerebral arteries are more common in women, blacks, and Asians [41]. The predominant mechanism of brain ischemia within the posterior circulation, as within the anterior circulation, is embolism [41,420,421]. Intra-arterial embolism is just as common and important a mechanism of stroke within the vertebrobasilar arterial system as it is within the carotid artery system.

Arterial dissections most often involve the pharyngeal portions of the extracranial carotid and vertebral arteries [41,75]. The pharyngeal portions of the neck arteries are relatively mobile, while the origins of the arteries and their penetrations into the cranial cavity are relatively anchored and much less mobile. Tearing seems to occur in portions of arteries which are flexible and stretch with motion. Within the ECVAs, the most common site of dissection is the most distal portion of the artery which emerges from the intervertebral foramina and courses around the atlas to penetrate the dura mater and enter the foramen magnum [392,422]. Dissections also occur in the mobile part of the proximal portion of the ECVAs above the origin of the arteries from the subclavian arteries but before the arteries enter the vertebral column at the intervertebral foramen of the sixth or fifth cervical vertebrae [41].

Intracranial dissections are much less common than extracranial dissections. In the anterior circulation, dissections most often affect the intracranial ICA and extend into the middle and anterior cerebral arteries. Within the posterior circulation the commonest site is the intracranial vertebral artery [422,423]. Dissections within the ICVAs often spread into the basilar artery. Occasionally the basilar artery is the primary site of dissection [422]. Dissecting aneurysms as well as large saccular and dolicocephalic fusiform aneurysms can serve as a source of thrombus formation with subsequent distal embolization.

EVALUATION OF POTENTIAL DONOR SOURCES OF EMBOLISM

In patients suspected of having brain embolic events, we believe that a thorough evaluation of all potential sources—cardiac, aortic, and cerebrovascular—is usually indicated. Atherosclerotic plaques and occlusive lesions often coexist in the heart, aorta, and brachiocephalic arteries. Furthermore, patients with cerebrovascular occlusive lesions have a very high frequency of coronary atherosclerotic heart disease, and their coronary disease is often a more serious threat for mortality and disability than their cerebrovascular disease. Also, of course, patients with coronary atherosclerotic heart disease have a high frequency of occlusive lesions within their extracranial and intracranial vascular beds. Prophylactic treatment to prevent subsequent thromboembolism should optimally consider measures to prevent embolism from *all* potential donor sources, not only the one that caused the present embolism.

All patients should have a thorough history concerning cardiac symptomatology followed by a careful physical examination of the chest and heart. An electrocardiogram and chest x-ray should ordinarily also be performed. Most patients with severe heart disease have abnormalities uncovered by these routine clinical procedures. A TTE including Doppler insonation and the injection of microbubbles searching for intracardiac shunts is ordinarily indicated. Some patients, especially youths and young adults, who have a well-defined vascular donor source of embolism such as a cervical dissection, will not need echocardiography because the yield of echocardiography is so low.

TTE is usually performed first, and the results may be definitive and thus a TEE would not be required. All observers agree that TEE shows many abnormalities not revealed by TTE. The utility of TEE in patients with strokes and TIAs has recently been extensively reviewed [424–429]. TEE is more accurate than TTE in showing atrial and ventricular thrombi and in detecting and quantifying intracardiac shunts, and it more often shows spontaneous echo contrast than TTE [426].

Even TEE can fail to identify some cardiac sources of emboli. Some thromboemboli are too small to be detected. An embolus that is 1 to 2 mm in size can produce a devastating neurological deficit, and this size particle might be beyond the resolution of echocardiography. The other major reason for failure is that thrombosis and embolism are dynamic processes. When a thrombus leaves the heart to go to the brain, echocardiography may not show a thrombus within the heart if performed soon after the clinical event. Later the thrombus may reform. Figure 33 shows an example of a disappearing cardiac thrombus. In this patient the initial TEE clearly showed a large intracardiac mass, but a repeat TEE showed that the mass was gone [289].

TEE also yields important information about the proximal aorta, a region not imaged by TTE. Figures 34 and 35 show aortic plaques detected by TEE. We believe that TEE is important in all patients in whom TTE suggests but does not adequately define the cardiac pathology, and in all patients in whom other studies (cerebrovascular, hematologic, and other cardiac investigations) do not satisfactorily show the cause of brain embolism and brain ischemia. A recent analysis showed that TEE was cost effective in patients with recent brain-hemorrhagic infarction [429].

Echocardiography can be accompanied by MRA of the extracranial and

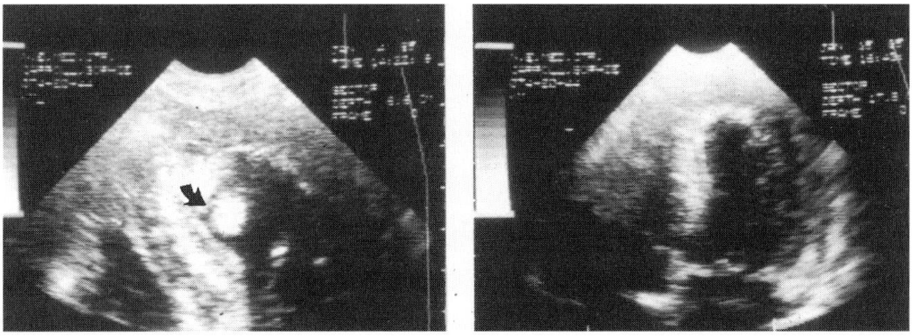

(a) (b)

Fig. 33 Transesophageal echocardiograms showing a disappearing thrombus. (A) The thrombus is clearly seen within the left ventricle (curved black arrow). (B) Repeat TEE shows that the previous lesion is gone. (From Ref. 289.)

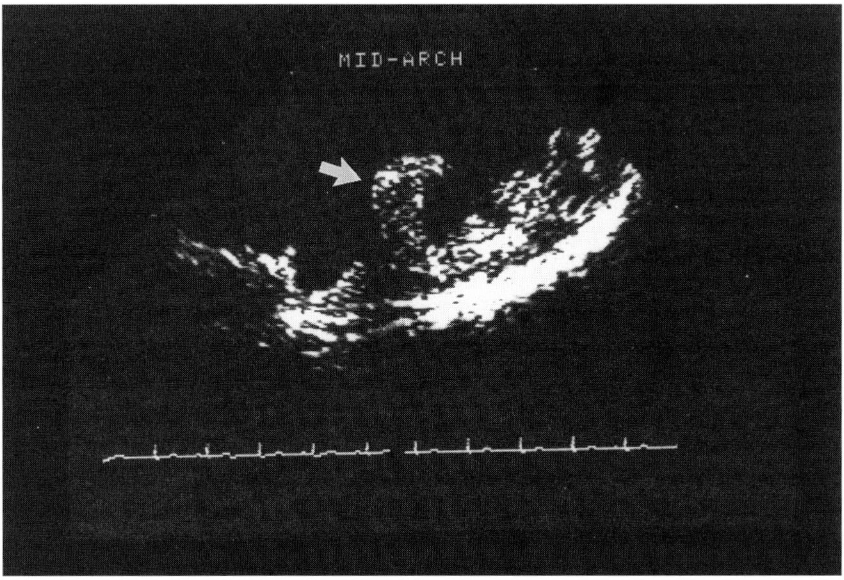

Fig. 34 Transesophageal echocardiogram through the midaortic arch showing a large pedunculated protruding mobile plaque (large white arrow).

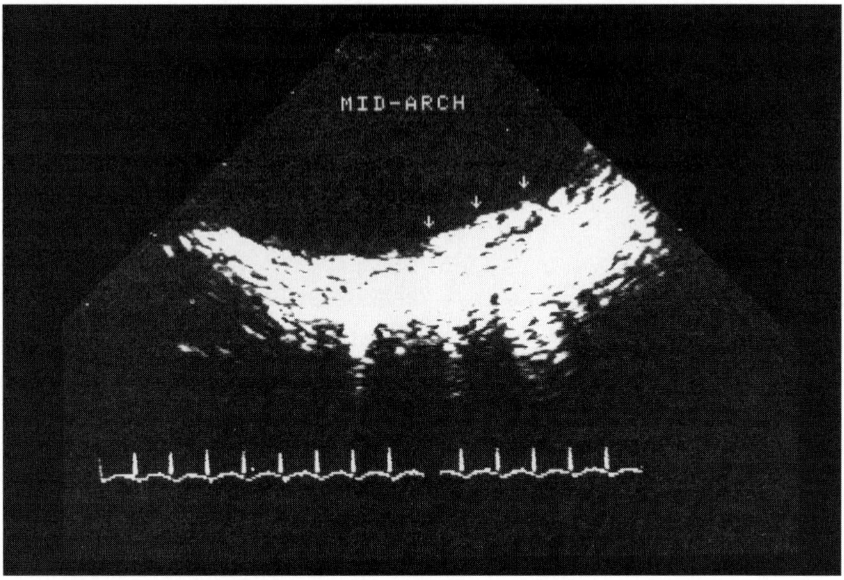

FIG. 35 Transesophageal echocardiogram through the midaortic arch showing an irregular relatively flat plaque (small white arrows).

intracranial arteries. MRA provides a good image of the extracranial carotid arteries but can overestimate the severity of the stenosis [434–436]. When stenosis is severe there is often a gap in the images, indicating a severe impediment to flow but not allowing accurate quantification of the severity of the stenosis or the presence of thrombi. MRA of the intracranial anterior circulation arteries is a good screening test for occlusion or severe stenosis of the major arterial branches of the intracranial ICAs [437–438]. Regions of tortuosity within the ICA siphon often are not imaged well and MRA does not show distal branch artery occlusions. When the ICA is occluded in the neck, there may be too little flow to provide good images of the intracranial carotid artery and its major branches, although often these vessels are well filled by collaterals.

MRA can also be used to screen for occlusive lesions within the vertebrobasilar circulation [41,439,440]. Unfortunately, the origins of the vertebral arteries from the subcalvian arteries are difficult to image unless a proximal view of the aortic arch arteries is included in the imaging. The extracranial and intracranial vertebral arteries are imaged using two different views—a neck and a head study. Sometimes the neck view is cut off too low and the head view is cut off too high so that the distal ECVA and the proximal ICVA are not shown on the images. Care must be taken to ensure that the entire vertebral artery is seen. The basilar and posterior cerebral arteries are well imaged using MRA [41].

In some centers that have the capability of echoplaner imaging, diffusion-weighted MR images and perfusion images taken after the intravenous infusion of contrast agent can yield important information about regions of brain ischemia and perfusion [441,442]. Comparing the findings on diffusion-weighted scans with those on T2-weighted images shows tissue that is stunned and ischemic but not yet infarcted. Matching perfusion images with those that show brain ischemia can detect areas that are underperfused but not yet ischemic [442]. The presence or absence of intracranial occlusions as shown by MRA coupled with information about brain ischemia and perfusion can help determine appropriate therapy. All of the MR testing can be performed using one machine in one sitting, and the time needed is not prohibitive (probably about 30 min using newer scanners).

The extracranial and intracranial arteries also can be accurately imaged by CTA [443,444]. This technique employs rapid filming using a spiral (helical) CT scanner after the intravenous injection of a dye load. Reformating of the CT images yields good reconstructions of the extracranial and intracranial vessels. The CT source films can be reviewed quickly to detect arterial occlusions, but time is needed to reproduce reformated arterial images. CT scans of the brain are also acquired, so both brain and vascular images are created using the same technology and at one sitting. CTA is accurate in showing large-artery occlusions, severe stenosis, and aneurysmal changes in both the anterior and posterior circulations [443,444].

Ultrasound capabilities have dramatically improved and are now an integral part of the evaluation of patients with brain embolism. Ultrasound has the advantages of being portable, noninvasive, and relatively inexpensive when compared to MR and CT, and ultrasound can be readily repeated sequentially to study the effects of spontaneous or therapeutic thrombolysis. Radionuclide testing including gated blood pool imaging (multigated acquisition [MUGA] scans) also may be helpful in selected patients, as might other cardiac imaging techniques [430]. Platelet scintigraphy is sometimes helpful in defining the presence of cardiac thrombi [431].

The aorta is an important potential source of embolism, especially during angiography and cardiac surgery. Presently TEE is the only effective established way to image the aorta for plaques and thrombi. The ascending aorta can be insonated using a Duplex ultrasound probe placed in the right supraclavicular fossa, and the arch and proximal descending thoracic aorta can be imaged using a left supraclavicular probe [432]. The results so far are preliminary but promising. Most plaques are located in the curvature of the arch from the distal ascending aorta to the proximal descending aorta, regions well shown using B-mode ultrasound [432].

The extracranial and intracranial arteries should be studied to define potential arterial donor sources of embolism and/or to provide information about blockage of reipient arteries by emboli. The four most common and effective means of studying the brachiocephalic arteries are by magnetic resonance angiography (MRA), computed tomographic angiography (CTA), ultrasound, and cerebral catheter dye angiography. Brain imaging should always accompany the vascular studies to show the location, severity, and distribution of related brain ischemia.

Probably, optimal information is provided by thorough magnetic resonance imaging. MRI scans of the brain, including fluid-attenuated inversion recovery (FLAIR) images [433] and T_1- and T_2-weighted images, show the extent of brain infarction and adequately show hemorrhages and reperfusion. In some centers ultrasound equipment is available at the bedside and can be used by examining physicians as an extension of the physical examination of the arteries. At present Doppler ultrasound is available in almost all intensive-care units to follow blood flow in various peripheral arteries. Duplex scanning (combined B-mode and multigated pulsed Doppler) is used to image the extracranial carotid and vertebral arteries. Both Duplex scans and CW Doppler give accurate information about the ICA in the neck [435,445,446].

Figure 36 is an artist's drawing of the findings from a B-mode ultrasound of a patient with an atherosclerotic plaque that extends from the common carotid artery along the posterior wall of the internal carotid artery. Figures 37 and 38 illustrate the capabilities of B-mode ultrasound in detecting and showing the location, size, and configuration of carotid artery plaques. Color-flow Doppler imaging is probably even more effective in grading the severity of ICA stenosis and depicts flow abnormalities and regions of turbulence [445–449]. The innominate, subclavian, and vertebral arteries can also be studied using Duplex and color-flow ultrasound [41,445,450,451]. Ultrasound of the carotid and vertebral arteries is also useful in suggesting dissections [451,453]. Figure 39 is a composite B-mode ultrasound picture that shows the extracranial arteries quite well. Figure 40 shows Doppler spectra from a patient with severe stenosis of the internal carotid artery, illustrating the utility of Doppler in quantitating stenosis.

Transcranial Doppler ultrasound (TCD) yields very important information about flow in the intracranial arteries [41,445,454]. TCD was discussed earlier in this chapter in the section on imaging recipient arteries. TCD has four main capabilities: (1) Detection of occlusive intracranial arterial lesions that could serve as a donor source of intrarterial embolism to distal branches of the stenotic artery. The intracranial ICAs, MCAs, ICVAs, basilar artery, and the posterior cerebral arteries (PCAs) are the major potential donor embolic sources. (2) Assessment of the impact of proximal stenotic and occlusive lesions on intracranial blood flow. Severe occlusive lesions decrease blood flow velocities in the major intracranial branches of that artery. (3) Detection and monitoring of occlusive

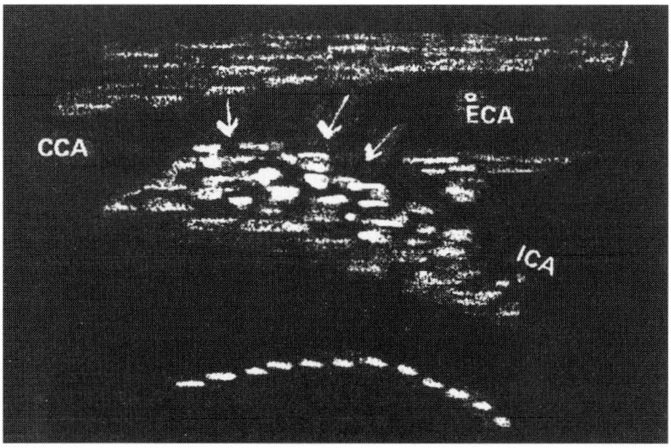

(a)

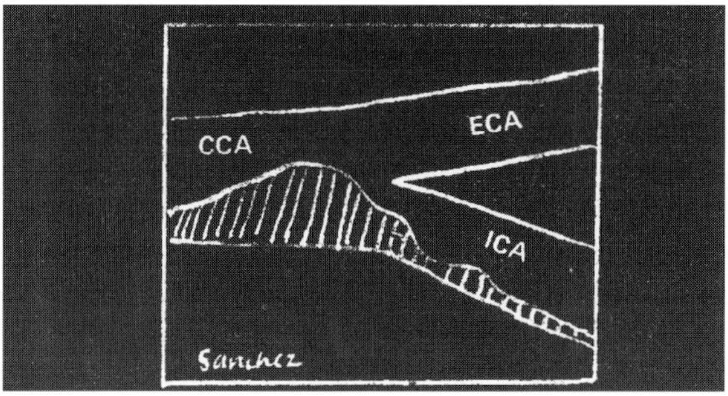

(b)

FIG. 36 Drawing from a B-mode ultrasound of the right internal carotid artery in a patient with an atherosclerotic plaque. (a) Echo (B-mode ultrasound) scan of the neck showing the plaque (white arrows). (b) Diagram of the scan showing the distribution of the plaque. The plaque begins in the common carotid artery and extends along the posterior wall of the internal carotid artery. Drawn by Dr. Juan Sanchez-Ramos. With permission. CCA, common carotid artery; ICA, internal carotid artery; ECA, external carotid artery. (Courtesy of Caplan LR, Stein RW. Stroke, a Clinical Approach. Boston: Butterworths, 1986.)

emboli to recipient intracranial arteries. (4) Emboli monitoring [16–21,78]. TCD machines are portable and insonation can be repeated sequentially or can be used as a continuous monitor as is often done during surgery or other procedures.

Angiography of the extracranial and intracranial arteries is still important. Angiography is performed in patients (1) in whom noninvasive vascular tests (CTA, MRA, extracranial and transcranial ultrasound) show lesions but not sufficiently to guide treatment; (2) when noninvasive testing shows a lesion that would be best treated by intra-arterial interventional radiology (intra-arterial

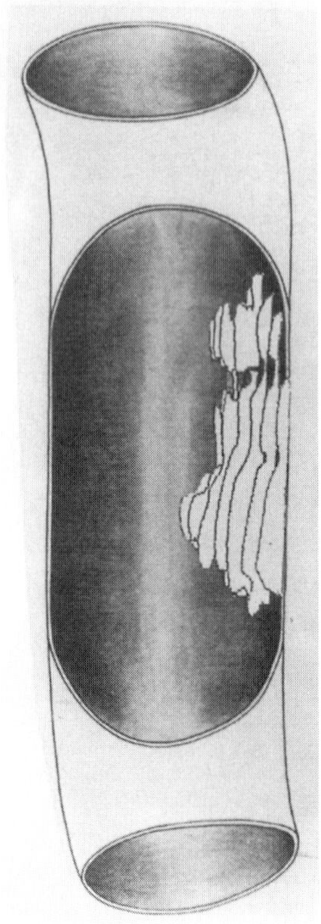

Fig. 37 Three-dimensional reconstruction of B-mode ultrasound showing the configuration, size, and extent of a plaque. (From Ref. 75.)

thrombolysis and/or angioplasty); and (3) in patients in whom noninvasive testing has not shown a donor source of embolism but an arterial source is suspected. Guidelines for the use of angiography in patients with brain ischemia have been published [74]. Figures 41 and 42 show thrombi within arteries detected only by angiography.

Hematological studies are also important in the evaluation of patients suspected of having brain embolism. Why does a patient with a chronic lesion such as an aortic protruding atheroma, atrial fibrillation, or ICA stenosis develop a superimposed thrombus or embolism at a given time? In many patients, the explanation lies in activation of platelets and/or the coagulation system [455]. The two processes—an intimal-endothelial lesion, and heightened coagulation—in-

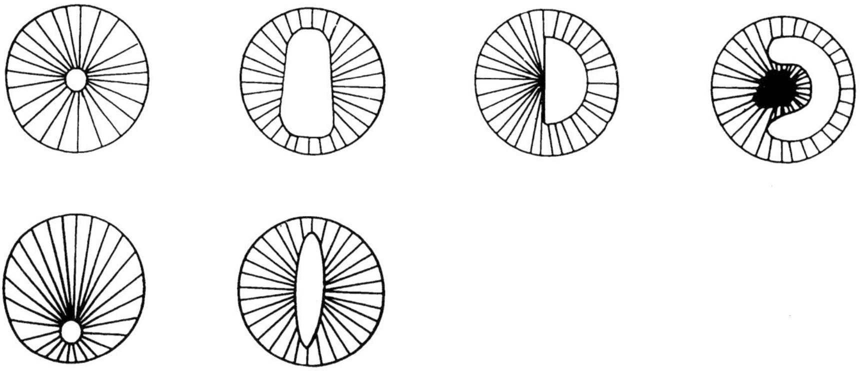

FIG. 38 Transverse sections through various types of plaques showing the size and shape of the residual lumina. The plaque on the upper right has an intramural hemorrhage. (From Ref. 75.)

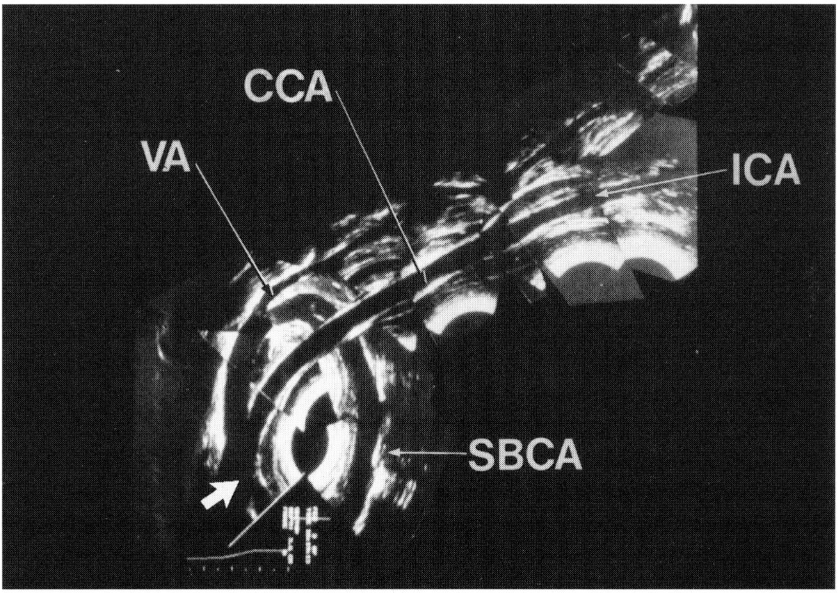

FIG. 39 Composite b-mode ultrasound image showing the innominate artery (large lower arrow to the left), subclavian artery (SBCA), right vertebral artery (VA), right common carotid artery (CCA), and right internal carotid artery (ICA). (From Ref. 41.)

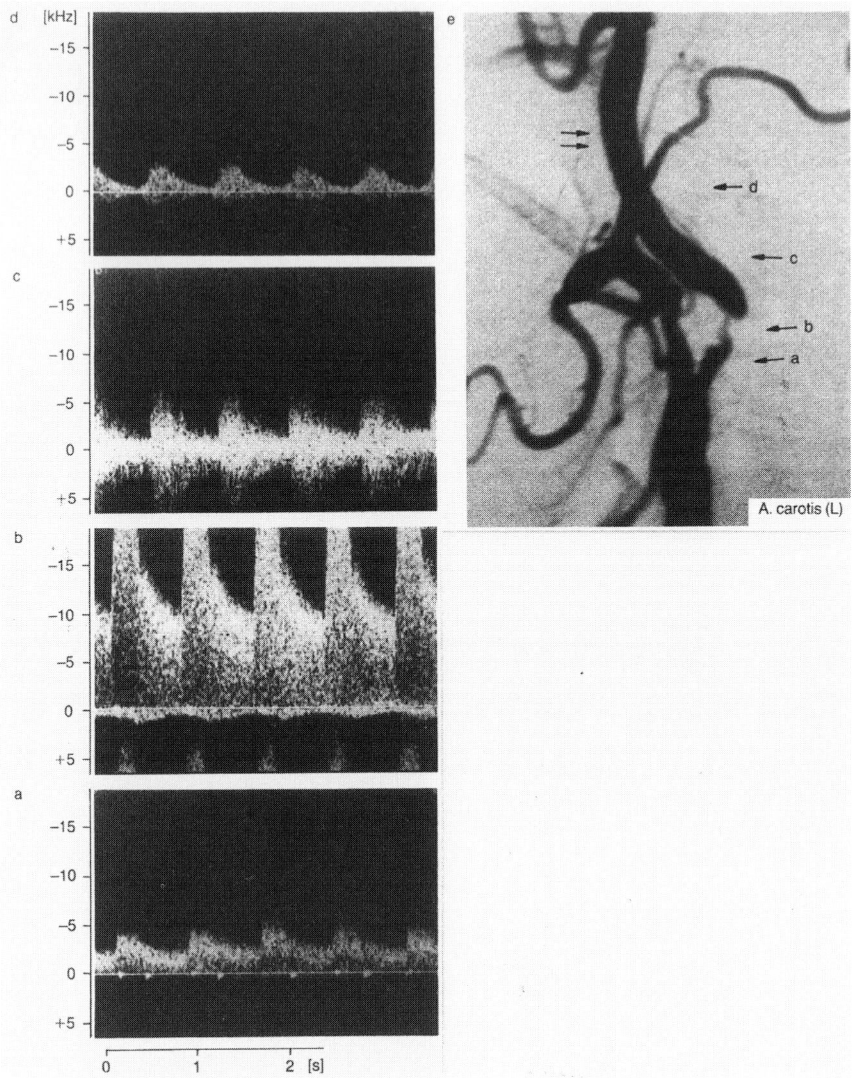

FIG. 40 Doppler spectra on the left of the figure (a–d) taken from various sites along the carotid artery from a patient whose arteriogram is shown on the right. At (a), a region just proximal to the severe stenosis, the maximal systolic frequency is reduced to 5 kHz; at (b), the region of maximal stenosis, there is increased velocity to a maximum of 20 kHz. (c, d) Velocities within the artery distal to the stenosis. These spectra are broadened and have decreased antegrade velocities. (e) Double arrows on the right show the internal carotid artery above the stenosis. (From Ref. 75.)

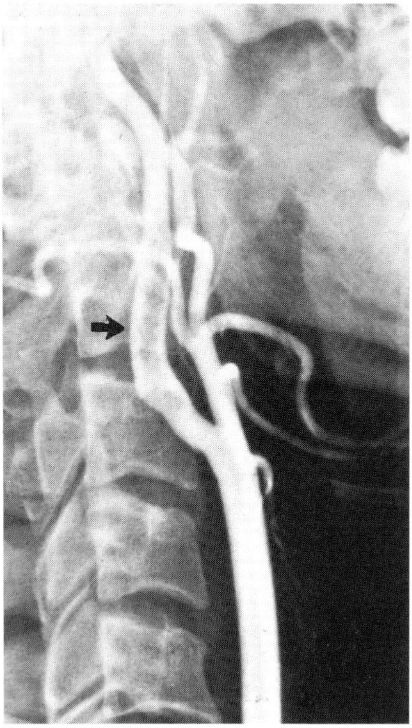

FIG. 41 Carotid angiogram. Lateral view. A large thrombus (black arrow) is seen within the proximal internal carotid artery. (From Ref. 75.)

teract to explain the thromboembolic event. A variety of different conditions activate the coagulation system. Coexisting infection, cancer, dehydration, congenital or acquired hypercoagulability (for example, in patients with resistance to activated protein C), trauma, all can cause activation of the coagulation cascade, which in the presence of a suitable lesion can lead to thrombus formation and embolism.

Two studies of hematological factors in patients with cardiogenic embolism should illustrate this point. Yasaka et al. detected eight intracardiac thrombi among 30 patients who had acute cardiac-origin embolism [456]. Enlargement of the cardiac thrombus was shown in four patients, and embolism recurred in three. Antithrombin III levels were low on admission in patients who later developed thrombi or had enlargement of thrombi on sequential echocardiography. An increase in the hematocrit also predicted thrombus formation or growth [456]. Takano and colleagues analyzed coagulation and fibrinolytic factors within 24

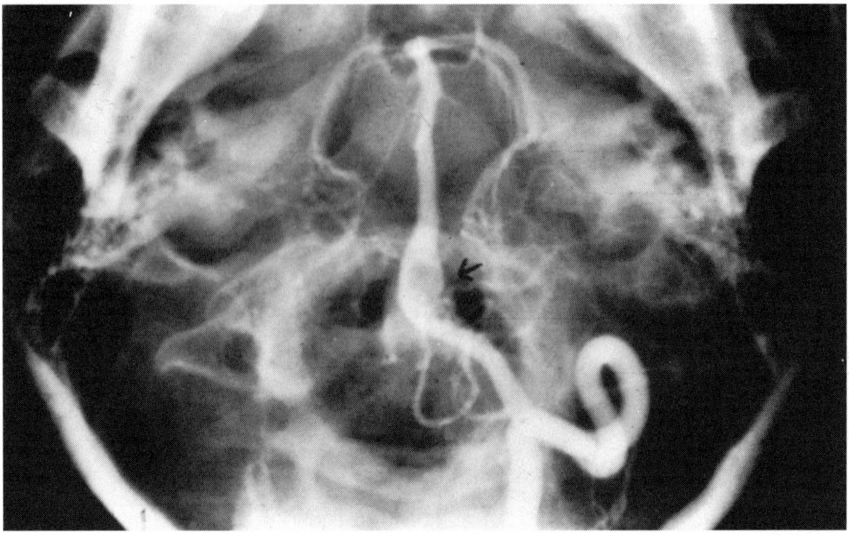

Fig. 42 Vertebral artery angiogram. Towns view. There is a thrombus (black arrow) within an aneurysm of the intracranial vertebral artery. (From Ref. 75.)

hours of stroke among 22 patients with cardiac-origin embolism and 25 age-matched controls [457]. The levels of antithrombin III, protein C, and alpha-2 plasmin inhibitor were significantly lower in embolic stroke patients than in controls. The plasma concentrations of thrombin-antithrombin III complex and cross-linked D-dimer were much higher in stroke patients than controls, indicating some degree of consumptive coagulopathy in patients with cardiac-origin embolism [457]. Coagulation studies should be an integral part of the evaluation of patients with suspected brain embolism and those with potential sources of embolism who have not yet had clinical events.

NONTHROMBOTIC EMBOLI

Some embolic materials that enter the systemic and brain circulations do not originate in the heart, aorta, or cervicocranial arteries and are not composed of blood elements or thrombi. The types of particles are diverse, as are the clinical syndromes and circumstances of brain embolization. These types of emboli are all very uncommon when compared to ordinary emboli that arise from the heart, aorta, and great vessels that have been discussed so far. Fat and gas bubbles cause microembolism to many small brain arteries, causing an encephalopathy-type syndrome, while tumor and foreign body emboli usually block single discrete arteries, causing stroke syndromes.

Fat Embolism

Fat embolism occurs most often after serious trauma that causes bone fractures. The long bones and pelvis are most frequently involved, especially the femurs; often there are multiple fractures resulting from vehicular accidents [458–462]. Occasionally the fat embolism syndrome develops after cardiac surgery when the atria or ventricles are entered [463,464] and in patients with sickle cell anemia (homozygous S-S or S-C disease) [465–468]. In sickle cell disease patients, the fat originates from bone and bone marrow infarcts. The exact mechanism of fat embolism after open heart surgery is unclear, but fat from sternotomy or the epicardium may directly enter the systemic circulation [464]. Other disorders that produce damage to bone marrow can occasionally give rise to fat embolism. One report described a patient with an aggressive lymphoma involving bone who died with massive fat embolism to the brain, lungs, and other viscera [468a].

There are two main hypotheses of the pathogenesis of the fat embolism syndrome; these are usually referred to as the mechanical and biochemical theories. According to the mechanical theory, the sources of fat are the bone marrow and other loci where fat is stored [462,469,470]. Bone or deposits of adipose tissue are injured and fat globules enter damaged blood vessels at the area of injury. Increase in local tissue pressure related to the trauma promotes fat entry into the intravascular compartment. According to the biochemical theory, intravascular fat is derived from lipid mobilized from fat deposits in the body. Catecholamine release, loss of chylomicra emulsion stability, and other biochemical perturbations that result from trauma and a variety of acute illnesses promote the formation and mobilization of fat globules.

Fat that embolizes to the lungs is converted metabolically to free fatty acids by pulmonary lipases. Free fatty acids are toxic to the lungs and damage capillaries and small arterioles and veins, causing lung edema, hemorrhage, and atelectasis [462]. Thromboplastin is also released after local tissue injury and induces platelet aggregation on injured surfaces and on fat globules, enhancing thromboembolism. Fat within the lungs enters pulmonary veins and passes through the left side of the heart into the systemic circulation. Some experimental evidence suggests that fat can travel through lymphatic ducts to enter the lungs [471]. In some cases, fat traverses a patent foramen ovale to enter the systemic circulation [472,473]. The two mechanisms, mechanical and biochemical, may in fact coexist and interact. Fat first mechanically enters into the vascular system in relation to local traumatic injury. The primary injury and embolization of fat and marrow into the lungs may set in motion biochemical changes which enhance fat globule formation, mobilization, and embolization.

The fat embolism syndrome usually develops after a delay of a few hours up to a few days after trauma. In one series of 14 patients, all of whom had traumatic injuries with long-bone fractures, the latency of onset of signs of fat embolism after trauma ranged from 12 to 72 hours (mean 41 hours) [461]. At times the clinical manifestations of fat embolism can be delayed for as long as 5 days [462]. Most patients have symptom onset between 24 and 72 hours after injury.

The major clinical manifestations of the fat embolism syndrome are confusion with delirium often followed by a decrease in the level of consciousness, dyspnea, tachypnea, fever, and tachycardia. Neurological symptoms and signs are present in >80% of patients. Most often patients develop an encephalopathy characterized by restlessness, agitation, confusion, poor memory, and decreased alertness. This state often passes into stupor or coma. Seizures are common at onset or early in the course of illness. Seizures can be focal or generalized. Focal neurological signs are also common and include hemiparesis, conjugate eye deviation to one side, aphasia, and visual field abnormalities. Motor abnormalities including increased tone in the lower extremities, Babinski signs, and decerebrate rigidity are often found. Focal neurological signs were noted in 33% of patients in one series [462]. Some patients have scotomas and other visual abnormalities related to retinal dysfunction caused by fat embolism.

Pulmonary symptoms usually develop shortly after or concurrent with the neurological symptoms. Dyspnea and tachypnea are prominent and patients may become cyanotic. Tachycardia, high fever, and circulatory collapse also occur; hypotension is often related to blood loss, hypoxemia, and hypovolemia. Renal failure can develop.

An important clue to the presence of fat microemboli is the presence on physical examination of petechiae. Petechiae are found in 50% to 75% of patients with the fat embolism syndrome. They are most often found in the lower palpebral conjunctivae and the skin of the neck, shoulder, and the axillary folds [459,460]. Another important clinical clue is the appearance of fat emboli within the arteries of the eye. Microinfarcts are sometimes visible in the optic fundus, especially in the perimacular regions. Small hemorrhages, sometimes with white pale centers, are also found. Fat globules can sometimes be seen within retinal arteries [459]. Papilledema is occasionally found. In one series, 11 of 24 (46%) patients with fat embolism had abnormalities of the ocular funduscopic examination [459].

Laboratory tests are also often helpful in diagnosis. Many patients develop abnormal chest x-rays. Fine stippling and fluffy lung infiltrates are common and are seen diffusely through both lung fields. Most patients have a drop in hemoglobin and hematocrit due to traumatic loss of blood and hemolysis. Thrombocytopenia and prolonged prothrombin and activated partial thromboplastin times are also common and are attributed to a consumptive coagulopathy. Frank disseminated intravascular coagulation may also occur. Brain imaging can show small hemorrhages, brain edema, or focal infarcts usually manifested by regions of gyral enhancement on CT or MRI scans. Lipid globules are sometimes found in the urine when fat stains are used. In one series nine of 19 (47%) patients had free fat in the urine, six of whom had lipuria within the first 48 hours after trauma [459]. Skin, renal, and muscle biopsies may show fat globules within small skin, muscle, and renal vessels and in renal glomeruli. Cryostat frozen sections of blood also can show the presence of neutral fat; in one series neutral fat was most often found in patients with hypoxemia and $PaCO_2$ of <60 mm Hg [460]. Hypoxemia is very common in patients with the fat embolism syndrome.

Probably the most effective and specific test for fat embolism is bronchopulmonary lavage [474,475]. The technique involves microscopic examination of cells recovered by lavage and stained with a specific stain for neutral fat—e.g., using oil red O dye. In one series, the five patients who had definite clinical evidence of the fat embolism syndrome all had very positive results from bronchopulmonary lavage [474]. Staining of bronchoalveolar cells in these five patients showed large intracellular fat droplets; the mean percentage of cells that contained fat droplets was 63% with a range of 31% to 82% [474]. Trauma patients who did not have signs of the fat embolism syndrome had <2% of cells that contained fat [474].

The mortality rate in patients with the fat embolism syndrome is quite high (as much as 50%), although it has declined over time [460,461]. When coma, severe blood loss, hypotension, high fever, and DIC are present, the mortality rate remains substantial. Necropsy of the brain of patients dying with the fat embolism syndrome shows many small ball, ring, and perivascular hemorrhages; brain edema; and regions of microinfarction [476]. Stains for fat reveal fat globules within hemorrhagic lesions and in small vessels throughout the brain [476]. Small hemorrhages, edema, and hyaline membranes are often found in the lungs [461]. Fat globules are also often visible in renal glomeruli, myocardium, liver, pancreas, spleen, and gastrointestinal mucosa.

Treatment of patients with the fat embolism syndrome has not been formally studied in therapeutic trials. Supportive care including oxygen administration often with assisted respiration and fluid and blood replacement is very important. Corticosteroids, heparin, and intravenous administration of 5% alcohol solutions have all been used but their effectiveness has not been well studied [459]. Heparin has been used in patients with consumptive coagulopathies and also because of its putative lipolytic effect. Alcohol is also believed to have a lipolytic capability. Among these treatments, corticosteroid administration has been most frequently used.

Air Embolism

Gas bubbles sometimes enter the systemic circulation and cause air embolism to the brain and other organs. In most cases air is introduced iatrogenically during procedures and surgery. Thoracentesis, pneumothorax, pneumo-orbitography perineal and peritoneal air insufflation, pneumoarthrography, and surgery on the heart, lungs, sinuses, neck, brain, and axilla offer opportunities for air to enter the circulation [477]. Venous and arterial catheterization and cardiopulmonary bypass are common causes of air embolism [477a]. The topic of embolism after cardiac procedures and surgeries will be discussed in Chapters 4 and 5. Less often, air embolism follows penetrating traumatic injuries to the thorax, lungs, or major blood vessels. Another circumstance that leads to air embolism is in relation to scuba diving and rapid ascents after descents into deep water [478].

Air bubbles in an artery supplying the brain cause an immediate but transient block in blood flow. Air quickly moves through the capillary bed into the venules and dissipates [477]. The gas bubbles cause arterial vasoconstriction followed by dilatation and stasis of blood flow [477].

During diving accidents, air becomes trapped in the alveoli of the lungs due to partial bronchial occlusion from mucous plugs and failure to exhale. Because the volume of a gas varies inversely with pressure (Boyle's law), pressurized air bubbles in the lungs increase dramatically in volume as the diver ascends and the ambient pressure around him falls [477]. The rapid expansion in the lungs causes entry of air into the pulmonary arterial and venous outflow systems [478]. Gas bubbles pass through the lung vasculature or through a patent foramen ovale into the systemic circulation. Similar to the situation in fat embolism, many small particles enter the circulation and block the microvasculature.

Symptoms and signs of brain gas embolism have been studied most thoroughly in individuals who have had diving-related incidents [478]. These occur during scuba diving and have been well studied in naval personnel who escape too quickly from submerged submarines [478]. Loss of consciousness often develops suddenly after the individual emerges onto the surface of the water. Dizziness, chest discomfort, paresthesias, weakness, blurred vision, nausea, and headache are also common symptoms reported and may precede the loss of consciousness. Seizures and focal neurological signs, especially related to dysfunction of the brainstem and cerebellum, are also quite common [478]. In several patients, discrete focal collections of gas were seen in the brain on cranial CT examination [477a,479]. Brain edema with compression of the ventricular system is another common and important finding on brain imaging examinations. Treatment has usually consisted of inhalation of 100% oxygen as well as the use of hyperbaric recompression chambers.

Tumor Embolism

Occasionally major arteries supplying the brain are occluded by tumor emboli. Most often the tumors are primary pulmonary neoplasms or tumors that have metastasized to the lungs [480]. At times the brain embolism has occurred after lung surgery for cancer. Necropsy has usually shown definite tumor invasion of pulmonary veins or invasion of the left atrium [480]. Surgical manipulation of the lungs in patients with lung tumors can promote systemic embolization of the tumor. Although most often the clinical syndrome is that of a stroke, embolism to other systemic organs also occurs. Tumor emboli also can pass through a patent foramen ovale or other cardiac septal defect. Passage through a patent dilated foramen ovale was documented in one patient with metastatic adenocarcinoma and bone metastases [473]. After a surgical intramedullary fixation of both femurs, the patient did not awaken from surgery and remained comatose and died. At necropsy, the patient had a patent foramen ovale and an embolus consisting of tumor cells admixed with bone marrow in the left middle cerebral artery and a large fatal infarct in the territory of the left middle cerebral artery [473]. Tumor emboli have also been reported in patients with thyroid and other neck cancers which have caused their effects by eroding into the neck vasculature [481].

Foreign Body Embolism

Occasionally foreign bodies enter the systemic vascular system and embolize to the brain. Kase and colleagues described the case of a patient who came to the emergency room because of shotgun blast wounds to the thorax and abdomen [482]. At thoracotomy, four small bullet wounds in the left ventricle were repaired. Initially he was alert and neurological screening examination was normal, but postoperatively he developed severe hypotension followed by cardiac arrest. External cardiac massage was initiated. After resuscitation he was comatose and had a severe hemiplegia. CT showed a 1- to 2-mm piece of shotgun pellet and a large middle cerebral artery territory infarct (Fig. 43). Angiography showed that there were two small shotgun pellets occluding the distal intracranial internal carotid artery and another fragment occluded the middle cerebral artery (Fig. 44) [482]. This case illustrates the small size of particles that can block a major intracranial artery, leading to devastating neurological deficits.

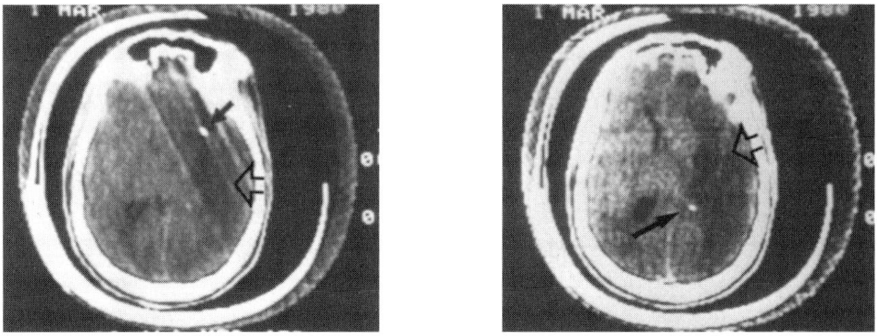

(a) (b)

Fig. 43 CT scans (a and b) showing a large middle cerebral artery territory infarct on the right of the scans (black open arrowheads). Black arrows point to the pieces of shotgun pellet seen within the brain images. (From Ref. 482.)

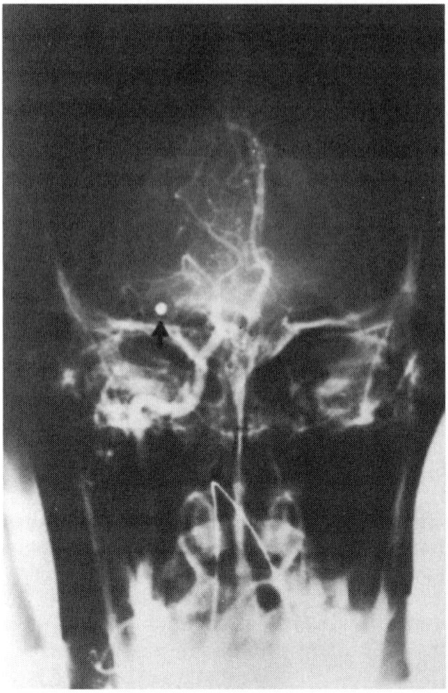

(a)

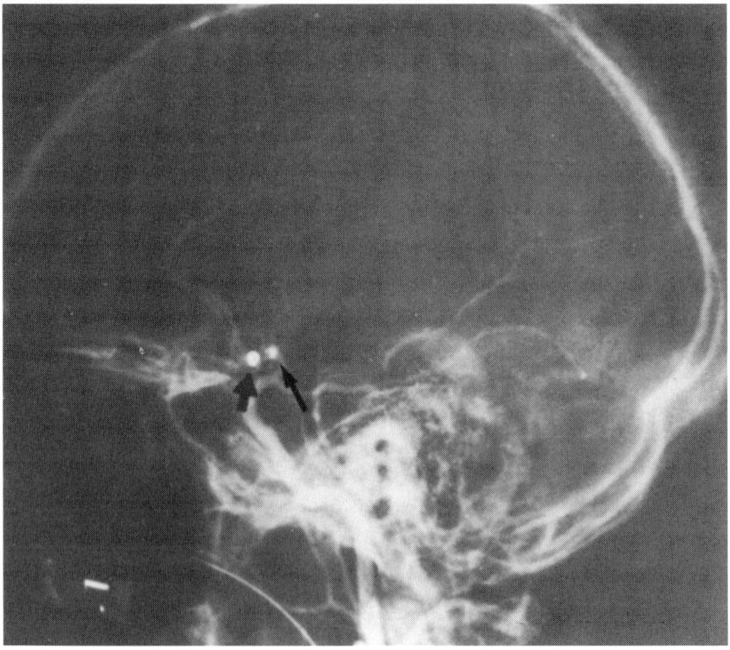

(b)

Langenbach et al. described the case of a 52-year-old man in whom a small metal particle penetrated his right neck while hammering [483]. He soon developed a severe left hemiplegia. Plain skull films showed a 2×7 mm metal-dense particle to the right of the pituitary fossa. CT showed a large right middle cerebral artery territory infarct, and angiography showed that the metal fragment was blocking the middle cerebral artery [483].

North and colleagues reported the case of a 9-year-old boy who was noted to have a severe right hemiplegia, right hemianopia, and right hemisensory loss detected immediately after awakening from surgical repair of a prosthetic heart valve [484]. CT showed a foreign body within the head and infarction of the left midbrain, thalamus, and temporal and occipital lobes in the distribution of the left posterior cerebral artery. He died after hemorrhage into the region of infarction. Necropsy showed that the foreign body within the proximal left posterior cerebral artery was a fragment of valve with surrounding fibrosis [484].

Retinal and brain arteries can become blocked by foreign particles in patients who mash drugs manufactured for oral use and inject the drugs intravenously [485–488]. The particles consist of talc and methylcellulose, which are used to bind drugs to maintain them in pill form. The particles first block lung vessels. Pulmonary vascular obliteration causes pulmonary hypertension, and arteriovenous shunting develops in the lungs, allowing the particles to enter the pulmonary veins and then the systemic circulation [485,486]. Talc and cornstarch emboli can be seen in the retinal arteries of some of these drug abusers [487]. Strokes have also been described in patients who have injected drugs directly into neck arteries [488,489]. Foreign bodies that embolize to the brain must either enter the lungs and pulmonary veins, enter or arise from the left side of the heart itself, enter the right side of the heart and traverse a defect in the cardiac septum, or penetrate the cervicocranial arteries that supply the brain.

TREATMENT OF PATIENTS WITH BRAIN EMBOLISM

The therapeutics of brain embolism can be divided into two main aspects—acute treatment of the embolic event, and prophylaxis to prevent further thromboembolism. Of course it is most important to prevent the first embolism. Prophylaxis of patients with atrial fibrillation using anticoagulants and prophylaxis of patients

---

FIG. 44 Carotid arteriograms. (a) Anteroposterior view, and (b) lateral view showing two pieces of buckshot (black arrows) blocking the middle cerebral artery. (From Ref. 482.)

very large study of the effectiveness of intravenous thrombolysis, the European Cooperative Acute Stroke Study (ECASS), all patients were treated within 6 hours [496]. However, salvageability of ischemic brain tissue varies considerably from patient to patient. After an embolic occlusion, there are three zones of brain tissue supplied by the recipient recently occluded artery. One zone, usually at the core center of blood supply, soon becomes irreversibly damaged (*infarcted*). Brain regions at the very periphery of supply often remain *normal* since they receive adequate blood supply through adjacent collateral channels. Between these two zones lies brain tissue that is in a state somewhere between infarcted and normal. This tissue has inadequate blood supply to function but is not irreversibly damaged. This state has been called ''stunned brain,'' or penumbral tissue. Infarcted brain tissue contains cells that are dead and blood vessels that may have also been damaged by ischemia. The major danger of thrombolysis (and of spontaneous reperfusion) is that reperfusion of these damaged vessels in the infarcted zone can cause major bleeding into the ischemic brain tissue. This process has been discussed in the section of this chapter on hemorrhagic infarction. Ideally the decision on whether to pursue thrombolysis should rest not on the time that has expired since symptom onset but instead on the presence of viable penumbral tissue that can be salvaged and the extent of brain that is already infarcted.

The extent of infarction determines the risk of treatment; the presence and size of penumbral, stunned tissue determines the potential benefit of thrombolysis that accomplishes reperfusion. The newer magnetic resonance techniques of diffusion-weighted and perfusion MR scans performed with echoplaner equipment, when coupled with MRA, should be able to give clinicians a quantitative estimate of these factors [441,442]. Alternatively, clinicians estimate the extent of normal, infarcted, and stunned brain supplied by the occluded artery by using brain imaging (CT and T_2-weighted MRI scans), vascular studies (CTA, MRA, TCD, angiography), and the neurological examination. If the patient has a severe neurological deficit and a large infarct is present on brain scans, then much of the brain is infarcted and there is little to gain by thrombolysis, which carries a substantial risk of hemorrhage in this circumstance. However, if the patient has a severe neurological deficit and brain scans are normal, then there could be considerable stunned, salvageable brain which could be restored to function if thrombolysis is successful.

Thrombolytic drugs can be given either intravenously or intra-arterially. Each has advantages and disadvantages [497]. Intravenous therapy can be given quickly and needs no special training to administer. The amount of drug that reaches large obstructed arteries is, however, more limited than intra-arterial infusion of drug, which can deliver the drug locally within the obstructing clot. Intra-arterial therapy requires a trained interventionalist. Arteriography is ordinarily required before, during, and after thrombolysis. This delays treatment. The major advantage of intra-arterial therapy is that the interventionalist can physically manipulate the clot, a process that facilitates thrombolysis, and can perform angioplasty at the same sitting if necessary [498–500]. Usually, less drug is used during intra-arterial therapy and the rate of hemorrhagic complications is lower than with intravenous therapy [497].

There are now considerable data from reports of patients treated with either intravenous or intra-arterial therapy after their occlusive lesions have been shown by angiography [497,501,502]. Embolic occlusions respond better than thrombi formed locally in vessels that have severe atherostenosis. Freshly formed thromboemboli lyse more often than older clots. Thrombi that block the extracranial or intracranial ICA do not respond to intravenous thrombolysis. An especially important and common situation is thrombosis of the ICA, which has caused neurological deficit by an embolus breaking off from the neck thrombus and embolizing intracranially to the middle cerebral artery (MCA). Intravenous thrombolysis in this situation is ineffective because the drug does not reach the MCA clot because of proximal obstruction. An interventionalist may be able to pass a catheter through the clot in the neck, then manipulate the catheter to and within the MCA clot to deliver the thrombolytic drug into the MCA clot. After lysing the intracranial clot, the catheter can be maneuvered back into the neck in order to lyse the neck clot and, if needed, perform an angioplasty with stenting of the atherostenotic ICA disease. MCA branch occlusions seem to lyse best with intravenous therapy.

To date, very few patients with basilar artery thromboemboli have been studied after intravenous thrombolysis [497,502], but intra-arterial therapy of patients with basilar artery occlusion is often effective, especially if the occlusion is embolic [503,504]. The most commonly used thrombolytic drugs for stroke patients are recombinant tissue plasminogen activator (rt-PA) and urokinase. Streptokinase has had an unacceptable rate of bleeding complications when used for stroke [502]. Ancrod, a substance derived from the purified protein fraction of venom from the Malayan pit viper, has defibrinolytic capabilities and has sometimes been given intravenously in acute stroke patients in order to lyse thrombi [505,506].

Heparin is also often prescribed as a treatment for patients with acute thromboembolism. The posited purpose of heparinization is to prevent propagation of thrombi and breakoff of the tail of existing thrombi and so prevent embolization. As far as is known, heparin does not actually lyse existing thrombi, although cardiac clots often disappear during heparin treatment. The decision whether or not to prescribe heparin acutely to prevent the next thromboembolic stroke depends on weighing the risk of acute reembolization vs. the risk of hemorrhage related to heparin therapy. In patients with lesions with high rates of reembolization—e.g., mitral stenosis with atrial fibrillation; atrial fibrillation, especially with large left atria and atrial thrombi; acute myocardial infarction with mural thrombi—then acute heparinization is probably warranted. In patients with a low risk of acute rembolization, such as chronic atrial fibrillation or mitral annulus calcification, heparin can be withheld during the acute period. If the patient has a large brain infarct then the risk of brain hemorrhage after heparin is higher than when there is no brain infarct or a small brain infarct. Heparin is often used after thrombolysis to maintain arterial patency.

Chronic Prophylactic Treatment to Prevent Reembolization

Once a cookie has been stolen from the jar, there is always a threat of a second and third cookie theft. Almost immediately physicians caring for patients with brain embolism must think of preventing the next embolus. The three strategies used for prophylaxis are (1) removal of the donor source of embolism when possible, (2) modification of risk factors that relate to disease at the donor site, and (3) modification of coagulation functions to prevent the formation of thromboemboli. Some donor site lesions can be corrected or at least ameliorated surgically or by using interventional radiologic techniques. Cardiac valve lesions, cardiac tumors, atrial septal defects, patent foramen ovales, and protruding mobile large aortic atheromas can be treated surgically. Newer interventional techniques may now or in the near future permit interventional percutaneous treatment of patent foramen ovale and aortic atheromas. Carotid and vertebral artery lesions can be corrected surgically (endarterectomy) [41,75,396,397,403] or by angioplasty, sometimes with stenting. Many patients with cardiac, aortic, and cerebrovascular donor site lesions have modifiable risk factors such as smoking, hyperlipidemia, hypertension, inactive sedentary life style, obesity, etc. Counseling and medical treatment of these risk factors is a very important part of the care of patients with brain embolism.

Manipulation of coagulation to prevent future thromboemboli is a strategy applicable to the great majority of patients with brain embolism. Embolic particles are diverse. White platelet thrombi, red erythrocyte-fibrin thrombi, cholesterol crystals, calcified particles from arteries and valves, myxomatous tissue, bacteria in patients with infective endocarditis, bland fibrous vegetations in patients with noninfective endocarditis, and fat in patients with bone fractures are the most important substances. Medical prophylactic treatment against reentry of these particles into the circulation depends very much on the ''stuff'' in the emboli rather than the source of the materials [22,507]. It's the bird rather than the nest that is important [507]. For example, the most effective prophylaxis for prevention of embolization in patients with bacterial endocarditis is effective antibiotic sterilization of the bacterial vegetations. Cholesterol crystal, calcific particle, bacterial vegetation, and myxomatous emboli do not, as far as is known, respond to treatment with anticoagulants or drugs that modify platelet function.

The two types of medicinal agents most often used to prevent thromboemboli are standard anticoagulants (heparin, low-molecular-weight heparins, heparinoids, and warfarin compounds) and agents that alter platelet adhesion, aggregation, and secretion such as aspirin, ticlopidine, clopidogrel, dipyridamole, omega-3 fish oils, etc. White platelet-fibrin thrombi are posited to form on irregular surfaces in fast-moving bloodstreams in widely patent arteries and cavities. Red erythrocyte-fibrin thrombi, on the other hand, tend to form in regions of stasis, such as leg veins, dilated cardiac atria, severely stenotic arteries, etc. At times both white and red thrombi coexist since activated platelets are a stimulus for activation of the coagulation cascade and subsequent red clot formation.

We choose anticoagulant treatment for prophylaxis, first with heparin or low-molecular-weight heparin and then with coumadin, in patients who have lesions that promote red clot formation and in patients whose imaging studies show thrombi. We continue coumadin as long as the situation that promotes red clots persists—for example, persistent atrial fibrillation, myocardial aneurysm, prosthetic valves, stenotic extracranial arteries. In patients with acute occlusive thrombi superimposed on preocclusive atherostenosis, we continue coumadin only for a short time (6 to 12 weeks), during which thrombi organize and no longer propagate or form fresh tails that embolize. During this time, collateral circulation has usually become maximal. Sometimes lesions that caused the original thrombosis later improve (e.g., arterial dissections, regressing atheromas, or corrected cardiac right-to-left shunts), so anticoagulation can be stopped and replaced with antiplatelet drugs.

We prescribe agents that alter platelet functions for patients with lesions posited to predispose to formation of white platelet-fibrin thrombi, and for patients with thrombocytosis. Irregular, nonstenosing atherosclerotic plaques, and irregular but nonstenotic valve surfaces are the commonest situations. In patients that tolerate aspirin, we usually prescribe 325 to 650 mg of coated aspirin daily. Smaller doses sometimes do not produce sufficient alterations in platelet function when tested in vitro [508]. The ability of aspirin to maintain its effect on platelet function sometimes diminishes with time and can be monitored in vitro [509]. High fibrinogen levels increase whole blood viscosity, increase platelet aggregability, and predispose to red clot formation. Increased fibrinogen levels are a risk factor for stroke and myocardial infarction [510]. Reducing serum fibrinogen levels might also help prevent thromboembolism. Omega-3 oils, ticlopidine, clopidogrel [511], atromid, and pentoxiphylline are all posited to have an effect in lowering serum fibrinogen levels and can be prescribed with antiplatelet aggregants or anticoagulants. In some situations in which both red and white clots are likely to form, a combination of platelet antiaggregants and coumadin might be more effective than either agent alone.

REFERENCES

1. Vesalius A. De Humani Corpis Fabrica. Basileae, J Oporini, 1543.
2. Fisher CM. The history of cerebral embolism and hemorrhagic infarction. In: Furlan A, ed. The Heart and Stroke. Berlin: Springer-Verlag, 1987:3–16.

3. Hunter J. Observations on the inflammation of the internal coats of veins. Trans Soc Improve Med Chirurg Knowledge 1793; 1:18–29.
4. Cruveilher J. Anatomie Pathologique du Corps Humain, Vol. I. Paris, 1829; Chap. 11, p. 7.
5. Virchow R. Uber die akut entzundung der arterien. Virchows Arch Pathol Anat 1847; 1:272–378.
6. Herrick JB. Clinical features of sudden obstruction of the coronary arteries. JAMA 1912; 59:2015–2020.
7. Blumgart HL, Schlesinger MJ, Davis D. Studies on the relation of the clinical manifestations of angina pectoris, coronary thrombosis, and myocardial infarction to the pathological findings. Am Heart J 1940; 19:1–9.
8. Chiari H. Uber das verhalten du teilungswinkels der carotis communis bei der endarteritis chronica deformans. Verhandl Deutsch Pathol Gesellsch 1905; 9:326–330.
9. Osler W. The Principles and Practice of Medicine. 5th ed. New York: D. Appleton and Co., 1903:1008–1009.
10. Fisher CM. Occlusion of the internal carotid artery. Arch Neurol 1951; 65:346–377.
11. Millikan C, Adams RD, Fang H, et al. A classification and outline of cerebrovascular diseases. Neurology 1958; 8:395–434.
12. Aring CD, Merritt HH. Differential diagnosis between cerebral hemorrhage and cerebral thrombosis. Arch Intern Med 1935; 56:435–456.
13. Whisnant JP. Fitzgibbons JP, Kurland LT, et al. Natural history of stroke in Rochester, Minnesota, 1945 through 1954. Stroke 1971; 2:11–22.
14. Matsumoto N, Whisnant JP, Kurland LT, et al. Natural history of stroke in Rochester, Minnesota, 1955 through 1969: an extension of previous study 1945 through 1954. Stroke 1973; 4:20–29.
15. Mohr JP, Caplan LR, Melski JW, et al. The Harvard Cooperative Stroke Registry: a propective registry. Neurology 1978; 28:754–762.
16. Markus HS. Transcranial Doppler detection of circulating cerebral emboli, a review. Stroke 1993; 24:1246–1250.
17. Markus HS, Harrison MJ. Microembolic signal detection using ultrasound. Stroke 1995; 26:1517–1519.
18. Tong DC, Albers GW. Transcranial Doppler-detected microemboli in patients with acute stroke. Stroke 1995; 26:1588–1592.
19. Sliwka U, Job F-P, Wissuwa D, et al. Occurrence of transcranial Doppler high-intensity transient signals in patients with potential cardiac sources of embolism, a prospective study. Stroke 1995; 26:2067–2070.
20. Daffertshofer M, Ries S, Schminke U, Hennerici M. High-intensity transient signals in patients with cerebral ischemia. Stroke 1996; 27:1844–1849.
21. Sliwka U, Lingnau A, Stohlmann W-D, et al. Prevalence and time course of microembolic signals in patients with acute strokes, a prospective study. Stroke 1997; 28:358–363.
22. Caplan LR. Brain embolism, revisited. Neurology 1993; 43:1281–1287.
23. Fisher CM, Perlman A. The nonsudden onset of cerebral embolism. Neurology 1967; 17:1025–1032.

24. Dalal P, Shah P, Sheth S, et al. Cerebral embolism: angiographic observations on spontaneous clot lysis. Lancet 1965; 1:61–64.
25. Liebeskind A, Chinichian A, Schechter M. The moving embolus seen during cerebral angiography. Stroke 1971; 2:440–443.
26. Fisher CM, Adams RD. Observations on brain embolism with special reference to the mechanism of hemorrhagic infarction. J Neuropathol Exp Neurol 1951; 10:92–94.
27. Fisher CM, Adams RD. Observations on brain embolism with special reference to hemorrhagic infarction. In: Furlan AJ, ed. The Heart and Stroke. London: Springer-Verlag, 1987:17–36.
28. Yamaguchi T, Minematsu K, Choki JI, Ikeda M. Clinical and neuroradiological analysis of thrombotic and embolic cerebral infarction. Jpn Circ 1984; 48:50–58.
29. Okada Y, Yamaguchi T, Minematsu K, et al. Hemorrhagic transformation in cerebral embolism. Stroke 1989; 20:598–603.
30. Pessin MS, Estol C, Lafranchise F, Caplan LR. Safety of anticoagulation after hemorrhagic infarction. Neurology 1993; 43:1298–1303.
31. Chaves CJ, Pessin MS, Caplan LR, et al. Cerebellar hemorrhagic infarction. Neurology 1996; 46:346–349.
32. Garcia J, Ho K-L, Caccamo DV. Intracerebral hemorrhage: pathology of selected topics. In: Kase CS, Caplan LR, eds. Intracerebral Hemorrhage. Boston: Butterworth-Heinemann, 1994:45–72.
33. Einhaupl KM, Villringer A, Meister W, et al. Heparin treatment in sinus venous thrombosis. Lancet 1991; 338:597–600.
34. Caplan LR. Venous and dural sinus thrombosis. In: Caplan LR, ed. Posterior Circulation Ischemia: Clinical Findings, Diagnosis, and Management. Boston: Blackwell Science, 1996:569–592.
35. Caplan LR, Hier DB, D'Cruz I. Cerebral embolism in the Michael Reese Stroke Registry. Stroke 1983; 14:530–536.
36. Bogousslavsky J, van Melle G, Regli F. The Lausanne Stroke Registry: Analysis of 1000 consecutive patients with first stroke. Stroke 1988; 19:1083–1092.
37. Gacs G, Merer FT, Bodosi M. Balloon catheter as a model of cerebral emboli in humans. Stroke 1982; 13:39–42.
38. Helgason C. Cardioembolic stroke topography and pathogenesis. Cerebrovasc Brain Metab Rev 1992; 4:28–58.
39. Caplan LR. Top of the basilar syndrome: selected clinical aspects. Neurology 1980; 30:72–79.
40. Mehler MF. The rostral basilar artery syndrome: diagnosis, etiology, prognosis. Neurology 1989; 39:9–16.
41. Caplan LR. Posterior Circulation Disease. Clinical Findings, Diagnosis, and Management. Boston, Blackwell Science, 1996.
42. Bogousslavsky J, Cachin C, Regli F, et al. Cardiac sources of embolism and cerebral infarction. Clinical consequences and vascular concomitants. Neurology 1991; 41:855–859.
43. Lodder J, Krijne-Kubat B, Broekman J. Cerebral hemorrhagic infarction at autopsy: cardiac embolic cause and the relationship to the cause of death. Stroke 1986; 17: 626–629.

intracardiovascular clotting in patients with chronic atrial fibrillation. J Am Coll Cardiol 1990; 16:377–380.
84. Wolf PA, Abbott RD, Kannel WB. Atrial fibrillation: a major contribution to stroke in the elderly. The Framingham Study. Arch Intern Med 1987; 147:1561–1564.
85. Cairns JA, Connolly SJ. Nonrheumatic atrial fibrillation. Risk of stroke and role of antithrombotic therapy. Circulation 1991; 84:469–481.
86. Wolf PA, Dawber TR, Thomas HE, Kannel WB. Epidemiologic assessment of chronic atrial fibrillation and risk of stroke. The Framingham Study. Neurology 1978; 28:973–977.
87. Tanaka H, Hayashi M, Date C, Imai K, Asada M, Shoji H, Okazaki Y, Yamamoto H, Yoshikawa K, Shimada T, Lee SI. Epidemiologic studies of stroke in Shibata, a Japanese provincial city: preliminary report on risk factors for cerebral infarction. Stroke 1985; 16:773–780.
88. Onundarsen PT, Thorgeirsson G, Jonmundsson E, Sigfusson N, Hardason T. Chronic atrial fibrillation—epidemiologic features and 14 year follow-up: a case control study. Eur Heart J 1987; 8:521–527.
89. Flegel KM, Shipley MJ, Rose G. Risk of stroke in nonrheumatic atrial fibrillation. Lancet 1987; 1:526–529.
90. Dunn MJ, Alexander R, DeSilva F, Hildner F. Antithrombotic therapy in atrial fibrillation. Chest 1989; 95:118S–127S.
91. Stroke Prevention in Atrial Fibrillation Investigators. Predictors of thromboembolism in atrial fibrillation: I. Clinical features of patients at risk. Ann Intern Med 1992; 116:1–5.
92. Atrial Fibrillation Investigators. Risk factors for stroke and efficacy of antithrombotic therapy in atrial fibrillation: analysis of pooled data from five randomized controlled trials. Arch Intern Med 1994; 154:1449–1457.
93. Caplan LR, D'Cruz I, Hier DB, Reddy H, Shah S. Atrial size, atrial fibrillation, and stroke. Ann Neurol 1986; 19:158–161.
94. Stroke Prevention in Atrial Fibrillation Investigators. Predictors of thromboembolism in atrial fibrillation: II. echocardiographic features of patients at risk. Ann Intern Med 1992; 116:6–12.
95. DiPasquale G, Urbinati S, Pinelli G. New echocardiographic markers of embolic risk in atrial fibrillation. Cerebrovasc Dis 1995; 5:315–322.
96. Black IW, Hopkins AP, Lee LCL, Walsh WF. Evaluation of transesophageal echocardiography before cardioversion of atrial fibrillation and flutter in nonanticoagulated patients. Am Heart J 1993; 126:375–381.
97. Vernhorst P, Kamp O, Visser CA, Verheught FWA. Left atrial appendage flow velocity assessment using transesophageal echocardiography in nonrheumatic atrial fibrillation and systemic embolism. Am J Cardiol 1993; 71:192–196.
98. Garcia-Fernandez MA, Torrecilla EG, San Roman D, et al. Left atrial appendage Doppler flow patterns: implications of thrombus formation. Am Heart J 1992; 124: 955–965.
99. Mugge A, Kuhn H, Nikutta P, Grote J, Lopez AG, Daniel WG. Assessment of left atrial appendage function by biplane transesophageal echocardiography in patients

with nonrheumatic atrial fibrillation: identification of a subgroup of patients at increased embolic risk. J Am Coll Cardiol 1994; 23:599–607.
100. Boston Area Anticoagulation Trial for Atrial Fibrillation Investigators. The effect of low-dose warfarin on the risk of stroke in patients with nonrheumatic atrial fibrillation. N Engl J Med 1990; 323:1505–1511.
101. Beppu S, Nimura Y, Sakakibara H. Smoke-like echo in the left atrial cavity in mitral valve disease: its features and significance. J Am Coll Cardiol 1985; 6:744–749.
102. Merino A, Hauptman P, Badiman L, et al. Echocardiographic 'smoke' is produced by an interaction of erythrocytes and plasma proteins modulated by shear forces. J Am Coll Cardiol 1992; 20:1661–1668.
103. Black IW, Stewart WJ. The role of echocardiography in the evaluation of cardiac sources of embolism. Echocardiography 1993; 10:429–439.
104. De Belder MA, Lovat LB, Tourikis L, Leech G, Camm A. Left atrial spontaneous contrast echoes—markers of thromboembolic risk in patients with atrial fibrillation. Eur Heart J 1993; 14:326–335.
105. Black IW, Hopkins AP, Lee LCL, et al. Left atrial spontaneous echo contrast: a clinical and echocardiographic analysis. J Am Coll Cardiol 1991; 18:398A.
106. Tsai LM, Chen JH, Fang CJ, Lin LJ, Kwan CM. Clinical implications of left atrial spontaneous echo contrast in nonrheumatic atrial fibrillation. Am J Cardiol 1992; 70:327–331.
107. Leung DY, Black IW, Cranney GB, Hopkins AP, Walsh WF. Prognostic implications of left atrial spontaneous echo contrast in nonvalvular atrial fibrillation. J Am Coll Cardiol 1994; 24:755–762.
108. Chimowitz MI, DeGeorgia MA, Poole RM, Hepner A, Armstrong WF. Left atrial spontaneous echo contrast is highly associated with previous stroke in patients with atrial fibrillation or mitral stenosis. Stroke 1993; 24:1015–1019.
109. Miller VT, Pearce LA, Feinberg WM, et al. Differential effect of aspirin versus warfarin on clinical stroke types in patients with atrial fibrillation. Neurology 1996; 46:238–240.
110. EAFT Study Group. Silent brain infarction in nonrheumatic atrial fibrillation. Neurology 1996; 46:159–165.
111. Bogousslavsky J, Van Melle G, Regli F, Kappenberger L. Pathogenesis of anterior circulation stroke in patients with nonvalvular atrial fibrillation: the Lausanne Stroke Registry. Neurology 1990; 40:1046–1050.
112. Petersen P, Godtfredsen J, Boysen G, et al. Placebo-controlled, randomized trial of warfarin and aspirin for prevention of thromboembolic complications in chronic atrial fibrillation: the Copenhagen AFASAK study. Lancet 1989; 1:175–179.
113. Stroke Prevention in Atrial Fibrillation Investigators. The stroke prevention in atrial fibrillation study: final results. Circulation 1991; 84:527–539.
114. EAFT (European Atrial Fibrillation Trial) Study Group. Secondary prevention in non-rheumatic atrial fibrillation after transient ischaemic attack or minor stroke. Lancet 1993; 342:1255–1262.
115. Stroke Prevention in Atrial Fibrillation Investigators. Warfarin versus aspirin for

prevention of thromboembolism in atrial fibrillation: Stroke Prevention in Atrial Fibrillation II Study. Lancet 1994; 343:687–691.

116. Stroke Prevention in Atrial Fibrillation Investigators. Adjusted-dose warfarin versus low-intensity, fixed-dose warfarin plus aspirin for high-risk patients with atrial fibrillation. Stroke Prevention in Atrial Fibrillation III randomised clinical trial. Lancet 1996; 348:633–638.
117. Stroke Prevention in Atrial Fibrillation Investigators. Prospective identification of patients with nonvalvular atrial fibrillation at low risk of stroke during treatment with aspirin: Stroke Prevention in Atrial Fibrillation III Study. Circulation 1997; 96(suppl):I–281. Abstract.
118. Connolly SJ, Laupacis A, Gent M. Canadian atrial fibrillation anticoagulation (CAFA) study. J Am Coll Cardiol 1991; 18:349–355.
119. European Atrial Fibrillation Trial Study Group. Optimal oral anticoagulation therapy in patients with nonrheumatic atrial fibrillation and recent cerebral ischemia. N Engl J Med 1995; 333:5–10.
120. Albers G. Atrial fibrillation and stroke. Three new studies, three remaining questions. Arch Intern Med 1994; 154:1443–1448.
121. Koudstaal PJ. Anticoagulation in very elderly patients (>80 years) with stroke and atrial fibrillation. Cerebrovasc Dis 1995; 5:8–9.
122. Bjerkelund CJ, Orning OM. The efficacy of anticoagulant therapy in preventing embolism related to D.C. electrical conversion of atrial fibrillation. Am J Cardiol 1969; 23:208–216.
123. Roy D, Marchand E, Gagne P, Chabot M, Cartier R. Usefulness of anticoagulant therapy in the prevention of embolic complications of atrial fibrillation. Am Heart J 1986; 112:1039–1043.
124. Gersh BJ, Gottdiener JS. Shadows on the cave wall: the role of transesophageal echocardiography in atrial fibrillation. Ann Intern Med 1995; 123:882–884.
125. Stoddard MF, Dawkins PR, Prince CR, Ammash NM. Left atrial appendage thrombus is not uncommon in patients with acute atrial fibrillation and a recent embolic event: a transesophageal echocardiographic study. J Am Coll Cardiol 1995; 25: 452–459.
126. Fatkin D, Kuchar DL, Thornburn CW, Fenely MP. Transesophageal echocardiography before and during direct current cardioversion of atrial fibrillation: evidence for "atrial stunning" as a mechanism of thromboembolic complications. J Am Coll Cardiol 1994; 23:307–316.
127. Fairfax AJ, Lambert CD, Leatham A. Systemic embolism in chronic sinoatrial disorder. N Engl J Med 1976; 295:190–192.
128. Rubenstein JJ, Schulman CL, Yurchak PM, et al. Clinical spectrum of the sick sinus syndrome. Circulation 1972; 46:5–13.
129. Orencia AJ, Hammill SC, Whisnant JP. Sinus node dysfunction and ischemic stroke. Heart Dis Stroke 1994; 3:91–94.
130. Lown B. Electrical reversion of cardiac arrythmias. Br Heart J 1967; 29:469–489.
131. Phillips SJ, Whisnant JP, O'Fallon WM, Frye RL. Prevalence of cardiovascular disease and diabetes mellitus in residents of Rochester, Minnesota. Mayo Clin Proc 1990; 65:344–359.
132. Koudstaal PJ, van Gijn J, Klootwijk APJ, van der Meche FGA, Kappelle LJ. Holter

monitoring in patients with transient and focal ischemic attacks of the brain. Stroke 1986; 17:192–195.
133. Stangl K, Seitz K, Wirtzfeld A, Alt E, Blomer H. Differences between atrial single chamber pacing (AAI) and ventricular single chamber pacing (VVI) with respect to prognosis and antiarrhythmic effect in patients with sick sinus syndrome. Pacing Clin Electrophysiol 1990; 13:2080–2085.
134. Rosenqvist M, Brandt J, Schuller H. Long-term pacing in sinus node disease: effects of stimulation mode on cardiovascular morbidity and mortality. Am Heart J 1988; 116:16–22.
135. Radford DJ, Julian DG. Sick sinus syndrome. Experience of a cardiac pacemaker clinic. Br Med J 1974; 3:504–507.
136. Rosenqvist M, Vallin H, Edhag O. Clinical and electrophysiologic course of sinus node disease: five year follow-up study. Am Heart J 1985; 109:513–522.
137. Bathen J, Sparr S, Rokseth R. Embolism in sinoatrial disease. Acta Med Scand 1978; 203:7–11.
138. Cerebral embolism task force. Cardiogenic brain embolism. Arch Neurol 1986; 43: 71–84.
139. Stein PD, Sabbah HN. Turbulent flow in the ascending aorta of humans with normal and diseased aortic leaflets. Circ Res 1976; 39:58–65.
140. Stein PD, Sabbah HN. Measured turbulence and its effect on thrombus formation. Circ Res 1974; 35:608–614.
141. Macagno EO, Hung TK. Computational and experimental study of a captive annular eddy. J Fluid Mech 1967; 28:43–64.
142. Stein PD, Sabbah HN, Pitha JV. Continuing disease process of calcific aortic stenosis. Am J Cardiol 1977; 39:159–163.
143. Harris AW, Levine SA. Cerebral embolism in mitral stenosis. Ann Intern Med 1941; 15:637–643.
144. Friedberg C. Diseases of the Heart. 3d ed. Philadelphia: W.B. Saunders, 1966.
145. Szekely P. Systemic embolism and anticoagulant prophylaxis in rheumatic heart disease. Br Med J 1964; 1:1209–1212.
146. Keen G, Leveaux VM. Prognosis of cerebral embolism in rheumatic heart disease. Br Med J 1958; 2:91–92.
147. Coulshed N, Epstein EJ, McKendrick CS, et al. Systemic embolism in mitral valve disease. Br Med J 1970; 32:26–34.
148. Daley R, Mattingly TW, Holt CL, et al. Systemic arterial embolism in rheumatic heart disease. Am Heart J 1951; 42:566–581.
149. Fleming HA, Bailey SM. Mitral valve disease, systemic embolism and anticoagulants. Postgrad Med J 1971; 47:599–604.
150. Adams GF, Merrett JD, Hutchinson WM, Pollock AM. Cerebral embolism and mitral stenosis: survival with and without anticoagulants. J Neurol Neurosurg Psychiatry 1974; 37:378–383.
151. Carter AB. The immediate treatment of cerebral embolism. Q J Med 1957; 26: 335–347.
152. Carter AB. prognosis of cerebral embolism. Lancet 1965; 2:514–519.
153. Carabello BA, Crawford FA. Valvular heart disease. N Engl J Med 1997; 337:32–41.

154. Goldman ME, Mora F, Guarino T, Fuster V, Mindich BP. Mitral valvuloplasty is superior to valve replacement for preservation of left ventricular function: an intraoperative two-dimensional echocardiographic study. J Am Coll Cardiol 1987; 10:568–575.
155. Edwards JE. On the etiology of calcific aortic stenosis. Circulation 1962; 26:817–818.
156. Pleet AB, Massey EW, Vengrow ME. TIA, stroke, and the bicuspid aortic valve. Neurology 1981; 31:1540–1542.
157. O'Donoghue ME, Dangond F, Burger AJ, et al. Spontaneous calcific embolization to the supraclinoid internal carotid artery from a regurgitant bicuspid aortic valve. Neurology 1993; 43:2715–2717.
158. Shanmugam V, Chhablani R, Gorelick PB. Spontaneous calcific cerebral embolus. Neurology 1997; 48:538–539.
159. Rancurel G, Marelle L, Vincent D, et al. Spontaneous calcific cerebral embolus from a calcific aortic stenosis in a middle cerebral artery infarct. Stroke 1989; 20:691–693.
160. Kapila A, Hart R. Calcific cerebral emboli and aortic stenosis: detection of computed tomography. Stroke 1986; 17:619–621.
161. Soulie P, Caramanian M, Soulie J, Bader JL, Colcher E. Les embolies calcaires des atteintes orificielles calcifees du coeur gauche. Arch Mal Coeur 1969; 12:1657–1684.
162. Holley KE, Bahn RC, McGoon DC, Mankin HT. Spontaneous calcific embolization associated with calcific aortic stenosis. Circulation 1963; 27:197–202.
163. Brockmeier LB, Adolph RJ, Gustin BW, et al. Calcium emboli to the retinal artery in calcific aortic stenosis. Am Heart J 1981; 101:32–37.
164. Wilson LA, Warlow CP, Ross-Russell RW. Cardiovascular disease in patients with retinal artery occlusion. Lancet 1979; 1:292–294.
165. Holley KE, Bahn C, McGoon DC, Mankin HT. Calcific embolization associated with valvulotomy for calcific aortic stenosis. Circulation 1963; 28:175–181.
166. Klues HG, Maron BJ, Dollar AL, Roberts WC. Diversity of structural mitral valve alterations in hypertrophic cardiomyopathy. Circulation 1992; 85:1651–1660.
167. Hardarson T, De la Calzada CS, Curiel R, Goodwin JF. Prognosis and mortality of hypertrophic obstructive cardiomyopathy. Lancet 1973; 2:1462–1467.
168. Glancy DL, O'Brien KP, Gold HK, Epstein SE. Atrial fibrillation in patients with idiopathic hypertrophic subaortic stenosis. Br Heart J 1970; 32:652–659.
169. Tajik AJ, Giuliani ER, Frye RL, et al. Mitral valve and/or annulus calcification associated with hypertrophic subaortic stenosis (IHSS). Circulation 1972; 16(suppl II):228.
170. Furlan AJ, Craciun AR, Raju NR, Hart N. Cerebrovascular complications associated with idiopathic hypertrophic subaortic stenosis. Stroke 1984; 15:282–284.
171. Barlow JB, Bosman CK. Aneurysmal protrusion of posterior leaflets of the mitral valve. An auscultatory-electrocardiographic syndrome. Am Heart J 1966; 71:166–178.
172. Lauzier S, Barnett HJM. Cerebral ischemia with mitral valve prolapse and mitral annular calcification. In: Furlan AJ, ed. The Heart and Stroke: Exploring Mutual

Cerebrovascular and Cardiovascular Issues. London: Springer-Verlag, 1987:63–100.
173. Markiewicz W, Stoner J, London E, Hunt SA, Popp RL. Mitral valve prolapse in one hundred presumably healthy young females. Circulation 1976; 53:464–473.
174. Cheitlin MD, Byrd RC. Prolapsed mitral valve: the commonest valve disease? Curr Prob Cardiol 1984; 8(10):3–53.
175. Ranganatham N, Silver MD, Robinson T, et al. Angiographic-morphological correlation in patients with severe mitral regurgitation due to prolapse of the posterior mitral valve leaflet. Circulation 1973; 48:514–518.
176. Kostuk WJ, Boughner DR, Barnett HJM, Silver MD. Strokes: a complication of mitral-leaflet prolapse? Lancet 1977; 2:313–316.
177. Hanson MR, Conomy JP, Hodgman JR. Brain events associated with mitral valve prolapse. Stroke 1980; 11:499–506.
178. Geyer SJ, Franzini DA. Myxomatous degeneration of the mitral valve complicated by nonbacterial thrombotic endocarditis with systemic embolization. Am J Clin Pathol 1979; 72:489–492.
179. Levine RA, Stathogiannis E, Newell JB, Harrigan P, Weyman AE. Reconsideration of echocardiographic standards for mitral valve prolapse. J Am Coll Cardiol 1988; 11:1010–1019.
180. Marks AR, Choong CY, Sanfillipo AJ, Ferre M, Weyman AE. Identification of high-risk and low-risk subgroups of patients with mitral-valve prolapse. N Engl J Med 1989; 320:1031–1036.
181. Nishimura RA, McGoon MD, Shub C, et al. Echocardiographically documented mitral-valve prolapse: long term follow-up of 237 patients. N Engl J Med 1985; 313:1305–1309.
182. Wynne J. Mitral-valve prolapse. N Engl J Med 1986; 314:577–578.
183. Barnett HJM. Transient cerebral ischemia: pathogenesis, prognosis, and management. Ann R Coll Phys Surg Can 1974; 7:153–173.
184. Barnett HJM, Jones MW, Boughner DR, Kostuk WJ. Cerebral ischemic events associated with prolapsing mitral valve. Arch Neurol 1976; 33:777–782.
185. Barnett HJM, Boughner DR, Taylor DW, et al. Further evidence relating mitral-valve prolapse to cerebral ischemic events. N Engl J Med 1980; 302:139–144.
186. Barletta GA, Gagliardi R, Benvenuti L, Fantini F. Cerebral ischemic attacks as a complication of aortic and mitral valve prolapse. Stroke 1985; 16:219–223.
187. Watson RT. TIA, stroke and mitral valve prolapse. Neurology 1979; 29:886–889.
188. Sandok BA, Giuliani ER. Cerebral ischemic events in patients with mitral valve prolapse Stroke 1982; 13:448–450.
189. Jones HR, Naggar CZ, Selijan MP, Downing ZZ. Mitral valve prolapse and cerebral ischemic events. A comparison between a neurology population with stroke and a cardiology population with mitral valve prolapse observed for five years. Stroke 1982; 13:451–453.
190. Kouvaras G, Bacoulos G. Association of mitral leaflet prolapse with cerebral ischemic events in the young and early middle-aged patient. J Med New Ser 1985; 55: 387–392.

191. McKeoun EF. De senectu: the FE Williams Lecture. J R Coll Physicians 1975; 10: 79.
192. Savage DD, Garrison RJ, Castelli WP, et al. Prevalence of submitral (annular) calcium and its correlates in general population-based sample (the Framingham Study). Am J Cardiol 1983; 51:1375–1378.
193. Korn D, DeSanctis R, Sell S. Massive calcification of the mitral valve, a clinicopathological study of fourteen cases. N Engl J Med 1962; 267:900–909.
194. DeBono D, Warlow C. Mitral annulus calcification and cerebral or retinal ischemia. Lancet 1979; 2:383–385.
195. Benjamin EJ, Plehn JF, D'Agostino RB, et al. Mitral annular calcification and the risk of stroke in an elderly cohort. N Engl J Med 1992; 327:374–379.
196. Pomerance A. Pathological and clinical study of calcification of the mitral valve ring. J Clin Pathol 1970; 23:354–361.
197. Fulkerson PK, Beaver BM, Auseon JC, Graver HL. Calcification of the mitral annulus—etiology, clinical associations, complications and therapy. Am J Med 1979; 66:967–977.
198. Ridolfi RL, Hutchins GM. Spontaneous calcific emboli from calcific mitral annulus fibrosus. Arch Pathol Lab Med 1976; 100:117–120.
199. Mouton P, Biousse V, Crassard I, Bousson V, Bousser M-G. Ischemic stroke due to calcific emboli from mitral valve annulus calcification. Stroke 1997; 28:2325–2326.
200. Stein JH, Soble JS. Thrombus associated with mitral valve calcification. A possible mechanism for embolic stroke. Stroke 1995; 26:1697–1699.
201. Vongpatanasin W, Hillis D, Lange RA. Prosthetic heart valves. N Engl J Med 1996; 335:407–416.
202. Edmunds LH Jr. Thromboembolic complications of current cardiac valvular prostheses. Ann Thorac Surg 1982; 34:96–106.
203. Metzdorff MT, Grunkemeier GL, Pinson CW, Starr A. Thrombosis of mechanical cardiac valves: a qualitative comparison of the silastic ball valve and the tilting disc valve. J Am Coll Cardiol 1984; 4:50–53.
204. Barnhorst DA, Oxman HE, Connolly DC, et al. Long-term follow-up of isolated replacement of the aortic or mitral valve with the Starr-Edwards prosthesis. Am J Cardiol 1975; 35:228–233.
205. Dudczak R, Niessner H, Thaler E, et al. Plasma concentration of platelet-specific proteins and fibrinopeptide A in patients with artificial heart valves. Haemostasis 1980; 10:229–238.
206. Pumphrey CW, Dawes J. Elevation of plasma-thromboglobulin in patients with prosthetic cardiac valves. Thromb Res 1981; 22:147–155.
207. Harker LA, Slichter SL. Studies of platelet and fibrinogen kinetics in patients with prosthetic heart valves. N Engl J Med 1970; 283:1302–1305.
208. Edmunds LH. Thrombotic and bleeding complications of prosthetic heart valves. Ann Thorac Surg 1987; 44:430–445.
209. Riddle JM, Magilligan DJ Jr, Stein PD. Surface morphology of degenerated porcine bioprosthetic valves four to seven years following implantation. J Thorac Cardiovasc Surg 1981; 81:279–287.
210. Thiene G, Bortolotti U, Pannizon G, Miland A, Gallucci V. Pathological substrates

of thrombus formation after heart valve replacement with the Hancock bioprosthesis. J Thorac Cardiovasc Surg 1980; 80:414–423.
211. Salgado ED, Furlan AJ, Conomy JP. Cardioembolic sources of stroke. In: Furlan AJ, ed. The Heart and Stroke: Exploring Mutual Cerebrovascular and Cardiovascular Issues. London: Springer-Verlag, 1987:47–61.
212. Cannegieter SC, Rosendaal FR, Briet E. Thromboembolic and bleeding complications in patients with mechanical heart valve prostheses. Circulation 1994; 89:635–641.
213. Cohn LH, Mudge GH, Pratter F, Collins JJ. Five to eight-year follow-up of patients undergoing porcine heart-valve replacement. N Engl J Med 1981; 304:258–262.
214. Braekken KS, Russell D, Brucher R, Svennevig J. Incidence and frequency of cerebral embolic signals in patients with a similar bileaflet mechanical heart valve. Stroke 1995; 26:1225–1230.
215. Sliwka U, Diehl RR, Meyer B, Schonhube F, Noth J. Transcranial Doppler 'high-intensity transient signals' in the acute phase and long-term follow-up of mechanical heart valve implantation. J Stroke Cerebrovasc Dis 1995; 5:139–146.
216. Georgiadis D, Grosset DG, Kelman AW, Faichney A, Lees KR. Incidence and characteristics of intracranial microemboli signals in patients with different types of prosthetic cardiac valves. Stroke 1994; 25:587–592.
217. Georgiadis D, Preiss M, Lindner A, et al. Doppler microemboli signals in children with prosthetic cardiac valves. Stroke 1997; 28:1328–1329.
218. Kaps M, Hansen J, Weiher M, et al. Clinically silent microemboli in patients with artificial prosthetic aortic valves are predominantly gaseous and not solid. Stroke 1997; 28:322–325.
219. Wingerchuk DM, Krecke KN, Fulgham JR. Multifocal brain MRI artifacts secondary to embolic metal fragments. Neurology 1997; 49:1451–1453.
220. Heras M, Chesebro JH, Fuster V, et al. High risk of thromboemboli early after bioprosthetic cardiac valve replacement. J Am Coll Cardiol 1995; 25:1111–1119.
221. Turpie AGG, Gunstensen J, Hirsh J, Nelson H, Gent M. Randomised comparison of two intensities of oral anticoagulant therapy after tissue heart valve replacement. Lancet 1988; 1:1242–1245.
222. Turpie AGG, Gent M, Laupacis A, et al. A comparison of aspirin with placebo in patients treated with warfarin after heart-valve replacement. N Engl J Med 1993; 329:524–529.
223. Sareli P, England MJ, Berk MR, et al. Maternal and fetal sequelae of anticoagulation during pregnancy in patients with mechanical heart valve prostheses. Am J Cardiol 1989; 63:1462–1465.
224. Hanania G, Thomas D, Michel PL, et al. Pregnancy and prosthetic heart valves: a French cooperative retrospective study of 155 cases. Eur Heart J 1994; 15:1651–1658.
224a. Altman R, Rouvier J, Gurfinkel E, et al. Comparison of two levels of anticoagulant therapy in patients with substitute heart valves. J Thorac Cardiovasc Surg 1991; 101:427–431.
224b. Butchart EG, Lewis PA, Bethel JA, Breckenridge IM. Adjusting anticoagulation to prosthesis thrombogenicity and patient risk factors: recommendations for the Medtronic Hall valve. Circulation 1991; 84(suppl 3):1161–1169.

224c. Horstkotte D, Schulte H, Bircks W, Strauer B. Unexpected findings concerning thromboembolic complications and anticoagulation after complete 10 year follow up of patients with St. Jude mechanical prostheses. J Heart Valve Dis 1993; 2:291–301.
224d. Acar J. Low-dose versus standard-dose anticoagulation for prosthetic heart valves. Circulation 1995; 92:2360.
224e. Tiede D, Nishimura RA, Gastineau D, et al. Modern management of prosthetic valve anticoagulation. Mayo Clin Proc 1998; 73:665–680.
225. Osler W. Gulstonian lectures on malignant endocarditis. Lancet 1885; 1:459–465.
226. Jones HR, Siekert RG, Geraci J. Neurologic manifestations of bacterial endocarditis. Ann Intern Med 1969; 71:21–28.
227. Salgado AV, Furlan AJ, Keys TF, Nichols TR, Beck GJ. Neurologic complications of endocarditis: a 12-year experience. Neurology 1989; 39:173–178.
228. Hart RG, Foster JW, Luther MF, Kanter MC. Stroke in infective endocarditis. Stroke 1990; 21:695–700.
229. Kanter MC, Hart RG. Neurologic complications of infective endocarditis. Neurology 1991; 41:1015–1020.
230. Keyser DL, Biller J, Coffman TT, Adams HP. Neurologic complications of late prosthetic valve endocarditis. Stroke 1990; 21:472–475.
231. Matsushita K, Kuriyama Y, Sawada T, et al. Hemorrhagic and ischemic cerebrovascular complications of active infective endocarditis of native valve. Eur Neurol 1993; 33:267–274.
232. Hart RG, Kagan-Hallet K, Joerns S. Mechanisms of intracranial hemorrhage in infective endocarditis. Stroke 1987; 18:1048–1056.
233. Masuda J, Yutani C, Waki R, et al. Histopathological analysis of the mechanisms of intracranial hemorrhage complicating infective endocarditis. Stroke 1992; 23: 843–850.
234. Morawetz RB, Karp RB. Evolution and resolution of intracranial bacterial (mycotic) aneurysms. Neurosurgery 1984; 15:43–49.
235. Moskowitz MA, Rosenbaum AE, Tyler HR. Angiographically monitored resolution of cerebral mycotic aneurysms. Neurology 1974; 24:1103–1108.
236. Bingham WF. Treatment of mycotic intracranial aneurysms. J Neurosurg 1977; 46: 428–437.
237. Salgado AV, Furlan AJ, Keys TF. Mycotic aneurysm, subarachnoid hemorrhage, and indications for cerebral angiography in infective endocarditis. Stroke 1987; 18: 1057–1060.
238. Bertorini TE, Laster RE, Thompson BF, Gelfand M. Magnetic resonance imaging of the brain in bacterial endocarditis. Arch Intern Med 1989; 149:815–817.
239. Gransden WR, Eykyn SJ, Leach RM. Neurological presentations of native valve endocarditis. Q J Med 1989; 73:1135–1142.
240. Berbari EF, Cockerill EF, Steckelberg JM. Infective endocarditis due to unusual or fastidious microorganisms. Mayo Clin Proc 1997; 72:532–542.
241. Libman E, Sacks B. A hitherto undescribed form of valvular and mural endocarditis. Arch Intern Med 1924; 33:701–737.
242. Klemperer P, Pollack AD, Baehr G. Pathology of disseminated lupus erythematosus. Arch Pathol 1941; 32:569–631.

243. Baehr G, Klemperer P, Schifrin A. A diffuse disease of the peripheral circulation usually associated with lupus erythematosus and endocarditis. Trans Assoc Am Physicians 1935; 50:139–155.
244. Gross L. The cardiac lesions in Libman-Sacks disease, with a consideration of its relationship to acute diffuse lupus erythematosus. Am J Pathol 1940; 16:375–407.
245. Fox IS, Spence AM, Wheelis RF, Healey LA. Cerebral embolism in Libman-Sacks endocarditis. Neurology 1980; 30:487–491.
246. Harvey AM, Shulman LE, Tumulty PA, Conley CL, Schoenrich EH. Systemic lupus erythematosus: review of the literature and clinical analysis of 138 cases. Medicine 1954; 33:291–437.
247. Johnson RT, Richardson EP. The neurological manifestations of systemic lupus erythematosus. Medicine 1968; 47:337–370.
248. Devinsky O, Petito CK, Alonso DR. Clinical and neuropathological findings in systemic lupus erythematosus: the role of vasculitis, heart emboli, and thrombotic thrombocytopenic purpura. Ann Neurol 1988; 23:380–384.
249. Galve E, Candell-Riera J, Pigrau C, et al. Prevalence, morphologic types, and evolution of cardiac valvular disease in systemic lupus erythematosus. N Engl J Med 1988; 319:817–823.
250. Roldan CA, Shively B, Crawford MH. An echocardiographic study of valvular heart disease associated with systemic lupus erythematosus. N Engl J Med 1996; 335:1424–1430.
251. Crozier I, Li E, Milne M, Nicholls MG. Valvular heart disease in systemic lupus erythematosus. (Letter.) N Engl J Med 1989; 320:739–740.
252. Brenner B, Blumenfeld Z, Markiewicz W, Reisner SA. Cardiac involvement in patients with primary antiphospholipid syndrome. J Am Coll Cardiol 1991; 18: 931–936.
253. Barbut D, Borer J, Gharavi A, et al. Prevalence of anticardiolipin antibody in isolated mitral or aortic regurgitation, or both, and possible relation to cerebral ischemic events. Am J Cardiol 1992; 70:901–905.
254. Barbut D, Borer J, Wallerson D, Ameisen O, Lockshin M. Anticardiolipin antibody and stroke: possible relation of valvular heart disease and embolic events. Cardiology 1991; 79:99–109.
255. Antiphospholipid Antibodies in Stroke Study Group. Clinical and laboratory findings in patients with antiphospholipid antibodies and cerebral ischemia. Stroke 1990; 21:1268–1273.
256. Amico L, Caplan LR, Thomas C. Cerebrovascular complications of mucinous cancer. Neurology 1989; 39:522–526.
257. Reagan TJ, Okazaki H. The thrombotic syndrome associated with carcinoma. Arch Neurol 1974; 31:390–395.
258. Kooiker JC, MacLean JM, Sumi SM. Cerebral embolism, marantic endocarditis, and cancer. Arch Neurol 1976; 33:260–264.
258a. Edoute Y, Haim N, Rinkevich D, Brenner B, Reisner SA. Cardiac valvular vegetations in cancer patients: a prospective echocardiographic study of 200 patients. Am J Med 1997; 102:252–258.
259. Connolly HM, Crary JL, McGoon MD, et al. Valvular heart disease associated with fenflurmine-phentermine. N Engl J Med 1997; 337:581–588.

295. Rice GP, Ebers GC, Newland F, Wysocki GP. Recurrent cerebral embolism in cardiac amyloidosis. Neurology 1981; 31:904–906.
296. Dyken ME, Biller J. Peripartum cardiomyopathy and stroke. Cerebrovasc Dis 1994; 4:325–328.
297. Hodgman MT, Pessin MS, Homans DC, et al. Cerebral embolism as the initial manifestation of peripartum cardiomyopathy. Neurology 1982; 32:668–671.
298. Sauer CM. Recurrent embolic stroke and cocaine-related cardiomyopathy. Stroke 1991; 22:1203–1205.
299. Ritter M, Oechslin E, Sutsch G, et al. Isolated noncompaction of the myocardium in adults. Mayo Clin Proc 1997; 72:26–31.
299a. Koniaris L, Goldhaber SZ. Anticoagulation in dilated cardiomyopathy. J Am Coll Cardiol 1998; 31:745–748.
299b. Fuster V, Gersh BJ, Giuliani ER, et al. The natural history of idiopathic dilated cardiomyopathy. Am J Cardiol 1981; 47:525–531.
300. Harthorne J. Case records of the Massachusetts General Hospital—case 46-1975. N Engl J Med 1975; 293:1138–1145.
301. Pritchard RW. Tumors of the heart: review of the subject and report of 150 cases. Arch Pathol Lab Med 1951; 51:98–128.
302. Reynen K. Cardiac myxomas. N Engl J Med 1995; 333:1610–1617.
303. McAllister HA Jr, Fenoglio JJ Jr. Tumors of the cardiovascular system. Atlas of Tumor Pathology, 2d ser, Fascicle 15. Washington, DC: Armed Forces Institute of Pathology, 1978:1–20.
304. St. John Sutton MG, Mercier L-A, Giuliani ER, Lie JT. Atrial myxomas: a review of clinical experience in 40 patients. Mayo Clin Proc 1980; 55:371–376.
305. Blondeau P. Primary cardiac tumors—French study of 533 cases. Thorac Cardiovasc Surg 1990; 38(suppl 2):192–195.
306. Silverman J, Olwin JS, Graettinger JS. Cardiac myxomas with systemic embolism: review of the literature and report of a case. Circulation 1962; 26:99–103.
307. Nishmura RN. Right atrial myxoma with a patent foramen ovale. Lancet 1977; 2: 1137–1138.
308. Duvernoy WFC, Drake EH, Reddy MS, et al. Right atrial myxomas: a review of 9 cases. Cardiology 1975; 60:206–219.
309. Butler MJ, Adams HP, Hiratzka LF. Recurrent cerebral embolism from a right atrial myxoma. Ann Neurol 1986; 19:608.
310. Sandok BA, von Estorff I, Giuliani E. CNS embolism due to atrial myxoma. Clinical features and diagnosis. Arch Neurol 1980; 37:485–488.
311. Hirose G, Kosoegawa H, Takado M, et al. Spinal cord ischemia and left atrial myxoma. Arch Neurol 1979; 36:439.
312. Thompson J, Kapoor W, Wechsler LR. Multiple strokes due to atrial myxoma with a negative echocardiogram. Stroke 1988; 19:1570–1571.
313. Hutton JT. Atrial myxoma as a cause of progressive dementia. Arch Neurol 1981; 38:533.
314. Browne WT, Wijdicks EFM, Parisi JE, Viggiano RW. Fulminant brain necrosis from atrial myxoma showers. Stroke 1993; 24:1090–1092.
315. Roeltgen DP, Weimer GR, Patterson LF. Delayed neurologic complications of left atrial myxoma. Neurology 1981; 31:8–13.

316. Damasio H, Seabra-Gomes R, daSilva JP, et al. Multiple cerebral aneurysms and cardiac myxoma. Arch Neurol 1975; 32:269–270.
317. Burton C, Johnstone J. Multiple cerebral aneurysms and cardiac myxoma. N Engl J Med 1970; 282:35–36.
318. Price DL, Harris JL, New PFJ, Cantu RC. Cardiac myxoma: a clinicopathologic and angiographic study. Arch Neurol 1970; 23:558–567.
319. Sandok BA, von Estorff I, Giuliani ER. Subsequent neurological events in patients with atrial myxoma. Ann Neurol 1980; 8:305–307.
320. Frank RA, Shalen PR, Harvey DG, et al. Atrial myxoma with intellectual decline and cerebral growths on CT scan. Ann Neurol 1979; 5:396–400.
321. Read RC, Whiter HJ, Murphy ML, et al. The malignant potential of left atrial myxoma. J Thorac Cardiovasc Surg 1974; 857–867.
322. Kasarskis EJ, O'Connor W, Earle G. Embolic stroke from cardiac papillary fibroelastomas. Stroke 1988; 19:1171–1173.
323. Brown RD, Khandheria BK, Edwards WD. Cardiac papillary fibroelastoma: a treatable cause of transient ischemic attack and ischemic stroke detected by transesophageal echocardiography. Mayo Clin Proc 1995; 70:863–868.
324. Fine G. Primary tumors of the pericardium and heart. Cardiovasc Clin 1973; 5: 207–238.
325. Guereta LG, Burgueros M, Elorza MD, et al. Cardiac rhabdomyoma presenting as fetral hydrops. Pediatr Cardiol 1986; 7:171–174.
326. Hall RJ, Cooley DA, McAllister HA, Frazier OH. Neoplastic heart disease. In: Schlant RC, Alexander RW, eds. Hurst's The Heart. 8th ed., New York: McGraw-Hill, 1994:2007–2029.
327. Mata M, Wharton M, Geisinger K, Pugh JE. Myocardial rhabdomyosarcoma in multiple neurofibromatosis. Neurology 1981; 31:1549–1551.
328. Hagen PT, Scholz DG, Edwards WD. Incidence and size of patent foramen ovale during the first 10 decades of life: an autopsy study of 965 normal hearts. Mayo Clin Proc 1984; 59:17–20.
329. Lechat Ph, Mas JL, Lascault G, et al. Prevalence of patent foramen ovale in patients with stroke. N Engl J Med 1988; 318:1148–1152.
330. Di Tullio M, Sacco RL, Gopal A, Mohr JP, Homma S. Patent foramen ovale as a risk factor for cryptogenic stroke. Ann Intern Med 1992; 117:461–465.
331. Petty GW, Khanderia BK, Chu C-P, Sicks JD, Whisnant JP. Patent foramen ovale in patients with cerebral infraction. A transesophageal echocardiographic study. Arch Neurol 1997; 54:819–822.
332. Jones HR, Caplan LR, Come PC, Swinton NW, Breslin DJ. Cerebral emboli of paradoxical origin. Ann Neurol 1983; 13:314–319.
333. Biller J, Adams HP, Johnson MR, Kerber RE, Toffol GJ. Paradoxical cerebral embolism: eight cases. Neurology 1986; 36:1356–1360.
334. Gautier JC, Durr A, Koussa S, Lascault G, Grosgogeat Y. Paradoxical cerebral embolism with a patent foramen ovale. A report of 29 patients. Cerebrovasc Dis 1991; 1:193–202.
335. Venketasubramanian N, Sacco RL, Di Tullio M, et al. Vascular distribution of paradoxical emboli by transcranial Doppler. Neurology 1993; 43:1533–1535.

336. Shuiab A. Cerebral infarction and ventricular septal defect. Stroke 1989; 20:957–958.
337. Harvey JR, Teague SM, Anderson JL, Voyles WF, Thadani U. Clinically silent atrial septal defects with evidence for cerebral embolism. Ann Intern Med 1986; 105:695–697.
338. Reguera JM, Colmenero JD, Guerrwro M, Pastor M, Martin-Palanca A. Paradoxical cerebral embolism secondary to pulmonary arteriovenous fistula. Stroke 1990; 21: 504–505.
339. Stollberger C, Slany J, Schuster I, et al. The prevalence of deep venous thrombosis in patients with suspected paradoxical embolism. Ann Intern Med 1993; 119:461–465.
340. Barbour SI, Izban KF, Reyes CV, McKiernan TL, Louie EK. Serpentine thrombus traversing the foramen ovale: paradoxical embolis shown by transesophageal echocardiography. Ann Intern Med 1996; 125:111–113.
341. Pell ACH, Hughes D, Keating J, et al. Brief report: fulminating fat embolism syndrome caused by paradoxical embolism through a patent foramen ovale. N Engl J Med 1993; 329:926–929.
342. Chimowitz MI, Nemec JJ, Marwick TH, et al. Transcranial Doppler ultrasound identifies patients with right-to-left cardiac or pulmonary shunts. Neurology 1991; 41:1902–1904.
343. Albert A, Muller HR, Hetzel A. Optimized transcranial Doppler technique for the diagnosis of cardiac right-to-left shunts. J Neuroimag 1997; 7:159–163.
344. Di Tullio M, Sacco RL, Venketasubramanian N, et al. Comparison of diagnostic techniques for the detection of a patent foramen ovale in stroke patients. Stroke 1993; 24:1020–1024.
345. Schminke U, Ries S, Daffertshofer M, Staedt U, Hennerici M. Patent foramen ovale: a potential source of cerebral embolism. Cerebrovasc Dis 1995; 5:133–138.
346. Klotzsch C, Janzen G, Berlit P. Transesophageal echocardiography and contrast-TCD in the detection of a patent foramen ovale. Experiences with 111 patients. Neurology 1994; 44:1603–1606.
347. Nemec JJ, Marwick TH, Lorig RJ, Davison MB, Chimowitz MI, Litowitz H, Salcedo EE. Comparison of transcranial Doppler ultrasound and transesophageal contrast echocardiography in the detection of intraatrial right-to-left shunts. Am J Cardiol 1991; 68:1498–1502.
348. Hanna JP, Sun JP, Furlan AJ, et al. Patent foramen ovale and brain infarct. Echocardiographic predictors, recurrence, and prevention. Stroke 1994; 25:782–786.
349. Homma S, Di Tullio MR, Sacco RL, et al. Characteristics of patent foramen ovale associated with cryptogenic stroke. A biplane transesophageal echocardiographic study. Stroke 1994; 25:582–586.
349a. Ay H, Buonanno FS, Abraham S, Kistler JP, Koroshetz W. An electrocardiographic criterion for diagnosis of patent foramen ovale associated with ischemic stroke. Stroke 1998; 29:1393–1397.
349b. Heller J, Hagege AA, Besse B, Desnos M, Marie FN, Guerot C. ''Crochetage'' (notch) on R wave in inferior limb leads: a new independent sign of atrial septal defect. J Am Coll Cardiol 1996; 27:877–882.

350. Lang FJ, Posselt A. Aneurysmatische Vorwolbung der Fossa Ovalis in den linken Vorhof. Wien Med Wochenschr 1934; 84:392–395.
351. Silver MD, Dorsey JS. Aneurysms of the septum primum in adults. Arch Pathol Lab Med 1978; 102:62–65.
352. Nater B, Bogousslavsky J, Regli F, Stauffer J-C. Stroke patterns with atrial septal aneurysms. Cerebrovasc Dis 1992; 2:342–346.
353. Belkin RN, Hurwitz BJ, Kisslo J. Atrial septal aneurysm: association with cerebrovascular and peripheral embolic events. Stroke 1987; 18:856–862.
354. Cabanes L, Mas JL, Cohen A, et al. Atrial septal aneurysm and patent foramen ovale as risk factors for cryptogenic stroke in patients less than 55 years of age. A study using transesophageal echocardiography. Stroke 1993; 24:1865–1873.
355. Grosgogeat Y, Lhermitte F, Carpenter A, et al. Aneurysme de la cloison interauriculaire revele par une embolie cerebrale. Arch Mal Coeur 1973; 66:169–177.
356. Bogousslavsky J, Garazi S, Jeanrenaud X, et al. Stroke recurrence in patients with patent foramen ovale: the Lausanne study. Neurology 1996; 46:1301–1305.
357. French Study Group on Patent Foramen Ovale and Atrial Septal Aneurysm. Recurrent cerebrovascular events in patients with patent foramen ovale or atrial septal aneurysms and cryptogenic stroke or TIA. Am Heart J 1995; 130:1083–1088.
358. Devuyst G, Bogousslavsky J, Ruchat P, et al. Prognosis after stroke followed by surgical closure of patent foramen ovale: a prospective follow-up study with brain MRI and simultaneous transesophageal and transcranial Doppler ultrasound. Neurology 1996; 47:1162–1166.
359. Bridges ND, Hellensbrand W, Catson L, et al. Transcatheter closure of patent foramen ovale after presumed paradoxical embolism. Circulation 1992; 86:1902–1908.
360. Meyer WW. Cholesterinkrystallembolie kleiner organarterien und ihre folgen. Virchows Arch Pathol Anat 1947; 314:616–638.
361. Winter WJ. Atheromatous emboli: a cause of cerebral infarction. Arch Pathol 1957; 64:137–142.
362. Fisher CM, Gore I, Okabe N, White PD. Atherosclerosis of the carotid and vertebral arteries—extracranial and intracranial. J Neuropathol Exp Neurol 1965; 24:455–476.
363. Tunick PA, Kronzon I. Protruding atherosclerotic plaque in the aortic arch of patients with systemic embolization: a new finding seen by transesophageal echocardiography. Am Heart J 1990; 120:658–660.
364. Tunick PA, Culliford AT, Lamparello PJ, Kronzon I. Atheromatosis of the aortic arch as an occult source of multiple systemic emboli. Ann Intern Med 1991; 114: 391–392.
365. Tunick PA, Perez JL, Kronzon I. Protruding atheromas in the thoracic aorta and systemic embolization. Ann Intern Med 1991; 115:423–427.
366. Karalis DG, Chandrasekaran K, Victor MF, Ross JJ, Mintz GS. Recognition and embolic potential of intraaortic atherosclerotic debris. J Am Coll Cardiol 1991; 17: 73–78.
367. Amarenco P, Duyckaerts C, Tzourio C, et al. The prevalence of ulcerated plaques in the aortic arch in patients with stroke. N Engl J Med 1992; 326:221–225.
368. Amarenco P, Cohen A, Baudrimont M, Bousser M-G. Transesophageal echocardio-

graphic detection of aortic arch disease in patients with cerebral infarction. Stroke 1992; 23:1005–1009.
369. Tobler HG, Edwards JE. Frequency and location of atherosclerotic plaques in the ascending aorta. J Thorac Cardiovasc Surg 1988; 96:304–306.
370. Horowitz DR, Tuhrim S, Budd J, Goldman ME. Aortic plaque in patients with brain ischemia. Neurology 1992; 42:1602–1604.
371. Di Tullio MR, Sacco RL, Gersony D, et al. Aortic atheromas and acute ischemic stroke: a transesophageal echocardiographic study in an ethnically mixed population. Neurology 1996; 46:1560–1566.
372. Toyoda K, Yasaka M, Nagata S, Yamaguchi T. Aortogenic embolic stroke: a transesophageal echocardiographic approach. Stroke 1992; 23:1056–1061.
373. Masuda J, Yutani C, Ogata J, Kuriyama Y, Yamaguchi T. Atheromatous embolism in the brain. A clinicopathologic analysis of 15 autopsy cases. Neurology 1994; 44:1231–1237.
374. French Study of Aortic Plaques in Stroke Group. Atherosclerotic disease of the aortic arch as a risk factor for recurrent ischemic stroke. N Engl J Med 1996; 334: 1216–1221.
375. Mitusch R, Doherty C, Wucherpfennig H, et al. Vascular events during follow-up in patients with aortic arch atherosclerosis. Stroke 1997; 28:36–39.
376. Wickremasinghe HR, Peiris J, Thenabadu PN, Sherifdeen AH. Transient emboligenic aortoarteritis. Noteworth new entity in young stroke patients. Arch Neurol 1978; 35:416–422.
377. Hirst AE, Johns VJ, Kime SW. Dissecting aneurysms of the aorta: a review of 505 cases. Medicine 1958; 37:217–279.
378. Zurbrugg HR, Leupi F, Schupbach P, Althaus U. Duplex scanner study of carotid artery dissection following surgical treatment of aortic dissection type A. Stroke 1988; 19:970–976.
379. Stecker M, Bavaria JE, Barclay DK, et al. Carotid dissection with acute aortic dissection. J Neurovasc Dis 1997; 2:166–171.
380. Bruns JL, Segel DP, Adler S. Control of cholesterol embolization by discontinuation of anticoagulant therapy. Am J Med Sci 1978; 275:105–108.
381. Blackshear JL, Jahangir A, Oldenberg WA, Safford RE. Digital embolization from plaque-related thrombus in the thoracic aorta: identification with transesophageal echocardiography and resolution with warfarin therapy. Mayo Clin Proc 1993; 68: 268–272.
382. Freedberg RS, Tunick PA. Culliform AT, Tatelbaum RJ, Kronzon I. Disappearance of a large intraaortic mass in a patient with prior systemic embolization. Am Heart J 1993; 125:1445–1447.
382a. Fine MJ, Kapoor W, Falanga V. Cholesterol crystal embolization: a review of 221 cases in the English literature. Angiology 1987; 38:769–784.
383. Hausmann D, Gulba D, Bargheer K, et al. Successful thrombolysis of an aortic-arch thrombus in a patient after mesenteric embolism. N Engl J Med 1992; 327: 500–501.
384. Belden JR, Caplan LR, Bojar RM, Payne DD, Blachman P. Treatment of multiple cerebral emboli from an ulcerated, thrombogenic ascending aorta with aortectomy and graft replacement. Neurology 1997; 49:621–622.

385. Duncan A, Rumbaugh C, Caplan LR. Cerebral embolic disease, a complication of carotid aneurysms. Radiology 1979; 133:379–384.
386. Fisher M, Davidson R, Marcus E. Transient focal cortical ischemia as a presenting manifestation of unruptured cerebral aneurysms. Ann Neurol 1980; 8:367–372.
387. Pessin MS, Chimowitz MI, Levine SR, et al. Stroke in patients with fusiform vertebrobasilar aneurysms. Neurology 1989; 39:16–21.
388. Caplan LR, Stein R, Patel D, et al. Intraluminal clot of the carotid artery detected radiographically. Neurology 1984; 34:1175–1181.
389. Hennerici M, Sitzer G, Weger H-D. Carotid Artery Plaques. Basel: Karger, 1987.
390. Fisher CM, Ojemann RG. A clinico-pathologic study of carotid endarterectomy plaques. Rev Neurol (Paris) 1986; 142:573–589.
391. Fisher CM, Ojemann R, Roberson G. Spontaneous dissection of cervicocerebral arteries. Can J Neurol Sci 1978; 5:9–19.
392. Caplan LR, Zarins C, Hemmatti M. Spontaneous dissection of the extracranial vertebral artery. Stroke 1985; 16:1030–1038.
393. Siebler M, Kleinschmidt A, Sitzer M, et al. Cerebral microembolism in symptomatic and asymptomatic high-grade internal carotid artery stenosis. Neurology 1994; 44:615–618.
394. Ries S, Schminke U, Daffertshofer M, et al. High-intensity transcranial signals in carotid artery disease. Cerebrovasc Dis 1995; 5:124–127.
395. Siebler M, Sitzer M, Rose G, et al. Silent cerebral embolism caused by neurologically symptomatic high-grade carotid stenosis: event rates before and after carotid endarterectomy. Brain 1993; 116:1005–1015.
396. North American Carotid Endarterectomy Trial Collaborators. Beneficial effect of carotid endarterectomy in symptomatic patients with high-grade carotid stenosis. N Engl J Med 1991; 325:445–453.
397. European Carotid Surgery Trialists Collaborator Group. MRC European Carotid Surgery Trial: interim results for symptomatic patients with severe (70–99%) and with mild (0–29%) carotid stenosis. Lancet 1991; 337:1235–1243.
398. Streifler JY, Eliasziw M, Benavente OR, et al. The risk of stroke in patients with first-ever retinal or hemispheral transient ischemic attacks and high-grade carotid stenosis. Arch Neurol 1995; 52:246–249.
399. Hennerici M, Hulsbower HB, Hefter K, et al. Natural history of asymptomatic extracranial disease: results of a long term prognostic study. Brain 1987; 110:777–791.
400. Norris JW, Zhu CZ. Silent stroke and carotid stenosis. Stroke 1992; 23:483–485.
401. Norris JW. Risks of cerebral infarction, myocardial infarction and vascular death in patients with asymptomatic carotid disease, transient ischemic attacks and stroke. Cerebrovasc Dis 1992; 2(suppl 1):2–5.
402. Norris JW, Zhu CZ, Bornstein N, Chambers BR. Vascular risks of asymptomatic carotid stenosis. Stroke 1991; 22:1485–1490.
403. Executive Committee for the Asymptomatic Carotid Atherosclerosis Study. Endarterectomy for asymptomatic carotid artery stenosis. JAMA 1995; 273:1421–1428.
404. Nicolaides A, Kalodiki E, Ramaswami G, et al. The significance of cerebral infarcts on CT scans in patients with transient ischemic attacks. In: Bernstein EF, Callow

AD, Nicolaides AJ, Shifrin EG, eds. Cerebral Revascularisation. London: Med-Orion, 1993:159–178.
405. Fazekas F, Fazekas G, Schmidt R, et al. Magnetic resonance imaging correlates of transient cerebral ischemic attacks. Stroke 1996; 27:607–611.
406. Lodder J, Hupperts R, Boreas A, Kessels F. The size of territorial brain infarction on CT relates to the degree of internal carotid artery obstruction. J Neurol 1996; 243:345–349.
407. Wechsler LR, Kistler JP, Davis KR, Kaminski MJ. The prognosis of carotid siphon stenosis. Stroke 1986; 17:714–718.
408. Craig DR, Meguro K, Watridge C, et al. Intracranial internal carotid artery stenosis. Stroke 1982; 13:825–828.
409. Chimowitz MI, Kokkinos J, Strong J, et al. The Warfarin-Aspirin Symptomatic Intracranial Disease Study. Neurology 1995; 45:1488–1493.
410. Imparato AM, Riles TS, Gorstein F. The carotid bifurcation plaque: pathological findings associated with cerebral ischemia. Stroke 1979; 10:238–245.
411. Gronholdt M-LM, Nordestgaard BG, Nielsen TG, Sillesen H. Echolucent carotid artery plaques are associated with elevated levels of fasting and postprandial triglyceride-rich lipoproteins. Stroke 1996; 27:2166–2172.
412. European Carotid Plaque Study Group. Carotid artery plaque composition: relationship to clinical presentation and ultrasound B-mode imaging. Eur J Vasc Endovasc Surg 1995; 10:23–30.
413. Geroulakos G, Ramaswami G, Nicolaides A, et al. Characterization of symptomatic and asymptomatic carotid plaques using high-resolution real-time ultrasonography. Br J Surg 1993; 80:1274–1277.
414. Caplan JR, Gorelick PB, Hier DB. Race, sex, and occlusive cerebrovascular disease: a review. Stroke 1986; 17:648–655.
415. Gorelick PB, Caplan LR, Hier DB, et al. Racial differences in the distribution of anterior circulation occlusive disease. Neurology 1984; 34:54–59.
416. Gorelick PB, Caplan LR, Hier DB, et al. Racial differences in the distribution of posterior circulation occlusive disease. Stroke 1985; 16:785–790.
417. Feldmann E, Daneault N, Kwan E, et al. Chinese-white differences in the distribution of occlusive cerebrovascular disease. Neurology 1990; 40:1541–1545.
418. Hutchinson EC, Yates PO. Carotico-vertebral stenosis. Lancet 1957; 1:2–8.
419. Hutchinson EC, Yates PO. The cervical portion of the vertebral artery. a clinico-pathological study. Brain 1956; 79:319–331.
420. Caplan LR. The E Graeme Robertson lecture. Vertebrobasilar embolism. Clin Exp Neurol 1991; 28:1–23.
421. Caplan LR, Tettenborn B. Vertebrobasilar occlusive disease: review of selected aspects. 2. Posterior circulation embolism. Cerebrovasc Dis 1992; 2:320–326.
422. Caplan LR, Tettenborn B. Vertebrobasilar occlusive disease: review of selected aspects. 1. Spontaneous dissection of extracranial and intracranial posterior circulation arteries. Cerebrovasc Dis 1992; 2:256–265.
423. Caplan LR, Baquis G, Pessin MS, et al. Dissection of the intracranial vertebral artery. Neurology 1988; 38:868–877.
424. Pop G, Sutherland GR, Koudstaal P, et al. Transesophageal echocardiography in

the detection of intracardiac embolic sources in patients with transient ischemic attacks. Stroke 1990; 21:560–565.
425. DeRook FA, Comess KA, Albers GW, Popp RL. Transesophageal echocardiography in the evaluation of stroke. Ann Intern Med 1992; 117:922–932.
426. Grullon C, Alam M, Rosman HS, et al. Transesophageal echocardiography in unselected patients with focal cerebral ischemia: when is it useful? Cerebrovasc Dis 1994; 4:139–145.
427. Daniel WG, Mugge A. Transesophageal echocardiography. N Engl J Med 1995; 332:1268–1279.
428. Horowitz DR, Tuhrim S, Weinberger J, et al. Transesophageal echocardiography: diagnostic and clinical applications in the evaluation of the stroke patient. J Stroke Cerebrovasc Dis 1997; 6:332–336.
429. McNamara RL, Lima JAC, Whelton PK, Powe NR. Echocardiographic identification of cardiovascular sources of emboli to guide clinical management of stroke: a cost-effectiveness analysis. Ann Intern Med 1997; 127:775–787.
430. Johnson LL, Pohost GM. Nuclear cardiology. In: Schlant RC, Alexander RW, eds. Hurst's The Heart. 8th ed. New York: McGraw-Hill, 1994:2281–2323.
431. Ezekowiz MD, Wilson DA, Smith EO, et al. Comparison of indium-111 platelet scintigraphy and two-dimensional echocardiography in the diagnosis of left ventricular thrombi. N Engl J Med 1982; 306:1509–1513.
432. Weinberger J, Azhar S, Danisi F, Hayes R, Goldman M. A new noninvasive technique for imaging atherosclerotic plaque in the aortic arch of stroke patients by transcutaneous real-time B-mode ultrasonography. Stroke 1998; 29:673–676.
433. Brant-Zawadzki M, Atkinson D, Detrick M, Bradley WG, Scidmore G. Fluid-attenuated inversion recovery (FLAIR) for assessment of cerebral infarction: initial clinical experience in 50 patients. Stroke 1996; 27:1187–1191.
434. Kido DK, Panzer RJ, Szumowski J, et al. Clinical evaluation of stenosis of the carotid bifurcation with magnetic resonance angiographic techniques. Arch Neurol 1991; 48:484–489.
435. Riles TS, Eidelman EM, Litt AW, et al. Comparison of magnetic resonance angiography, conventional angiography, and Duplex scanning. Stroke 1992; 23:341–346.
436. Anderson CM, Saloner D, Lee RE, et al. Assessment of carotid artery stenosis by MR angiography: comparison with x-ray angiography and color-coded Doppler ultrasound. AJNR 1992; 13:989–1003.
437. Gillard JH, Oliverio P, Barker PB, Oppenheimer SM, Bryan RN. MR angiography in acute cerebral ischemia of the anterior circulation: a preliminary report. AJNR 1997; 18:343–350.
438. Johnson BA, Heiserman JE, Drayer BP, Keller P. Intracranial MR angiography: its role in the integrated approach to brain infarction. AJNR 1994; 15:901–908.
439. Rother J, Wentz K-U, Rautenberg W, et al. Magnetic resonance angiography in vertebrobasilar ischemia. Stroke 1993; 24:1310–1315.
440. Bogousslavsky J, Regli F, Maeder P, et al. The etiology of posterior circulation infarcts: a prospective study using magnetic resonance imaging and magnetic resonance angiography. Neurology 1993; 43:1528–1533.
441. Warach S, Chien D, Li W, et al. Fast magnetic resonance diffusion-weighted imaging of acute human stroke. Neurology 1992; 42:1717–1723.

442. Sorenson AG, Buonanno FS, Gonzales RG, et al. Hyperacute stroke: evaluation with combined multisection diffusion-weighted and hemodynamically-weighted echo-planar MR imaging. Radiology 1996; 199:391–401.
443. Schwartz RB, Jones KM, Chernoff DM, et al. Common carotid artery bifurcation: evaluation with spiral CT. Radiology 1992; 185:513–519.
444. Alberico RA, Patel M, Casey S, et al. Evaluation of the circle of Willis with three-dimensional CT angiography in patients with suspected intracranial aneurysms. AJNR 1995; 16:1571–1578.
445. von Reutern G-M, von Budingen HJ. Ultrasound diagnosis of cerebrovascular disease. Doppler sonography of the extra- and intracranial arteries, Duplex scanning. New York: Thieme, 1993.
446. Hennerici M, Freund H-J. Efficacy of C-W Doppler and Duplex system examinations for the evaluation of extracranial carotid disease. J Clin Ultrasound 1984; 12: 155–161.
447. Steinke W, Kloetzsch C, Hennerici M. Carotid artery disease assessed by color Doppler flow imaging: correlation with standard Doppler sonography and angiography. AJNR 1990; 11:259–266.
448. Steinke W, Hennerici M, Rautenberg W, Mohr JP. Symptomatic and asymptomatic high-grade carotid stenosis in Doppler color-flow imaging. Neurology 1992; 42: 131–138.
449. Sitzer M, Furst G, Fischer H, et al. Between-method correlation in quantifying carotid stenosis. Stroke 1993; 24:1513–1518.
450. Ackerstaff RGA. Duplex scanning of the aortic arch and vertebral arteries. In: Bernstein EF, ed. Vascular Diagnosis. 4th ed. St. Louis: Mosby, 1993:315–321.
451. Touboul PJ, Bousser M-G, LaPlane D, Castaigne P. Duplex scanning of the vertebral arteries. Stroke 1986; 17:921–923.
452. Sturzenegger M. Ultrasound findings in spontaneous carotid artery dissection: the value of Duplex sonography. Arch Neurol 1991; 48:1057–1063.
453. Sturzenegger M, Mattle HP, Rivon A, et al. Ultrasound findings in spontaneous extracranial vertebral artery dissection. Stroke 1993; 24:1910–1921.
454. Caplan LR, Brass LM, DeWitt LD, et al. Transcranial Doppler ultrasound: present status. Neurology 1990; 40:696–700.
455. Caplan LR, Feinberg WM, Fisher MJ, del Zoppo GJ. The Blood in Brain Ischemia. Basic Concepts and Clinical Relevance. Caplan LR, ed. London: Springer-Verlag, 1995:83–126.
456. Yasaka M, Yamaguchi T, Miyashita T, et al. Predisposing factors of recurrent embolization in cardiogenic cerebral embolism. Stroke 1990; 21:1000–1007.
457. Takano K, Yamaguchi T, Kato H, Omae T. Acivation of coagulation in acute cardioembolic stroke. Stroke 1991; 22:12–16.
458. Sevitt S. Fat Embolism. London, Butterworth & Co., 1962.
459. Thomas JE, Ayyar DR. Systemic fat embolism. A diagnostic profile in 24 patients. Arch Neurol 1972; 26:517–523.
460. Dines DE, Linscheid RL, Didier EP. Fat embolism syndrome. Mayo Clin Proc 1972; 47:237–240.
461. Dines DE, Burgher LW, Okazaki H. The clinical and pathological correlation of fat embolism syndrome. Mayo Clin Proc 1975; 50:407–411.

462. Jacobson DM, Terrence CF, Reinmuth OM. The neurologic manifestations of fat embolism. Neurology 1986; 36:847–851.
463. Hill JD, Aguilar MJ, Baranco AP, Gerbode F. Neuropathological manifestations of cardiac surgery. Ann Thorac Surg 1969; 7:409–517.
464. Ghatal NR, Sinnenberg RJ, DeBlois GG. Cerebral fat embolism following cardiac surgery. Stroke 1983; 14:619–621.
465. Charache S, Page DL. Infarction of bone marrow in sickle cell disorders. Ann Intern Med 1967; 67:1195–1200.
466. Hutchinson RM, Merrick MV, White JM. Fat embolism in sickle cell disease. J Clin Pathol 1973; 26:620–622.
467. Vichinsky E, Williams K, Das M, et al. Pulmonary fat embolism: a distinct cause of severe acute chest syndrome in sickle cell anemia. Blood 1994; 83:3107–3112.
468. Shelley WM, Curtis EM. Bone marrow and fat embolism in sickle cell anemia and sickle cell–hemoglobin C disease. Bull Johns Hopkins Hosp 1958; 103:8–25.
468a. Rosen JM, Mark EJ. Case records of the Massachusetts General Hospital: case 23–1998. N Engl J Med 1998; 339:254–261.
469. Oh WH, Mital MA. Fat embolism: current concepts of pathogenesis, diagnosis, and treatment. Orthop Clin North Am 1978; 9:769–779.
470. Ing HR, Pellegrini VD. Fat embolism syndrome: a review of the pathophysiological basis of treatment. Clin Orthop 1982; 165:68–82.
471. Fuchsig P, Brucke P, Blumel G, Gottlob R. Current concepts. A new clinical and experimental concept on fat embolism. N Engl J Med 1967; 276:1192–1193.
472. Pell AC, Hughes D, Keating J, et al. Brief report. Fulminating fat embolism syndrome caused by paradoxical embolism through a patent foramen ovale. N Engl J Med 1993; 329:926–929.
473. Oostenbrugge RJ, Freling G, Lodder J, Lalisang R, Twijnstra A. Fatal stroke due to paradoxical fat embolism. Cerebrovasc Dis 1996; 6:313–314.
474. Chastre J, Fagon J-Y, Soler P, et al. Bronchoalveolar lavage for rapid diagnosis of the fat embolism syndrome in trauma patients. Ann Intern Med 1990; 113:583–588.
475. Godeau B, Schaeffer A, Bachir D, et al. Bronchoalveolar lavage in adult sickle cell patients with acute chest syndrome: value for diagnostic assessment of fat embolism. Am J Respir Care Med 1996; 153:1691–1696.
476. Kamenar E, Burger PC. Cerebral fat embolism: a neuropathological study of a microembolic state. Stroke 1980; 11:477–484.
477. Menkin M, Schwartzman RJ. Cerebral air embolism. Report of five cases and review of the literature. Arch Neurol 1977; 34:169–170.
477a. Wijman CAC, Kase CS, Jacobs AK, Whitehead RE. Cerebral air embolism as a cause of stroke during cardiac catheterization. Neurology 1998; 51:318–319.
478. Gillen HW. Symptomatology of cerebral gas embolism. Neurology 1968; 18:507–512.
479. Hwang T-L, Fremax R, Sears ES, et al. Confirmation of cerebral air embolism with computerized tomography. Ann Neurol 1983; 13:214–215.
480. Lefkovitz NW, Roessman U, Kori S. Major cerebral infarction from tumor embolus. Stroke 1986; 17:555–557.

3

Encephalopathies and Neurological Effects of Drugs Used in Cardiac Patients

INTRODUCTION

Confusion, decreased state of alertness, diminished intellectual functioning, and focal neurological signs are very common in patients with heart disease, especially those who have congestive heart failure. Some of these neurological abnormalities are explained by brain embolism arising from the heart, aorta, and occlusive lesions within the cervicocranial arteries, a topic that was thoroughly discussed in Chapter 2. Occasionally, the neurological abnormalities relate to episodes of hypotension and systemic hypoperfusion, a topic discussed in Chapter 1. In many other patients the neurological symptoms and signs are caused by various physiological and biochemical perturbations that develop in patients with cardiac disease and congestive heart failure. Sometimes the neurological findings are side effects or complications of medicines used to treat patients with cardiovascular disease. This chapter considers non-stroke-related complications of cardiac diseases and congestive heart failure and their medical treatments.

ENCEPHALOPATHY

Definition of Encephalopathy

Brain function depends to a great extent on the milieu in which the brain exists. Just as a freshwater fish cannot swim, or even survive, in ocean waters, the brain is quite sensitive to any alteration in its chemical or physical environment. A very common example of this sensitivity is provided by experience with alcohol. Inebriation and drunkedness are examples of altered brain functioning hopefully reversed completely by a sober interval of abstention from alcohol. Most biochemical perturbations affect the brain globally, often first affecting the most complex intellectual functions which are most vulnerable. Diffuse brain dysfunction related to potentially reversible biochemical and physiological changes is usually referred to as *encephalopathy*. When the dysfunction relates to endogenous abnormalities in various body organs, the term *metabolic encephalopathy* is often used, while dysfunction due to exogenous factors such as drugs and toxic substance exposure is usually called *toxic encephalopathy*.

Although the brain accounts for only about 2% of body mass, it is a disproportionate consumer of resources. The brain receives about 20% of cardiac output, consumes about 65% of the glucose used by the body, and uses about 20% of the body's oxygen supply [1]. Cerebral cortical gray matter nerve cells metabolize about 75% of the oxygen used by the brain although gray matter accounts for only 20% of brain mass [1]. The brain has enormous needs and demands for nutritional substrates and blood flow, explaining the vulnerability of this very complex and precise organ to metabolic perturbations. Most of the metabolism of the brain is aerobic (utilization of sugars in the presence of oxygen) and much of the energy produced in the brain is used to maintain normal ionic gradients between brain cells and the extracellular space [1]. The most important of these gradients across cell membranes are those for sodium, potassium, hydrogen ion, and calcium [1].

The first metabolic encephalopathy that was studied and described in clinical detail was hepatic encephalopathy [2,3]. Adams and Foley analyzed the clinical findings in patients with liver failure, usually due to alcoholism, who were hospitalized at the Boston City Hospital [2]. They emphasized the presence of a wide variety of intellectual and behavioral abnormalities, personality changes, and reduced states of alertness as prominent findings [2]. Table 1 lists the findings during various stages of hepatic encephalopathy. Sometimes the patients studied by Adams and Foley had acute and severe neurological deterioration (acute encephalopathy), and in other patients the neurological symptoms and signs were more chronic and fluctuated from time to time. Since recognition of the hepatic encephalopathy syndrome during the 1950s, similar encephalopathic findings have been recognized in patients who have a wide variety of metabolic and biochemical disorders. The chronicity and reversibility of the neurological signs depend on the nature, severity, and course of the causative metabolic disorder.

Recognition of the Presence of an Encephalopathy

All encephalopathies have six features in common:

Altered state of alertness and consciousness
Global decrease in all intellectual functions

TABLE 1 Clinical Stages of Liver Encephalopathy

Stage I	Mild confusion
	Euphoria or depressed feelings
	Decreased ability to sustain attention
	Slowing of performance of mental tasks
	Untidiness
	Slurred speech
	Irritability
	Altered sleep patterns
Stage II	Drowsiness and lethargy
	Gross deficits in ability to perform mental tasks
	Personality changes and inappropriate behaviors
	Intermittent disorientation, especially to time
	Incontinent on occasion
Stage III	Somnolent but arousable
	Cannot perform mental tasks
	Persistent disorientation to time and place
	Amnesia
	Incoherent speech
Stage IV	Coma with or without response to painful stimuli

Source: Ref. 3.

Variability from minute to minute and from hour to hour in the neurological findings
Asterixis—a metabolic ''flap''
Diffuse slowing of rhythms on electroencephalograms (EEGs)
Reversibility after correction of the biochemical and physiological abnormalities

Metabolic abnormalities usually depress brain functions, explaining the depressed state of alertness, limb hypotonia, and decreased respirations that develop in patients with encephalopathies. Some metabolic abnormalities cause heightened excitability of neural structures, explaining hallucinations, seizures, and increased muscle contractions [1]. Regional differences in tissue metabolism and metabolic requirements explain why some chemical changes affect some brain regions more than others [1]. For example, the cerebellum is especially vulnerable to the effects of high levels of blood alcohol.

Decreased alertness is a universal finding in encephalopathic patients. The earliest stage of altered alertness is drowsiness. Patients may need prodding or stimulation to remain fully awake and alert. They often sleep when left unstimulated. Loss of consciousness and restlessness with agitation and sometimes delirium follow if the encephalopathy worsens. Patients may be unable to remain still, move restlessly in bed, and become unable to hold and continue a coherent conversation. They flit from one topic to another and become quite unable to concentrate on queries or directions. Stupor and coma ensue as the encephalopathy becomes more severe.

All intellectual functions are usually compromised to some extent. The most complex and difficult functions, e.g., mathematical computations, abstractions, and writing, are affected earliest and most severely. Memory, language, planning, concentration, persistence in tasks, visual-spatial abilities, and computational skills are all affected to some degree. Stroke and other focal brain disorders such as tumors and abscesses, in contrast, usually affect only isolated cognitive and behavioral functions depending on the side and region of the brain involved by the focal process. Perceptual abilities are also affected and patients may have visual illusions and frank hallucinations. Testing of intellectual functions is an integral part of the physical examination, at least as important as testing of strength, sensation, and vision.

Screening of cognitive abilities can usually be performed during a short period of time using rather simple tests. *Language should always be checked first*, because the ability of patients to follow and understand spoken and written questions and directions and patients' ability to communicate answers and follow directions depend on preservation of language. When the patient speaks another language, either because their native tongue is different or because of aphasia, other intellectual functions are very difficult to assess. Table 2 lists bedside tasks used to check the intactness of language abilities. The brain's language zones are located in the parasylvian region of the dominant cerebral hemisphere.
Visual-spatial abilities are also very important to assess. Patients are asked to draw simple objects such as a house, clock, daisy, or bicycle. Then they are asked to copy a simple diagram such as that shown in Figure 1 or the Reye figure shown in Figure 2. Depicting accurately the shape, size, angles, symmetry, and proportions on spontaneous drawings and in making copies of objects is mostly

TABLE 2 Screening of Language Functions

1. Write a few sentences about: your work, the town in which you now live, the last or next election, etc.
2. Read aloud a paragraph from the newspaper or a magazine
3. Name common objects present in the room or in the examiner's doctor bag or pockets, e.g., keys, coin, pen, button, buttonhole, tie, shoelace, watch, ring, etc.
4. Name from recall 5 items in given categories, e.g., articles of clothing, means of travel, zoo animals, fruits, vegetables, articles of apparrel
5. Name or identify 5 famous individuals from photographs

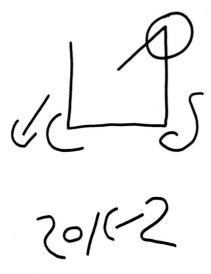

Fig. 1 A complex figure for the patient to copy.

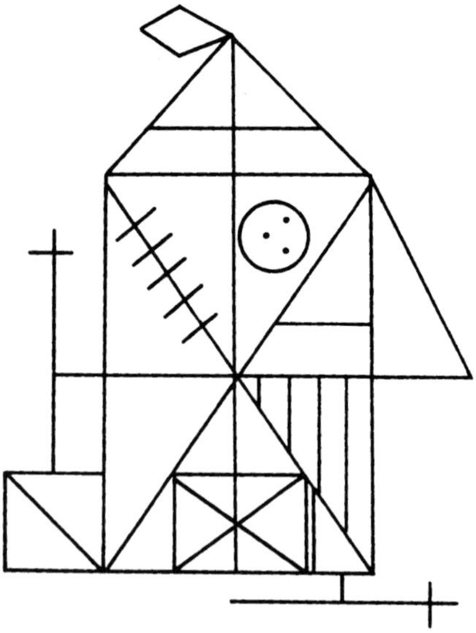

Fig. 2 The Reye figure for the patient to copy.

a function of the inferior parietal lobe on the right side of the brain. Another very useful strategy for screening visual-spatial functions as well as observational facility and language is to show patients pictures or cartoons in magazines. The examiner watches the patient scan the picture. Do they search the picture carefully and systematically or instead direct their gaze randomly or in a cursory fashion? After the picture has been removed from the patient's vision, the patient is asked to describe what he or she saw. Specific queries can then be posed depending on the patient's initial responses, such as, how many people are shown in the picture? How many are men and how many women? What are the people doing? Where do you think the scene took place? Memory retention can then be tested later by asking the patients to recall the pictures shown earlier.

Memory should always be tested actively by giving the patient items to be recalled later. Passive memory testing, that is, asking the patient to describe recent personal activities such as meals and occurrences, is very unreliable because patients with severe amnesia such as those with Korsakoff's syndrome, often confabulate answers which the examiner usually has no way to verify. To save time, the patient can be asked to recall items used in previous tests. Ask patients to tell you about the paragraph that they read, the items that you had asked them to name, the picture scenes that you had already shown them, and the names of famous people that they had been asked to identify from pictures shown earlier. Alternatively, patients are told a brief story that contains five or more facts, and 5 to 10 minutes later they are asked to recall the story. Testing is more effective if patients are told at the time of the original tests that they will be asked later to recall the items shown as a test of their memory.

Encephalopathic patients have difficulty *maintaining concentration on tasks*. Although they may understand the nature of a request and can begin to answer correctly, they are unable to persevere and finish the task. For example, ask the patient to name 10 colors, zoo animals, articles of clothing, fruits, etc. If they can begin by producing two or three correct names then they clearly understand the directions and the nature of the task and have sufficient language abilities to supply items within the category requested. The inability to persevere and give further items usually means that they cannot sustain attention long enough to finish the task. The frontal lobes and their reciprocal connections with the basal ganglia and thalamus are the anatomical structures most responsible for initiating and persevering with tasks. These structures are quite vulnerable to metabolic perturbations. Alternative tests of concentration and attention are: counting backward quickly from 20 to 0; reciting numbers after the examiner both forward and backward; crossing off all the letter A's on a printed page; counting backward from 100 by threes or sevens.

Valuable data about patients' functioning can be gained from others. Visitors, family, roommates, and the nursing staff should be asked about the state of alertness of patients. Do they spend most of the day sleeping or dozing off periodically? Are they alert enough to read, watch television, carry on conversations with visitors, etc.? Are they difficult to arouse in the morning or after naps? Are they alert enough to fill out their menu requests and to eat the food served on their tray?

Asterixis, a metabolic flap, is an important sign in patients with encephalopathy. Although asterixis was first described in patients with hepatic encephalopathy, it is a nonspecific sign and is present in patients with encephalopathy of diverse causes. Asterixis is most often elicited by asking the patient to hold the upper limbs outstretched in front of them with the wrists and fingers held in full extension. After a short latency, side-to-side movements of the fingers, and flexion/extension movements of the fingers at the metacarpophalangeal joints and at the wrist appear [4,5]. The flexion movements are quick; the flexion phase is much more rapid than the extension movements used to return the fingers and wrists to their former positions. Asterixis can also be elicited in the lower limbs by having patients dorsiflex the feet with the legs elevated and extended [4]. Alternatively the examiner can use his or her arms placed under the patient's knees to gently lift the lower extremities off the bed while the patient's thighs and legs are flexed. Flapping movements of the legs and feet appear. Electrical studies during asterixis show an absence of electrical activity during the flapping movements followed by compensatory muscle contractions as the extensor muscles restore the posture of the limbs [4,5]. Asterixis is really a failure to maintain a sustained posture [1,4–6]. It represents a central nervous system disorder of the mechanisms that sustain muscle contractions. Just as the patient cannot sustain concentration on mental tasks, they also cannot sustain attention to hold a fixed limb posture. Asterixis usually can be elicited when some degree of reduced alertness develops. Some degree of attention and wakefulness is required. When patients become frankly stuporous, asterixis may not be elicitable.

Differential Diagnosis of Toximetabolic Encephalopathy in Cardiac Patients

Cardiac patients, especially those who are acutely ill with congestive heart failure, have a wide variety of potential explanations for encephalopathy. Most often encephalopathy is related to perturbations of the biochemical makeup of the body's internal milieu. In fact, encephalopathies are often referred to as "toximetabolic" to capture the biochemical nature of the disorder. Acute and rapidly developing metabolic changes are more likely to cause an encephalopathy than disorders that develop slowly. The most common causes of encephalopathy in cardiac patients are: (1) dysfunction of other systemic organs especially the kidneys, lungs, and liver; (2) effects of pharmacologic agents used to treat cardiovascular abnormalities or used for pain control or sedation/tranquilization; (3) hypovolemia; and (4) electrolyte and acid-base abnormalities. The differential diagnosis of toximetabolic encephalopathies can be thought of in terms of whether the condition is *endogenous* or *exogenous* and whether the abnormality involves *too little* or *too much* of a biochemical/metabolic ingredient. Endogenous disorders arise from changes within the biochemical milieu of the body whereas exogenous conditions include various deficiency states and exposure to potentially toxic substances. Table 3 lists the differential considerations using these categories. The effects of drugs used to treat cardiac patients are discussed in more detail in the second half of this chapter.

Organ dysfunctions and organ failures are common in patients with cardiac decompensation. All organs are dependent on the heart to supply an adequate amount of blood. Organ dysfunction is often related to poor perfusion or congestion with increased venous pressure, or a combination of decreased perfusion and congestion. In order to adequately perfuse organs that have increased venous pressures and impaired venous drainage, the perfusion pressure supplying that organ with blood must increase in order to maintain an effective arterio-venous pressure differential. Circulatory compromise due to cardiac dysfunction may impair the ability to augment perfusion. The nutritive contents of the blood, espe-

TABLE 3 Differential Diagnosis of Toximetabolic Encephalopathies

Too much	Too little
Endogenous	
Liver failure—substances not detoxified in the liver	O_2
Renal failure—urea and other excreta	Na^+
Pulmonary failure—CO_2	Thyroid
Na^+	Blood (anemia)
Ca^{2+}	Intravascular volume
Thyroid	Sugar
Adrenal corticosteroids	Phosphate
Viscosity	
Sugar	
Ketone bodies	
Acid (reduced pH)	
Osmolarity	
Exogenous	
Alcohol	B_{12}
Psychotropic drugs	Thiamine
haloperidol	Niacin
benzodiazepines	Pyridoxine
barbiturates	
Morphine	

cially oxygen, sugar, and ketone bodies, also effects the delivery of needed metabolic substrates to each organ. Although most organs can utilize a variety of substrates, neurons in the brain are quite dependent on sugar and oxygen for survival.

Pulmonary congestion, pulmonary edema, and pleural effusions are all common in patients with cardiac decompensation. Patients with heart disease very often also have concurrent chronic bronchopulmonary disease, especially if they smoke cigarettes. Depression of alertness and toximetabolic disorders of all causes can depress respiratory function causing hypoventilation [1]. Hypoventilation can lead to hypoxia and CO_2 retention. Morphine, sedatives, and psychotropic agents that are often used to treat cardiac pain and anxiety can depress ventilatory drive and further decrease ventilation. Pulmonary embolism, an important complication of congestive heart failure, can further compromise ventilation and perfusion within the lung.

Liver congestion is another very frequent accompaniment of congestive heart failure, especially in patients with right heart disease and tricuspid valve incompetence. Increased pressure in the inferior vena cava and hepatic veins is caused by the heart's inability to efficiently pump blood coming to it from the systemic venous system. The increased pressure in veins draining the liver leads to an increase in pressure in the intrahepatic veins with compression and necrosis of hepatic lobules. Abnormalities of liver enzymes may occur in patients with congestive heart failure but frank hepatic coma is rare. Some patients with chronic congestive heart failure or constrictive pericarditis may develop cardiac cirrhosis related to chronic liver congestion. These patients may develop signs of liver failure when acute heart failure is superimposed on the chronic state.

Renal dysfunction with elevation of blood urea nitrogen and blood creatinine levels may also occur in patients with acute cardiac decompensation. Many patients with hypertension and atherosclerotic coronary artery disease have nephrosclerosis and chronic kidney disease due to concurrent involvement of the small and large renal arteries. Changes in blood and serum volume and acid-base components are common in patients with congestive heart failure and are often related to the use of diuretics and other pharmacologic agents. Kidney congestion and reduced perfusion also occur. Renal failure is especially common in patients who have transient or persistent hypotension during cardiac decompensation and its treatment. Renal and hepatic dysfunction affect the metabolism and excretion of drugs. The serum level of drugs excreted by the kidneys increases and remains higher in patients when they have renal failure. Toxic effects of drugs previously well tolerated may develop in the presence of renal failure even when the dose of the drugs is not changed.

Patients with *fever, infection, and pain* often develop confusion and an encephalopathic clinical picture without any definite abnormality of metabolic parameters measured by blood tests. Of course, pneumonia, urinary infections, and other septic complications are common in patients with cardiac decompensation. Chest pain is also common and may be multifactoral. The release of substances into the circulation such as cytokines, endorphins, and other agents, some as yet undiscovered and unidentified, are probably responsible for the encephalopathy of infectious illnesses and pain.

Patients who are acutely ill because of congestive heart failure frequently have more than one metabolic abnormality. For example, a patient with congestive heart failure who has an encephalopathy may have slight hypoxemia, slight hyponatremia, modest elevation of blood urea nitrogen, and a low-grade fever. Each of these problems may be insufficient alone to explain the encephalopathy, but when added together the combined effect of all the metabolic changes may be enough to cause important brain dysfunction. If a person takes two shots of Scotch, one shot of bourbon, three glasses of wine, and two cans of beer, he or she would become "drunk." Yet the level of Scotch, bourbon, beer, or wine, if separately measurable, would not be very high. When summed, the effect of all of these alcohol-containing drinks can be profound.

The clinical neurological findings are very similar in patients with encephalopathies of all causes with some minor differences. Patients with *hepatic encephalopathy* nearly always have tachypnea and a respiratory alkalosis. Abnormal movements, myoclonic jerks, dystonic posturing of the limbs, and choreoathetotic movements of the arms are often present in patients with hepatic encephalopathy but are less common in other encephalopathies. Most patients with liver failure have important abnormalities of motor and reflex function found on examination, including weakness, stiffness, limb ataxia and incoordination, increased deep tendon reflexes, and Babinski signs.

Uremic patients and those with severe hypoventilation ("CO_2 narcosis") are usually apathetic, abulic, and inactive and have less motor abnormalities and abnormal limb movements than those with hepatic encephalopathy. Abulic patients have a markedly reduced amount of speech and spontaneous activity. When asked questions or directed to do an action, they often fail to respond or do so only after a long latent interval. Their responses are brief. They have difficulty persevering with tasks. Abulic patients are described as generally inactive, disinterested, and quiet. Seizures and twitching movements of the limbs are common in patients with renal failure and those with hyponatremia and severe hyperglycemia. Uremic patients often have fine muscular twitching resembling fasciculations and may also have multifocal myoclonic muscle contractions especially involving facial muscles [4,6]. Patients with chronic renal insufficiency are invariably pale and anemic and have a polyneuropathy characterized by burning feet, absent ankle reflexes, reduced knee jerks, and diminished vibration and position sensation in the feet.

The chemical makeup of the brain and cerebrospinal fluid (CSF) is quite different from other body tissues. Equilibration of brain metabolism with restoration of normal brain function often takes time even after blood tests return to normal. Patients with electrolyte and acid-base abnormalities, and hyperosmolar states may take a particularly long time to regain their baseline neurological functions. We have cared for patients who, for weeks after correction of hyponatremia, acidosis, and nonketotic hyperosmolar coma, remain confused, hallucinate, and show prominent intellectual and behavioral abnormalities. These neurological signs often return to normal slowly over days to weeks after correction of the metabolic abnormality.

Cardiac Encephalopathies Without Apparent Other Causes

Some patients with acute and chronic congestive heart failure have the clinical neurological findings of an encephalopathy without any recognized liver, renal, pulmonary, or definite biochemical or metabolic abnormality detected by blood tests sufficient to explain the encephalopathy. These patients are often sleepy, confused, inattentive, and unable to consistently sustain intelligent conversations. There are two different clinical syndromes found in patients with cardiac encephalopathy—one that resembles in every way the findings discussed in patients with systemic organ failures and metabolic perturbations, and a different clinical syndrome that closely mimics that found in patients with hydrocephalus.

The mechanisms of brain dysfunction in patients with congestive heart failure are multifactorial. Systemic venous pressure is increased causing pari passu an increase in pressure in the venous dural sinuses and veins in the cranial cavity. Increased intracranial venous pressure diminishes absorption of CSF and so an increased amount of fluid accumulates in the cisterns around the brain, in the subarachnoid spaces, and sometimes within the ventricles. The CSF pressure may be elevated when measured by lumbar puncture. Brain edema may result from the increased venous pressure and increased amounts of CSF. In order to perfuse the brain and maintain an effective arteriovenous pressure difference adequate for brain perfusion, arterial pressure and cerebral blood flow must be maintained and even augmented in patients with elevated intracranial venous pressures. Cardiac decompensation can limit the ability of the heart and systemic circulation to augment cerebral blood flow. Hypoxia related to pulmonary dysfunction and hypoventilation reduces the oxygen content of the blood that reaches neurons in the brain. Of course, dysfunction of other organs, and electrolyte, blood volume, acid-base abnormalities, and drugs also can compound the cardiac encephalopathy. Neurological abnormalities occur when cardiac failure is most severe and the clinical signs are indistinguishable from those found in patients with renal failure and CO_2 narcosis.

A somewhat different clinical picture, similar to that found in patients with hydrocephalus, can also be found in patients with congestive heart failure. This syndrome can develop during treatment of congestive heart failure and may occur even after cardiac compensation when the patient is recovering from heart failure. The major feature of this syndrome is *abulia*. Abulic patients have severely reduced spontaneous behavior. They seem content to sit or lie about without doing much. They show little or no interest in television, reading, listening to the radio, conversations, or any other activity. The quantity of spontaneous initiated speech is much reduced. When asked questions or urged to perform tasks, abulic patients often fail to respond or do so only after a relatively long interval. When questions or directions are repeated, patients often say that they had heard you the first time but just couldn't get rolling to reply or act. Responses, when they are forthcoming, are generally short, laconic, and terse. Patients don't persist with familiar tasks—for example, name 10 zoo animals, 10 articles of clothing; count backward from 20 to 1. Intellectual functions including memory, language, and ability to draw and copy are preserved although these functions take longer than usual to perform and require frequent prodding to complete. The patients remain alert despite their inactivity and slowness in contrast to all other encephalopathies that are invariably accompanied by drowsiness and later stupor. Friends and family describe abulic patients as ''bumps on a log'' or ''couch potatoes.''

A clinical example of this syndrome may serve to illustrate the findings. Several years ago one of the authors (L.R.C.) was asked to consult on a patient because of a change in behavior. A 67-year-old woman, the wife of a former governor of the state, had entered the Michael Reese Hospital in severe congestive heart failure. She was known to have severe aortic and mitral valve disease and had lower-extremity edema, ascites, and pleural effusions. She was vigorously treated with diuretics, bed rest, and thoracentesis and her congestive heart failure greatly improved. As her heart failure improved, her husband and family noted a marked personality change. Usually gregarious, outgoing, friendly, and talkative, now she had become very quiet, uninterested, and inert. When asked, she said that she was not discouraged or depressed. She seemed not to heed questions. Her replies were usually one or two words—yes, no, or single-word names—which were usually correct. Her motor, sensory, visual, and reflex examinations were normal except that she had bilateral Babinski signs. After lumbar punctures that removed CSF, she returned to her former self and her plantar responses became flexor.

The abulic syndrome is most likely caused by retention of CSF within the intracranial cavity. Pericardial, pleural, and peritoneal effusions are quite common and well known in patients with congestive heart failure. Effusions within the cranial cavity probably have the same explanation as pleural and peritoneal effusions. The meninges are connective tissue structures very similar in structure and function to the pleura, pericardium, and peritoneum. CSF effusions can develop similarly to pleural effusions. Increased venous pressure leads to decreased absorption of CSF at the same time that production of CSF continues unchanged.

The amount of CSF increases and fluid accumulates in the cisterns around the brain, in the subarachnoid space, and sometimes in the ventricles. As is well known, compensation and correction of congestive heart failure do not necessarily result in full reabsorption of pleural and pericardial effusions and ascites. The pressure in the intracranial venous sinuses and neck and cranial veins that drain the head may normalize sufficiently to prevent further CSF effusions but not enough to allow absorption and clearing of the effusions already present. Similarly, thoracentesis and abdominocentesis may be required to remove persistent pleural fluid and ascites even after treatment with diuretics and cardiac drugs.

Computed tomography (CT) scans in patients with the hydrocephalic, abulic syndrome are often read as showing ''brain atrophy.'' Radiologists see increased CSF between cerebral and cerebellar gyri and interpret the widening of the sulci as indicating loss of brain tissue. Of course, increased quantity of intracranial CSF can expand the sulci and cause an increased amount of fluid outside the brain (so-called external hydrocephalus) as well as some enlargement of the ventricular system (internal hydrocephalus). Usually there is not a major enlargement of the cerebral ventricles. Lumbar puncture in patients with the abulic syndrome is often followed by clinical improvement and normalization of the ''brain atrophy'' shown by CT. Sulci become smaller and the gyri widen. CT scans may take time to normalize after lumbar puncture and after treatment of congestive heart failure.

Some reports of patients with severe heart disease, syncope, and congestive heart failure have noted a high frequency of cognitive abnormalities although none has defined the pathogenesis of the loss of intellectual function. Zuccala et al. studied 57 consecutive patients with chronic congestive heart failure [7]. The average age of these patients was 76.7 years. More than half (53%) had low scores on a battery of tests that quantitate cognitive functions, and the presence of low scores was highly correlated with left ventricular ejection fractions of $<30\%$ [7]. Rosenberg and colleagues performed detailed neuropsychological testing on seven patients with recurrent cardiogenic syncope, six of whom had documented arrythmias [8]. The patients with syncope had abnormalities on tests of memory function not found in age- and education-matched control subjects [8]. Garcia et al. performed neuropsychological testing on 100 consecutive cardiac patients admitted to a rehabilitation hospital, and found that 4/24 (16.7%) patients with ischemic heart disease but no known strokes had significant cognitive impairment [9].

The most detailed information about cognitive and intellectual functions in patients with severe heart disease comes from studies of patients considered for cardiac transplantation [10,11]. Neuropsychological tests are often included as part of the routine battery of testing before transplantation, and these tests are occasionally repeated after transplantation. Schall and colleagues studied 54 patients, among whom 20 had idiopathic myocardiopathies and 25 had ischemic cardiomyopathies [10]. The mean left ventricular ejection fraction of these patients was 20% and the mean cardiac index was 2.6 L/min/m^2. The major impairments were in tests of memory and visual and tactile perception; 56% of patients were moderately impaired on logical memory tests and this increased to 61% when 30-minute delays were introduced into the testing [10]. Among the 54 patients, 20 were retested, (mean of 7.7 months after cardiac transplantation) and were found to have only slight improvements [10]. Bornstein et al. studied 62 patients (mean age 44.7 years) who were evaluated extensively for cardiac transplantation [11]; 45% of the patients had dilated cardiomyopathies and 40% had ischemic cardiomyopathies. The patients were impaired on 50% of the neuropsychological measures, and 58% of patients met the criteria for overall impairment that 45% or more of the cognitive test scores fell into the impaired range. The highest rates of impairment were on tests of memory, speed of motor activity, and measures of attention, reasoning, and concept formation. Impaired intellectual functioning correlated with elevated right atrial pressure. Better performance correlated with higher stroke volume, stroke volume index, and cardiac index. Pulmonary capillary wedge pressures and left ventricular ejection fractions did not correlate with results of neuropsychological testing in this series. Only 11 of these patients were retested (seven who had transplantation and four who did not) a mean of 36 months after the initial test battery. In general, the transplant patients showed improvement, and patients who did not have transplantation usually did worse than they had before [11]. The authors considered that elevated right atrial pressure was probably a marker for biventricular failure and low cardiac output and that the cognitive deficits might relate to chronically reduced brain blood flow [11].

Nontoximetabolic Encephalopathies

It is important for cardiologists to know that some conditions that effect the brain multifocally and diffusely, or involve the meninges, can cause clinical syndromes indistinguishable from toximetabolic disorders.

Bacterial endocarditis is well known to cause an encephalopathic syndrome. Symptoms include lethargy and decreased level of consciousness, confusion, agitation, poor concentration, and poor memory. In some patients encephalopathy is a toxic effect related to fever and to acute infection. Patients who have *Staph. aureus* acute endocarditis are more likely to develop encephalopathy than patients with endocarditis caused by other organisms. Necropsy and CT/MRI studies of patients with endocarditis and encephalopathy often show multiple small, scatterred brain infarcts and/or microabscesses [12–14]. Encephalopathy usually develops during uncontrolled infection with more virulent organisms supporting the role of microscopic-size septic emboli as the cause [12–14].

Hypercoagulable states can also be associated with scatterred small regions of brain infarction, edema, and hemorrhage. The clinical syndrome is that of an encephalopathy. Thrombotic thrombocytopenic purpura [15,16], cancer, especially mucinous adenocarcinomas [17,18], and disseminated intravascular coagulation (DIC) [19,20] are often associated with multiple small brain infarcts and hemorrhages. Some patients with leukemia who have very high leukocyte counts and high leukocrits, and some patients with thrombocytosis (counts of over 1,000,000 platelets) can develop encephalopathic syndromes due to altered blood flow and multiple small hemorrhages and infarcts.

Occlusion of venous dural sinuses can present clinically as a syndrome that mimics an encephalopathy. Occlusion of the deep venous system including usually the vein of Galen and the straight sinus cause edema and ischemia bilaterally in the thalamus, basal ganglia, and deep white matter of the brain [21–23]. Headache and decreased consciousness ensue, often with bilateral motor abnormalities. Because the brain dysfunction is bilateral and often relatively symmetrical, there may not be prominent focal signs. Similarly, occlusion of the superior sagittal sinus, or the transverse sinuses bilaterally, can cause bilateral brain edema, infarction, and hemorrhage and can be accompanied by a syndrome that mimics an encephalopathy [21,24].

Increased whole-blood viscosity can lead to reduced brain and retinal blood flow, causing a syndrome closely resembling a toximetabolic encephalopathy. The two most important contributors to whole-blood viscosity are the hematocrit and the fibrinogen levels [25]. Patients with severe polycythemia develop headache, drowsiness, and confusion, symptoms that improve after the hematocrit is lowered. Waldenstrom's macroglobulinemia, other disorders such as multiple myeloma which involve an overabundance of abnormal globulins, and occasionally severe hyperlipidemia can be associated with a hyperviscosity syndrome. The neurologic findings in patients with hyperviscosity syndromes include somnolence, stupor, headache, seizures, confusion, ataxia, and blurred vision [26]. The retinal vessels usually provide an important clue to the presence of hyperviscosity. Retinal veins are dilated and may show segmentation of blood columns within the vessels. Occasionally, retinal hemorrhages, exudates, microaneurysms, and even papilledema are found in patients with severe hyperviscosity.

Encephalitis is, of course, included within the differential diagnosis of encephalopathies since infections and inflammatory disorders can affect the brain diffusely. During the summer months gastrointestinal viruses such as Coxsackie and echovirus are common pathogens. During the winter months, herpes simplex is the most important viral cause. Viral infections, especially childhood exanthems, can be followed by a postinfectious diffuse perivenous demyelinating disorder often called acute postinfectious encephalomyelitis. Fever and other signs of infection and cerebrospinal fluid abnormalities are invariably present in patients with encephalitis.

Various types of *arteritis* can cause a diffuse, usually subacute, disorder that can mimic an encephalopathy [27,28]. Central nervous system arteritis is extremely rare. The diagnosis is probably considered in 1000 patients for every one that actually has the condition. Arteritis or a subacute encephalitis can follow herpes zoster infection, especially herpes zoster opthalmicus.

Patients with *systemic lupus erythematosis, polyarteritis nodosa, severe rheumatoid arthritis, Wegener's granulomatosis, lymphomatoid granulomatosis, and other collagen and systemic inflammatory disorders* can develop central nervous system findings. The signs and symptoms in patients with these conditions can mimic an encephalopathy but diagnosis of the underlying inflammatory disease almost always precedes brain involvement.

Laboratory Investigations of Patients Suspected of Having an Encephalopathy

The most important diagnostic tests are usually biochemical analyses of the blood. Complete blood counts including quantification of platelets should be routinely ordered. Blood electrolytes, pO_2, pCO_2, pH, blood urea nitrogen, Ca^{2+}, and PO^4 are also important to assess and monitor. B_{12}, folate, and iron levels are important in appropriate patients, especially those with anemia. Measurement of prothrombin time, partial thromboplastin time, and other coagulation testing is important, especially in patients taking anticoagulants and those with clinical evidence of bleeding. Liver enzymes, thyroid hormone and TSH levels, and early-morning levels of corticosteroids are often helpful in patients with suspected liver, thyroid, and adrenal cortical disease. Levels of drugs such as digitalis and antidepressants are also important in patients who are taking these medications. Blood levels of various potential exogenous toxins are sometimes useful when patients are suspected of using potentially toxic substances and drugs surreptitiously.

Since bronchopulmonary problems are extremely common in patients with congestive heart failure, assessment of lung functions is often useful. Monitoring of blood gasses should be routine in encephalopathic patients. Ordinarily, pulse oximetry is adequate but periodic measurements of pO_2, pCO_2, and O_2 saturation are also important since circulatory factors and peripheral vasoconstriction in the limbs can affect the pulse oximetry readings. Even when lung disease is not the initial cause of the encephalopathy, any disorder that clouds alertness can be complicated by secondary ventilatory abnormalities, most often hypoventilation. Measurement of lung volumes, tidal volume, and other respiratory functions is often helpful in quantitating the role of pulmonary factors in causing or contributing to an encephalopathy. Some patients who breathe quite normally during the day, while they are awake, develop severe hypoventilation during sleep. Nighttime measurement of blood gases can be diagnostically very helpful in these patients.

Electroencephalography (EEG) can be very helpful in diagnosing encephalopathies and in following their clinical course. The EEG is invariably diffusely abnormal in encephalopathic patients in contrast to focal or multifocal abnormalities usually found in patients with localized structural central nervous system disease. In patients with a variety of different toximetabolic conditions sufficient to cause an encephalopathy, the background activity is slow and there is an excess of theta (four to six cycles per second) and delta waves (one to three cycles per second). Alpha rhythms are suppressed. There may be a loss of amplitude of waves [3,29]. Paroxysmal triphasic waves may appear, especially in patients with hepatic encephalopathy. Evoked potentials after visual, auditory, or somatosensory stimuli may also be altered in patients with encephalopathy but these electrophysiologic tests are seldom required to make the diagnosis. Occasional patients with encephalopathy will have spike discharges or frank seizures recorded by EEG. The severity of the EEG abnormalities does not always parallel clinical findings. The EEG may become abnormal even before clinical neurological symptoms and signs develop. On the other hand, the EEG may remain abnormal for some time after the patient seems to have clinically recovered well. In some patients it is useful to perform sleep EEG studies in search of sleep apnea or hypoventilation during sleep.

Brain imaging using CT or magnetic resonance imaging (MRI) is sometimes helpful, especially in patients who are unconscious or heavily sedated or narcotized. Such patients are difficult to examine clinically and of course they cannot tell us of any neurological or other symptoms. In patients with severe atherosclerotic disease, vascular imaging studies (magnetic resonance angiography [MRA], computed tomography angiography [CTA], or extracranial and transcranial ultrasound) may be useful in detecting and quantifying occlusive cerebrovascular disease. Similarly, echocardiography will define the ejection fraction, myocardial dysfunction, and potential cardiac and aortic donor sources of emboli. Vascular testing has been described in detail in Chapter 2 on brain embolism.

Lumbar puncture is occasionally helpful in encephalopathic patients. The most common indication for a spinal tap is fever. Meningitis, encephalitis, and bacterial endocarditis can yield diagnostic cerebrospinal fluid findings even when brain imaging tests are normal. In patients with cardiac encephalopathy and a hydrocephalic-like syndrome, lumbar puncture with measurement of the opening pressure and removal of a large quantity of cerebrospinal fluid can be both diagnostic and therapeutic. After the opening pressure is obtained, fluid can be removed in 5-mL increments. Each time fluid is removed, the pressure should be rechecked. In general, when there is a large volume of cerebrospinal fluid, as is the case in patients with subarachnoid effusions related to congestive heart failure, the spinal fluid pressure will not change very much when a small volume of fluid is removed. Removing enough fluid to halve the opening spinal fluid pressure may be quite therapeutic in patients with subarachnoid effusions.

NEUROLOGIC SIDE EFFECTS AND TOXICITIES OF DRUGS

Who would choose to practice medicine today or tomorrow without pharmacological drugs? In fact, the word *medicine* is used as a synonym for drug as well as the designation of our profession. More and more medicines and more potent medicines are introduced each year, making it quite difficult for practicing physicians to keep up with the rapidly expanding drug armamentarium available. Among patients with cardiovascular diseases, polypharmacy is the rule rather than the exception. Ask an elderly cardiac patient to show you the medicines he or she is taking, and soon their pocketbooks or sacks will be emptied of many bottles that have been prescribed.

Drugs are clearly two-edged swords. Although some have great therapeutic potentials when used appropriately, many drugs are not prescribed or taken correctly, and many have important side effects and potential toxicity. Old, sick, frail patients, many of whom have multiple system abnormalities and multiple organ failure, tolerate medicines poorly.

In this section, we will attempt to summarize concisely the nervous system side effects of drugs commonly used by cardiac patients. We will emphasize the most common and most important neurological side effects. Larger reviews should be consulted for more details, discussions, and references [30,31]. We will first discuss medicines primarily used to treat cardiovascular disease. We will then turn to pharmacological agents that are frequently used in cardiac patients (e.g., antibiotics, anti–peptic ulcer drugs, sedatives, psychotropic drugs, antidepressants, neuromuscular blocking drugs) but are not directed primarily at the cardiovascular problems.

Interpretation of published reports of drug side effects are often difficult to interpret. Some symptoms mentioned, such as headache, dizziness, light-headedness, depression, sleep abnormalities, and tinnitus, are quite common in older patients who have cardiovascular diseases. In most studies, the authors simply report symptoms mentioned by patients who are taking the drugs studied, but no attempt has been made to compare the frequencies of these symptoms with comparable patients who are not taking these or other drugs. Moreover, it is difficult to find patients with important cardiovascular disease who are not taking any medication. Herein we simply note side effects prominently mentioned, some of which may more probably be attributed to the nature of the patients and their diseases than to the drug or drugs used.

Digitalis

Digitalis and its derivatives have long been used for the treatment of congestive heart failure and to control rapid ventricular rates in patients with atrial fibrillation. Drug activity on the heart is related to inhibition of sodium- and potassium-activated adenosine triphosphatase, but the drug also affects neuronal sodium-potassium ATPase, accounting for neurological side effects [32]. Neurological side effects are dose related and are more common in elderly patients. Hyperactive, restless states characterized by agitation, excitement, insomnia, irritability, euphoria, and manic psychoses and delirium have been reported [33]. In other patients, decreased alertness, somnolence, apathy, and depression occur. Visual and auditory hallucinations have been described [34]. Visual symptoms are especially prominent and characteristic of digitalis toxicity. Some patients describe white borders around dark objects and altered color perception; most often yellow tints are reported but green, red, blue, and brown discoloration have also been described. Some patients describe rather vivid visual hallucinations such as seeing friends dressed in unusually bright colored clothes, butterflies, bird houses, and Confederate soldiers [34]. Optic neuropathy with persistent visual loss has also been reported [30]. Neuropsychological side effects can occur in patients with plasma levels of digoxin within the accepted therapeutic range.

Diuretics

Most of the neurological side effects of diuretics are related to decreased plasma volume, hyponatremia, and hypokalemia. Patients treated with *thiazide diuretics* (e.g., chlorothiazide, hydrochlorothiazide, chlorthalidone, methylclothiazide) often report fatigue and dizziness soon after starting the diuretic therapy. Blurred vision can occur in relation to fluid changes in the retina or lens [30]. Vertigo and neuropsychiatric symptoms are especially frequent in patients treated with indapamide [30]. Headache, limb paresthesias, and muscle cramps are often reported. Depression and decreased sexual desire and function have also been described [2,35].

Carbonic anhydrase inhibitors (e.g., acetazolamide, dichlorphenamide, methazolamide) can cause a metabolic acidosis with resultant confusion and seizures. Headaches, limb paresthesias, tremor, and altered taste are also reported. *Loop diuretics* (e.g., furosemide, buthetanide, ethacrynic acid) can cause deafness probably related to electrolyte changes in the labyrinthine endolymph [30]. Hearing loss can persist even after the loop diuretics have been stopped. These drugs can cause acute hyperglycemia. Loop diuretic use can decrease the renal clearance of lithium and salicylates, resulting in toxic levels of these drugs and accompanying toxic side effects [30]. Syncope can result from volume depletion.

The toxicity of potassium-sparing diuretics (e.g., spironolactone, triamterene, amiloride) is mostly related to hyperkalemia. Muscle cramps, muscle weakness, and cardiac rhythm abnormalities are attributed to elevated serum potassium levels. Hyperkalemic complications are especially common in patients who have renal or hepatic failure and in patients who take potassium supplements or angiotensin-converting enzyme (ACE) inhibitors [30].

Antiarrythmic Drugs

Quinidine

Derived from the cinchona plant and used even in the 18th century to treat palpitations, quinidine has long been recognized as causing neuropsychiatric symptoms as a manifestation of toxicity. The toxic symptoms of quinine and quinidine are often referred to as cinchonism. The proarrhythmic and potential toxic effects of the drug severely limit its usefulness. The most common side effects are tinnitus, dizziness, nausea, and headache. Some patients become restless and excited and may develop a manic type of delirium. Confusion and even a reversible dementia have been described [36,37]. One patient who had been taking quinidine for 14 years and was considered quite demented, had greatly improved mental functioning within 24 hours of stopping quinidine [36]. Visual blurring and distortion also occur but could be at least partially attributable to concurrent use of digitalis [38]. Fisher reported five patients who had recurrent visual aberrations; especially prominent was visual dimming or other visual obscuration soon after exposure to bright light [38]. Four of these five patients were also taking digitalis derivatives, and quinidine is known to elevate digitalis levels. Quinidine is also known to potentiate neuromuscular blocking agents, and its use can cause increased muscle weakness in patients who have mysthenia gravis.

Procainamide

This drug can cause increased muscle weakness in patients with myasthenia gravis and peripheral neuropathies [30,39,39a]. Procainamide has also been reported to cause an immune-mediated form of chronic inflammatory demyelinating polyradiculoneuropathy, usually accompanied by other serological and clinical manifestations of drug-induced systemic lupus erythematosis [39b,39c]. The anticholinergic effects of the drug can cause blurred vision, dry mouth, and tremors. Cerebellar type ataxia [40] and mental abnormalities including frank psychosis have been reported but rarely [41,42]. The proarrhythmic and toxic side effects of this drug limit its clinical usefulness.

Lidocaine

Lidocaine toxicity is especially likely to occur when rapid intravenous infusions of drug are given. Paresthesias in the lips and fingers, tinnitus, decreased hearing, and lethargy are very common during infusions [43]. Central nervous system side effects are prominent and are estimated to occur in 6% to 20% of treated patients [43,44]. In a review of 750 patients treated with lidocaine, 31 (4%) had important neurological toxicity including agitation, confusion, dysarthria, tremulousness, visual disturbances, seizures, respiratory depression, and coma [44]. Muscle twitching also occurs. Hyperactive states characterized by agitation, confusion, hallucinations, and delirium have been reported [45]. One of the authors (L.R.C.)

has seen several patients who developed coma with absent ocular and limb movements while receiving lidocaine infusions through automatic pumps. Brainstem hemorrhage or infarction was suspected until it was discovered that lidocaine had been infused very quickly in larger-than-desired quantities due to faulty function of the infusion pumps. Coma and muscle paralysis were reversible, but the respiratory depression that occurred during the paralysis led to some cortical brain damage. One reported patient who had liver disease with ascites developed coma and decerebrate rigidity while receiving lidocaine [45]. Since the liver is responsible for the catabolism of the drug, lidocaine must be used very cautiously or not at all in patients with liver disease.

Tocainide and Mexiletine

These drugs are chemically similar to lidocaine and are associated with similar neurologic toxicity. Dizziness, headache, and fatigue are common. Patients often report paresthesias, especially around the mouth, and altered taste. Tremors and incoordination are especially common after mexilitine [30]. Blurred vision, seizures, hallucinations, vivid nightmares, confusion, paranoia, and psychosis have all been reported in patients given these drugs [31,46].

Disopyramide

The side effects of this antiarrhythmic agent are dose related and are explained primarily by anticholinergic side effects. Dizziness, dry mouth, fatigue, headache, urinary retention, and blurred vision are prominent. Nervousness and agitation have been described and can progress to psychosis [30]. Impotence is also an important side effect of this drug [47].

Flecainide

Dizziness, headache, and blurred vision are common side effects [30]. Visual hallucinations, dysarthria, and seizures have been reported [48].

Amiodarone

This drug blocks sodium channels as well as potassium and calcium currents. Neurological toxicity is very common and can be severe. Many parts of the nervous system are affected by amiodarone as well as the skin, lungs, thyroid glands, and other vital organs. Weakness, fatigue, tremors, and unsteady gait are very common side effects. Tremor is probably the most frequent symptom and begins soon after starting the drug. Other types of abnormal movements can also occur. Some patients develop a Parkinsonian syndrome; the Parkinsonian tremors and stiffness can persist in patients treated with long-term amiodarone even after the drug is stopped [49].

Amiodarone often causes a clinically significant peripheral polyneuropathy

[50,51]. Sensory symptoms of numbness and paresthesias are prominent; loss of deep tendon reflexes and gait ataxia are part of the neuropathy. Weakness, especially of the lower extremities, may also be found and can be caused by the sensori-motor neuropathy or to a toxic myopathy. Myopathic weakness can be severe. Visual symptoms are due to corneal deposits of lipofuchsin or to an optic neuropathy. Feiner et al. reported 13 patients who developed an optic neuropathy related to amiodarone [52]. The onset of acute sudden-onset visual loss occurred on average 10 months after starting the drug. In five patients the visual loss was bilateral and in eight unilateral. Visual loss usually persisted even after stopping amiodarone [52]. Abnormal taste and smell function, decreased libido and sexual function, confusion, delirium [53], pseudotumor cerebri, and psychosis have also been attributed to amiodarone.

Moricizine

Headache, dizziness, and fatigue are commonly reported in patients who take this antiarrhythmic drug. Psychosis and seizures have been reported to occur but rarely [30].

Propafenone

Neurologic side effects occur in about 20% of patients who take propafenone [30]. Symptoms include headache, dizziness, abnormal taste, blurred vision, drowsiness, and paresthesias. Psychiatric side effects and seizures are rare.

Drugs Used to Treat Hypertension

Centrally Acting Drugs (Clonidine, Methyldopa, Guanabenz)

Common side effects include sleepiness, dry mouth, fatigue, and headache. Sedation is the most frequent side effect noted in patients who take these drugs. *Clonidine* has been reported to cause sleep disturbances, confusion, and paranoia [31,54]. A withdrawal syndrome has been described after abruptly stopping clonidine in patients who have been taking the drug for a long period [54–56]. Symptoms of the withdrawal syndrome include tremor, sweating, anxiety, headache, vivid dreams, and rebound hypertension. These findings have been explained by sympathetic overactivity and increased catecholamine production [54–56]. *Methyldopa* has been known to precipitate or exacerbate Parkinson's disease [54,57–59]. Depression and psychosis are other side effects of methyldopa administration [54,57]. Taste alterations and sexual dysfunction are also reported in patients who take methyldopa or clonidine [30,54, 60,61].

Ganglionic Blocking Sympatholytic Drugs (Mecamylamine, Trimethaphan)

Mecamylamine has been associated with limb paresthesias, abnormal movements of the limbs, and seizures [30]. Depression, hallucinations, and delirium have occasionally been reported but most often in patients who are taking mecamylamine with other drugs [54,62]. Pupillary dilatation, blurred vision, sedation, and restlessness are reported in patients taking these ganglionic blocking drugs.

Postganglionic Blocking Sympatholytic Drugs (Guanethidine, Reserpine, Guanadrel)

Headache occurs in about 30% of patients taking guanethidine [63]. Postural syncope, impotence, failure to ejaculate, and muscle fasciculations and weakness are common after guanethidine use [64,65].

Parkinsonian side effects are common after *reserpine* use and improve when the drug is stopped. Reserpine worsens Parkinson's disease. Depression, often severe, is a very important and serious side effect of reserpine use [66]. Sedation, decreased concentration, decreased intellectual functions, hallucinations, and psychosis have also been described in patients taking reserpine [67].

Alpha-Adrenergic Blocking Sympatholytic Drugs (Prazosin, Phentolamine, Phenoxybenzamine, Doxazosin, Tarazosin, Tolazoline)

Postural light-headedness, headache, fatigue, and weakness are the major complaints in patients taking these drugs. Hallucinations and psychosis can develop in patients taking doxazosin, prazosin, and terazosin [30]. These agents can significantly exacerbate narcolepsy.

ACE Inhibitors (Captopril, Enalapril, Lisinopril, Losartan, Benazepril)

Altered taste and a nonproductive cough are common in patients taking ACE inhibitors. Mood elevation and euphoria sometimes occur in patients taking captopril and this drug may have some antidepressant effect [31]. Visual hallucinations, psychosis, and manic behavior have occasionally been reported [68–70]. Peripheral neuropathy and a Guillain-Barré-type syndrome have also been attributed to captopril [71,72].

Metyrosine

Metyrosine quite often causes sedation. Tremor, Parkinsonian symptoms, depression, hallucinations, and confusion occasionally occur [30].

Hydralazine

Hydralazine can cause paresthesias and a peripheral polyneuropathy. The neuropathy is dose dependent and responds well to the administration of pyridoxine [30]. Headache, tremor, dizziness, and muscle cramps are relatively common side effects. Occasional patients have had psychiatric side effects including anxiety, depression, and manic behavior [54]. Although hydralazine is well known to cause a lupus erythematosis–like syndrome, this invariably spares the nervous system [30,54].

Diazoxide

Diazoxide can cause tinnitus and decreased hearing, symptoms that are usually reversible when the drug is stopped [30]. Headache, dizziness, altered taste and smell sensations, and sleepiness are also complained of in patients taking diazoxide. Diazoxide administration frequently causes significant hyperglycemia which can progress to ketoacidosis even in nondiabetic patients.

Sodium Nitroprusside

Sodium nitroprusside given in high doses can lead to an accumulation of cyanide and thiocyanate which can cause a toxic encephalopathy and psychosis [30]. Nitroprusside is a cerebral vasodilator which can increase intracranial pressure, a potential problem in patients with brain tumors and large strokes.

Beta-Adrenergic-Blocking Drugs (Propanolol, Atenolol, Labetalol, Metoprolol, Esmolol, Nadolol, Pindolol, Solatol, Timolol)

Fatigue and reduced exercise tolerance are very common side effects in patients taking beta blockers. Sedation and drowsiness are also often reported in patients taking relatively high doses. Depression is usually thought to be an important potential side effect of treatment [73–75]. In a review of 31 studies of patients treated with propanolol, the frequencies of neuropsychiatric symptoms were: drowsiness and fatigue (3.5%); depression (1.1%); hallucinations and illusions (0.6%); nightmares (1.6%); and sleep abnormalities (0.7%) [31]. After reviewing the 19 reports of depression attributed by the authors to beta-blocker treatment, Paykel et al. concluded that the frequency of depression reported was similar to controls with hypertension and felt that the data "did not indicate that propanolol causes depression" [54].

Impaired coordination severe enough to affect driving has been reported [30]. Dimsdale and colleagues summarized the results reported among 55 studies of neuropsychological tests in patients taking beta blockers and noted that slightly impaired memory functions and delayed motor reaction times were the most common abnormalities found [73]. Transient memory loss, hallucinations, and psychosis are described but are rare complications of beta-blocker drugs [73–75]. Pindolol often causes tremor and impaired hearing; diplopia, muscle weakness, and impotence are occasionally noted.

Although propanolol and other beta-blocking agents have been used to prevent migraine headaches, there is concern that these drugs could potentiate stroke in migraineurs [76,77]. James Lance, a noted headache expert, concludes, ''Beta-blockers are best avoided in patients with a prolonged aura or severe focal neurologic symptoms because there have been reports of migrainous stroke with their use in such instances'' [77].

Calcium Channel Blockers (Diltiazem, Verapamil, Nifedipine, Nimodipine, Nicardipine, Amlodipine, Flunarizine, Cinnarizine, Lidoflazine)

Dizziness, paresthesias, and headache are common side effects reported by patients taking calcium channel blockers. Restlessness, tremors, dysequilibrium, nervousness, tinnitus, and insomnia are relatively common side effects, especially in patients taking high doses. Serious neuropsychiatric toxicity has been reported but is relatively rare. Depression, delirium, confusion, mania, and psychosis have occasionally been reported [31,78,79]. Muscle weakness can occur and may be due to hypokalemia. Parkinson's disease can be exacerbated during treatment with calcium channel blockers [80]. Parkinsonism is an especially important toxic side effect in older patients who take cinnarizine or flunarazine [80].

Coronary Dilating Drugs

Organic nitrates (nitroglycerin, isosorbide dinitrate, isosorbide mononitrate, erythityl tetranitrate, pentaerythritol) are very often prescribed for patients with coronary artery disease and angina pectoris. Headache is the most common side effect and can be a severe problem in patients who have migraine headaches before taking nitrates. In fact, nitroglycerin has been used to induce headache to test the effectiveness of various antimigraine agents [81]. Headaches are usually diffuse and throbbing, and begin shortly after nitrates are taken, especially when nitrates are used sublingually. Some patients taking isosorbide mononitrate report restlessness, insomnia, decreased concentration, and depression, but these symptoms are also common in patients with coronary artery disease who do not take nitrates [30]. An overdose of nitrates can cause methemaglobinemia with all of its complications.

Lipid-Lowering Drugs

Fibrates (Clofibrate, Gemfibrozil)

Myopathy is an important complication of treatment especially when fibrates are used along with hydroxymethylglutaryl (HMG) coenzyme A–reductase inhibitors or in patients with hypothyroidism or renal insufficiency [30]. The onset of myopathy varies from days to weeks after fibrates are begun [82]. The onset of myalgias in the lower limbs and back is usually abrupt. Muscle tenderness and weakness are often present [82]. The severity of myopathy can range from elevation of creatine kinase with few or no symptoms, to slight muscle cramps and weakness, to acute rhabdomyolysis with myoglobinuria [30,82]. Headache is an important side effect of gemfibrozil treatment [83,84]. Impotence has also been reported in patients who take clofibrate or gemfibrozil [85].

Ion Exchange Resins (Cholestyramine, Colestipol)

Important neurological side effects are rare in patients taking ion exchange resins. Myalgia, headache, paresthesias, and dizziness are occasionally reported. Malabsorption of vitamins K, D, and A can result in bleeding, muscle weakness, and impaired vision.

Hydroxymethylglutaryl Coenzyme A–Reductase Inhibitors (Lovostatin, Pravastatin, Simvastatin, Atorvastatin)

Myopathy can develop in patients taking HMG Co-A reductase inhibitor drugs especially when these agents are used with fibrates, cyclosporine, erythromycin, or niacin [30]. Serious neurological side effects are very rare. Some patients complain of headache, insomnia [86], altered taste, and tremor.

Probucol

Probucol, a promotor of the clearance of lipoproteins, has rarely been associated with important neurological toxicity. Paresthesias, headache, and blurred vision do occasionally occur [30].

Nicotinic Acid

Visual loss can occur either due to a toxic amblyopia or to reversible macular edema [87]. The cystoid maculopathy that is often responsible for the visual loss usually improves when the drug is stopped [87]. Myopathy has been reported especially when nicotinic acid is used with HMG Co-A reductase inhibitors [88,89]. Flushing, headache, and syncope are common transient symptoms in patients taking nicotinic acid.

Drugs That Modify Platelet Functions

A number of substances including aspirin, dipyridamole, ticlopidine, clopidogrel, abciximab, and the omega-3 oils are used to modify platelet adhesion, aggregation, and secretion. These drugs are most often used to prevent the formation of white platelet-fibin thrombi that develop on the surfaces of irregular atherosclerotic plaques. They have been used to prevent myocardial infarction and ischemic stroke, and to treat patients with occlusive peripheral vascular disease.

Dipyridamole use often causes headaches, especially when 300 mg or more of drug is taken each day [89]. Recently drugs that inhibit the platelet glycoprotein IIb/IIIa complex and its binding to fibrinogen have been developed such as abciximab (ReoPro), which consists of monoclonal antibodies to this complex. These platelet IIb/IIIa inhibitors show promise for lysing and preventing the development of white platelet-fibrin thrombi. Abciximab when given intravenously can cause dizziness and difficulty concentrating and thinking [30]. Myopathy may also be an unusual side effect of abciximab therapy [30]. Because antiplatelet aggregants are known to precipitate and exacerbate bleeding in various parts of the body, physicians have naturally been concerned that intracranial bleeding might be an important complication of the use of these agents. There is to date very little evidence on this subject. In the Physicians Health Study there was a slightly increased frequency of hemorrhagic strokes in patients taking aspirin that was of borderline statistical significance [90]. In other studies, the frequency of hemorrhagic stroke has not been increased in patients taking antiplatelet aggregants. There is reason for concern that patients who have subarachnoid or intracerebral bleeding or bleeding at other sites may have more extensive hemorrhaging if they are taking antiplatelet aggregants.

Anticoagulants

Anticoagulant drugs (heparin, heparinoids, low-molecular-weight heparins, warfarins) have most often been given to patients with cardiovascular disease to prevent brain and systemic embolism. These drugs all have the potential to cause serious bleeding. Heparin also can cause a syndrome of thrombocytopenia and disseminated thrombosis of small blood vessels (the ''white clot syndrome'') [92,93]. This syndrome can be associated with brain infarction and hemorrhages. Warfarin can also cause a disseminated vascular occlusion syndrome, perhaps related to activation of protein C, that is characterized by skin necrosis, muscle pain, and infarction of the kidneys, spleen, liver, pancreas, brain, and spinal cord [94,95].

The most important complication of anticoagulant therapy is bleeding. The frequency of bleeding depends heavily on the quality and consistency of the supervision of anticoagulant therapy. Older age, higher intensity of treatment, variability of the parameters used (International Normalized Ratios [INR] or prothrombin time ratios [PTR]), use of substances known to affect warfarin metabolism, and the presence of serious comorbid conditions clearly increase the likelihood of bleeding [96–98]. In one review of complications of warfarin anticoagulation, among 928 patients who had 1103 courses of anticoagulant therapy, there were 1332 bleeding events, 261 severe and 1071 classified as minor [97]. Among the severe bleeding episodes nine (3%) were intracranial including three categorized as serious, two as life-threatening, and four as fatal [97]. In another large series of anticoagulated patients, among 2376 patients treated for 3702 patient-years, there were 812 first bleeding episodes including four fatal, 33 life-threatening, and 222 serious bleeds [98]. Intracranial bleeding was responsible for 20% of the bleeds judged to be either life-threatening or fatal [98]. In these two very large series, all fatal hemorrhages (eight in all) were intracranial. Intracranial bleeding is most often directly into the brain substance but also can be subdural or subarachnoid.

All of the medications described so far have been used directly or indirectly to treat the primary cardiac and cardiovascular diseases and their risk factors. The drugs discussed below are also commonly used in patients with cardiovascular diseases but they are most often not primarily directed at the cardiovascular disorders. Narcotics and other analgesics, sedatives, and psychotropic agents are often used to treat the pain, anxiety, and fear that often accompany myocardial infarction and other severe, life-threatening disorders. Antibiotics are most often used to treat coexisting infections, especially of the respiratory and genitourinary systems. Neuromuscular blocking agents are used in patients with hypoxia and pulmonary insufficiency. Histamine H_2 antagionists are now widely used both in and outside the hospital to prevent or treat peptic ulcer disease and gastric hyperacidity. Neurological complications and side effects related to the use of these drugs are very important to recognize.

Antibiotics

Sulfonamides and *trimethoprim* occasionally cause an allergic type of aseptic meningitis [99]. High doses of trimethoprim can cause headache, difficulty concentrating, and confusion. *Quinolone* antibiotics (nalidixic acid, ciprofloxacin, cinoxacin, norfloxacin, lomefloxacin, ofloxacin, enoxacin, levofloxacin, sparfloxacin, pefloxacin, trouafloxacin) can cause headache, anxiety, and abnormal visual and sensory perception. Increased brightness of lights, changed colors, double vision, and difficulty focusing vision are described [30]. Fluorinated -4-quinolones (norfloxacin, ofloxacin, pefloxacin) can exacerbate muscle weakness in patients with myasthenia gravis and have been shown to have an effect on neuromuscular transmission by decreasing the amplitude of miniature endplate potentials and currents [99a]. *Nalidixic acid* is more likely than ciprofloxacin and other, newer quinolones to cause these sensory aberrations. *Nitrofurantoin* often causes a peripheral neuropathy, especially when taken over a prolonged period of time and in patients with impaired kidney function [100]. High doses of *penicillin* can cause or potentiate seizures [101]. In experimental conditions using tissue slices, cloxacillin, ampicillin, gentamicin, chloramphenicol, ciprofloxacin, and erythromycin, all decrease the seizure threshold, indicating a possible risk clinically for seizure development in patients treated with these antibiotics [101] *Cephalosporin* antibiotics (e.g., cephalexin, cefaclor, cefuroxime, cefixime) can also cause or potentiate seizures especially in patients with renal dysfunction [101]. Cefuroxime can cause an encephalopathy characterized by stupor, myoclonic jerks, and confusion, especially when given in high doses or in patients with renal disease [101a]. Altered taste and muscle cramps are occasionally noted in patients given cephalosporins.

Aminoglycoside antibiotics (amikacin, gentamicin, kanamycin, streptomycin, tobramycin, paramomycin, neomycin) have hearing loss and tinnitus as important side effects. The effects on hearing are dose related; hearing loss often persists even with cessation of the antibiotic. The aminoglycosides also have a curarelike action which can potentiate neuromuscular blocking agents and can lead to increased muscle weakness, especially in patients with myasthenia gravis and other neuromuscular diseases [102].

Macrolide antibiotics (erythromycin, clarithromycin, azithromycin, troleandomycin, dirithromycin) cause hearing loss which is reversible when the drugs are stopped. Paranoia and hallucinations are occasionally reported in patients given macrolides. *Lincomycin* and *clindamycin* have a curare effect similar to but quantitatively less than that of the aminoglycosides, and should be used very cautiously in patients with myasthenia gravis and patients given neuromuscular blocking agents [102]. *Vancomycin* can cause hearing loss. Similar to the situation with the aminoglycosides, hearing loss is dose related, more likely to occur in patients with renal insufficiency, and often not reversible when the drug is stopped [103]. Hearing loss is more apt to occur if vancomycin is used with an aminoglycoside antibiotic.

Analgesic, Sedative, and Psychotropic Medications

These types of medications are often given to patients with cardiogenic pain and anxiety in an attempt to alleviate discomfort and allay anxiety and agitation. *Opioid drugs* can cause drowsiness and difficulty concentrating as well as feelings of euphoria [104]. Respiratory depression is the most important neurological side effect of morphine use [104]. Opioids can increase intracranial pressure, so these agents should be used cautiously in patients with large strokes or brain tumors. *Meperidine* can cause delirium, myoclonus, and seizures when administered in high doses [30]. *Fentanyl* administered in high doses can cause muscular rigidity as a side effect [105].

Barbiturates were formerly the most common drug used for sedation. Unfortunately, barbiturates can cause paradoxical excitement that can progress to delirium and hallucinations, especially in older patients [30,106]. Barbiturates are also likely to cause respiratory depression. *Benzodiazepines* (alprazolam, chlordiazepoxide, clonazepam, chlorazepate, diazepam, lorazepam, oxazepam, triazolam) are probably the most common drugs now used for sedation and tranquilization [106,107]. These drugs also occasionally cause paradoxical excitement and delirium. Hypotension is an important side effect, especially when *diaz-*

epam is given intravenously. Amnesia has been described, especially after *triazolam* [108]. Abnormal movements have also been described including dystonia, restless movements, and tardive dyskinesia-like movements of the mouth, lips, and tongue [30,109,110]. Respiratory depression is less apt to occur with benzodiazepines than with barbiturates. In caring for cardiac patients, short-acting benzodiazepines such as triazolam and midazolam, and intermediate-duration drugs such as alprazolam, lorazepam, and oxazepam are preferred over long-acting (30 to 100 hours) drugs such as diazepam, chlordiazepoxide, flurazepam, and chlorazepate. *Buspirone* is less likely to produce drowsiness or excitement or memory loss than the benzodiazepines, but tremors, abnormal movements, and dystonia sometimes occur [111].

Among psychotropic agents, *haloperidol* is the only drug used frequently in previously nonpsychotic cardiac patients. In our opinion, the side effects and adverse reactions associated with this drug far outweigh any potential benefits. *We believe that haloperidol should not be used in elderly nonpsychotic patients for sedation or tranquilization.* When haloperidol is given to animals undergoing physical therapy after strokes, their recovery rate is greatly retarded for nearly 3 weeks compared to animals not given haloperidol [112,113]. There is some evidence that haloperidol also retards recovery from strokes in humans, especially when given as part of polypharmacy [112–114]. Haloperidol produces a ''wooden'' feeling, stiffness, rigidity, and Parkinsonian-like extrapyramidal signs. Excretion is slow, so Parkinsonian signs can last for weeks after haloperidol is stopped. Other neuroleptic drugs also often cause Parkinsonian side effects [30,115,116]. The neuroleptic malignant syndrome can occur with the use of haloperidol, especially if given in high doses parenterally. This disorder is life-threatening and consists of bradykinesia, rigidity, stupor, high fever, myoglobinuria, renal failure, labile pulse and blood pressure [30,117,118]. Neuroleptic drugs should generally be avoided, especially in older, frail, sick patients.

Restlessness, hyperactivity, and agitation often follow withdrawal from analgesics, sedatives, and psychotropic agents. The higher the doses of medicines, the more likely there are to be rebound effects of agitation. Unfortunately, all too often a self-perpetuating cycle occurs in which rebound excitation is treated each time it occurs with more sedatives or psychotropics. Agitation is a natural response to being knocked down artificially with drugs. With time and reassurance and nursing supervision the agitation usually can be calmed without prescribing more sedatives or psychotropics. Overuse of narcotics, sedatives, and psychotropic agents is an important cause of morbidity and mortality in our hospitals today, especially in intensive care units.

Antidepressants

Depression often develops in the hospital in patients with acute cardiac disorders, and many patients are treated as outpatients for depression. *Tricyclic and tetracy-*

clic antidepressants (amitriptyline, imipramine, desipramine, doxepin, maprotiline, nortriptyline, protriptyline, trimipramine) often cause sedation [119,120]. Anticholinergic side effects such as blurred vision, dry mouth, urinary retention, and constipation cause problems in older patients. Nightmares, delusions, hallucinations, and delirium are occasionally described [119,120]. Tremor has also been noted. These antidepressant drugs lower seizure threshold, which can be a problem in patients with epilepsy or known brain lesions. Sexual dysfunction including decreased libido, impotence, and delayed ejaculation are common.

Serotonin uptake inhibitors (fluoxetine, fluvoxamine, paroxetine, sertraline, venlafaxine) [121,122], like the tricyclic antidepressants, lower seizure threshold [123] and cause sexual dysfunction. Sedation characterized by drowsiness and fatigue is common. Excitation with agitation and manic delirium are occasionally described. The ''acute serotonin syndrome'' is a serious complication of the use of these drugs and includes restlessness, rigidity, myoclonus, agitation, diarrhea, sweating, fever, and rhabdomyolysis, and can progress to coma and death [30,124]. Abnormal movements and exacerbation of Parkinsonism has been noted with *fluoxetine* and other serotonin uptake inhibitors [30,125,126]. The concurrent use of fluoxetine and tricyclic antidepressants can cause serious side effects since fluoxetine may result in a two- to fivefold increase in levels of tricyclic drugs, benzodiazepines, and trazadone; seizures, confusion, and mania can result [127,128].

Trazadone commonly causes drowsiness. Some patients develop priapism [30]. *Bupropion* sometimes causes amphetaminelike nervous system stimulation, and both anticholinergic and Parkinsonian side effects have been described [30]. *Lithium* has a host of neurologic complications and is probably best avoided in older patients who have not been taking the drug previously. Tremors, abnormal movements and dystonia, ataxia, peripheral neuropathy, and impaired intellectual functions are relatively common after lithium use, especially when the dose or blood levels are high [30,129]. Sometimes the neurologic symptoms develop even when blood levels are within therapeutic range. Sometimes the neurologic signs are not reversible even when lithium is stopped [130]. Lithium toxicity has been reported in patients who take drugs that cause excretion of sodium, including ACE inhibitors [131]. When lithium is used in elderly patients, therapeutic blood levels are lower than those used in younger patients and should be very carefully and frequently monitored.

Neuromuscular Blocking Drugs

Patients with respiratory insufficiency are often given neuromuscular blocking drugs, with respiration being controlled mechanically. Heavy sedation often accompanies the institution of artificial respiration. Neuromuscular blocking drugs are either depolarizing (succinylcholine) or nondepolarizing, curarelike drugs (e.g., pancuronium, tubocurarine, vercuronium). It is now well recognized that the use of these drugs is often followed by prolonged paralysis even after the drugs are stopped. Factors that potentiate these drugs include cholinesterase deficiency (either hereditary or acquired) renal disease, and liver disease. A host of other drugs exert an effect on the neuromuscular blocking action of these drugs including estrogens, glucocorticoids, lithium, quinidine, verapamil, aminoglycoside antibiotics, lincomycin, clindamycin [30,102].

Drugs Used for Gastrointestinal Symptoms

Histamine H_2 antagonists (cimetidine, ranitidine, nizatidine, famotidine) are now very often used in the community at large and so are often prescribed to patients with cardiac disorders. Some of these drugs are now available over the counter. Hallucination, psychosis, and choreiform movements are occasionally reported after cimetidine use [132]. *Cimetidine* also can cause decreased libido and impotence. Occasional patients develop a myopathy or peripheral neuropathy [30]. Hydrogen ion pump inhibitors (omeprazole and lansoprazole) can cause headache, dizziness, somnolence, myalgias, and paresthesias. *Misoprostol* use is associated with headache. *Metoclopramide* often causes sedation, restlessness, and fatigue. Extrapyramidal side effects also occur [133].

For ease of reference, we close this chapter with tables that list drugs that are well known to cause specific important neurological side effects. Table 4 shows those drugs that cause headache as a prominent symptom. Table 5 lists the drugs known to cause agitation, delusions, and psychosis. Table 6 lists those drugs that are recognized as causing decreased intellectual function—a dementialike presentation. Table 7 lists those drugs that cause or potentiate seizures.

TABLE 4 Drugs That Cause Headache as a Prominent Side Effect

Nitroglycerin and other organic nitrates
Dipyridamole
Caffeine withdrawal
Alcohol and sedative drug withdrawal
Guanethidine
Hydralazine
Gemfibrozil
Nicotinic acid
Omeprazole
Calcium channel blockers
Flecainide
Mexiletine

TABLE 5 Drugs That Cause Agitation, Delirium, and Psychosis

Amiodarone	Procainamide
Amphetamines	Tocainide
Anticholinergics	Reserpine
Antihistamines	Hydralazine
Bupropion	Alcohol and sedative drug withdrawal
Calcium channel blockers	L-dopa
Caffeine	Lidocaine
Captopril	Lithium
Cimetidine	Theophylline
Cocaine	Methyldopa
Digitalis	
Quinidine	

Source: Ref. 134.

TABLE 6 Drugs That Cause Prominent Loss of Cognitive Function (a Dementialike Presentation)

Alcohol
Barbiturates
Antihistamines
Neuroleptic antipsychotic drugs
Cimetidine
Digitalis
Quinidine
L-dopa
Lithium
Narcotics
Anticonvulsants
Sedative/tranquilizing drugs
Reserpine
Trimethoprim
Anticholinergics

Source: Ref. 134.

TABLE 7 Drugs That Potentiate or Cause Seizures

Amoxapine	Insulin
Amphetamines	Isoniazid
Flecainide	Neuroleptics
Mecamylamine	Lidocaine
Cephalosporin antibiotics	Lithium
Tricyclic antidepressants	Meperidine
Serotonin uptake inhibitors	Penicillins
Cocaine	Phenylpropanolamine
Dextropropoxyphene	Salicylates
Ethanol and sedative drug withdrawal	Theophylline

Source: Ref. 134.

REFERENCES

1. Arieff AI, Griggs RC. General considerations in metabolic encephalopathies and systemic disorders affecting the nervous system. In: Arieff AI, Griggs RC, eds. Metabolic Brain Dysfunction in Systemic Disorders. Boston: Little Brown & Co., 1992:1–20.
2. Adams RD, Foley JM. The neurological disorders associated with liver disease. Proc Assoc Res Nerv Ment Dis 1952; 32:198–237.
3. Jones EA, Weisenborn K. Neurology and the liver. J Neurol Neurosurg Psychiatry 1997; 63:279–293.
4. Raskin NH. Neurological complications of renal failure. In: Aminoff M, ed. Neurology and General Medicine. The Neurological Aspects of Medical Disorders. 2d ed. New York: Churchill Livingstone, 1995:303–316.
5. Leavitt S, Tyler HR. Studies in asterixis. Arch Neurol 1964; 10:360.
6. Raskin NH, Fishman RA. Neurologic disorders in renal failure. N Engl J Med 1976; 294:143, 204.
7. Zuccala G, Cattel C, Manes-Gravina E, Di Niro MG, Cocchi A, Bernabei R. Left ventricular dysfunction: a clue to cognitive impairment in older patients with heart failure. J Neurol Neurosurg Psychiatry 1997; 63:509–512.
8. Rosenberg GA, Haaland KY. Cardiogenic dementia. Lancet 1981; 2:1171.
9. Garcia CA, Tweedy JR, Blass JP. Underdiagnosis of cognitive impairment in a rehabilitation setting. J Am Geriatr Soc 1984; 32:339–342.
10. Schall RR, Petrucci RJ, Brozena SC, Cavarocchi NC, Jessup M. Cognitive function in patients with symptomatic dilated cardiomyopathy before and after cardiac transplantation. J Am Coll Cardiol 1989; 14:1666–1672.
11. Bornstein RA, Starling RC, Myerowitz P, Haas GJ. Neuropsychological function in patients with end-stage heart failure before and after cardiac transplantation. Acta Neurol Scand 1995; 91:260–265.
12. Kanter MC, Hart RG. Neurologic complications of infective endocarditis. Neurology 1991; 41:1015–1020.

53. Trohman RG, Castellanos D, Castellanos A, Kessler KM. Amiodarone induced delirium. Ann Intern Med 1988; 108:68–69.
54. Paykel ES, Fleminger R, Watson JP. Psychiatric side effects of antihypertensive drugs other than reserpine. J Clin Psychopharmacol 1982; 2:14–39.
55. Hunyor SN, Hansson L, Harrison TS, Hoobler SW. Effects of clonidine withdrawal: possible mechanisms and suggestions for management. Br Med J 1973; 2:209–211.
56. Hansson L, Hunyor SN, Julius S, Hoobler SW. Blood pressure crisis following withdrawal of clonidine (Catapres, Catapresan) with special reference to arterial and urinary catecholamine levels and suggestions for acute management. Am Heart J 1973; 85:605–610.
57. Raftos J, Julian DG, Valentine PA. The prolonged use of alpha methyldopa in the treatment of hypertension. Med J Aust 1964; 1:837–842.
58. Strang RR. Parkinsonism occurring during methyldopa therapy. Can Med Assoc J 1966; 95:928–929.
59. Prescott LF. Methyldopa and Parkinsonism. Br Med J 1964; 2:687.
60. Newman RJ, Salerno HR. Sexual dysfunction due to methyldopa. Br Med J 1974; 4:106.
61. Alexander WD, Evans JI. Side effects of methyldopa. Br Med J 1975; 1:501.
62. Harrington M, Kincaid-Smith P. Psychosis and tremor due to mecamylamine. Lancet 1958; 1:499–501.
63. Lowther CP, Turner RWD. Guanethidine in the treatment of hypertension. Br Med J 1963; 3:776–781.
64. Seedat YK, Pillay VKG. Further experiences with guanethidine—a clinical assessment of 103 patients. S Afr Med J 1966; 40:140–143.
65. Dollery CT, Emslie-Smith D, Milne MD. Guanethidine in the treatment of hypertension. Lancet 1960; 3:381–387.
66. Fries ED. Mental depression in hypertensive patients treated for long periods with large doses of reserpine. N Engl J Med 1954; 251:1006–1008.
67. Kass I, Brown EC. Treatment of hypertensive patients with rauwolfia compounds and reserpine. JAMA 1959; 159:1513–1516.
68. Haffner CA, Smith BS, Pepper C. Hallucinations as an adverse effect of angiotensin-converting enzyme inhibition. Postgrad Med J 1993; 69:240.
69. Gillman MA, Sandyk R. Reversal of captopril-induced psychosis with naloxone. Am J Psychiatry 1985; 142:270.
70. Patten SB, Brager N, Sanders S. Manic symptoms associated with the use of captopril. Can J Psychiatry 1991; 36:314–315.
71. Samanta A, Burden AC. Peripheral neuropathy due to captopril. Br Med J 1985; 291:1172.
72. Chakrabarty TK, Ruddell WS. Guillain-Barré neuropathy during treatment with captopril. Postgrad Med J 1987; 63:221–222.
73. Dimsdale JE, Newton RP, Joist T. Neuropsychological side effects of beta blockers. Arch Intern Med 1989; 149:514–525.
74. Kostis JB, Rosen RC. Central nervous system effects of beta-adrenergic-blocking drugs: role of ancillary properties. Circulation 1987; 75:204–212.
75. McAinsh J, Cruikshank JM. Beta-blockers and central nervous system side effects. Pharmacol Ther 1990; 46:163–197.

76. Bardwell A, Trott JA. Stroke in migraine as a consequence of propanolol. Headache 1987; 27:381–383.
77. Lance JW. Preventive treatment in migraine. In: Goadsby PJ, Silberstein SD, eds. Headache. Boston: Butterworth-Heinemann, 1997:131–141.
78. Kahn JK, Nifedipine-associated psychosis. Am J Med 1986; 81:705–706.
79. Palat GK, Movaled A. Secondary mania associated with diltiazem. Clin Cardiol 1986; 9:39.
80. Garcia-Ruiz PJ, Garcia de Yebanes FJ, Jiminez-Jiminez A, et al. Parkinsonism associated with calcium channel blockers: a prospective follow-up study. Clin Neuropharmacol 1992; 15:19–26.
81. Iversen HK, Olesen J, Tfelt-Hansen P. Intravenous nitroglycerine as an experimental model of vascular headache: basic characteristics. Pain 1989; 38:17–24.
82. Magarian GL, Lucas LM, Colley C. Gemfibrozil-induced myopathy. Arch Intern Med 1991; 151:1873–1874.
83. Alvarez-Sabin J, Codina A, Rodriquez C, Laporte JR. Gemfibrozil induced headache. Lancet 1988; 2:1246.
84. Arellano F, De Cos MA, Valiente R, Quiros C. Gemfibrozil-induced headache. Lancet 1988; 1:705.
85. Pizzaro S, Bargay J, D'Agosto P. Gemfibrozil-induced impotence. Lancet 1990; 336:1135.
86. Black DM, Lamkin G, Olivera EH, et al. Sleep disturbance and HMG CoA reductase inhibitors. JAMA 1990; 264:1105.
87. Millay RH, Klein ML, Illingworth DR. Niacin maculopathy. Opthalmology 1988; 95:930–936.
88. Reaven P, Witztum JL. Lovostatin, nicotinic acid and rhabdomyolysis. Ann Intern Med 1988; 109:597–598.
89. Litin SC, Andersewn DF. Nicotinic acid-associated myopathy. A report of three cases. Am J Med 1989; 86:481–483.
90. Schafer AI. Antiplatelet therapy. Am J Med 1996; 101:199–209.
91. Steering Committee of the Physician's Health Study Research Group. Final report on the aspirin component of the ongoing Physicians' Health Study. N Engl J Med 1989;321:129–135.
92. Rankin JA. Heparin-induced thrombosis (white clot syndrome) secondary to prophylactic subcutaneous administration of heparin. Can J Surg 1988; 31:33–34.
93. Laster J, Cikrit D, Walker N, Silver D. The heparin-induced thrombocytopenia syndrome: an update. Surgery 1987; 102:763–770.
94. Sallah S, Thomas DP, Roberts HR. Warfarin and heparin-induced necrosis and the purple toe syndrome: infrequent complications of anticoagulant treatment. Thromb Haemost 1997; 78:785–790.
95. Raskob GE, George JN. Thrombotic complications of antithrombotic therapy: a paradox with implications for clinical practice. Ann Intern Med 1997; 127:839–841.
96. Gurwitz JH, Avorn J, Ross-Degnan D, Choodnovskiy I, Ansell J. Aging and the anticoagulant response to warfarin therapy. Ann Intern Med 1992; 116:901–904.
97. Fihn SD, McDonell M, Martin D, Henikoff J, Vermes D, Kent D, White RH, for the Warfarin Optimized Outpatient Follow-up Study Group. Risk factors for com-

plications of chronic anticoagulation. A multicenter study. Ann Intern Med 1993; 118:511–520.
98. Fihn SD, Callahan C, Martin D, McDonell MB, Henikoff JG, White RH, for the National Consortium of Anticoagulation Clinics. The risk for and severity of bleeding complications in elderly patients treated with warfarin. Ann Intern Med 1996; 124:970–979.
99. Joffe AM, Farley JD, Linden D, et al. Trimethoprim-sulfamethoxazole associated aseptic meningitis: case report and review of the literature. Am J Med 1989; 87: 332–338.
99a. Sieb JP. Fluoroquinolone antibiotics block neuromuscular transmission. Neurology 1998; 50:804–807.
100. Toole JF, Parrish ML. Nitrofurantoin polyneuropathy. Neurology 1973; 23:554–559.
101. Grondahl TO, Langmoen IA. Epileptogenic effect of antibiotic drugs. J Neurosurg 1993; 78:938–943.
101a. Herishanu YO, Zlotnik M, Mostoslavsky M, et al. Cefuroxime-induced encephalopathy. Neurology 1998; 50:1873–1875.
102. Howard JF. Adverse drug effects on neuromuscular transmission. Semin Neurol 1990; 10:89–102.
103. Kavanagh KT, McCabe BF. Ototoxicity of oral neomycin and vancomycin. Laryngoscope 1983; 93:649–653.
104. Brust JCM. Opioids. In: Neurological Aspects of Substance Abuse. Boston: Butterworth-Heinemann, 1993:16–59.
105. Christian CM, Waller JL, Moldenhauer CC. Postoperative rigidity following fentanyl anaesthesia. Anesthesiology 1983; 58:275–277.
106. Brust JCM. Barbiturates and other hypnotics and sedatives. In: Neurological Aspects of Substance Abuse. Boston: Butterworth-Heinemann, 1993:115–130.
107. Woods JH, Katz JL, Winger G. Benzodiazepines. Use, abuse, and consequences. Pharmacol Rev 1992; 44:151–347.
108. Morris HH, Estes ML. Traveler's amnesia: transient global amnesia secondary to triazolam. JAMA 1987; 258:945–946.
109. Stolarek IH, Ford MJ. Acute dystonia induced by midazolam and abolished by flumazenil. Br Med J 1990; 300:614.
110. Rosenbaum AH, De la Fuente JR. Benzodiazepines and tardive dyskinesia. Lancet 1979; 2:900.
111. Boylan K. Persistent dystonia associated with buspirone. Neurology 1990; 40:1904.
112. Davis JN, Crisostomo EA, Duncan P, Propst M, Feeney DM. Amphetamine and physical therapy facilitate recovery of function from stroke: correlative animal and human studies. In: Raichle ME, Powers WJ, eds. Cerebrovascular Diseases. New York: Raven Press, 1987:297–304.
113. Feeney DM, Gonzales A, Law WA. Amphetamine, haloperidol, and experience interact to affect the rate of recovery after motor cortex injury. Science 1982; 217: 855–857.
114. Goldstein LB, Acute Stroke Study Investigators. Common drugs may influence motor recovery after stroke. Neurology 1995; 45:865–871.
115. Hardie RJ, Lees AJ. Neuroleptic-induced Parkinson's syndrome: clinical features

and results of treatment with levodopa. J Neurol Neurosurg Psychiatry 1988; 51: 850–854.
116. Levinson DF, Simpson GM. Neuroleptic-induced extrapyramidal symptoms with fever. Arch Gen Psychiatry 1986; 43:839–848.
117. Keck PE, Pope HG, McElroy SL. Frequency and presentation of neuroleptic malignant syndrome: a prospective study. Am J Psychiatry 1987; 144:1344–1346.
118. Levenson JL. Neuroleptic malignant syndrome. Am J Psychiatry 1985; 142:1137–1145.
119. Preskorn SH, Jerkovich GS. Central nervous system toxicity of tricyclic antidepressants: pharmacology, course, risk factors, and role of therapeutic drug monitoring. J Clin Psychopharmacol 1990; 10:88–95.
120. Bryant SG, Fisher S, Kluge RM. Long-term vs short-term amitryptilline side effects as measured by a post-marketing surveillance system. J Clin Psychopharmacol 1987; 7:78–82.
121. Gram LF. Fluoxetine. N Engl J Med 1994; 331:1354–1361.
122. Grimsley SR, Jann MW. Paroxetine, sertraline, and fluvoxamine, new selective serotonin reuptake inhibitors. Clin Pharm 1992; 11:930–957.
123. Weber JJ. Seizure activity associated with fluoxetine therapy. Clin Pharm 1989; 8:296–298.
124. Bodner RA, Lynch T, Lewis L, Kahn D. Serotonin syndrome. Neurology 1995; 45:219–223.
125. Choo V. Paroxetine and extrapyramidal reactions. Lancet 1993; 341:624.
126. Steur ENHS. Increase of Parkinsonian disability after fluoxetine medication. Neurology 1993; 43:211–213.
127. Preskorn SH, Beber JH, Faul JC, Hirschfeld RMA. Serious adverse effects of combining fluoxetine and tricyclic antidepressants. Am J Psychiatry 1990; 147:532.
128. Aranow RB, Hudson JL, Pope HG Jr, et al. Elevated antidepressant plasma levels after addition of fluoxetine. Am J Psychiatry 1989; 146:911–913.
129. Ananth J, Ghadirian AM, Engelsmann F. Lithium and memory: a review. Can J Psychiatry 1987; 32: 312–316.
130. Schou M. Long-lasting neurological sequellae after lithium intoxication. Acta Psychiatr Scand 1984; 70:594–602.
131. Ruddy, MC, Kostis JB, Frishman WH. Drugs that affect the renin-angiotensin system. In: Frishman WH, Sonnenblick EH, eds. Cardiovascular Pharmacotherapeutics. New York: McGraw-Hill, 1997:131–192.
132. Colin Jones D, Langman MJS, Lawson DH, Vessey MP. Postmarketing surveillance of the safety of cimetadine: twelve-month morbidity report. Q J Med 1985; 54:253–268.
133. Bateman DN, Darling WM, Boys R, Rawlins MD. Extrapyramidal reactions to metoclopramide and prochlorperazine. Q J Med 1989; 71:307–311.
134. Benowitz NL. Central nervous system manifestations of toxic disorders In: Arieff AI, Griggs RC, eds. Metabolic Brain Dysfunction in Systemic Disorders. Boston: Little Brown & Co., 1992:409–436.

4

Neurological Complications of Cardiac Surgery

INTRODUCTION

Central and peripheral nervous system complications are a major cause of morbidity following cardiac surgery. This chapter focuses on the frequency, cause, and prevention of these complications. The data presented largely apply to coronary artery bypass graft surgery (CABG) since our knowledge of these neurological complications is derived mostly from studies of this operation. Complications of valvular heart surgery are similar to CABG, but the frequency of complications may be lower with valvular surgery [1].

HISTORICAL BACKGROUND

After extensive laboratory work, Gibbon performed the first successful intracardiac operation using extracorporeal circulation on a patient in 1953 [2]. Several oxygenating techniques were subsequently used during open heart surgery until 1955, when DeWall and Lillihei developed a bubble oxygenator that became the method of choice for oxygenation during cardiopulmonary bypass [3]. In the early 1960s, Ehrenhaft and others published the first clinical reports on the neurological complications of open heart surgery [4–7]. These reports on patients undergoing valvular procedures suggested that the frequency of persistent brain dysfunction after open heart surgery was as high as 23%. Most of these events were attributed to air embolization or inadequate cerebral blood flow during cardiopulmonary bypass.

The introduction of membrane oxygenators and arterial line filters (20 to 40 μm) greatly reduced the risk of air and particulate-matter microemboli during cardiopulmonary bypass. This development, along with improvements in surgical and anesthetic techniques, led to a reduction in the risk of stroke and encephalopathy during cardiac surgery. The first aorto-coronary bypass in man was performed by David C. Sabiston in 1962 following an unsuccessful right coronary endarterectomy [119]. Two years later, again as a result of difficulties during coronary endarterectomy, Garret, Dennis, and DeBakey performed an aorto-coronary bypass to the left anterior descending artery [8]. The procedure was later popularized by Favaloro [9]. Subsequently, CABG has become one of the most commonly performed operations in the United States, with approximately 400,000 operations performed annually. Despite the improvements in bypass, surgical, and anesthetic techniques, recent data suggest that neurological morbidity and mortality from CABG is increasing, largely because the percentage of sicker and older patients undergoing CABG has increased substantially [10].

PATHOPHYSIOLOGY OF CARDIOPULMONARY BYPASS AND POTENTIAL IMPACT ON THE BRAIN

Considering the number of potential threats to the brain during heart surgery, it is remarkable that the frequency of neurological complications from CABG is not substantially higher than reported. The major threats to the brain include embolization and hypoperfusion, which are related in part to the myriad effects of the heart-lung machine on blood constituents. Plasma proteins, particularly fibrinogen, are adsorbed onto the synthetic surfaces of the bypass machine [11]. Activation of platelets by blood-synthetic surface contact leads to uncovering of fibrinogen receptors on the platelet membrane [12,13]. In some patients, increased levels of thromboxane A_2 and B_2 have been detected in plasma during bypass [14]. These events promote adherence of platelets on synthetic surfaces of the bypass machine despite heparinization. Erythrocytes and leucocytes are also affected by bypass. Osmotic stresses, turbulence, and trauma from the cardiotomy suction system induce hemolysis and impede the ability of erythrocytes to change shape during passage through capillaries [15]. This predisposes to erythrocyte sludging in areas of reduced blood flow. Leucocytes are activated largely by the complement cascade and accumulate in pulmonary capillaries [16,17]. Plasma proteins and lipoproteins are denatured, which leads to an increase in plasma viscosity, a decrease in protein solubility, and formation of macromolecules. Chylomicrons and lipid aggregates are formed and fat droplets may coalesce to form fat emboli as large as 100 μm [18,19]. The net effect of these changes in blood constituents during bypass is to predispose to thromboembolism and hypoperfusion.

There are numerous potential sources of emboli during bypass. These include platelet-fibrin aggregates from the aorta or the synthetic surfaces of the bypass machine; atherosclerotic or calcified emboli from the aorta; thrombus from the cardiac chambers; air emboli introduced during the operation or generated by the oxygenator (particularly bubble oxygenators); and fat emboli formed by the effects of bypass on serum lipids or introduced into the circulation from direct trauma to mediastinal and epicardial fat. Additionally, talc, silicone antifoam products, and other foreign material can be introduced during bypass and act as a source of emboli [20]. Modern surgical techniques and bypass technology, including the use of arterial line filters (20 to 40 μm), have reduced but not eliminated the risk of embolization during open heart surgery [20]. In fact, there is substantial evidence that the brain is constantly bombarded by microemboli during cardiopulmonary bypass, and accumulating evidence that these microemboli may cause encephalopathy and cognitive disorders following cardiopulmonary bypass.

As early as 1965, Austen and Howry used ultrasound to detect gaseous and particulate microemboli in the arterial line during bypass [21]. In more recent years, the development of transcranial Doppler ultrasound has enabled the evaluation of cerebral hemodynamics during CABG [22]. This technique permits quantification of cerebral blood flow velocity in the major intracranial arteries and detection of microemboli to the brain (Fig. 1). The use of transcranial Doppler to monitor brain embolization has been discussed at length in Chapter 2, on brain embolism.

Using transcranial Doppler ultrasound, several investigators have shown that microemboli to the cerebral circulation are detectable in virtually all patients undergoing CABG [22–25]. In one study, in which transcranial Doppler ultrasound was compared to transesophageal echocardiography for detecting microemboli during CABG, the mean number of emboli detected by transcranial Doppler of a middle cerebral artery was 133 $\pm$ 28 per patient, and the mean number of emboli detected by transesophageal echocardiography of the aortic arch was 535 $\pm$ 109 per patient [26]. Since the smallest particle size detectable is at least 50 μm for transcranial Doppler ultrasound and 200 μm for transesophageal echocardiography, it is probable that an even higher number of microemboli (i.e., $<$50 μm) travel to the brain during CABG. Most of the microemboli are detected during manipulation of the aorta, i.e., during aortic cannulation, cross clamping of the aorta, and particularly when aortic cross clamps are released [23,25]. Although transcranial Doppler ultrasound and transesophageal echocardiography enable detection of microemboli, these techniques cannot reliably distinguish subtypes of microemboli, i.e., air, fat, platelet-fibrin emboli, etc. Headway is being made in this area with recent studies suggesting that gaseous emboli are associated with high amplitude and intense, bidirectional signals whereas par-

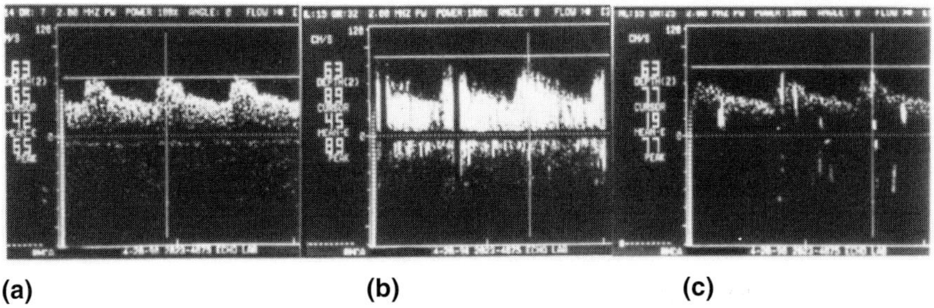

FIG. 1 Example of air emboli detected in the middle cerebral artery by transcranial Doppler ultrasound during a bubble test in a patient with pulmonary A-V fistulae. (a) Normal middle cerebral artery signal before intravenous contrast injection. (b) Multiple micro air emboli initially detected in the middle cerebral artery after contrast injection. (c) Thirty to 60 seconds later, individual air emboli detected in the middle cerebral artery. Note that gaseous emboli are associated with high-amplitude, intense, bidirectional signals whereas particulate microemboli detected during CABG are more likely to be associated with less intense, lower-amplitude, unidirectional signals. From Ref. 120.

ticulate microemboli are more likely to be associated with less intense, lower-amplitude, unidirectional signals [27].

Other evidence that microemboli travel to the brain during CABG is provided by retinal microvascular studies using fluorescein angiography during bypass, and neuropathological studies of patients dying following bypass. Blauth et al. performed retinal fluorescein angiograms preoperatively and again 5 minutes before bypass was discontinued in 21 patients [28]. All patients developed retinal microvascular occlusions indicative of microembolism during bypass. The mean number of blocked arterioles <50 μm in size was 3.5 per patient and the mean microembolic count was 12.6 per patient. Repeat studies at 30 minutes showed a reduced mean microembolic count of 4.8 per patient. The use of a 40-μm arterial filter in 11 patients did not reduce the total microembolic count [28].

In an elegant neuropathological study that utilized an alkaline phosphatase histochemical stain to visualize brain arterioles and capillaries in patients dying after cardiopulmonary bypass or noncardiac operations, Moody et al. [29] provided strong evidence that numerous microemboli travel to the brain during bypass. Four of five patients undergoing bypass and none of 34 patients undergoing noncardiac operations had numerous small-capillary and arteriolar dilatations (SCADs) scattered throughout the brain (Fig. 2). These SCADs were typically 10 to 40 μm in size and the lumina were clear and free of blood products. They were found most commonly in areas of high cerebral blood flow (i.e., the cerebral cortex and deep gray matter), and in one patient the density of SCADs was estimated at 11,760/cm^3, suggesting a total brain load of 15.3 million SCADs [29]. The authors speculated that SCADs are caused by air or fat emboli.

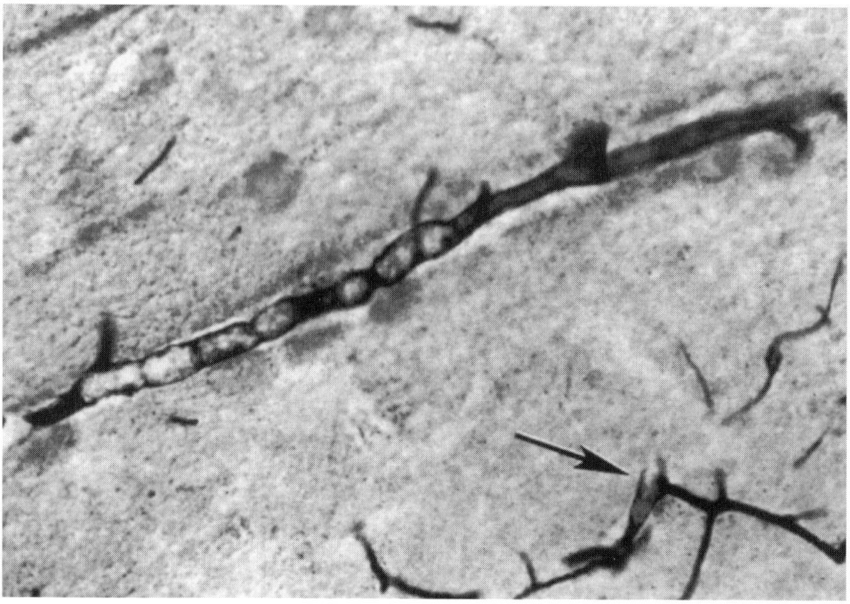

FIG. 2 Sausagelike dilatations in a medium-sized arteriole from white matter of a patient dying following CABG. These putative emboli are 40 μm in diameter. Another of these emboli is seen in a smaller arteriole (arrow). From Ref. 29.

Hypoperfusion is also a potential threat to the brain during bypass. Most studies have shown a substantial reduction in cerebral blood flow (CBF) that is coupled to a decrease in the cerebral metabolic rate during hypothermic bypass [30,31]. Factors other than metabolic rate also have an impact on CBF during CABG. The most important factors include mean arterial pressure (MAP), carbon dioxide levels, and pump flow rate. In normotensive normothermic humans, cerebral autoregulation maintains a constant CBF between MAPs of 50 to 150 mm Hg. At MAPs below or above this range, CBF is directly proportional to MAP. Based on these data, MAP during CABG is typically maintained above 50 mm Hg. One study suggested that CBF is preserved at MAPs as low as 30 mm Hg during hypothermic bypass [30]; i.e., the lower limit of cerebral autoregulation is extended during bypass. However, there are conflicting data on cerebral autoregulation during bypass, with some studies showing a poor correlation between CBF and MAP [30,32] (i.e., preservation of autoregulation) and other studies showing a strong correlation between CBF and MAP [33,34] (i.e., loss of autoregulation). This is a critical issue because if cerebral autoregulation is abolished, it is possible that prolonged hypotension ($MAP < 50$ mm Hg) during bypass could cause brain ischemia. Hypertensive patients may be at highest risk of ischemia from low MAPs because the lower and upper limits of MAP at which autoregulation is abolished are higher in hypertensive patients.

Clues to the effectiveness of cerebral autoregulation during bypass are provided by clinical studies that have correlated neurological outcome to CBF or CBF velocity during bypass. While some studies have not shown a correlation between neurologic outcome and MAP during bypass [35,36], other studies have shown a strong correlation [32,37–39]. Tufo et al. [37] observed that 78% of patients whose MAP was maintained at <40 mm Hg had a neurological deficit, compared with 27% whose MAP was maintained >60 mm Hg. In a recent prospective study, 248 patients undergoing CABG were randomized to a MAP of 50 to 60 mm Hg or 80 to 100 mm Hg during bypass [39]. The impact of MAP on mortality, cardiac morbidity, stroke, cognitive dysfunction, and functional status was evaluated in the postoperative period and at 6 months. The overall incidence of postoperative cardiac and neurological complications was 4.8% in the higher pressure group vs. 12.9% in the lower pressure group ($P = .03$). At 6 months, the two groups had the following event rates (higher-pressure group first): mortality 1.6% vs. 4%; stroke 2.4% vs. 7.2%; cardiac complications 2.4% vs. 4.8%. Cognitive and functional status did not differ between the two treatment groups [39].

Maintaining normal $PaCO_2$ levels during bypass is important because the response of the cerebral circulation to changes in CO_2 tension is maintained during hypothermic bypass, i.e., a fall (rise) in $PaCO_2$ is associated with lower (higher) CBF. Since CO_2 is more soluble at lower temperatures, it exerts a lower partial pressure. Therefore, maintaining a $PaCO_2$ of 40 mm Hg at a body temperature of 28°C (the pH-stat technique) is approximately equivalent to a $PaCO_2$ of 60 mm Hg at normal body temperature. Use of the pH-stat technique increases total CO_2 and CBF, which carries the risk of hyperemia and cerebral edema. Therefore, $PaCO_2$ is typically maintained at a level of approximately 26 mm Hg at 28°C during bypass (the alpha-stat method), which is equivalent to 40 mm Hg at normal body temperature [40]. The effect of pump flow rates on CBF during bypass is also controversial. Govier et al. found that varying pump flow rates between 1.0 and 2.0 L/min/m^2 in 10 patients did not significantly affect CBF [30]; however, other investigators have suggested that pump flow rates are an important determinant of CBF [41].

Cooling of body temperature to 28°C during cardiac surgery became routine after Bigelow and others employed this technique in the 1950s, to protect the brain from ischemia [42]. The neuroprotective effects of hypothermia include reducing cerebral oxygen metabolism, inhibiting the release of toxic excitatory neurotransmitters (e.g., glutamate, aspartate) in response to ischemia, and reducing the hyperglycemic response to cerebral ischemia [43]. Typically, coronary artery bypass grafting is performed during cooling and rewarming. Hypothermic

of multiple simultaneous emboli, it is likely that multiple territorial infarcts occurring during CABG are probably related to a "shower of emboli" produced by manipulation of an atherosclerotic aorta (e.g., aortic arch cannulation, cross clamping). Support for this is provided by pathological studies of patients dying from multiple strokes following CABG that have shown multiple lipid laden intracerebral emboli [55].

Microembolization and hypoperfusion may interact to compound brain infarction acquired during cardiopulmonary bypass. Reduced systemic and brain perfusion associated with low mean arterial pressures may reduce clearance (washout) of microemboli, especially in border zone regions where cerebral blood flow is most compromised. [55a] The poor washout of emboli can lead to more prolonged obstruction of small brain arteries and more extensive brain infarction than if perfusion were well maintained.

In patients with a single, unilateral territorial infarct that occurs during CABG, the mechanism is most likely embolic with potential sources including the cervical carotid and vertebral arteries, aorta, and heart. The heart is the most common source of such macroemboli. Many patients undergoing CABG surgery have regions of myocardial damage that are associated with thrombi within the heart. Unfortunately, many patients undergoing CABG have not had recent echocardiography which could assess the presence of myocardial thrombi or myocardial lesions that might predispose to thrombus formation within the heart during or immediately after surgery.

Small deep infarcts are also sometimes noted after surgery. Most studies have shown that small (<1.5 cm) subcortical or brainstem infarcts (lacunar infarcts) are uncommon following CABG, although one study showed that 16% of post-CABG strokes were lacunar [53]. These infarcts are typically caused by stenosis or occlusion of one of the small branches of the middle cerebral artery (lenticulostriate arteries) or basilar artery (paramedian penetrators, thalamogeniculate arteries, thalamoperforators) that penetrates the substance of the brain. Narrowing of these small arteries is typically caused by microatheroma or lipohyalinosis, an occlusive hypertensive-related vasculopathy. The mechanism of lacunar infarction during CABG is uncertain but may be related to hypoperfusion of the subcortical or brainstem region perfused by a diseased penetrating artery. Another possible cause of lacunar infarction following CABG is microembolism.

Most studies have shown that patients with *previous stroke* are at increased risk of recurrent stroke during CABG. The mechanisms of recurrent stroke during CABG have been evaluated in a few studies. In a retrospective study of 127 patients with a history of stroke, 17 (13%) had a new stroke or worsening of their prior neurological deficit. In patients whose initial stroke was within 3 months of surgery, 60% of recurrent strokes were extensions of previous strokes, 80% of recurrent strokes occurred in patients whose MAP was <50 mm Hg at some point during bypass, and 0% had perioperative atrial fibrillation or flutter [56].

The authors suggested that patients with recent stroke have peri-infarction hemodynamic vulnerability which may lead to extension of infarction during bypass induced hypotension. In patients with more remote infarcts (i.e., >3 months old), 75% of recurrent strokes were in a different vascular territory and 50% had perioperative atrial fibrillation or flutter [56]. These findings suggest that embolism, in particular cardioembolism related to atrial fibrillation, was the cause of most of these strokes. In a prospective study of 71 patients with previous stroke who underwent CABG, 31 (44%) had a focal neurological deficit postoperatively. These deficits were a new stroke in six patients (9%) and reappearance or worsening of a previous deficit without a new infarct on brain imaging in 25 (35%) [57]. These findings confirm the vulnerability of previously ischemic brain to cardiopulmonary bypass.

CAROTID ARTERY DISEASE AND RISK OF STROKE DURING CABG

Extracranial carotid artery disease is frequently suggested as an important cause of stroke during CABG. This has prompted the practice of performing prophylactic staged or combined carotid endarterectomy/CABG in asymptomatic patients who are discovered to have carotid stenosis (usually through the detection of a bruit) during the preoperative evaluation. Since up to 10% of patients undergoing CABG have coexistent moderate or severe asymptomatic carotid stenosis [58], clarification of the role of endarterectomy in this setting is important. Unfortunately, most of the studies that have evaluated the risk of peri-CABG stroke in patients with carotid stenosis [48,59–64] have one or more of the following design flaws: retrospective study design; no control groups; low power; neurologists not involved in determining whether a stroke occurred; neurological evaluation not blinded to the presence of carotid disease; strokes contralateral to carotid stenosis included in some series; evaluation for other potential causes of stroke not performed; accuracy of techniques used for documenting degree of carotid stenosis not validated.

Given the differences in the design of these studies, it is not surprising that the results of these studies are discordant. Some studies have shown no increase in the risk of peri-CABG stroke in patients with *asymptomatic* carotid stenosis [48,59,65], whereas other studies suggest that the risk of stroke in patients with carotid stenosis is significantly increased [58,60–64]. In a retrospective study in which angiography was used to document percent stenosis of the carotid artery, Furlan et al. [66] identified 155 stenotic (>50%) or occluded carotid arteries in 144 patients undergoing CABG. Ipsilateral stroke occurred in 1 of 90 patients (1%) with 50% to 90% stenosis, 1 of 16 (6%) with 90% to 99% stenosis, and in 1 of 49 (2%) with carotid occlusion. Other studies using ultrasound have also found a low risk of ipsilateral stroke in patients with carotid stenosis undergoing CABG. In one prospective study, the frequency of ipsilateral TIA or stroke in patients with carotid stenosis not repaired during CABG was 2%; however, the rate of ipsilateral TIA or stroke in patients with carotid occlusion was 17% [67].

Other studies have suggested that the risk of stroke during CABG is related to the degree of carotid occlusive disease. In one study of 582 veterans who had a high frequency (22%) of carotid stenosis (>50%) or occlusion, Schwartz et al. [63] found that none of the 52 patients with unilateral 50% to 79% carotid stenosis had a stroke, but that 4 of 75 patients (5.3%) with unilateral 80% to 99% stenosis, bilateral 50% to 99% stenosis, or unilateral occlusion with contralateral stenosis >50% had a stroke. In a well-designed prospective study of 1631 consecutive patients, Mickleborough et al. [68] showed that the risk of stroke was 0% in patients without carotid stenosis, 3.2% in patients with >70% stenosis, and 27% in patients with carotid occlusion. Faggioli et al. [58] reported that 4 of 28 patients (14%) had a stroke ipsilateral to carotid stenosis >75%; however, Ricotta et al. [62] found no increased risk of stroke in patients with >75% stenosis.

Since the risk of peri-CABG stroke in patients with asymptomatic carotid stenosis is uncertain, the role of carotid endarterectomy for asymptomatic carotid stenosis before or combined with CABG is controversial. In a single-center prospective, randomized trial of 129 patients with asymptomatic carotid stenosis >70% who underwent CABG, Hertzer et al. [69] reported a stroke rate of 7% in patients undergoing CABG alone (i.e., without prophylactic endarterectomy) versus 3% in patients undergoing combined CABG/carotid endarterectomy. The difference between the two groups was not statistically significant; however, a benefit from carotid endarterectomy cannot be excluded because of the very low power of the study. The most comprehensive data available on the role of staged or combined carotid endarterectomy/CABG comes from a meta-analysis of 56 studies [70] (virtually all retrospective; only 19 had >50 patients) that evaluated three operative strategies: simultaneous endarterectomy and CABG, endarterectomy followed by CABG, and CABG followed by endarterectomy. Stroke rates for these three groups were 6%, 5%, and 10%, respectively. The frequency of stroke was significantly higher ($P < .05$) if CABG preceded endarterectomy. Myocardial infarction rates for the three groups were 5%, 11%, and 3%, respectively, and death rates were 6%, 9%, and 4%. The frequency of myocardial infarction ($P = .01$) and death ($P = .02$) was higher when carotid surgery preceded CABG [70]. Combining all endpoints shows that endarterectomy followed by CABG is associated with the worst outcome of the three strategies, with similar outcomes in the other two groups. Clarification of the optimal strategy for managing asymptomatic carotid stenosis in patients undergoing CABG will require an adequately powered, multicenter, randomized clinical trial. However, the design of such a trial is challenging since it will require standardization of the surgical and bypass techniques (e.g., management of aortic atherosclerosis) to ensure that differences in the outcome of the treatment groups can be attributed to the performance of carotid endarterectomy.

In summary, the available data on the risk of stroke associated with asymptomatic carotid stenosis in patients undergoing CABG suggests that (1) there is no increase in the risk of peri-CABG stroke in patients with moderate carotid stenosis i.e., 50% to 75%; (2) it is probable that a subgroup of patients with severe asymptomatic carotid stenosis (>75%) are at increased risk of stroke during CABG; (3) patients with carotid occlusion or bilateral carotid stenosis (especially if high grade) are at increased risk of stroke; (4) currently available data do not support the strategy of prophylactic endarterectomy prior to CABG in patients with asymptomatic carotid stenosis >75%.

The management of *symptomatic* carotid stenosis in patients undergoing CABG is also challenging. There are limited data on the risk of peri-CABG stroke in patients with symptomatic high-grade carotid stenosis. In one study, Hertzer et al. [69] reported that 2 of 23 patients (9%) with symptomatic or bilateral carotid

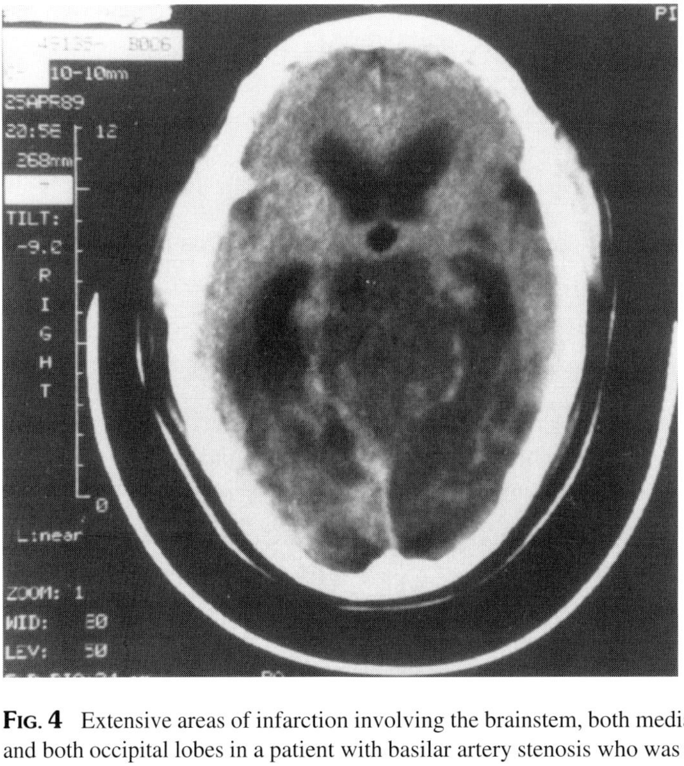

FIG. 4 Extensive areas of infarction involving the brainstem, both medial temporal lobes, and both occipital lobes in a patient with basilar artery stenosis who was comatose following CABG. From Ref. 121.

stenosis $\geq$ 70% who underwent CABG had a stroke. In another study, 3 of 10 patients with symptomatic carotid stenosis >50% had ipsilateral perioperative stroke [60]. Although there are no studies on the safety and efficacy of staged or simultaneous endarterectomy/CABG in patients with symptomatic carotid stenosis, most surgeons and neurologists advocate endarterectomy prior to CABG (if the cardiac symptoms are stable) or during CABG (if the cardiac symptoms are active) in these patients. This strategy is based on the North American Symptomatic Carotid Endarterectomy Trial, which showed a 17% absolute reduction in the risk of ipsilateral stroke over 2 years in patients with symptomatic carotid stenosis $\geq$70% treated surgically compared with patients treated medically (2-year ipsilateral stroke rates were 26% in the medical arm and 9% in the surgical arm; $P < .001$) [71]. There are virtually no data on the risk of stroke during CABG in patients with vertebrobasilar occlusive disease. Anecdotal experience of the authors suggests that the risk of stroke may be high in patients with symptomatic intracranial vertebral artery or basilar artery stenosis undergoing CABG (Fig. 4).

AORTIC ATHEROSCLEROSIS AND THE RISK OF STROKE DURING CABG

While carotid artery disease has received considerable attention as a potential cause of stroke during CABG, it is important to recognize that the vast majority of strokes in the setting of CABG occur in patients without carotid stenosis. Moreover, strokes that occur in patients with carotid stenosis are frequently in a different territory from the stenotic carotid artery or are bilateral. These data imply that other vascular pathologies must be responsible for these strokes. Over the last few years, aortic atherosclerosis has emerged as an important cause of peri-CABG stroke. Studies in which transesophageal echocardiography or epiaortic ultrasound have been used to image the aorta during CABG have shown that embolism produced by surgical manipulation of the aorta (i.e., cannulation for bypass, cross clamping, insertion of vein grafts or the cardioplegia needle) is probably the most common cause of stroke during CABG (Fig. 5). One of the first studies to suggest a correlation between aortic arch disease and peri-CABG stroke was an autopsy study by Blauth et al. [72]. These investigators performed autopsies in 221 patients who died following CABG or valvular surgery. Atheroemboli were found in 48 patients (22%) and were most common in the brain (16% of patients). Multiple embolic sites were found in 63% of patients. Emboli were significantly more common in patients undergoing CABG (26%) than in patients undergoing valve procedures (9%) ($P = .008$). There was a high correlation between atheroemboli and severity of atherosclerosis of the ascending aorta: atheroemboli were found in 46 (37%) of 123 patients with severe aortic athero-

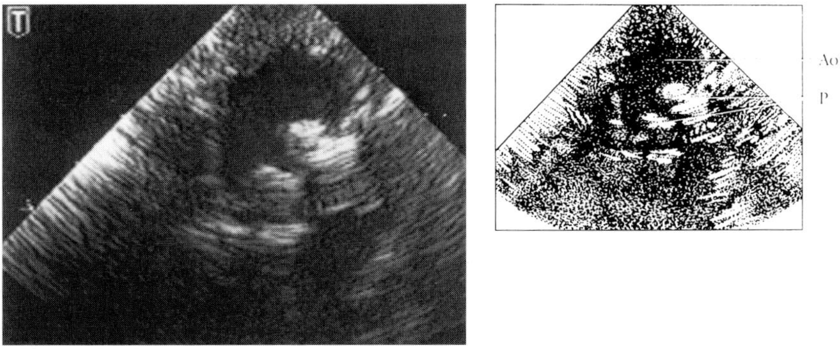

FIG. 5 Aortic arch atheroma detected by transesophageal echocardiography. Insert on the right is a diagram of the TEE on the left. Aol., aortic lumen; P, plaque. From Ref. 122.

sclerosis but in only 2 (2%) of 98 patients who did not have severe aortic atherosclerosis ($P < .0001$) [72].

Other studies using transesophageal echocardiography have consistently confirmed the importance of atherosclerosis of the aorta as a cause of stroke during CABG. Hosoda et al. [73] reported that 3 of 13 (23%) patients with severe atherosclerosis of the ascending aorta had a peri-CABG stroke, compared to 0 of 87 with mild or moderate aortic disease. In another transesophageal echocardiography study, 3 of 9 patients (33%) with mobile plaques of the aortic arch had peri-CABG stroke versus 2 of 74 patients (2.7%) with nonmobile plaque ($P = .01$) [74]. In another study, in which atherosclerosis of the descending aorta was classified into one of five grades (I = normal; V = >5 mm intraluminal plaque with mobile component), no strokes occurred in 123 patients with grade I or II atheroma, while 9 of 66 patients (14%) with grades III to V atheroma had a stroke ($P = .00001$). In patients with grade V atheroma, 5 of 11 patients (46%) had a stroke [75]. Although the atheromas in the descending aorta were probably not responsible for the strokes, it is likely that patients with severe atherosclerosis of the descending aorta also had atherosclerosis of the ascending aorta.

The emergence of aortic atherosclerosis as a major cause of stroke has led to studies on the appropriate diagnosis and management of aortic atherosclerosis during CABG. These studies show that the traditional technique of inspection/palpation of the ascending aorta during CABG is insensitive for detecting aortic atherosclerosis. Davila-Roman et al. [76] performed inspection/palpation and epiaortic ultrasonography of the ascending aorta during CABG in 100 consecutive patients. Moderate or severe aortic atherosclerosis was diagnosed by ultrasound in 29% of patients. Palpation of the aorta significantly underestimated the presence ($P < .001$) and severity ($P < .001$) of aortic atherosclerosis compared with ultrasound. Age and diabetes were shown to be independently associated with severe aortic atherosclerosis [76]. In another study by the same group, palpation identified only 38% of patients with significant aortic atherosclerosis [77].

Management of aortic atherosclerosis during CABG has also been evaluated by a few investigators. Wareing et al. [77] used intraoperative ultrasound to identify 68 (14%) of 540 consecutive patients undergoing CABG who had significant atherosclerosis of the ascending aorta. The authors applied Doppler probes to the external surface of the aorta after the chest was opened, and surveyed the aorta for regions of severe plaque disease. A total of 168 modifications in the standard technique for cannulation and clamping of the aorta were made in the 68 patients. These included changing the sites of aortic cannulation, aortic clamping, insertion of vein grafts, and insertion of the cardioplegic needle. Additionally, 10 patients with severe diffuse atheromatous aortic arch disease underwent graft replacement of the ascending aorta with hypothermic circulatory arrest without aortic clamping. Remarkably, none of the 68 patients with significant aortic atherosclerosis in whom surgical modifications were performed had a stroke [77]. In a subsequent study by the same group, 47 patients with atheromatous aortic arch disease underwent graft replacement of the ascending aorta during CABG. Two patients (4.3%) died within 30 days of CABG, both from myocardial infarction, and none of the surviving patients had a perioperative stroke [78].

In a case control study, Duda et al. [79] performed intraoperative surface aortic ultrasonography on 195 consecutive patients (study group) undergoing CABG and compared their outcome with a historical control group of 164 consecutive patients in whom the ascending aorta was assessed during CABG by inspection and palpation alone. Based on the presence of aortic atherosclerosis, changes in the operative technique (hypothermic fibrillatory arrest with no cross clamping of the aorta and left ventricular venting, single cross clamping, modification in aortic cannulation site or placement of arterial grafts) were made in both groups. The frequency of moderate/severe aortic atherosclerosis was 14% in patients having epiaortic ultrasound versus 2% in the control group. Surgery was modified in 19 study patients (10%) and 3 control patients (2%). None of the study patients had a perioperative stroke, versus 5 (3%) in the control group ($P < .02$) [79].

In summary, these studies suggest that (1) 14% to 29% of patients undergoing epiaortic ultrasound during CABG have moderate or severe atherosclerosis of the ascending aorta, and that age is the most important predictor of aortic atherosclerosis; (2) patients with severe aortic atherosclerosis may have a 23% to 46% risk of peri-CABG stroke; (3) modifications of the operative technique (e.g., changing the sites of aortic cannulation, aortic clamping, insertion of vein grafts, and insertion of cardioplegic needle) may substantially reduce the risk of peri-CABG stroke; and (4) more invasive techniques (e.g., hypothermic fibrillatory arrest with no cross clamping of the aorta and left ventricular venting, graft replacement of the ascending aorta with hypothermic circulatory arrest without aortic clamping) may also have a role in patients with severe diffuse aortic arch atherosclerosis. However, these techniques need further study.

The importance of aortic disease as a cause of postoperative neurological complications has been one of the factors that has favored the use of minimally invasive coronary artery bypass grafting, and coronary artery grafting without the use of cardiopulmonary bypass. Minimally invasive coronary artery bypass grafting can be performed with or without cardiopulmonary bypass and does not use a median sternotomy incision [79a,79b]. Coronary artery bypass grafting has also now been performed quite effectively off cardiopulmonary bypass using a number of techniques to obtain cardioplegia during the grafting [79c,79d]. When cardiopulmonary bypass is not used, cannulation of the aorta is avoided.

POST-CABG ATRIAL FIBRILLATION AND THE RISK OF STROKE

Another important treatable condition that may cause stroke following CABG is atrial fibrillation (AF). AF occurs in up to 32% of patients after CABG and in up to 64% of patients after CABG and aortic valve replacement [80]. AF occurs most commonly 24 to 72 hours after surgery [81]. Risk factors for the development of post-CABG AF include advanced age, preoperative withdrawal of β blockers, chronic obstructive pulmonary disease, and prolonged aortic cross clamp time [80]. Post-CABG AF usually resolves in a few days in most patients who do not have a history of preoperative AF. Most studies have shown a three- to fivefold increase in stroke risk post-CABG in patients who develop AF [61,80-82]. However, one study showed similar stroke rates in patients with AF (3.6%) compared with patients without AF (3.5%) [83].

In view of the increased risk of post-CABG stroke and prolonged hospital stay in patients who develop AF, the role of prophylactic therapy to prevent post-CABG AF has been studied extensively. In a meta-analysis of 12 placebo-controlled trials, β blockers alone or in combination with digoxin was effective for preventing post-CABG AF whereas digoxin alone was not [84]. In another meta-analysis, the frequency of post-CABG AF was 8.7% in patients given β blockers preoperatively, compared to 34% in patients not prescribed β blockers. This meta-analysis also showed that digoxin or verapamil alone were not effective for preventing post-CABG AF [85]. Other medications that are effective for preventing post-CABG AF are procainamide [86] and amiodarone [87]. In a recent double-blind randomized study, patients were given either oral amiodarone or placebo for a minimum of 7 days before elective cardiac surgery (CABG or valvular surgery). The dose of amiodarone was 600 mg/day for 7 days, then 200 mg/day until the day of discharge from the hospital. Postoperative AF occurred in 25% of patients given amiodarone, compared with 53% given placebo ($P = .003$).

Additionally, the length of stay was significantly lower in the amiodarone group than the placebo group (6.5 ± 2.6 vs. 7.9 ± 4.3 days; $P = .04$) [87].

The management of post-CABG AF is similar to the treatment of AF in other settings. Pires et al. [81] have suggested the following approach that we have found useful in clinical practice. If postoperative AF causes hemodynamic instability, urgent electrical cardioversion is required. If postoperative AF is not associated with hemodynamic instability, control of the ventricular response can be achieved using digoxin, β blockers, or calcium channel blockers. The use of digoxin in this situation is controversial. Since most episodes of post-CABG AF resolve within a few days of surgery, antiarrhythmic agents that convert AF to sinus rhythm (quinidine, procainamide, amiodarone, sotalol) are usually not instituted unless the episode of AF lasts longer than 48 to 72 hours. When this occurs, anticoagulation is also recommended. Since it is unknown whether patients who have a brief episode of post-CABG AF are at higher risk of developing chronic AF in the future, long-term anticoagulation is not warranted after post-CABG AF lasting less than 72 hours.

COGNITIVE ABNORMALITIES FOLLOWING CABG

Cognitive abnormalities that are not associated with focal motor, sensory, or visual dysfunction are the most common neurological complication of CABG. The spectrum of cognitive problems is wide: some patients have obvious cognitive problems that are detectable at the bedside whereas others may have subtle problems that are only detectable by detailed neuropsychological testing. Estimates of the incidence of cognitive problems post-CABG range from 30% [88] to 88% [89], depending on the type and timing of the neuropsychological diagnostic tests performed. Advanced age and length of bypass appear to be the most important risk factors for cognitive abnormality following CABG [90].

The most common cognitive abnormalities are disturbances of memory, concentration, and attention, and rapidity of responses to stimuli [89]. Although these cognitive problems resolve within a few months in a substantial number of patients, a few studies have shown that cognitive problems persist in up to 35% of patients at 1 year [91] and in 20% of patients at 3 years after surgery [92]. In a recent well-designed prospective study, testing of eight cognitive domains was performed preoperatively, at 1 month, and 1 year postoperatively in 127 patients undergoing CABG [89]. Only 12% of patients showed no decline across all domains tested. Of the 88% with abnormalities in at least one domain, 10% had persistent decline in the domains of verbal memory, visual memory, attention, and visuoconstruction at 1 year [89]. Depression was also evaluated in this study using a validated depression measure. In patients who were not depressed preoperatively, the frequency of postoperative depression was 13% at 1 month and 9% at 1 year. There was no correlation between depression and cognitive decline, suggesting that depression did not account for the cognitive abnormalities [93].

The causes of cognitive decline following CABG are uncertain. Abnormalities of intellectual function and behavior are frequently attributed to cerebral hypoperfusion during bypass, medications (analgesics, sedatives), and metabolic disturbances. Studies of the relationship between hypoperfusion and cognitive problems have produced discordant results. Tufo et al. [37] found neurological deficits (stroke or cognitive problems) in 78% of patients whose mean arterial pressure was maintained at <40 mm Hg during bypass, compared with 27% of patients whose mean arterial pressure was maintained >60 mm Hg. However, in a recent prospective randomized study comparing mean arterial pressures of 50 to 60 versus 80 to 100 mm Hg during bypass, neuropsychological testing revealed no differences in the incidence of cognitive problems in the two groups, whereas the incidence of stroke was higher (7.2%) in the lower-pressure group than in the higher-pressure group (2.4%) [39]. Other studies have also failed to show a correlation between cerebral hypoperfusion during CABG and cognitive dysfunction [35,94]. Although medications or metabolic disorders may account for some cases of cognitive decline following CABG, they do not account for the high incidence of persistent cognitive problems at 1 and 5 years after surgery.

Recent prospective studies provide accumulating evidence that microembolism is probably the most important cause of cognitive decline following CABG. Using transcranial Doppler or carotid ultrasound to detect brain microemboli during CABG, several investigators have shown that patients with cognitive deficits post-CABG have a significantly higher frequency of microemboli during surgery than patients with no cognitive decline. In a study of 395 patients, Hammon et al. [95] found that more than 100 cerebral emboli per case was significantly ($P < .04$) associated with postoperative neurobehavioral abnormalities. Pugsley et al. [96] found that 43% of patients with intraoperative embolic counts >1000 had cognitive decline at 8 weeks after CABG, versus only 8.6% of patients with <200 emboli.

In a study of 20 patients, Barbut et al. [23] showed a correlation between the number of emboli at cross clamp removal and severity of aortic arch disease ($P < .04$). Additionally, the mean number of embolic events at clamp removal was 166 in six patients with cognitive deterioration, compared with 73 in 11 patients without deterioration ($P < .05$). This study suggests that in addition to being a source of macroemboli, aortic arch atheroma is an important source of microemboli during CABG. This implies that embolization from aortic arch disease may be the most important cause of cognitive decline (from microembolization) as well as stroke (from macroembolization) during CABG.

Encephalopathy, which is characterized by obtundation or delirium without focal neurological signs, also occurs after CABG but it is substantially less common than cognitive dysfunction. In one study of 59 patients, delirium occurred within the first 5 postoperative days in 4 patients (6%), but resolved by the sixth postoperative day in all patients [97]. The cause of post-CABG encephalopathy is usually multifactorial and is typically related to one or more of the following problems: medications (particularly sedatives and narcotics), fever, sepsis, hypoxia, metabolic abnormalities, and hypotension. Microemboli might also cause reversible encephalopathy following CABG, but this needs further study.

OTHER POST-CABG NEUROLOGICAL PROBLEMS

Complications involving the *peripheral nervous system* occur in up to 13% of patients following CABG [98]. In the most comprehensive study to date, Lederman et al. [98] prospectively evaluated 421 patients following CABG and found that 55 patients (13%) developed 63 new problems involving the peripheral nervous system. These included brachial plexopathy (23 patients), saphenous neuropathy (13), common peroneal palsy (8), phrenic nerve palsy (6), ulnar neuropathy (5), recurrent laryngeal nerve palsy (5), radial sensory neuropathy (1), Horner's syndrome (1), and facial palsy (1). Most of these deficits were transient but two patients, one with a brachial plexopathy and another with peroneal palsy, had persistent weakness. Risk factors for the development of peripheral nervous system complications in this study were hypothermia and male sex. The predominance of men is difficult to explain, but hypothermia is a recognized cause of neuropathy [99,100]. Surprisingly, diabetes was not associated with peripheral nervous problems despite the well-recognized risk of stretch and compressive nerve injuries in diabetics [98].

Brachial plexopathy is the most common and potentially serious peripheral nervous lesion after CABG. Typically, the lower trunk or C8-T1 nerve roots are involved resulting in the syndrome of pain (which may be very severe), dysesthesias, and weakness of the hand. In one study, 85% of brachial plexus injuries involved the lower trunk and 73% of plexus lesions correlated with the side of internal jugular vein cannulation [101]. These findings suggest that trauma of the lower trunk of the brachial plexus during jugular vein cannulation is a common mechanism of brachial plexus injury during CABG. Another mechanism of brachial plexus injury during CABG is stretching of the plexus from chest wall retraction. Harvesting the internal mammary artery for use as a donor vessel for bypass carries the highest risk because this typically requires more chest wall retraction. Patients with weakness of the hand (lower trunk) or arm (more extensive brachial plexopathy) may be misdiagnosed as having had a stroke following CABG. A careful history and neurological examination and brain imaging (if necessary) will distinguish between these two disorders. Ulnar and peroneal palsies are typically caused by compression of these nerves at the elbow and knee from poor positioning of the patient during anesthesia or in the postoperative period. Foot drop (weakness of foot dorsiflexion) is the usual presentation of a peroneal palsy whereas numbness of the fourth and fifth digits is the typical presentation of ulnar neuropathy. Saphenous neuropathy is related to injury to the nerve during harvesting of the saphenous vein and typically presents with sensory loss of the medial calf. Some patients develop meralgia paresthetica, a disorder due to pressure on the lateral femoral cutaneous nerve, during or more likely after surgery. These patients complain of paresthesias and burning in the lateral upper thigh without any accompanying motor or reflex abnormalities. Compression of the nerve in the groin near the inguinal ligament is the presumed cause of this minor disorder.

Coma is a rare complication of CABG, occuring in <1% of patients. The cause of coma is not always apparent. In one study of 34 patients who failed to awaken following open heart surgery, the cause of coma was uncertain in 19 patients (56%). In the other patients, the causes of coma were well-documented episodes of global cerebral ischemia or hypoxia (7 patients), large hemispheric infarction with brain herniation (5), and multifocal infarctions (3) [102]. It is likely that global ischemia is responsible for the majority of cases of coma of uncertain cause. Although severe hypotension (e.g., mean arterial pressure < 40 mm Hg) may not have occurred in these cases, it is probable that cerebral blood flow was inadequate in some patients (e.g., those with impaired autoregulation) at levels of mean arterial pressure that are commonly used during bypass, i.e., 40 to 60 mm Hg. The absence of infarcts on brain imaging does not prove that ischemia was not the cause of coma because the pathology associated with cerebral hypoperfusion may be limited to diffuse cortical laminar necrosis that is typically not detected by CT and may not be detected by MRI.

A few other rare neurological complications of CABG have been reported. These include intracranial hemorrhage [103], unilateral hearing loss [104], and pituitary apoplexy [105]. Intracerebral hemorrhage may be due to anticoagulation during bypass, unilateral hearing loss has been attributed to embolism to end arteries that supply the cochlea, and pituitary apoplexy is typically caused by infarction (less commonly, hemorrhage) of a preexisting pituitary adenoma. Pituitary apoplexy may be misdiagnosed in the postoperative setting. Obtundation may be attributed to medications or metabolic problems, and the visual loss and ophthalmoplegia may be missed. If ophthalmoplegia and visual loss are recognized, a diagnosis of brainstem/occipital infarcts from a top of the basilar artery embolus may be made. Awareness that pituitary apoplexy may occur in this setting, coupled with a careful neurological examination and detection of the pituitary mass on brain imaging, leads to the correct diagnosis.

PREVENTION OF NEUROLOGICAL COMPLICATIONS FROM CABG

Since specific causes of stroke, neuropsychological problems, and peripheral nerve lesions following CABG have been identified, prophylactic measures can be taken in the preoperative, intraoperative, and postoperative periods to lower the risk of these complications. *Preoperative* evaluation should include a detailed neurological history and examination to determine if the patient has had previous TIAs or stroke. Given the increased risk of extending a recent stroke during cardiopulmonary bypass [56], we suggest delaying CABG for 3 months unless the patient has unstable cardiac symptoms. All patients with TIA or stroke should have an extensive diagnostic evaluation to determine the cause of the symptoms. At a minimum this should include a carotid ultrasound (if the symptoms are in the distribution of a carotid artery), MRA or transcranial Doppler ultrasound (if intracranial stenosis is suspected), and transesophageal echocardiography (if a cardioembolic source is suspected).

Patients with symptomatic high-grade carotid stenosis should undergo carotid endarterectomy before CABG if the coronary symptoms are stable; otherwise, endarterectomy should be combined with CABG. The evaluation and management of asymptomatic carotid stenosis in the setting of CABG is controversial. In the absence of a prospective, randomized clinical trial on the efficacy of carotid endarterectomy in this setting, the following approach is recommended. Patients with carotid bruits detected preoperatively should undergo carotid ultrasound. If the degree of stenosis is $<75\%$, endarterectomy is not recommended in the peri-CABG setting. If the degree of carotid stenosis is $>75\%$, one approach is to determine cerebral perfusion reserve ipsilateral to the carotid stenosis using transcranial Doppler ultrasound or single-photon emission computed tomography (SPECT) after the administration of acetazolamide [106]. In patients with normal ipsilateral reserve, acetazolamide produces arteriolar vasodilation and a marked increase in ipsilateral CBF or CBF velocity. In patients with impaired reserve, the cerebral arterioles are already maximally dilated to maintain CBF. Therefore the administration of acetazolamide does not produce the expected increase in CBF or CBF velocity. Since autoregulation is impaired in these patients, they are probably at high risk of stroke during bypass induced hypotension and therefore should be considered for simultaneous carotid endarterectomy/CABG. However, this hypothesis remains untested. For patients with bilateral carotid stenosis $>75\%$, we usually recommend simultaneous CABG and carotid endarterectomy on the side of the most severe stenosis. If the degree of stenosis is similar on both sides, endarterectomy is performed on the side ipsilateral to the brain hemisphere responsible for language, i.e., usually the left side.

Patients with TIA or stroke caused by high-grade intracranial stenosis are probably at increased risk of stroke during CABG. Identification of symptomatic intracranial stenosis will sometimes lead to a decision to cancel CABG, e.g., a patient with 90% basilar artery stenosis whose coronary disease is asymptomatic. If CABG is deemed necessary, preoperative angioplasty of the stenotic intracranial artery is an option. If this is not available, maintaining mean arterial pressures between 80 and 100 mm Hg during bypass is recommended, followed by anticoagulation postoperatively. Another option to consider before surgery is the use of pharmacological agents (e.g., beta blockers, amiodarone) to prevent post-CABG atrial fibrillation [84,87]. This is especially true for high-risk patients such as those of advanced age with chronic obstructive pulmonary disease [80].

Several measures should be taken *intraoperatively* to lower the risk of neurological complications. Available data favor the use of high mean arterial pressure (at least 60 mm Hg; preferably 80 to 100 mm Hg) during bypass to lower the risk of stroke [39]. Until the last decade, moderate hypothermia was used routinely in patients undergoing CABG. Recently, normothermic bypass has gained some support on the basis of a few randomized studies, suggesting that neurological outcome is similar in patients undergoing normothermic versus hypothermic bypass [10,46]. However, other randomized studies have suggested that normothermia is associated with a significantly higher rate of stroke [45]. Some centers now use ''tepid'' cardiopulmonary bypass in which the temperature is allowed to remain at between 28 and 32°C but no active cooling is employed. Further studies are needed to clarify whether the rates of stroke and encephalopathy are similar or higher in patients undergoing normothermic bypass versus hypothermic bypass.

Several techniques are used intraoperatively to minimize the risk of embolization during CABG. These include using arterial filtration and membrane oxygenators [20], epiaortic ultrasound or transesophageal echocardiography [76], and transcranial Doppler ultrasound [22,24]. Since the aortic arch is an important source of both macroemboli and microemboli during CABG, we recommend, when possible, performing transesophageal echocardiography in all patients before CABG to scan the aorta for atherosclerosis. The information gained from echocardiography can be used by the cardiac surgeon and cardiologist to plan the optimal procedure for the patient. This would permit the best site for cannulation and cross clamping of the aorta to be planned in advance of the operation, and to detect potential cardiac sources of emboli (e.g., left atrial appendage thrombus in a patient with atrial fibrillation). The ascending aorta can also be insonated using a Duplex ultrasound probe placed in the right supraclavicular fossa, and the arch and proximal descending thoracic aorta can be imaged using a left supraclavicular probe [107a]. The results so far are preliminary but promising. Most plaques are located in the curvature of the arch from the distal ascending aorta to the proximal descending aorta, regions well shown using B-mode ultrasound. When transesophageal echocardiography is not feasible before surgery, insonation of the aorta using Duplex ultrasound can be performed at the same time as ultrasound study of the carotid and vertebral arteries. In some patients, minimally invasive surgery and surgery off bypass could be selected when the risk of aortic cannulation appears to be very high.

Alternatively, many surgeons rely on epiaortic ultrasound after the heart is exposed intraoperatively to make these decisions. Palpation of the aorta is an unreliable technique for detecting aortic atherosclerosis [77]. If focal aortic atherosclerosis is identified, relatively simple modifications of the operative technique should be made. These include changing the sites of aortic cannulation, aortic clamping, insertion of vein grafts, and insertion of cardioplegic needle, the use of a single aortic clamp, or cannulation of the femoral artery instead of the aorta [77,107]. In patients with severe diffuse aortic arch atherosclerosis, more invasive techniques may need to be considered, e.g., hypothermic fibrillatory arrest without cross clamping of the aorta and left ventricular venting, graft replacement of the ascending aorta with hypothermic circulatory arrest without aortic clamping [78]. Coronary artery bypass grafting without cardiopulmonary bypass is another option in selected patients [79c,79d,108]. In one nonrandomized study, the frequency of stroke in 378 patients who underwent CABG without cardiopulmonary bypass was 1.1%, compared with 3.8% in 689 patients who underwent CABG with cardiopulmonary bypass [108].

Some investigators are currently using transcranial Doppler ultrasound intraoperatively for microemboli detection and to monitor cerebral perfusion. Detection of a fall in cerebral blood flow velocities or microemboli in the middle cerebral arteries enables corrective action to be taken. If a drop in cerebral blood flow velocities is detected, pump flow rates can be increased to maintain cerebral perfusion. Detection of multiple emboli when the aorta is not being manipulated should raise suspicion of another source of emboli, e.g., gaseous emboli from the cardiac chambers. Using transesophageal echocardiography, pockets of air in the cardiac chambers can be detected and removed by irrigation or balloting [109]. Barbut et al. [110] have shown the prognostic value of intraoperative embolic counts detected during CABG by comparing embolic counts in patients with and without various complications following CABG. The mean number of embolic counts was 449 in patients with stroke, versus 169 in patients without stroke; the major cardiac complication rate was 4.3% in patients with <400 emboli, versus 30.7% in patients with > 400 emboli; and the mean length of hospitalization was 8.6 days in patients with <100 emboli, versus 55.8 days in patients with >500 emboli. The relationship between embolic counts and hospital stay was similar even in the absence of cardiac complications or stroke.

Pharmacological therapies have also been used to prevent or ameliorate the effects of cerebral ischemia during CABG. There is some evidence that prostacyclin infusion prevents adhesion of platelets to the extracorporeal tubing, thereby lowering blood loss and platelet-fibrin embolization during cardiopulmonary bypass [111,112]. However, prostacyclin may also cause hypotension [111,113] and therefore is not routinely used during CABG. Although barbiturates have been shown to protect the brain during CABG in a sheep model of hypothermic cardiopulmonary bypass [114], the efficacy of barbiturates in humans undergoing bypass has yet to be established. In one study in which 300 patients were randomized to thiopental or saline infusion beginning with the administration of heparin and ending after aortic decannulation, the thiopental group required more inotropic drugs during separation from bypass and required a significantly longer time for awakening and for tracheal extubation than the placebo group. Moreover, the frequency of stroke was 5 of 149 (3.3%) in the thiopental group, versus 2 of 151 (1.3%) in the saline group [115]. Recent development of other neuroprotective pharmacological agents (e.g., glutamate antagonists, GM1 ganglioside) that have ameliorated the effects of cerebral ischemia in animal models has led to the suggestion that these agents should be tested as neuroprotective agents during CABG [116,117]. Efforts to prevent peripheral nerve injuries during CABG include paying special attention to positioning the patient during anesthesia, using guards to protect against compression neuropathies at the elbows and knees, avoiding excessive chest wall retraction, and improving techniques of jugular vein cannulation and harvesting of the saphenous veins.

In the *postoperative* period, it is important to monitor patients closely for post-CABG atrial fibrillation and hypotension, both of which can lead to stroke. The management of post-CABG atrial fibrillation is described above, in the section ''Post-CABG Atrial Fibrillation and the Risk of Stroke.'' Postoperative hypotension should be treated promptly with intravenous fluids, pressors, or an intra-aortic balloon pump if necessary. Neurological symptoms or signs following CABG should prompt consultation with a neurologist. Diagnostic evaluation usually involves brain CT or MRI, carotid ultrasound (if stroke is in the territory of a carotid artery), transcranial Doppler ultrasound or MRA, and consideration of echocardiography (mandatory following valvular surgery). Fever and stroke following valvular surgery should always raise the suspicion of bacterial endocarditis.

The management of acute stroke following CABG is similar to the routine management of stroke, with a few exceptions. Since one of the contraindications of intravenous thrombolytic therapy for acute ischemic stroke is major surgery within 14 days of the stroke [118], intravenous thrombolytic therapy is not an option in the post-CABG setting. Intra-arterial thrombolysis has been used occasionally in the postoperative setting (e.g., for acute stroke following carotid endarterectomy), but the safety and efficacy of this approach remain to be established. Intravenous heparin can be used to prevent recurrent brain embolization in a patient with cardioembolic stroke following CABG (e.g., in a patient with atrial fibrillation or an intracardiac thrombus) as long as the patient has no evidence of an intracerebral hematoma on brain imaging or active systemic bleeding.

REFERENCES

1. Kuroda Y, Uchimoto R, Kaieda R, Shinkura R, Shinohara K, Miyamoto S, Oshita S, Takeshita H. Central nervous system complications after cardiac surgery: a com-

parison between coronary artery bypass grafting and valve surgery. Anesth Analg 1993; 76:222–227.
2. Gibbon JH Jr. Application of mechanical heart and lung apparatus to cardiac surgery. Minn Med 1954; 37:171–180.
3. Lillehei CW. A personalized history of extracorporeal circulation. Trans Am Soc Artif Intern Organs 1982; 28:5–16.
4. Gilman S. Cerebral disorders after open-heart operations. N Engl J Med 1965; 272: 489–498.
5. Brierley J. Neuropathological findings in patients dying after open-heart surgery. Thorax 1963; 18:291–304.
6. Ehrenhaft J, Claman M. Cerebral complications of open-heart surgery. J Thorac Cardiovasc Surg 1961; 41:503–506.
7. Ehrenhaft J, Claman M, Layton J, Zimmerman G. Cerebral complications of open-heart surgery: further observations. J Thorac Cardiovasc Surg 1961; 42:514–526.
8. Garrett H, Dennis E, DeBakey M. Aortocoronary bypass with saphenous vein graft. Seven-year follow-up. JAMA 1973; 223:792–794.
9. Favaloro R. Saphenous vein autograft replacement of severe segmental coronary artery occlusion: operative technique. Ann Thorac Surg 1968; 5:334–339.
10. Warm Heart Investigators. Randomised trial of normothermic versus hypothermic coronary bypass surgery. Lancet 1994; 343:559–563.
11. Gorman JH, Edmunds LH. Blood anesthesia for cardiopulmonary bypass. J Card Surg 1995; 10:270–279.
12. Rinder CS, Mathew JP, Rinder HM, Bonan J, Ault KA, Smith BR. Modulation of platelet surface adhesion receptors during cardiopulmonary bypass. Anesthesiology 1991; 75:563–570.
13. Lindon J, McManama G, Kushner L, Merrill E, Salzman E. Does the confirmation of absorbed fibrinogen dictate platelet-surface interaction? Blood 1986; 68:355–362.
14. Hashimoto K, Miyamoto H, Suzuki K, Horikoshi S, Matsui M, Arai T, Kurosawa H. Evidence of organ damage after cardiopulmonary bypass. The role of elastase and vasoactive mediators. J Thorac Cardiovasc Surg 1992; 104:666–673.
15. Tsai SK, Chan P, Lee TY, Yung J, Hong CY. Trilinolein improves erythrocyte deformability during cardiopulmonary bypass. Br J Clin Pharmacol 1994; 37:457–459.
16. Chenoweth D, Cooper S, Hugli T, Stewart R, Blackstone E, Kirklin J. Complement activation during cardiopulmonary bypass. N Engl J Med 1981; 304:497–503.
17. Mosre DS, Adams D, Magnani B. Platelet and neutrophil activation during cardiac surgical procedures: impact of cardiopulmonary bypass. Ann Thorac Surg 1998; 65:691–695.
18. Wright E, Sarkozy E, Dobell A, et al. Fat globulinemia in extracorporeal circulation. Surgery 1963; 63:500–504.
19. Clark R, Magraf H, Beauchamp R. Fat and solid filtration in clinical perfusion. Surgery 1975; 77:216–224.
20. Edmunds L, Williams W. Microemboli and the use of filters during cardiopulmonary bypass. In: Utley J, ed. Pathophysiology and Techniques of Cardiopulmonary Bypass. Baltimore: Williams and Wilkins, 1983:101–114.
21. Austen WG, Howry DH. Ultrasound as a method to detect bubbles or particulate

matter in the arterial line during cardiopulmonary bypass. J Surg Res 1965; 5:283–284.
22. Padayachee T, Parsons S, Theobold R, Linley J, Gosling R, Deverall P. The detection of microemboli in the middle cerebral artery during cardiopulmonary bypass: a transcranial Doppler ultrasound investigation using membrane and bubble oxygenators. Ann Thorac Surg 1987; 44:298–302.
23. Barbut D, Hinton R, Szatrowski T, Hartman G, Bruefach M, Williams-Russo P, Charlson M, Gold J. Cerebral emboli detected during bypass surgery are associated with clamp removal. Stroke 1994; 25:2398–2402.
24. Georgiadis D, Wenzel A, Zerkowski HR, Zierz S, Lindner A. Automated intraoperative detection of Doppler microemboli signals using the bigate approach. Stroke 1998; 29:137–139.
25. Van der Linden J, Casimir-Ahn H. When do cerebral emboli appear during open heart operations? A transcranial Doppler study. Ann Thorac Surg 1991; 51:237–241.
26. Barbut D, Yao F, Hager D, Kavanaugh P, Trifiletti R, Gold J. Comparison of transcranial Doppler ultrasonography and transesophageal echocardiography to monitor emboli during coronary artery bypass surgery. Stroke 1996; 27:87–90.
27. Ringelstein E, Droste D, Babikian V, Evans D, Grosset D, Kaps M, Markus H, Russell D, Siebler M. Consensus on microembolus detection by TCD. International Consensus Group on Microembolus Detection. Stroke 1998; 29:725–729.
28. Blauth C, Arnold J, Schulenberg W, McCartney A, Taylor K. Cerebral microembolism during cardiopulmonary bypass: retinal microvascular studies in vivo with fluorescein angiography. J Thorac Cardiovasc Surg 1988; 95:668–676.
29. Moody D, Bell M, Challa V, Johnston W, Prough D. Brain microemboli during cardiac surgery or aortography. Ann Neurol 1990; 28:477–486.
30. Govier A, Reves J, McKay R, Karp R, Zorn G, Morawetz R, Smith L, Adams M, Freeman A. Factors and their influence on regional cerebral blood flow during nonpulsatile cardiopulmonary bypass. Ann Thorac Surg 1984; 38:592–599.
31. Nevin M, Adams S, Colchester A, Pepper J. Evidence for involvement of hypocapnia and hypoperfusion in aetiology of neurological deficit after cardiopulmonary bypass. Lancet 1987; 2:1493–1495.
32. Brusino F, Reves J, Smith L, Prough D, Stump D, McIntyre R. The effect of age on cerebral blood flow during hypothermic cardiopulmonary bypass. J Thorac Cardiovasc Surg 1989; 97:541–547.
33. Lundar T, Lindegaard K-F, Froysaker T, Aaslid R, Wiberg J, Nornes H. Cerebral perfusion during nonpulsatile cardiopulmonary bypass. Ann Thorac Surg 1985; 40: 144–150.
34. Lundar T, Lindegaard K-F, Froysaker T, Aaslid R, Grip A, Nornes H. Dissociation between cerebral autoregulation and carbon dioxide reactivity during nonpulsatile cardiopulmonary bypass. Ann Thorac Surg 1985; 40:582–587.
35. Slogoff S, Girgis K, Keats A. Etiologic factors in neuropsychiatric complications associated with cardiopulmonary bypass. Anesth Analg 1982; 61:903–911.
36. Kolkka R, Hilberman M. Neurologic dysfunction following cardiac operation with low-flow, low-pressure cardiopulmonary bypass. J Thorac Cardiovasc Surg 1980; 79:432–437.

37. Tufo H, Ostfeld A, Shekelle R. Central nervous system dysfunction following open-heart surgery. JAMA 1970; 212:1333–1340.
38. Stockard J, Bickford R, Schauble J. Pressure-dependent cerebral ischemia during cardiopulmonary bypass. Neurology 1973; 23: 521–529.
39. Gold J, Charlson M, Williams-Russo P, Szatrowski T, Peterson J, Pirraglia P, Hartman G, Yao F, Hollenberg J, Barbut D. Improvement of outcomes after coronary artery bypass: a randomized trial comparing intraoperative high vs. low mean arterial pressure. J Thorac Cardiovasc Surg 1995; 110:1302–1314.
40. Prough D, Stump D, Roy R, Gravlee G, Williams T, Mills S, Hinshelwood L, Howard G. Response of cerebral blood flow to changes in carbon dioxide tension during hypothermic cardiopulmonary bypass. Anesthesiology 1986; 64:576–581.
41. Barbut D, Lo Y, Trifiletti R, et al. Cerebral perfusion is determined by cardiopulmonary bypass flow rate. Outcomes '97, Key West 1997. Abstract.
42. Bigelow W, Callaghan J, Hopps J. General hypothermia for experimental intracardiac surgery: the use of electrophrenic respirations, an artificial pacemaker for cardiac standstill, and radio-frequency rewarming in general hypothermia. Ann Surg 1950; 132:531–539.
43. Conroy B, Lin C, Jenkins L, DeWitt D, Zornow M, Uchida T, Johnston W. Hypothermic modulation of cerebral ischemic injury during cardiopulmonary bypass in pigs. Anesthesiology 1998; 88:390–402.
44. Rohrer M, Natale A. Effect of hypothermia on the coagulation cascade. Crit Care Med 1992; 20:1402–1405.
45. Martin T, Craver J, Gott J, Weintraub W, Ramsay J, Mora C, Guyton R. Prospective, randomized trial of retrograde warm blood cardioplegia: myocardial benefit and neurologic threat. Ann Thorac Surg 1994; 57:298–304.
46. McLean R, Wong B, Naylor C, Snow W, Harrington E, Gawel M, Fremes S. Cardiopulmonary bypass, temperature, and central nervous system dysfunction. Circulation 1994; 90(5 part 2):II250–II255.
47. Roach G, Kanchuger M, Mangano C, Newman M, Nussmeier N, Wolman R, Aggarwal A, Marschall K, Graham S, Ley C. Adverse cerebral outcomes after coronary bypass surgery. Multicenter Study of Perioperative Ischemia Research Group and the Ischemia Research and Education Foundation Investigators. N Engl J Med 1996; 335:1857–1863.
48. Breuer A, Furlan A, Hanson M, Lederman R, Loop F, Cosgrove D, Greenstreet R, Estafanous F. Central nervous system complications of coronary artery bypass graft surgery: prospective analysis of 421 patients. Stroke 1983; 14:682–687.
49. Shaw P, Bates D, Cartlidge N, Heaviside D, Julian D, Shaw D. Early neurological complications of coronary artery bypass surgery. Br Med J 1985; 291:1384–1387.
50. Mangano D. Multicenter outcome research. J Cardiothorac Vasc Anesth 1994; 8: 10–12.
51. McKhann G, Goldsborough M, Borowicz L, Mellits E, Brookmeyer R, Quaskey S, Baumgartner W, Cameron D, Stuart R, Gardner T. Predictors of stroke risk in coronary artery bypass patients. Ann Thorac Surg 1997; 63:516–521.
52. Gardner T, Horneffer P, Manolio T, Pearson T, Gott V, Baumgartner W, Vorkon A, Watkins L, Reitz B. Stroke following coronary artery bypass grafting: a ten-year study. Ann Thorac Surg 1985; 40:574–581.

53. Libman R, Wirkowski E, Neystat M, Barr W, Gelv S, Graver M. Stroke associated with cardiac surgery. Determinants, timing, and stroke subtypes. Arch Neurol 1996; 54:83–87.
54. Barbut D, Grassineau D, Heier L, et al. Radiologic appearances in CABG-related strokes are characteristic of embolic infarction predominantly affecting the posterior circulation. Outcomes '97, Key West 1997. Abstract.
55. Masuda J, Yutani C, Ogata J, Kuriyama Y, Yamaguchi T. Atheromatous embolism in the brain: a clinicopathologic analysis of 15 autopsy cases. Neurology 1994; 44: 1231–1237.
55a. Caplan LR, Hennerici M. Impaired clearance of emboli is an important link between hypoperfusion, embolism, and ischemic stroke. Arch Neurol 1998; 55: 1475–1482.
56. Rorick M, Furlan A. Risk of cardiac surgery in patients with prior stroke. Neurology 1990; 40:835–837.
57. Redmond J, Greene P, Goldsborough M, Cameron D, Stuart R, Sussman M, Watkins L, Laschinger J, McKhann G, Johnston M, Baumgartner W. Neurologic injury in cardiac surgical patients with a history of stroke. Ann Thorac Surg 1996; 61: 42–47.
58. Faggioli G, Curl G, Ricotta J. The role of carotid screening before coronary artery bypass. J Vasc Surg 1990; 12:724–729.
59. Ropper A, Wechsler L, Wilson L. Carotid bruit and the risk of stroke in elective surgery. N Engl J Med 1982; 307:1388–1390.
60. Gerraty R, Gates P, Doyle J. Carotid stenosis and perioperative stroke risk in symptomatic and asymptomatic patients undergoing vascular or coronary surgery. Stroke 1993; 24:1115–1118.
61. Reed G, Singer D, Picard E, DeSanctis R. Stroke following coronary artery bypass surgery: a case control estimate of the risk from carotid bruits. N Engl J Med 1988; 319:1246–1250.
62. Ricotta J, Faggioli G, Castilone A, Hassett J. Risk factors for stroke after cardiac surgery. Buffalo Cardiac-Cerebral Study Group. J Vasc Surg 1995; 21:359–363.
63. Schwartz L, Bridgman A, Kieffer R, Wilcox R, McCann R, Tawil M, Scott S. Asymptomatic carotid artery stenosis and stroke in patients undergoing cardiopulmonary bypass. J Vasc Surg 1995; 21:146–153.
64. Dashe J, Pessin M, Murphy R, Payne D. Carotid occlusive disease and stroke risk in coronary artery bypass graft surgery. Neurology 1997; 49:678–686.
65. Hart R, Easton J. Management of cervical bruits and carotid stenosis in preoperative patients. Stroke 1983; 14:290–297.
66. Furlan A, Craciun A. Risk of stroke during coronary artery bypass graft surgery in patients with internal carotid artery disease documented by angiography. Stroke 1985; 16:797–799.
67. Brener B, Brief D, Alpert J, Goldendranz R, Parsonnet V, Feldman S, Gielchinsky I, Abel R, Hochberg M, Hussain M. A four-year experience with preoperative noninvasive carotid evaluation of two thousand twenty-six patients undergoing cardiac surgery. J Vasc Surg 1984; 1:326–338.
68. Mickleborough L, Walker P, Takagi Y, Ohashi M, Ivanov J, Tamariz M. Risk

factors for stroke in patients undergoing coronary artery bypass grafting. J Thorac Cardiovasc Surg 1996; 112:1250–1258.
69. Hertzer N, Loop F, Beven E, O'Hara P, Krajewski L. Surgical staging for simultaneous coronary and carotid disease: a study including prospective randomization. J Vasc Surg 1989; 9:455–463.
70. Moore W, Barnett H, Beebe H, Bernstein E, Brener B, Brott T, Caplan L, Day A, Goldstone J, Hobson R. Guidelines for carotid endarterectomy. A multidisciplinary consensus statement from the Ad Hoc Committee, American Heart Association. Stroke 1995; 26:188–201.
71. North American Symptomatic Carotid Endarterectomy Trial Collaborators. Beneficial effect of carotid endarterectomy in symptomatic patients with high-grade carotid stenosis. N Engl J Med 1991; 325:445–453.
72. Blauth C, Cosgrove D, Webb B, Ratliff N, Boylan M, Piedmonte M, Lytle B, Loop F. Atheroembolism from the ascending aorta. An emerging problem in cardiac surgery. J Thorac Cardiovasc Surg 1992; 103:1104–1111.
73. Hosoda Y, Watanabe M, Hirooka Y, Ohse Y, Tanaka A, Watanabe T. Significance of atherosclerotic changes of the ascending aorta during coronary bypass surgery with intraoperative detection by echography. J Cardiovasc Surg 1991; 32:301–306.
74. Barbut D, Lo Y, Hartman G, Yao F, Trifiletti R, Hager D, Hinton R, Gold J, Isom O. Aortic atheroma is related to outcome but not numbers of emboli during coronary bypass. Ann Thorac Surg 1997; 64:454–459.
75. Hartman G, Yao F, Bruefach M, Barbut D, Peterson J, Purcell M, Charlson M, Gold J, Thomas S, Szatrowski T. Severity of aortic atheromatous disease diagnosed by transesophageal echocardiography predicts stroke and other outcomes associated with coronary artery surgery: a prospective study. Anesth Analg 1996; 83:701–708.
76. Davila-Roman V, Barzilai B, Wareing T, Murphy S, Kouchoukos N. Intraoperative ultrasonographic evaluation of the ascending aorta in 100 consecutive patients undergoing cardiac surgery. Circulation 1991; 84(suppl 5):III47–III53.
77. Wareing T, Davila-Roman V, Barzilai B, Murphy S, Kouschoukos N. Management of the severely atherosclerotic ascending aorta during cardiac operations. A strategy for detection and treatment. J Thorac Cardiovasc Surg 1992; 103:453–462.
78. Kouchoukos N, Wareing T, Daily B, Murphy S. Management of the severely atherosclerotic aorta during cardiac operations. J Card Surg 1994; 9:490–494.
79. Duda A, Letwin L, Sutter F, Goldman S. Does routine use of aortic ultrasonography decrease the stroke rate in coronary artery bypass surgery? J Vasc Surg 1995; 21: 98–107.
79a. Acuff TE, Landreneau RJ, Griffith BP, Mack MJ. Minimally invasive coronary artery bypass grafting. Ann Thorac Surg 1996; 61:135–137.
79b. Ribakove GH, Miller JS, Andersen RV, et al. Minimally invasive port-access coronary artery bypass grafting with early angiographic follow-up: initial clinical experience. J Thorac Cardiovasc Surg 1998; 115:1101–1110.
79c. Jansen EWL, Boest C, Lahpor JR, et al. Coronary artery bypass grafting without cardiopulmonary bypass using the octopus-method: results in the first one hundred patients. J Thorac Cardiovasc Surg 1998; 116:60–67.
79d. Tasdemir O, Vural K, Kasragoz H, Bayazit K. Coronary artery bypass grafting on

the beating heart without the use of extracorporeal circulation: review of 2052 cases. J Thorac Cardiovasc Surg 1998; 116:68–73.

80. Creswell L, Schuessler R, Rosenbloom M, Cox J. Hazards of postoperative atrial arrhythmias. Ann Thorac Surg 1993; 56:539–549.
81. Pires L, Wagshal A, Lancey R, Huang S. Arrhythmias and conduction disturbances after coronary artery bypass graft surgery: epidemiology, management, and prognosis. Am Heart J 1995; 129:799–808.
82. Taylor G, Malik S, Colliver J, Dove J, Moses H, Mikell F, Batchelder J, Schneider J, Wellons H. Usefulness of atrial fibrillation as a predictor of stroke after isolated coronary artery bypass grafting. Am J Cardiol 1987; 60:905–907.
83. O'Neill BJ III, Furlan AJ, Hobbs RD. Risk of stroke in patients with transient postoperative atrial fibrillation/flutter. Stroke 1983; 14:133.
84. Kowey P, Taylor J, Rials S, Marinchak R. Meta-analysis of the effectiveness of prophylactic drug therapy in preventing supraventricular arrhythmia early after coronary artery bypass grafting. Am J Cardiol 1992; 69:964–965.
85. Andrews T, Reimold S, Berlin J, Antman E. Prevention of supraventricular arrhythmias after coronary artery bypass surgery. Circulation 1991; 84(Suppl III):III236–III243. Abstract.
86. Gold M, O'Gara P, Buckley M, DeSanctis R. Efficacy and safety of procainamide in preventing arrhythmias after coronary artery bypass surgery. Am J Cardiol 1996; 78:975–979.
87. Daoud E, Strickberger S, Man K, Goyal R, Deeb G, Bolling S, Pagani F, Bitar C, Meissner M, Morady F. Preoperative amiodarone as prophylaxis against atrial fibrillation after heart surgery. N Engl J Med 1997; 337:1785–1791.
88. Sotaniemi K, Mononen H, Hokkanen T. Long-term cerebral outcome after open-heart surgery. Stroke 1986; 17:410–416.
89. McKhann G, Goldsborough M, Borowicz L, Selnes O, Mellits E, Enger C, Quaskey S, Baumgartner W, Cameron D, Stuart R, Gardner T. Cognitive outcome after coronary artery bypass: a one-year prospective study. Ann Thorac Surg 1997; 63:510–515.
90. Borowicz L, Goldsborough M, Selnes O, McKhann G. Neuropsychologic change after cardiac surgery: a critical review. J Cardiothorac Vasc Anesth 1996; 10:105–111.
91. Venn G, Klinger L, Smith P. Neuropsychologic sequelae of bypass twelve months after coronary artery surgery. Br Heart J 1987; 57:565.
92. Martzke J, Murkin J, Baird D, et al. Perioperative predictors of neuropsychological outcome 3 years after coronary artery bypass surgery. Anesth Analg 1996; 82: SCA37.
93. McKhann G, Borowicz L, Goldsborough M, Enger C, Selnes O. Depression and cognitive decline after coronary artery bypass grafting. Lancet 1997; 349:1282–1284.
94. Freeman A, Folks D, Sokol R, Govier A, Reves J, Fleece E, Hall K, Zorn G, Karp R. Cognitive function after coronary bypass surgery: effect of decreased cerebral blood flow. Am J Psychiatry 1985; 142:110–112.
95. Hammon J, Stump D, Kon N, Cordell A, Hudspeth A, Oaks T, Brooker R, Rogers A, Hilbawi R, Coker L, Troost B. Risk factors and solutions for the development

of neurobehavioral changes after coronary artery bypass grafting. Ann Thorac Surg 1997; 63:1613–1618.
96. Pugsley W, Klinger L, Paschalis C, Treasure T, Harrison M, Newman S. The impact of microemboli during cardiopulmonary bypass on neuropsychological functioning. Stroke 1994; 25:1393–1399.
97. Calabrese J, Skwerer R, Gulledge A, Gill C, Mullen J, Rodgers D, Taylor P, Goding L, Lytle B, Cosgrove D, Bazarel M, Loop F. Incidence of postoperative delirium following myocardial revascularization. Cleve Clin J Med 1987; 54:29–32.
98. Lederman R, Breuer A, Hanson M, Furlan A, Loop F, Cosgrove D, Estafanous F, Greenstreet R. Peripheral nervous system complications of coronary artery bypass graft surgery. Ann Neurol 1982; 12:297–301.
99. Denny-Brown D, Adams R, Brenner C, et al. The pathology of injury to nerve induced by cold. J Neuropathol Exp Neurol 1945; 4:305–323.
100. Swan H, Virtue R, Blount G, et al. Hypothermia in surgery: analysis of 100 clinical cases. Ann Surg 1955; 142:382–400.
101. Hanson M, Breuer A, Furlan A, Lederman R, Wilbourn A, Cosgrove D, Loop F, Estafanous F. Mechanism and frequency of brachial plexus injury in open-heart surgery: a prospective analysis. Ann Thorac Surg 1983; 36:675–679.
102. Furlan A, Craciun A. Central nervous system complications of open heart surgery. Stroke 1984; 15:912–915.
103. Humphreys R, Hoffman H, Mustard W, Trusler G. Cerebral hemorrhage following heart surgery. J Neurosurg 1975; 43:671–675.
104. Plasse H, Mittleman M, Frost J. Unilateral sudden hearing loss after open heart surgery: a detailed study of seven cases. Laryngoscope 1981; 91:101–109.
105. Cooper D, Bazaral M, Furlan A, Seuilla E, Ghatias M, Sheeler L, Little J, Hahn J, Sheldon W, Loop F. Pituitary apoplexy: a complication of cardiac surgery. Ann Thorac Surg 1986; 41:547–550.
106. Chimowitz M, Furlan A, Jones S, Sila C, Lorig R, Paranandi L, Beck G. Transcranial Doppler assessment of cerebral perfusion reserve in patients with carotid occlusive disease and no evidence of cerebral infarction. Neurology 1993; 43:353–357.
107. Aranki S, Sullivan T, Cohn L. The effect of the single aortic cross-clamp technique on cardiac and cerebral complications during cardiac bypass surgery. J Card Surg 1995; 10:498–502.
107a. Weinberger J, Azhar S, Danisi F, Hayes R, Goldman M. A new noninvasive technique for imaging atherosclerotic plaque in the aortic arch of stroke patients by transcutaneous real-time B-mode ultrasonography. Stroke 1998; 29:673–676.
108. Buffolo E, deAngrade C, Branco J, Teles C, Aguiar L, Gomes W. Coronary artery bypass grafting without cardiopulmonary bypass. Ann Thorac Surg 1996; 61:63–66.
109. Topol E, Humphrey L, Borkon A, Baumgartner W, Dorsey D, Reitz B, Weiss J. Value of intraoperative left ventricular microbubbles detected by transesophageal two-dimensional echocardiography in predicting neurologic outcome after cardiac operations. Am J Cardiol 1985; 56:773–775.
110. Barbut D, Lo Y, Gold J, Trifiletti R, Yao F, Hager D, Hinton R, Isom O. Impact

of embolization during coronary artery bypass grafting on outcome and length of stay. Ann Thorac Surg 1997; 63:998–1002.

111. Fish K, Sarnquist F, van Steennis C, Mitchell P, Hilberman M, Jamieson S, Linet O, Miller D. A prospective, randomized study of the effects of prostacyclin on platelets and blood loss during coronary bypass operations. J Thorac Cardiovasc Surg 1986; 91:436–442.
112. Pokar H, Bleese N, Fischer-Dusterhoff H, et al. Prevention of postoperative psychic and neurological disturbances after open-heart surgery using prostacyclin: a clinical study. In: Becker R, Katz J, Plonius M-J, Speidel H, eds. Psychopathological and Neurological Dysfunction Following Open-Heart Surgery. New York: Springer-Verlag, 1982:312–319.
113. Aren C, Blomstrand C, Wikkelso C, Radegran K. Hypotension induced by prostacyclin treatment during cardiopulmonary bypass does not increase the risk of cerebral complications. J Thorac Cardiovasc Surg 1984; 88(5 pt 1):748–753.
114. Swain J, Anderson R, Siegman M. Low-flow cardiopulmonary bypass and cerebral protection: a summary of investigations. Ann Thorac Surg 1993; 56:1490–1492.
115. Zaidan J, Klochany A, Martin W, Ziegler J, Harless D, Andrews R. Effect of thiopental on neurologic outcome following coronary artery bypass grafting. Anesthesiology 1991; 74:406–411.
116. Fisher M, Jonas S, Sacco R. Prophylactic neuroprotection for cerebral ischemia. Stroke 1994; 25(5):1075–1080.
117. Grieco G, d'Hollosy M, Culliford A, Jonas S. Evaluating neuroprotective agents for clinical anti-ischemic benefit using neurological and neuropsychological changes after cardiac surgery under cardiopulmonary bypass: methodological strategies and results of a double-blind, placebo-controlled trial of GM_1 ganglioside. Stroke 1996; 27:858–874.
118. National Institute of Neurological Disorders and Stroke rt-PA Stroke Study Group. Tissue plasminogen activator for acute ischemic stroke. N Engl J Med 1995; 333: 1581–1587.
119. Baldwin J, Sanchez J, Bing RJ. Coronary Artery Surgery. In: Bing RJ, ed. Cardiology: The evolution of the science and the art. Switzerland: Harwood Academic Publishers, 1992:173.
120. Chimowitz MI, Nemec JJ, Marwick TH, Lorig RJ, Furlan AJ, Salcedo EE. Transcranial Doppler ultrasound identifies patients with right-to-left cardiac or pulmonary shunts. Neurology 1991; 41:1902–1904.
121. Chimowitz MI, Furlan AJ. Preventing cerebral complications of cardiac surgery. In: Norris JW, Hachinski VC, eds. Prevention of Stroke. New York: Springer-Verlag, 1991:222.
122. Poole RM, Chimowitz MI. Cardiac imaging for stroke diagnosis. In: Fisher M, Bogousslavsky J, eds. Current Review of Cerebrovascular Disease. Philadelphia: Current Medicine, 1996:195.

5

Neurological Complications of Nonsurgical Cardiac Interventions

INTRODUCTION

Neurological complications of nonsurgical cardiac interventions are relatively uncommon but their occurrence may lead to death or major disability. This chapter focuses on the neurological complications of common cardiac interventions such as coronary angiography and angioplasty, valvuloplasty, cardiac assist devices, thrombolytic therapy, and cardioversion.

PERCUTANEOUS CORONARY ANGIOGRAPHY AND ANGIOPLASTY

Modern percutaneous coronary angiography was pioneered by Seldinger in 1953 [1] and Sones in 1959 [2]. Subsequently it has become one of the most commonly performed invasive diagnostic tests in the United States. In an early study of 46,904 patients undergoing coronary angiography at 173 hospitals, stroke occurred in 106 patients (0.23%) [3]. Subsequent studies that have incorporated modern catheter design have shown an even lower stroke rate following coronary angiography (0.07% to 0.11%) [4,5]. Initial concern about the possibility of higher thrombotic events with the use of nonionic contrast has largely abated because of studies showing no difference in the rates of cerebral embolic events when nonionic vs. ionic contrast agents are used [6,7]. Predisposing risk factors for neurological complications following coronary angiography have been evaluated in one case control study. Using multiple logistic regression analysis, Lazar et al. found that female gender, left ventricular hypertrophy, depressed ejection fraction, and presence of >50% stenosis of two or more coronary arteries were independent predictors of neurological events [8].

The risk of embolism during transeptal left heart catheterization has also been evaluated. With this technique, a catheter is threaded into the right atrium via a femoral vein. Subsequently, the atrial or ventricular septum is punctured to gain access to the left atrium or left ventricle. Indications for this procedure are direct measurement of left atrial pressure, mitral valvuloplasty, or access to the left ventricle in patients with prosthetic aortic or mitral valves. In one study of 1279 patients undergoing transeptal left heart catheterization, only one patient (0.08%) had a systemic embolus [9].

Most [5,10,11], but not all [8], studies show that the majority of strokes following coronary angiography occur in the vertebrobasilar circulation. In contrast, ischemic stroke usually involves the vertebrobasilar circulation in approximately 10% to 20% of cases. One possible explanation for the preponderance of vertebrobasilar strokes is injury to the proximal vertebral artery when the brachial artery approach (Sones technique) is used. However, centers using the Seldinger technique (femoral artery approach) have also reported that the majority of events occurred in the posterior circulation [12]. One explanation for the high frequency of vertebrobasilar symptoms is that many of these events may not be ischemic in origin. The preponderance of transient visual symptoms suggests migraine may be the cause in many patients.

Postangiography strokes involving the vertebrobasilar circulation typically manifest as combinations of a confusional state with memory difficulties (medial temporal lobe ischemia), visual field defects such as hemianopia or cortical blindness (occipital lobe ischemia), and a brainstem syndrome. Carotid territory strokes occur in approximately 30% to 40% of patients and typically manifest as combinations of hemiparesis, hemisensory loss, hemianopia, and aphasia (left hemisphere) or neglect (right hemisphere). Some series have shown that >50% of patients have mild or no residual neurological signs following cerebral ischemia related to coronary angiography [5,8,12]. In one series of 30,000 patients who underwent coronary angiography, 35 patients had a stroke (0.11%). The neurological deficit resolved within 48 hours in 19 patients but persisted in 16 patients, two of whom died [5].

Invariably the cause of stroke following coronary angiography is embolization related to guidewire or catheter manipulation. The most common embolic sources are protruding atheromas in the aorta [13] or at the origins of the brachiocephalic trunk, left common carotid artery, or left subclavian artery. Other potential embolic sources are thrombus forming on the catheter tip, valvular material (e.g., calcification) [14], subintimal dissection [15], and intracardiac thrombi dislodged by guidewire or catheter manipulation. Several techniques have been employed to prevent embolization during coronary angiography; however, none of these approaches have been evaluated in controlled studies. The strategies include pretreatment with aspirin, use of heparin during the procedure, and the use of frequent, small test injections of contrast to establish the presence of rapid runoff. This runoff indicates that the catheter tip is properly placed and not trapped or subintimal [15]. It has also been suggested that transesophageal echocardiography or spiral CT should be used before angiography to detect protruding atheromas in the aortic arch [13]; however, this is unlikely to be a cost-effective approach given the low rate of stroke following coronary angiography.

Until recently there was little to offer patients with stroke related to coronary angiography. However, recent evidence that thrombolytic therapy is effective for patients presenting within 3 hours of an ischemic stroke [16] provides a strong rationale for using thrombolytic therapy in this setting [17]. Frequently the stroke is recognized during the procedure, when the arterial sheath is still in place. This provides a unique opportunity to perform selective cerebral intra-arterial thrombolysis (rather than intravenous thrombolysis) and thereby limit the risk of hemorrhage from the site of cannulation. Immediately after recognition of a significant neurological deficit, a brain CT should be performed to rule out a cerebral hemorrhage. Although cerebral hemorrhage is rare in this setting, the authors have personally seen such cases. If the brain CT does not show a hemorrhage, a diagnostic cerebral angiogram is performed to determine if a cerebral artery is occluded. If so, selective intra-arterial thrombolysis can be performed. Since most mild neurological deficits resolve spontaneously following coronary angiography, we reserve intra-arterial thrombolysis for those patients with a disabling deficit (hemiplegia, aphasia, cortical blindness) and occlusion of a major intracranial artery (middle cerebral artery, basilar artery).

Other central nervous system complications of coronary angiography include migraine, encephalopathy, and occasionally seizures [10]. Many of these complications probably occur as a reaction to the contrast agent, and use of nonionic agents may lower the incidence of these events. Elderly, dehydrated patients may be particularly susceptible to developing encephalopathy if a large volume of contrast agent is used. Hypotension or microemboli may also be responsible for encephalopathy following coronary angiography. In a neuropathological study of patients dying after cardiopulmonary bypass or invasive diagnostic procedures, Moody et al. [18] reported that two patients who underwent coronary angiography or aortography without cardiopulmonary bypass had numerous small capillary and arteriolar dilatations (SCADs) scattered throughout the brain (see Fig. 2 in Chapter 4). These SCADs were typically 10 to 40 μm in size and the lumina were clear and free of blood products. They were found most commonly in areas of high cerebral blood flow (i.e., the cerebral cortex and deep gray matter). The authors speculated that SCADs are caused by air or fat microemboli.

Peripheral nerve injury is an uncommon complication of coronary angiography. In a prospective study of coronary angiography performed via the femoral approach, Kent et al. [19] reported that 20 of 9585 patients (0.2%) had damage to the femoral nerve. The neurological symptoms in most of these patients resolved. Kennedy et al. [20] reported five patients with high median neuropathy following coronary angiography via the brachial route. All patients were followed for 6 to 22 months and had persistent sensory disturbance or weakness of the hand. One patient developed reflex sympathetic dystrophy. The authors estimate that median neuropathy may occur in 0.2% to 1.4% of patients undergoing coronary angiography via the brachial route [20]. Possible mechanisms of nerve injury during coronary angiography include compression of a peripheral nerve by a hematoma at the site of cannulation, direct trauma to the nerve by cutdowns, cannulation of the nerve sheath, incorrectly placed sutures, ischemia to the nerve from local arterial thrombosis, and tight arm boards. Rare cases of brachial plexopathy complicating axillary cannulation have also been reported [20].

Percutaneous transluminal coronary angioplasty, which was performed first by Gruntzig in 1977 [21], is performed in more than 500,000 patients per year worldwide [22]. The neurological complications of coronary angioplasty are similar to those of coronary angiography. Dorros et al. [23] reported that 5 of 1500 patients (0.3%) undergoing coronary angioplasty had a central nervous system complication (one stroke, three TIAs, and one anoxic encephalopathy). Galbreath et al. [24] reported that four of 1968 patients (0.2%) had cerebrovascular complications (three stroke, one TIA). Two patients had strokes while the angiographer was searching the ascending aorta for the sites of aortosaphenous vein grafts. One patient had a stroke during a hypotensive episode following technically successful angioplasty, and one patient had a TIA that was attributed to injection of a small quantity of air through the guiding catheter.

VALVULOPLASTY

Percutaneous balloon valvuloplasty is an alternative to surgery in selected patients with mitral stenosis or aortic stenosis. The technique was developed by Kan et al. [25] in 1982 for the treatment of pulmonary valve stenosis and subsequently refined for the treatment of mitral stenosis and aortic stenosis by Inoue [26] and others [27–29].

There are several variations of the technique used for *mitral valvuloplasty*, but the cardiac outcome and complication rates of the various techniques are similar [30]. The transeptal antegrade approach is most commonly used. A catheter is threaded into the right atrium via the right femoral vein. Subsequently, the atrial septum is punctured in the area of the fossa ovalis, a sheath is placed across the septum, and a heparin bolus is given. The partially inflated dilating balloon is positioned across the mitral valve and inflated briefly, thereby splitting the mitral commissures [31].

The major neurological risk of mitral valvuloplasty is cerebral embolism. The typical sources of embolism are left atrial thrombus or calcification of the mitral valve. Hence, mitral valve calcification and left atrial thrombus are contraindications to the procedure. In order to lower the risk of embolism during the procedure, transesophageal echocardiography (TEE) is performed before the procedure to rule out left atrial thrombus [32]. If thrombus is found, the procedure is delayed and anticoagulation is instituted for 2 to 3 months [31]. Subsequently, TEE is repeated to ensure that the left atrium is free of thrombus. Some authors have also advocated using online TEE during the procedure to guide the transeptal puncture and the positioning of the balloon catheter across the mitral valve [33].

By paying close attention to patient selection and use of anticoagulation during the procedure, experienced operators have reported relatively low rates of neurological complications from mitral valvuloplasty. Early studies reported embolic rates of up to 4% [31], but recent studies report lower rates. Fu et al. [30] reported that 3 of 262 patients (1.1%) had embolic events (two cerebral, one coronary), Chioin et al. [34] reported that 2 of 235 patients (0.85%) had TIAs, and Demirtas et al. [35] reported that 1 of 50 patients (2%) had systemic embolism related to mitral valvuloplasty. In a very large study of 4832 patients with rheumatic mitral stenosis from 120 medical centers in China, the rate of thromboembolism associated with mitral valvuloplasty was 0.48% [36].

Aortic valvuloplasty is usually performed in patients with symptomatic aortic stenosis who are not candidates for aortic valve replacement. The procedure is performed retrograde from one of the femoral arteries. A balloon catheter is advanced over a guidewire traversing the aortic valve. The balloon catheter must be large enough to cause transient hypotension with full dilatation. Multiple dilatations of the balloon are typically performed [31].

Transcranial Doppler (TCD) has been used to monitor cerebral hemodynamics during aortic valvuloplasty. Karnik et al. [37] performed TCD of a middle cerebral artery during valvuloplasty in 12 elderly patients. In three patients whose systolic blood pressure fell to <75 mm Hg during balloon inflation, middle cerebral artery mean blood flow velocity fell to <35 cm/sec (normal range, 45 to 65 cm/sec). Deflation and retraction of the balloon resulted in restoration of systemic blood pressure and middle cerebral artery blood flow velocity. In patients whose blood pressure remained >75 mm Hg during balloon inflation, middle cerebral artery mean blood flow velocity did not drop significantly.

The risk of neurological events from aortic valvuloplasty is higher than that of mitral valvuloplasty. Most series have shown stroke rates of approximately 2% to 3% from aortic valvuloplasty [28,31,38]; however, in one small study of 26 patients cerebral infarction occurred in 2 patients (8%) [39]. Both of these patients had calcific bicuspid aortic stenosis. Stroke from aortic valvuloplasty is probably related to embolism rather than hypotension, which is usually transient. Since many of the elderly patients undergoing this procedure have calcific aortic stenosis, it is likely that calcium deposits are the substrate of emboli that occur during the procedure. Younger patients with congenital, noncalcific aortic stenosis appear to have a low risk of embolism during aortic valvuloplasty. In one series of 18 patients between the ages of 17 and 40 years undergoing aortic valvuloplasty, none had an embolic event [40].

CARDIAC ASSIST DEVICES

Intra-aortic Balloon Pump

The intra-aortic balloon pump, which was developed in 1962 by Moulopoulos et al. [41], provides mechanical circulatory support in a number of life-threatening cardiovascular conditions, e.g., difficulty weaning from cardiopulmonary bypass and cardiogenic shock. The balloon catheter is usually inserted percutaneously through the femoral artery. Given the relatively large size of the balloon pump catheters (French 8.5 or 9.5), a dilator is used to expand the artery before a 10 French arterial sheath is inserted over a guidewire. A French balloon catheter is then inserted over the guidewire through the sheath and advanced up the descending thoracic aorta so that the tip is distal to the left subclavian artery. The balloon is rapidly inflated in diastole and deflated in systole, producing an increase in diastolic pressure and a decrease in peak systolic left ventricular pressure. Patients are anticoagulated with heparin while the balloon is in place [42].

The major neurological complications of the intra-aortic balloon pump are myelopathy and lower extremity nerve injury. Myelopathy from spinal cord ischemia is rare, occurring in 8 of 100,000 patients with an intra-aortic balloon pump according to a report by Riggle and Oddi [43]. Potential mechanisms of spinal cord ischemia include aortic dissection [44], hypoperfusion of the spinal cord, and thromboembolism to the spinal cord. Peripheral nerve injury may occur as a result of trauma to the femoral nerve during insertion of the balloon catheter or ischemic injury to a lower-extremity peripheral nerve (monomelic neuropathy) as a consequence of limb ischemia. Lower-extremity ischemia, which accounts for 80% of all complications of intra-aortic balloon pump, may result from reduction of the functional size of the femoral artery by the balloon catheter or from distal thromboembolism [42]. In one study of 77 patients with an intra-aortic balloon pump, 12 developed limb ischemia and 3 developed permanent foot drop [44]. Patients at highest risk of limb ischemia are those with peripheral vascular disease, obesity, and diabetes, and females, who tend to have smaller arteries [42].

Left Ventricular Assist Devices

These devices are used as a bridge to cardiac transplantation in patients with end stage cardiac failure. The first successful bridge to transplantation was performed by Reemtsma et al. [45] in 1978 using an intra-aortic balloon pump. Subsequently, left ventricular assist devices or a pneumatic total artificial heart were used for this purpose. The typical assist device consists of a pneumatically driven implantable blood pump connected via a drive line to a portable external console. The pump consists of a housing that holds a pusher-plate diaphragm. One side of the diaphragm is in contact with the blood chamber and the other side is in contact with the air chamber. Pulses of air from the external console are delivered to the pump air chamber, which propels the blood out of the pump into the arterial system. During cardiopulmonary bypass, the pump inflow cannula is passed through the apex of the left ventricle, and the outflow cannula is inserted into the proximal aorta. Bioprosthetic valves are placed in the inflow and outflow cannulas to ensure unidirectional flow [46].

The use of early left ventricular assist devices was associated with a high frequency of thromboembolism, despite the use of anticoagulation. A study using transcranial Doppler ultrasound to detect microemboli in the middle cerebral artery in six patients with a Novacor left ventricular assist device showed that multiple microemboli were detected in all six patients and in 143 of 170 (84%) monitoring periods (typically lasting 30 minutes). Although most of these microemboli were asymptomatic, the six study patients had a total of 12 clinically detectable embolic events (10 cerebral, 2 peripheral) during a total observation period of 177 days [47]. Other, larger studies have shown that the use of the early left ventricular assist devices were associated with at least a 30% risk of thromboembolism despite adequate anticoagulation [48–50]. Additionally, the rate of anticoagulation-associated hemorrhage was high, approaching 31% in one study [48].

In recent years, a new left ventricular assist device has been developed to lower the rate of thromboembolism. The HeartMate 1000 device contains textured interior surfaces to promote formation of a densely adherent pseudointima [46,51] when the device comes into contact with blood. This biological lining derived from blood acts as an interface between blood and the device and obviates the need for anticoagulation. Electron microscopic studies have shown the various steps that occur in the formation of the pseudointima. When the surface of the device initially comes into contact with blood, a fibrin-cellular layer forms over the surface. Subsequently, thrombus forms over the surface and is anchored by fibrin deposition within the textured surface [46]. The pseudointimal lining is ultimately composed of fibrin, collagen, endothelial cells, and mononucleated cells [52–56]. Despite the presence of the pseudointima, a recent study has shown that the coagulation and fibrinolytic systems are activated by the HeartMate device, but the low rate of thromboembolism associated with the use of the device suggests that these pathways are well balanced [57].

The most comprehensive evaluation of the HeartMate 1000 was reported by Slater et al. [46], who described the risk of thromboembolism in 223 patients who were supported by the device at 22 centers. Antithrombotic therapy (anticoagulation or antiplatelet therapy) was allowed but not mandated in the study. Transcranial Doppler ultrasound was performed on selected patients to detect microemboli in the middle cerebral artery. Overall, the total time of support by the device was 531.2 patient-months during which warfarin was used for a total of 42.4 months, i.e., 8.2% of the total support time. Despite the limited anticoagulation used in the study, only six patients (2.7%) had a clinically detectable thromboembolic event (four strokes, one seizure, one axillary artery thrombus). This represents 0.011 clinically detectable thromboembolic events per patient-month use of the device [46].

Autopsy studies, which were performed in 69 patients who died during the study, revealed previously undetected evidence of thromboembolism in another eight patients (3.6%): four of these patients had disseminated intravascular coagulopathy from sepsis and multiple splenic infarcts; two patients who had been managed preoperatively with an intra-aortic balloon pump had thrombi in the distal aorta and common iliac arteries; one patient had a peripheral renal artery thrombus; and another patient had an internal carotid artery thrombus [46]. Given the clinical settings and location of the thrombi, it is unlikely that the HeartMate device was responsible for most of these previously undetected thrombi. Transcranial Doppler of the middle cerebral artery detected a mean of 0.52 ± 1.0 microemboli per 30-minute evaluation in each of the eight patients tested during left ventricular assist support [46]. This rate of microemboli with the HeartMate device is substantially lower than the 3 to 40 microemboli per 30-minute session detected by Nabavi et al. [47] in their evaluation of the Novacor device.

THROMBOLYTIC THERAPY FOR MYOCARDIAL INFARCTION (MI)

The most common neurological complication of thrombolytic therapy for acute MI is intracerebral hemorrhage. Spinal epidural hematoma has also been reported but is rare [58]. In the prethrombolytic era, virtually all strokes that occurred following acute MI were ischemic in origin. The mechanism of ischemic stroke in this setting is typically cardioembolism, with left ventricular mural thrombus the usual source of the embolus. Other possible causes of cardioembolism following acute MI include atrial fibrillation and cardiac failure. Typically, ischemic stroke occurs within the first week of MI, with most occurring within 6 weeks.

Early use of thrombolytic therapy for acute MI raised concern that the frequency of stroke (hemorrhagic and ischemic combined) following MI would increase because of the higher risk of intracranial hemorrhage. The results of randomized, placebo-controlled thrombolytic trials suggest that this may be the case. Analysis of aggregate stroke rates (ischemic and hemorrhagic combined) in six placebo-controlled thrombolytic trials show that 161 of 18,824 (0.86%) patients treated with placebo and 195 of 18,806 (1.04%) patients treated with thrombolysis had a stroke following MI [59]. While thrombolysis increased the risk of stroke following MI, the additional risk was small and was far outweighed by the substantial reduction in mortality.

A recent community-based study by Longstreth et al. [60] suggests that thrombolysis actually lowers the risk of ischemic stroke while increasing the risk of hemorrhagic stroke following MI. In this study of 5635 patients, thrombolysis was used in 1413 (25%) patients and was associated with relative risks of 3.6 (95% confidence interval 1.7 to 8.0) for hemorrhagic stroke and 0.4 (95% confidence interval 0.2 to 0.9) for ischemic stroke. Overall, thrombolysis was not associated with an increased risk of ischemic and hemorrhagic stroke combined (relative risk 1.0; 95% confidence interval 0.6 to 1.7); however, the risk of death following stroke was significantly higher in patients treated with thrombolysis (relative risk 3.0; 95% confidence interval 1.4 to 6.4). Thrombolysis may lower the risk of ischemic stroke after MI by reducing the size of MI and by preserving left ventricular function. The higher rate of death from stroke in the thrombolytic group reflects the fact that hemorrhagic stroke has a worse prognosis than ischemic stroke.

Frequency and Risk Factors for Thrombolysis-related Intracranial Hemorrhage

The risk of intracranial hemorrhage has varied between 0.2% and 1.3% [61–67] in most trials of thrombolysis for acute MI. Most of these hemorrhages are parenchymal, i.e., occur within the brain. Subdural hematoma is much less common, occurring in approximately 0.01% of patients receiving thrombolytic therapy for acute MI [59]. In one study, subdural hematoma was significantly associated with head trauma within 2 weeks of treatment and syncope within 48 hours of treatment [87].

Factors that have been associated with an increased risk of parenchymal intracranial hemorrhage following thrombolysis include advanced age, severe hypertension, previous stroke, dose and type of thrombolytic agent, concomitant use of antithrombotic therapy, small body size, and female sex. In one case control study of 150 patients with intracranial hemorrhage and 294 matched controls who underwent thrombolysis, four factors were independently associated with intracranial hemorrhage in a multivariate analysis: age over 65 (odds ratio 2.2; 95% confidence interval 1.4 to 3.5); weight <70 kg (odds ratio 2.1; 95% confidence interval 1.3 to 3.2); hypertension on admission (odds ratio 2.0; 95% confidence interval 1.2 to 3.2); and treatment with tissue plasminogen activator (tPA) (odds ratio 1.6; 95% confidence interval 1.0 to 2.5). With a 0.75% risk of intracranial hemorrhage overall, patients with one, two, or three of these four risk factors had the following rates of intracranial hemorrhage: 0.96%, 1.32%, and 2.17% [68].

Advanced age has consistently been associated with increased risk of intracranial hemorrhage in thrombolytic trials. Nevertheless, studies have clearly shown the benefit of thrombolytic therapy in this subgroup. A recent meta-analysis of five large thrombolytic trials shows that the mortality rate in elderly patients is 17.9% if treated with thrombolysis, compared with 22.1% if untreated ($P < .0001$) [69]. In this meta-analysis, the magnitude of the reduction in mortality was highest in the elderly subgroup. Decision analysis performed in another study showed that for a 10% relative risk reduction in mortality from the use of thrombolysis, the maximal acceptable nonfatal intracranial hemorrhage rate for elderly patients is 5.9%, which far exceeds the rate of intracranial hemorrhage in the elderly in thrombolytic trials [70].

Severe hypertension (systolic > 180 mm Hg or diastolic > 110 mm Hg) is also associated with an increased risk of intracranial hemorrhage following thrombolytic therapy and is considered a relative contraindication for the use of thrombolysis [71]. In TIMI-II, 2 of 22 patients (9.1%) with severe hypertension had intracranial hemorrhage following thrombolysis, compared with 9 of 647 patients without severe hypertension [65]. In GUSTO-I, the rate of ischemic and hemorrhagic stroke combined was 3.4% in patients with systolic blood pressure ≥ 175 mm Hg, compared with 1.2% in patients with systolic pressure between 100 and 124 mm Hg. Nevertheless, patients with systolic blood pressure ≥ 175 mm Hg who received accelerated tPA had a lower rate of death within 30 days (4.3% versus 7.8%; $P = .04$) and a lower rate of death plus disabling stroke (4.9% versus 8.9%; $P = .031$) despite having a higher rate of hemorrhagic stroke (2.3% versus 1.5%) than patients treated with streptokinase [72]. Further analysis of the GUSTO-I data showed that in hypertensive patients who have a low risk of cardiac death (no previous MI, Killip class I), the risk/benefit ratio with thrombolysis is 1, with approximately 13 lives saved per 1000 persons treated at the risk of about 13 intracranial hemorrhages [72]. However, in hypertensive patients at high risk of cardiac death following MI, the reduction in mortality with the use of thrombolysis outweighs the increased risk of intracranial hemorrhage. A subgroup analysis of patients with systolic blood pressure ≥ 175 mm Hg in ISIS-2 also supports the use of thrombolysis in patients with severe hypertension. In this study, the mortality rate was 5.7% in patients treated with streptokinase, compared with 8.7% in untreated patients [63].

The results of a case control study suggest that high pulse pressure is a better predictor of intracranial hemorrhage following thrombolysis than systolic, diastolic, or mean blood pressure. Using logistic regression, the relative risk of intracranial hemorrhage was increased by 1.76 (95% confidence interval 1.26 to

2.46) for each 10-point increase in pulse pressure after adjusting for age [73]. Further studies are needed to determine risk/benefit ratios of thrombolysis in patients with severe hypertension and to determine the effects of lowering blood pressure before initiation of thrombolytic therapy on the subsequent risk of death and intracranial hemorrhage.

It is paradoxical that stroke beyond 3 months is not a contraindication to thrombolytic therapy for acute stroke, yet stroke within 6 to 12 months is often recommended as a contraindication to thrombolytic therapy for acute MI [71,74]. Recent guidelines have gone as far as suggesting that any history of stroke should be a contraindication to thrombolysis [75,76], and some thrombolytic trials for acute MI have excluded patients with any history of stroke or TIA [66]. Clarification of the risk/benefit of thrombolysis in this setting is important since 6% to 10% of patients presenting with MI have a history of stroke [75,77,78].

The evidence that prior stroke is a significant risk for intracranial hemorrhage following thrombolytic therapy is based on sparse data. In the TIMI-II trial, in which patients with stroke within 6 months of MI were excluded, 3 of 89 patients (3.4%) with a history of stroke, TIA, or "neurological disease" had an intracranial hemorrhage, compared with 20 of 3835 patients (0.5%) without neurological problems [65]. Although the difference in intracranial hemorrhage rates between the two groups was significant, the increased risk is based on only three events. The results of a more recent case control study suggests that thrombolytic therapy for MI may be advantageous in patients with a remote cerebral ischemic event [75]. In this study, 29 patients with an acute MI and previous cerebral ischemic event who were treated with thrombolysis were compared to 46 patients with a previous cerebral ischemic event who were not treated with thrombolysis. Approximately 80% of cerebral events had occurred beyond 1 year of the MI in both groups. Despite the fact that patients treated with thrombolysis were older, had a higher rate of anterior wall infarction, and received aspirin and anticoagulation more often than the control group, the rates of intracranial hemorrhage were zero in both groups and the 1-year mortality rate was twice as high in patients not receiving thrombolysis (33% versus 18%; odds ratio 2.4; 95% confidence interval 0.78 to 7.64). The authors conclude that patients with previous cerebral ischemic events should not categorically be excluded from receiving thrombolytic therapy [75]. Further studies are needed to clarify the risk/benefit of thrombolysis for acute MI in patients with recent (3 to 6 months) or remote (>6 months) strokes.

The dose and type of thrombolytic agent have also been linked to risk of intracranial hemorrhage. In the TIMI-II trial the dose of tPA was reduced from 150 mg tPA to 100 mg tPA because of concern about the intracranial hemorrhage rate at the higher dose. Of 908 patients treated with 150 mg tPA, 12 (1.3%) had an intracranial hemorrhage. Subsequently, 11 of 3016 (0.004%) patients treated with 100 mg of tPA had an intracranial hemorrhage ($P < .01$) [65]. More recent trials have used weight-based doses of tPA that do not exceed a total dose of 90 to 100 mg tPA [66].

Several studies have suggested that intracranial hemorrhage rates are higher in patients treated with tPA than in those treated with streptokinase. Simoons et al. [68] have estimated that the relative risk of intracranial hemorrhage from the use of tPA compared with streptokinase is 1.6 (95% confidence interval 1.0 to 2.5). In ISIS-3 definite or probable intracranial hemorrhage occurred in 0.24% of patients treated with streptokinase, compared with 0.66% of patients treated with tPA [67]. In GISSI-2, the rates of intracranial hemorrhage in streptokinase- versus tPA-treated patients were 0.3% vs. 0.4% in patients $\leq$ 70 years and 0.3% vs. 0.7% in patients >70 years [79]. Since brain imaging was not routinely performed as part of the protocol in patients who had a neurological event in these trials, the true rate of intracranial hemorrhage in patients treated with tPA versus streptokinase is uncertain.

The most compelling evidence that tPA is associated with a higher rate of intracranial hemorrhage comes from GUSTO-I, in which 93% of patients with stroke had brain imaging. In GUSTO-I, four different thrombolytic regimens were used: streptokinase and subcutaneous heparin, streptokinase and intravenous heparin, accelerated tPA and intravenous heparin, or a combination of streptokinase, tPA, and intravenous heparin. The rates of intracranial hemorrhage in these four groups were 0.49%, 0.54%, 0.72%, and 0.94%, respectively, which represents a significant increase in intracranial hemorrhages for accelerated tPA ($P = .03$) and for combined tPA/streptokinase ($P < .001$) compared with streptokinase only. Moreover, total hemorrhage volume was significantly higher ($P = .03$) in the combined tPA/streptokinase group than in the other treatment groups. Despite the increased risk of intracranial hemorrhage with accelerated tPA compared with streptokinase, the combined endpoint of death or disabling stroke was significantly lower in patients treated with accelerated tPA group than in patients treated with streptokinase only (6.9% vs. 7.8%; $P = .006$) [66].

Concomitant use of antithrombotic agents (aspirin, heparin) with thrombolysis is a standard part of the care of patients with acute MI. The rationale for these agents is to maintain coronary artery patency after successful thrombolysis by preventing rethrombosis while the ruptured plaque is stabilizing. Concomitant use of aspirin and/or heparin with thrombolysis has been shown to lower mortality compared with thrombolytic therapy alone [63,80]. Therefore, most patients with acute MI are given a combination of a thrombolytic agent, 160 to 325 mg of chewable aspirin, and intravenous heparin to maintain the activated partial thromboplastin time (aPTT) at 1.5 to 2 times control for 24 to 72 hours. Although the role of heparin is uncertain in patients treated with streptokinase or urokinase, heparin is usually recommended in patients treated with tPA [66].

It is uncertain whether concomitant antithrombotic therapy increases the risk of thrombolytic-related intracranial hemorrhage. In an animal model of experimental intracranial hemorrhage, the incidence and severity of intracranial hemorrhage was significantly increased when heparin was given in conjunction with tPA in spontaneously hypertensive rats. Furthermore, the potentiation of intracranial hemorrhage by heparin was dose dependent and proportional to the prolongation of the aPTT [81]. In humans, one study showed that patients taking anticoagulation before admission had a higher risk of intracranial hemorrhage [64]; however, in TIMI-II, patients treated with tPA alone had a similar rate of intracranial hemorrhage to patients treated with tPA and heparin [65]. Moreover, in TIMI-II there was no correlation between aPTT and risk of intracranial hemorrhage. In GUSTO-I, patients treated with streptokinase and subcutaneous heparin had a slightly lower (but not significantly so) rate of intracranial hemorrhage than patients treated with streptokinase and intravenous heparin (0.49% vs. 0.54%) [66]. Mahaffey et al. [82] have recently compared the frequency of intracranial hemorrhage in patients treated with heparin versus no heparin in six randomized controlled thrombolytic trials. The frequency of intracranial hemorrhage was 0.6% in 878 patients allocated to heparin versus 0.3% in 857 patients not receiving heparin. This difference was not statistically significant; however, this may have been due to low power.

Recent studies have compared the efficacy and safety of hirudin, a new thrombin inhibitor, with heparin as adjunctive therapy with thrombolysis. These studies have produced discordant results. In HIT-III, the study was terminated early because of the higher rate of intracranial hemorrhage in the hirudin group—5 of 148 (3.4%), versus 0 of 154 (0%) in the heparin group [83]. On the other hand, in TIMI-9A the rates of intracranial hemorrhage were 1.7% in the hirudin group and 1.9% in the heparin group [84], and in TIMI-9B the rates of intracranial hemorrhage were 0.4% in the hirudin group and 0.9% in the heparin group [85].

Most studies have shown a correlation between low body weight and increased risk of intracranial hemorrhage. Simoons et al. [68] have estimated that the relative risk of body weight below 70 kg for intracranial hemorrhage following thrombolysis is 2.1 (95% confidence interval 1.3 to 3.2). Weight-adjusted dosing of thrombolytic therapy may lower the risk of intracranial hemorrhage. Females appear to have a higher risk of thrombolytic-related intracranial hemorrhage. In one study intracranial hemorrhage occurred in 5.3% of females and 0.7% of males ($P = .04$), and mortality was also significantly higher in females (14% vs. 3.5%, $P = .006$) [86]. However, it is uncertain whether the higher intracranial hemorrhage rate in females is largely explained by lower body weight.

Radiological Features of Thrombolysis-related Hemorrhages

The GUSTO-I trial provides the most comprehensive data on the radiological features of intracranial hemorrhages following thrombolysis for acute MI. In this trial, brain imaging was performed in 93% of patients who were classified as having a hemorrhagic stroke [87]. There were 298 hemorrhages in 244 patients in GUSTO-I, of which 81% were parenchymal hemorrhages alone, 15% were parenchymal and subdural, 3% were subdural alone, and 1% were intraventricular. Subarachnoid hemorrhage was present in 11% of patients, all of whom had parenchymal hemorrhage as well. In another, smaller study of 13 patients with 33 hemorrhages, 36% of hemorrhages were parenchymal, 33% were subdural, 24% were subarachnoid, and 6% were intraventricular [88]. The high frequency of subarachnoid and intraventricular hemorrhages in these series is explained by the tendency of large parenchymal hemorrhages to decompress into the subarachnoid space.

In GUSTO-I the locations of parenchymal hemorrhages were lobar (i.e., involving frontal, parietal, temporal, or occipital lobes) in 77%, cerebellar in 9%, putaminal or capsular in 8%, and thalamic in 3%. The brainstem was involved in 3% [87]. Other studies have also found that thrombolytic-related intracranial hemorrhages are usually lobar [88]. This pattern is distinct from that of hypertensive parenchymal hemorrhages, which are most common in the basal ganglia, brainstem, and cerebellum and are lobar in only 10% of cases.

Other characteristic features of parenchymal intracranial hemorrhages in GUSTO-I were the large volume of the hemorrhages, multiple hemorrhages (30% of patients in GUSTO-I), and the high percentage of hemorrhages with a blood/fluid level (82% in GUSTO-I) (Fig. 1) [87]. This last finding, which is probably related to ongoing fibrinolysis within the hemorrhage, is unusual in spontaneous hypertensive parenchymal hemorrhage. In GUSTO-I, the median volume of parenchymal hemorrhage was 48 mL (range 21 to 85 mL), which is substantially larger than the average volume of spontaneous parenchymal hemorrhages. Features that were significantly associated with large-volume hemorrhages were elevated diastolic blood pressure, treatment with combined streptokinase/tPA, older age, hemorrhages occurring $\leq$ 13 hour after treatment (median time to hemorrhage was 14 hours; range 8 to 30 hours), hydrocephalus, mass effect, and blood/fluid level within the hematoma [87].

It is common to find preexisting lesions (e.g., brain atrophy, periventricular white matter lesions, infarcts) in patients with thrombolytic-related intracranial hemorrhage (44% of cases in GUSTO-I) [87]. However, the significance of these lesions is unknown since none of the thrombolytic trials provided brain imaging data in patients who did not have intracranial hemorrhage.

Etiology of Thrombolysis-related Hemorrhages

The broad spectrum of risk factors and radiological features of parenchymal hemorrhage following thrombolysis suggest that heterogeneous vascular pathologies may underlie these hemorrhages. While rupture of a Charcot-Bouchard aneurysm of a small penetrating artery to the basal ganglia or brainstem is the most common

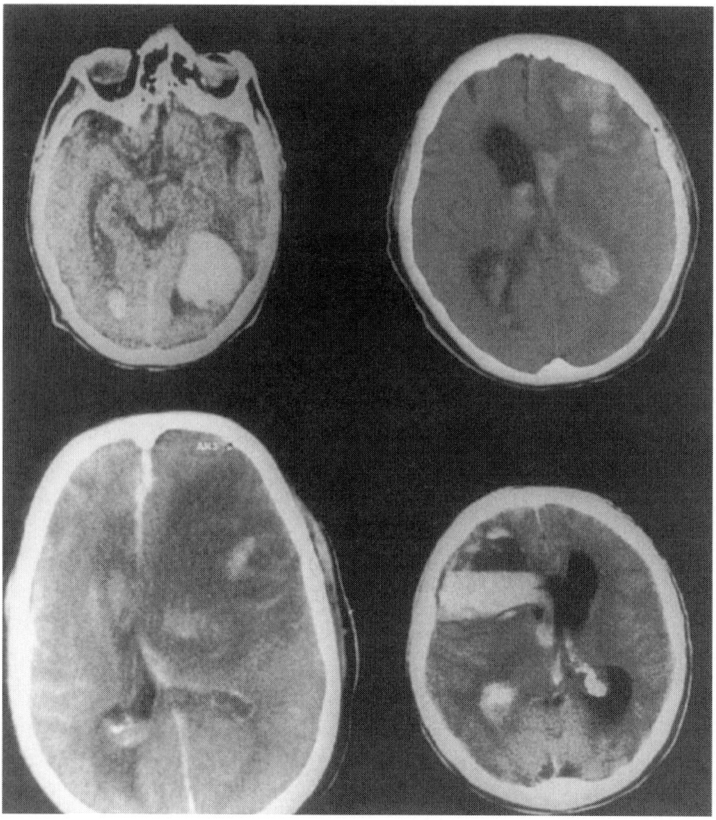

FIG. 1 CT scan examples of intracerebral hematoma following thrombolysis for acute myocardial infarction (top left, top right, bottom right). Note intraventricular extension (top right, bottom right) and blood fluid level (bottom right). The bottom left image shows a large area of hypodensity (a cerebral infarct with mass effect) within which there are scattered areas of hyperdensity (hemorrhagic infarction). Hemorrhagic infarction frequently occurs with cardioembolic stroke regardless of whether anticoagulation or thrombolytic therapy is used. (From Ref. 87.)

cause of spontaneous hypertensive intracranial hemorrhage [89], this is probably responsible for a minority of parenchymal hemorrhages following thrombolysis. The strongest evidence for this is the lobar location of most thrombolytic-related hemorrhages versus the deep (basal ganglia or brainstem) location of most hypertensive hemorrhages. Some of the deep hemorrhages following thrombolysis are probably related to acute or chronic hypertension since high systolic blood pressure prior to neurological symptoms was significantly associated ($P = .02$) with a deep location of hemorrhage compared with other locations in GUSTO-I [87].

The predominance of lobar hemorrhages, multiple hemorrhages in up to 30% of patients, and the strong association of advanced age with increased risk of hemorrhage suggests that amyloid angiopathy may be an important pathological substrate of thrombolytic-related intracranial hemorrhages. Neuropathological studies in patients who have died from intracerebral hemorrhage following thrombolysis for acute MI have confirmed that amyloid angiopathy is responsible for some of these hemorrhages [90,91]. Amyloid angiopathy affects the cerebral vasculature selectively and is not seen in combination with systemic amyloidosis. The neuropathology consists of amyloid infiltration of the walls of small and medium-size arteries of the cerebral cortex and leptomeninges [92]. The frequency of amyloid angiopathy increases with age, as demonstrated in an autopsy study showing that approximately 10% of patients aged 60 to 69 years, 20% of patients aged 70 to 79 years, 37% of patients aged 80 to 89 years, and 44% of patients 90 years and older having the disorder [93]. There is an association between Alzheimer's disease and amyloid angiopathy, with approximately 80% of demented patients having the angiopathy. The mechanism of intracranial hemorrhage associated with amyloid angiopathy is uncertain but may be associated with fibrinoid necrosis of the vessels infiltrated with amyloid [92]. Another suggested mechanism of intracranial hemorrhage is that amyloid beta protein precursor is a potent inhibitor of coagulation factors XIa and IXa [94].

Other neuropathological lesions that have been identified in patients with intracerebral hemorrhage following thrombolysis are arteriovenous malformations, hemorrhagic transformation of an ischemic infarct, and cerebral vasculitis. Srinivasan et al. [95] recently reported a 49-year-old who died of multiple intracranial hemorrhages following thrombolytic therapy. Autopsy showed polyarteritis nodosa of the coronary arteries and cerebral vasculitis.

Diagnosis, Treatment, and Prognosis of Thrombolysis-related Hemorrhages

Most (70% to 83%) intracerebral hemorrhages occur within 24 hours of thrombolysis [65,87]. The initial symptoms and signs depend on the location of the hemorrhage. Lobar hemorrhages typically present with one or more of the following: hemiparesis, hemisensory loss, hemianopia, aphasia, neglect, eye deviation, confusion, headache, seizure, vomiting, and decrease in level of consciousness, which is an ominous sign. Basal ganglia or internal capsule hemorrhages typically present with contralateral hemiparesis and eye deviation to the side of the hemorrhage. Confusion, somnolence, aphasia, and hemisensory loss may also occur if the hemorrhage is large. Small thalamic hemorrhages present with hemisensory loss and sensory ataxia; larger thalamic hemorrhages may also cause hemiparesis (by involving the adjacent internal capsule), vertical gaze palsy with eyes deviated down and in, and somnolence. Cerebellar hemorrhages typically present with vertigo, ipsilateral ataxia of the limbs, inability to walk, and vomiting. Most brainstem hemorrhages occur in the pons and present with long tract signs (hemiparesis, quadraparesis, hemisensory loss), abnormal eye movements (sixth-nerve palsy, unilateral horizontal gaze palsy, bilateral horizontal gaze palsy with vertical ocular bobbing, the one-and-a-half syndrome), and cerebellar signs (ataxia, nystagmus). Crossed sensory or motor signs, e.g., ipsilateral face weakness (or sensory loss) and contralateral arm and leg weakness (or sensory loss) always imply a brainstem location.

Since many of the neurological syndromes associated with intracranial hemorrhage are similar to ischemic stroke syndromes, it is difficult on clinical grounds alone to be certain of the diagnosis. Clinical signs favoring a hemorrhage include markedly elevated blood pressure (i.e., >220/120), early somnolence, vomiting, and seizure at onset. Coma at onset is invariably caused by hemorrhage. Early severe headache suggests intraventricular or subarachnoid extension of the hemorrhage. Brain imaging (preferably CT) should be performed in any patient with suspected stroke following thrombolysis to distinguish between hemorrhagic and ischemic stroke.

The management of intracranial hemorrhage following thrombolysis is challenging. Sloan [59] has suggested the following approach which we have found useful in clinical practice. As soon as a stroke is suspected, thrombolytic agents and anticoagulation should be stopped. At a minimum, the following coagulation studies should be sent for urgent testing: aPTT, PT INR, platelets, bleeding time, hematocrit, and fibrinogen. An urgent CT of the brain must be performed. Early involvement of a neurologist, hematologist, and neurosurgeon will facilitate optimal care for the patient. If any intracranial hemorrhage is detected by CT, cryoprecipitate is given to increase the fibrinogen and factor VIII levels. If the aPTT is elevated, 1 mg of protamine for every 100 units of heparin administered in the preceding 4 hours should be given intravenously. If the PT INR is elevated, fresh frozen plasma should be given. If the bleeding time is prolonged, an infusion of platelets is given. Even though these treatments may increase the risk of coronary reocclusion, they should be administered because of the risk of continuing intracranial hemorrhage and fibrinolysis of the intracranial hematoma.

The optimal treatment for blood pressure control in this setting is controversial. We usually attempt to maintain a mean arterial pressure of 90 to 100 mm Hg in the setting of intracranial hemorrhage but permit higher blood pressures if the patient develops raised intracranial pressure. All patients should be managed in an intensive care unit (preferably a neurointensive care unit), and insertion of a Camino catheter to measure intracranial pressure should be considered. The role of craniotomy with evacuation of the hematoma is controversial. While evacuation of a large hematoma may be life saving, most of these patients are left with severe disability. Ventriculostomy is essential in patients with hydrocephalus.

Given the radiological features (large volume, multiplicity, frequent intraventricular and subarachnoid extension), it is not surprising that the prognosis of thrombolytic-related intracranial hemorrhages is very poor. Mortality from intracranial hemorrhage has varied between 36% and 83% in previous thrombolytic studies [60,65,87]. Of patients that survive, up to 54% have major or moderate disability [70].

Cardioversion

Direct-current cardioversion (DC cardioversion) was first used to restore sinus rhythm in patients with atrial fibrillation in 1962 by Lown et al. [96]. Subsequent studies have shown that DC cardioversion restores sinus rhythm in 80% of patients with recent-onset atrial fibrillation, whereas the success rate with pharmacological therapy may be as low as 40% [97]. Following successful cardioversion, sinus rhythm at 1 year is maintained in 50% to 70% of patients on antiarrhythmic therapy, compared to 30% to 50% in patients without antiarrhythmic therapy [97,98]. Features that are associated with failure of DC cardioversion or a high recurrence rate of atrial fibrillation include untreated thyrotoxicosis, mitral valve disease, congestive heart failure, atrial fibrillation lasting >1 year, left atrial enlargement, and increased body size [98].

The major risk of cardioversion (electrical or pharmacological) in patients with atrial fibrillation is embolic stroke, which occurs in 0.6% to 5.6% of patients [96,99,100]. Stroke occurs when thrombus is dislodged from the left atrium or left atrial appendage following cardioversion. Since left atrial thrombus may be detected by transesophageal echocardiography (TEE) in 10% to 15% of patients with atrial fibrillation lasting at least 48 hours [16,18,48], it is possible that early cardioversion (i.e., within 48 hours) may be associated with a lower risk of embolism. This inference is supported by a recent study in which only 3 of 375 patients (0.8%) had a thromboembolic event after converting from atrial fibrillation to sinus rhythm within 48 hours [101].

While most strokes following cardioversion probably occur when preexisting thrombus is dislodged from the left atrium, recent studies have shown that left atrial thrombus may also develop *after* sinus rhythm is restored. This occurs because left atrial contractile function may be compromised for up to a week after cardioversion [99,102–104]. Echocardiographic features of left atrial contractile dysfunction (''atrial stunning'') include diminished left atrial appendage ejection fraction, diminished left atrial appendage peak systolic velocity, and the presence of left atrial spontaneous echo (Fig. 2). In one study of 20 patients undergoing TEE after successful cardioversion, spontaneous echo contrast developed de novo in four patients and increased in intensity in three patients following the procedure [104]. One study suggests that patients who undergo DC cardioversion have a greater degree and longer duration of ''atrial stunning'' than patients who convert to sinus rhythm pharmacologically or spontaneously [102].

To lower the risk of stroke following DC cardioversion in patients with atrial fibrillation, the American College of Chest Physicians developed specific

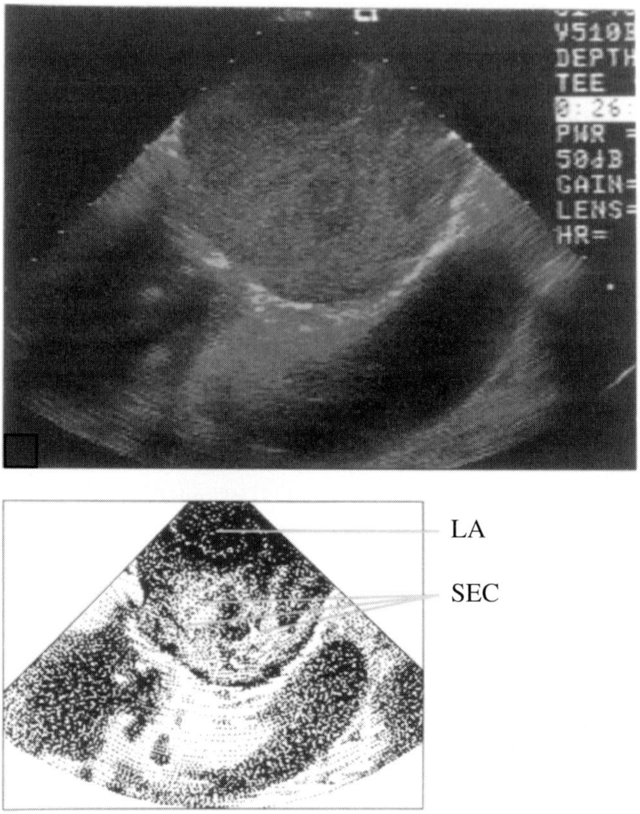

FIG. 2 Transesophageal echocardiography showing prominent left atrial (LA) spontaneous echo contrast (SEC) in a patient with atrial fibrillation. Spontaneous echo contrast has the appearance of smoke swirling and circulating through the atrial chamber (From Ref. 112.)

recommendations regarding the use of anticoagulation before and after cardioversion [105]. These recommendations are to use warfarin (INR 2-3) for 3 weeks before and 4 weeks after cardioversion. One study, which evaluated cardioversion practice patterns at a tertiary care teaching hospital, showed that physicians failed to follow the American College of Chest Physicians recommendations in 18 of 51 cases (35%) [106].

Another protocol, which incorporates the use of TEE to screen for left atrial thrombus before DC cardioversion, has recently been recommended [100,107–109]. This protocol involves anticoagulating patients with warfarin (outpatients)

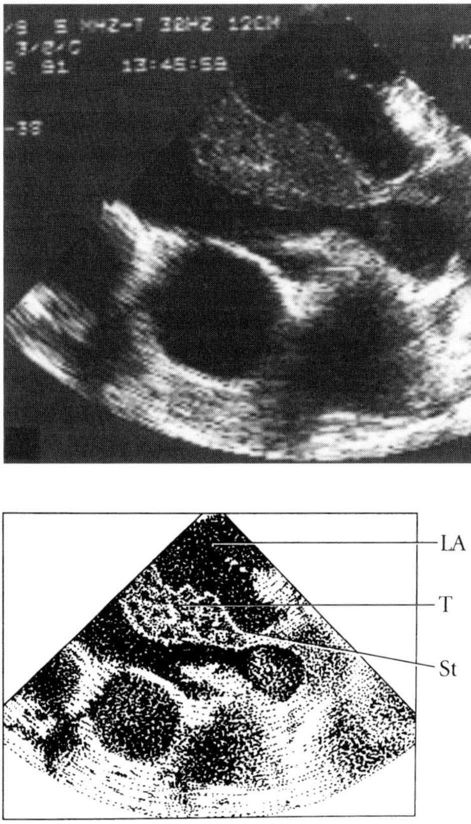

FIG. 3 Transesophageal echocardiography showing thrombus (T) in the left atrium (LA) in a patient with atrial fibrillation. The thrombus is attached to the atrial wall by a stalk (St). (From Ref. 112.)

or heparin (inpatients). TEE is scheduled as soon as a therapeutic level of anticoagulation is achieved (INR 2-3 or partial thrombolplastin time of 1.5 to 2.5). DC cardioversion is performed within 24 hours of TEE if there is no evidence of left atrial thrombus and anticoagulation is continued for 4 weeks. If thrombus is detected at TEE (Fig. 3), cardioversion is postponed, warfarin is continued for 4 weeks, and TEE is repeated. If the thrombus has resolved, cardioversion is performed and warfarin is continued for 4 more weeks. If a thrombus is still present, warfarin is continued and cardioversion is not done [107].

The potential advantages of the TEE guided approach over the conventional approach include: (1) lowering the risk of embolism by avoiding cardioversion in patients with left atrial thrombus; (2) lowering the risk of hemorrhagic complications by decreasing the duration of anticoagulation; (3) increasing the rate of successful cardioversion and maintenance of sinus rhythm because cardioversion is performed earlier; and (4) decreasing health care costs associated with the procedure. A recent study employing decision analysis suggests that the TEE-guided approach is more cost effective than the conventional approach if the risk of stroke from cardioversion after TEE is slightly less than that of conventional therapy. The decision analysis showed that the TEE approach is most cost effective in patients with an increased risk of hemorrhagic complications of anticoagulation [110].

Only one randomized study has compared the feasibility and safety of the TEE-guided approach to the conventional approach for performing DC cardioversion. In a multicenter pilot study of patients with atrial fibrillation lasting >2 days, 62 patients were randomized to the TEE-guided protocol for DC cardioversion and 64 patients were randomized to the conventional protocol [107]. The two groups were compared with respect to the following outcome variables: frequency of DC cardioversion, frequency of conversion to sinus rhythm, time to convert to sinus rhythm, embolic events, hemorrhagic complications, and hemodynamic instability. The patients in both groups were well matched with respect to clinical and echocardiographic features such as age, hypertension, coronary artery disease, valvular heart disease, duration of atrial fibrillation, prior DC cardioversion, concomitant antiarrhythmic therapy, left atrial size, and left ventricular ejection fraction. At the time of cardioversion, heparin was used significantly more frequently ($P < .01$) in the TEE-guided group, whereas warfarin was used significantly more frequently ($P < .01$) in the conventional group [107].

Of the 62 patients randomized to the TEE group, 6 (10%) did not undergo TEE because of spontaneous conversion to sinus rhythm (3 patients), patient refusal (1 patient), technical reasons (1 patient), and clinical instability (1 patient). The latter 2 patients subsequently underwent successful DC cardioversion. Of the 56 patients who underwent TEE, left atrial thrombus was detected in 6 patients (11%), right atrial thrombus was detected in 1 patient (1%), and spontaneous echo contrast was detected in the left atrium or left atrial appendage in 44 patients (79%). DC cardioversion was performed in 45 patients undergoing TEE with immediate achievement of sinus rhythm in 38 (84%). DC cardioversion was not performed after the first TEE in 11 patients because of the presence of left atrial thrombus in 6 patients, right atrial thrombus in 1 patient, or conversion to sinus rhythm (spontaneous, pharmacological, or pacemaker overdrive) in 4 patients. The 7 patients with atrial thrombus underwent repeat TEE after a mean period of 6 weeks on anticoagulation. The atria were free of thrombus in 4 of these patients who underwent DC cardioversion (3 successful), whereas left atrial thrombus persisted in 3 patients who did not undergo DC cardioversion. Overall, sinus rhythm was achieved early in 47 of the 62 patients (76%) in the TEE-guided group at a mean of 1 week after enrollment in the study, and was achieved later (at least 6 weeks after enrollment) in 3 patients who had atrial thrombus on the initial TEE. The frequency of sinus rhythm at 8 weeks after enrollment was 34 of 62 (55%) in the TEE-guided group. None of the TEE-guided group had an embolic event and 1 patient (1.6%) had ''hemodynamic instability and bleeding,'' but the clinical details were not provided [107].

In the conventional therapy group, 37 of 64 patients (58%) had DC cardioversion which was successful in 28 patients (76%). DC cardioversion was not performed in 27 patients because of spontaneous or pharmacological conversion to sinus rhythm in 20 patients or other reasons in 7 patients. Overall, sinus rhythm was achieved in 48 of the 64 patients (75%) in the conventional therapy group at a mean of 4.3 weeks after enrollment in the study. The frequency of sinus rhythm at 8 weeks after enrollment was 37 of 64 (56%) in the conventional group. One patient (1.6%) in the conventional-therapy group had an embolic event (to an upper extremity), and five patients (7.8%) had ''hemodynamic instability and bleeding'' [107].

Comparison of the two groups shows that the TEE-guided group had a significantly shorter mean time to sinus rhythm (1 week vs. 4.3 weeks; $P < .01$), a significantly shorter mean duration of anticoagulation (5.7 weeks vs 7.7 weeks; $P < .01$), and lower (but not significant) rates of embolism (0% vs. 1.6%) and hemodynamic instability and bleeding (1.6% vs. 7.8%). Despite the longer time to achieve sinus rhythm in the conventional group, the frequency of sinus rhythm at 8 weeks was virtually identical in the two groups (56% conventional, 55% TEE guided). Moreover, significantly fewer patients in the conventional group had to undergo DC cardioversion [37 of 64 (58%)] in the conventional group, versus 51 of 62 (82%) in the TEE group ($P < .05$) because of the high rate of spontaneous or pharmacological conversion while awaiting DC cardioversion [107].

Overall, this pilot study suggests that the TEE-guided approach is feasible and may result in fewer embolic and hemorrhagic events than the conventional approach; however, a larger randomized study with sufficient power is needed to confirm or refute this hypothesis. Such a trial, which will involve 3000 patients at 65 sites, is currently being planned [111].

REFERENCES

1. Seldinger SI. Catheter replacement of needle in percutaneous arteriography; new technique. Acta Radiol 1953; 39:368–376.
2. Sones FM Jr. Cine-cardio-angiography. Pediatr Clin North Am 1958; 4:945–979.
3. Adams D, Fraser D, Abrams J. The complications of coronary arteriography. Circulation 1973; 48:609–617.
4. Johnson L, Lozner E, Johnson S, Krone R, Pichard A, Vetrovec G. Noto T. Coro-

nary angiography 1984–1987: a report of the registry of the Society for Cardiac Angiography and Interventions. I. Results and Complications. Cathet Cardiovasc Diagn 1989; 17:5–10.
5. Lockwood K, Capraro J, Hanson M, Conomy J. Neurologic complications of cardiac cathetherization. Neurology 1983; 33(suppl 2):143.
6. Levorstad K, Vatne K, Brodahl U, Aakhus T, Simonsen S, Vik H. Cerebral thromboembolic complications associated with the use of a nonionic contrast medium in coronary angiography. Acta Radiol 1995; 36:69–71.
7. Davidson C, Mark D, Peiper K, Kisslo K, Hlatky M, Gabriel D, Bashore T. Thrombotic and cardiovascular complications related to nonionic contrast media during coronary angiography: analysis of 8,517 patients. Am J Cardiol 1990; 65:1481–1484.
8. Lazar J, Uretsky B, Denys B, Reddy P, Counihan P, Ragosta M. Predisposing risk factors and natural history of acute neurologic complications of left-sided coronary angiography. Am J Cardiol 1995; 75:1056–1060.
9. Roelke M, Smith A, Palacios I. The technique and safety of transeptal left heart catheterization: the Massachusetts General Hospital experience with 1,279 procedures. Cathet Cardiovasc Diagn 1994; 32:332–339.
10. Dawson D, Fischer E. Neurologic complications of coronary angiography. Neurology 1977; 27:496–497.
11. Kosmorsky G, Hanson M, Tomsak R. Neuroophthalmologic complications of coronary angiography. Neurology 1988; 38:483–485.
12. Keilson G, Schwartz W, Recht L. The preponderance of posterior circulatory events is independent of the route of coronary angiography. Stroke 1992; 23:1358–1359.
13. Shmuely H, Zoldan J, Sagie A, Maimon S, Pitlik S. Acute stroke after coronary angiography associated with protruding mobile thoracic aortic atheromas. Neurology 1997; 49:1689–1691.
14. Kirk G, Johnson J. Computed tomography detection of a cerebral calcific embolus following coronary catheterization. J Neuroimag 1994; 4:241–242.
15. Clements S. Prevention and treatment of complications in coronary angiography. In: Lutz J, ed. Complications of Interventional Procedures. New York: Igaku-Shoin, 1995:64–71.
16. National Institute of Neurological Disorders and Stroke rt-PA Stroke Study Group. Tissue plasminogen activator for acute ischemic stroke. N Engl J Med 1995; 333: 1581–1587.
17. Dwivedi S, Bansal S, Atrawal A, Saran R. Thrombolysis for stroke complicating cardiac catheterisation. Indian Heart J 1997; 49:545–546.
18. Moody D, Bell M, Challa V, Johnston W, Prough D. Brain microemboli during cardiac surgery or aortography. Ann Neurol 1990; 28:477–486.
19. Kent K, Moscucci M, Gallagher S, DiMattia S, Skillman J. Neuropathy after cardiac catherization: incidence, clinical patterns, long term outcome. J Vasc Surg 1994; 19:1008–1014.
20. Kennedy A, Grocott M, Schwartz M, Modarres H, Scott M, Schon F. Median nerve injury: an underrecognised complication of brachial artery cardiac catheterisation? J Neurol Neurosurg Psychiatry 1997; 63:542–546.
21. Gruntzig A. Transluminal dilatation of coronary artery stenosis. Lancet 1978;1: 263.

22. Douglas J. Complications of percutaneous transluminal coronary angioplasty. In: Lutz J, ed. Complications of Interventional Procedures. New York: Igaku-Shoin, 1995:173–185.
23. Dorros G, Cawley M, Simpson J, Bentivaglio L, Block P, Bourassa M, Detre K, Gosselin A, Grunteig A, Kelsey S, Kent K, Mock M, Mullin S, Meyer R, Passamani E, Stertzer S, Williams D. Percutaneous transluminal coronary angioplasty: report of complications from the National Heart, Lung, and Blood Institute PTCA registry. Circulation 1983; 67:723–730.
24. Galbreath C, Salgado E, Furlan A, Hollman J. Central nervous system complications of percutaneous transluminal coronary angioplasty. Stroke 1986; 17:616–619.
25. Kan J, White R, Mitchell S, Gardner T. Percuatneous balloon valvuloplasty: a new method for treating congenital pulmonary-valve stenosis. N Engl J Med 1982; 307: 540–542.
26. Inoue K, Owaki T, Nakamura T, Kitamura F, Miyamoto N. Clinical application of transvenous mitral commissurotomy by a new balloon catheter. J Thorac Cardiovasc Surg 1984; 87:394–402.
27. Lock J, Khalilullah M, Shrivastava S, Bahl V, Keane J. Percutaneous catheter commissurotomy in rheumatic mitral stenosis. N Engl J Med 1985; 313:1515–1518.
28. Letac B, Cribier A, Koning R, Bellefleur J-P. Results of percutaneous transluminal valvuloplasty in 218 adults with valvular aortic stenosis. Am J Cardiol 1988; 62: 598–605.
29. Cribier A, Scroudi N, Besland J, Savin T, Rocha P, Letac B. Percutaneous transterminal valvuloplasty of acquired aortic stenosis in elderly patients: an alternative to valve replacement? Lancet 1986; 1:63–67.
30. Fu X, Zhang D, Schiele F, Anguenot T, Bernard Y, Bassand J. Complications of percutaneous mitral valvuloplasty; comparison of the double balloon and the Inoue techniques. Arch Mal Coeur Vaiss 1994; 87:1403–1411.
31. Block P. Complications of valvuloplasty. In: Lutz J, ed. Complications of Interventional Procedures. New York: Igaku-Shoin, 1995:164–172.
32. Li S, Yang H, Liu H, Dai R. Role of transesophageal echocardiography in pre- and post-percutaneous balloon mitral valvuloplasty. Chin Med J 1994; 107:897–902.
33. Goldstein S, Campbell A. Mitral stenosis. Evaluation and guidance of valvuloplasty by transesophageal echocardiography. Cardiol Clin 1993; 11:409–425.
34. Chioin R, Ramondo A, DeConti F, Isabella G, Cardaioli P, Marchiori M, LoPresti A, Campisi F, Razzolini R. Percutaneous mitral valvuloplasty: the immediate and long-term results. G Ital Cardiol 1995;25:409–420.
35. Demirtas M, Usal A, Birand A, San M, Batyraliev T, Niyazova Z. A serious complication of percutaneous mitral valvuloplasty: systemic embolism. How can we decrease it? Case history. Angiology 1996; 47:285–289.
36. Chen C, Cheng T. Percutaneous balloon mitral valvuloplasty by the Inoue technique: a multicenter study of 4832 patients in China. Am Heart J 1995; 129:1197–1203.
37. Karnik R, Valentin A, Bonner G, Ziegler B, Slany J. Transcranial Doppler monitoring during percutaneous transluminal aortic valvuloplasty. Angiology 1990; 41: 106–111.

38. Drobinski G, Lechat P, Metzger J, Lepailleur C, Vacheron A, Grosgogeat Y. Results of percutaneous catheter valvuloplasty for calcified aortic stenosis in the elderly. Eur Heart J 1987; 8(4):322–328.
39. Davidson C, Skelton T, Kisslo K, Kong Y, Peter R, Simonton C, Phillips H, Behar V, Bashore T. The risk for systemic embolization associated with percutaneous balloon valvuloplasty in adults. A prospective comprehensive evaluation. Ann Intern Med 1988; 108:557–560.
40. Rosenfeld H, Landzberg M, Perry S, Colan S, Keane J, Lock J. Balloon aortic valvuloplasty in the young adult with congenital aortic stenosis. Am J Cardiol 1994; 73:1112–1117.
41. Moulopoulos S, Topaz S, Kolff W. Diastolic balloon pumping (with carbon dioxide) in the aorta—a mechanical assistance to the failing circulation. Am Heart J 1962;63:669–675.
42. Smith A. Complications of the intraaortic balloon pump. In: Lutz J, ed. Complications of Interventional Procedures. New York: Igaku-Shoin, 1995:80–85.
43. Riggle K, Oddi M. Spinal cord necrosis and paraplegia as complications of the intra-aortic balloon. Crit Care Med 1989; 17:475–476.
44. Harvey J, Goldstein J, McCabe M, Hoover E, Gay W, Subramanian V. Complications of percutaneous intraaortic balloon pumping. Circulation 1981; 64(2 Pt 2): II114–II117.
45. Reemtsma K, Drusin R, Edie R, Bregman D, Dobelle W, Hardy M. Cardiac transplantation for patients requiring mechanical circulatory support. N Engl J Med 1978; 298:670–671.
46. Slater J, Rose E, Levin H, Frazier O, Roberts J, Weinberg A, Oz M. Low thromboembolic risk without anticoagulation using advanced-design left ventricular assist devices. Ann Thorac Surg 1996; 62:1321–1328.
47. Nabavi D, Georgiadis D, Mumme T, Schmid C, Mackay T, Scheld H, Ringelsten E. Clinical relevance of intracranial microembolic signals in patients with left ventricular assist devices: a prospective study. Stroke 1996; 27:891–896.
48. Pennington D, McBride L, Peigh P, Miller L, Swartz M. Eight years experience with bridging to cardiac transplantation. J Thorac Cardiovasc Surg 1994; 107:472–481.
49. Icenogle T, Smith R, Cleavinger M, Vasu M, Williams R, Sethi G, Copeland J. Thromboembolic complications of the symbion AVAD system. Artif Organs 1989; 13:532–538.
50. Didisheim P, Olsen D, Farrar D, Portner P, Griffith B, Pennington D, Joist J, Schoen F, Gristina A, Anderson J. Infection and thromboembolism with implantable cardiovascular devices. ASAIO Trans 1989; 35:54–70.
51. McGee M, Myers T, Abou-Awdi N, Dasse K, Radovancevic B, Lonquist J, Duncan J, Frazier O. Extended support with a left ventricular assist device as a bridge to heart transplantation. ASAIO Trans 1991; 37(3):M425–M426.
52. Graham T, Dasse K, Coumbe A. Neo-intimal development on textured biomaterial surfaces during clinical use of an implantable left ventricular assist device. Eur J Cardiothorac Surg 1990; 4:182–190.
53. Salih V, Graham T, Berry C, et al. The lining of textured surfaces in implantable left ventricular assist devices. An immunocytochemical and electronmicroscopic study. Am J Cardiovasc Pathol 1993; 4:317–325.

54. Rafii S, Oz M, Seldomridge J, et al. Characterization of hematopoietic cells arising on the textured surface of left ventricular assist devices. Ann Thorac Surg 1995; 60:1627–1632.
55. Menconi M, Pockwinse S, Owen T, Dasse K, Stein G, Lian J. Properties of blood-contacting surfaces of clinically implanted cardiac assist devices: gene expression, matrix composition, and ultrastructural characterization of cellular linings. J Cell Biochem 1995; 57:557–573.
56. Menconi M, Owen T, Dasse K, Stein G, Lian J. Molecular approaches to the characterization of cell and blood/biomaterial interactions. J Cardiac Surg 1992; 7:177–187.
57. Spanier T, Oz M, Levin H, Weinberg A, Stamatis K, Stern D, Rose E, Schmidt A. Activation of coagulation and fibrinolytic pathways in patients with left ventricular assist devices. J Thorac Cardiovasc Surg 1996; 112:1090–1097.
58. Connolly E, Winfree C, McCormick P. Management of spinal epidural hematoma after tissue plasminogen activator. A case report. Spine 1996; 21:1694–1698.
59. Sloan M. Stroke associated with thrombolytic therapy for acute myocardial infarction. Heart Dis Stroke 1992; 1:287–294.
60. Longstreth W, Litwin P, Weaver W. Myocardial infarction, thrombolytic therapy, and stroke. A community-based study. Stroke 1993; 24:587–590.
61. Maggioni A, Franzosi M, Farina M, Santoro E, Celani M, Ricci S, Tognoni G. Cerebrovascular events after myocardial infarction: analysis of the GISSI trial. BMJ 1991; 302:1428–1431.
62. Schroder R, Neuhaus K-L, Leizorovicz A, Linderer T, Tebbe U. A prospective placebo-controlled double-blind multicenter trial of intravenous streptokinase in acute myocardial infarction (ISAM): long-term mortality and morbidity. J Am Coll Cardiol 1987; 9:197–203.
63. ISIS-2 (Second International Study of Infarct Survival) Collaborative Group. Randomised trial of intravenous streptokinase, oral aspirin, both, or neither among 17,187 cases of suspected acute myocardial infarction. Lancet 1988; 2:349–360.
64. DeJaegere P, Arnold A, Balk A, Simoons M. Intracranial hemorrhage in association with thrombolytic therapy: incidence and clinical predictive factors. J Am Coll Cardiol 1992; 19:289–294.
65. Gore J, Sloan M, Price T, Young-Randall A, Bovill E, Collen D, Forman S, Knatterud G, Sopko G, Terrin M. Intracerebral hemorrhage, cerebral infarction, and subdural hematoma after acute myocardial infarction and thrombolytic therapy in the thrombolysis in myocardial infarction study; thrombolysis in myocardial infarction. Phase II. Pilot and and clinical trial. Circulation 1991; 83:448–459.
66. GUSTO Investigators. An international randomized trial comparing four thrombolytic strategies for actue myocardial infarction. N Engl J Med 1993; 329:673–682.
67. ISIS-3 (Third International Study of Infarct Survival) Collaborative Group. ISIS-3: A randomised comparison of streptokinase vs tissue plasminogen activator vs anistreplase and of aspirin plus heparin vs aspirin alone among 41,299 cases of suspected acute myocardial infarction. Lancet 1992; 339:753–770.
68. Simoons M, Maggioni A, Knatterud G, Leimberger J, de Jaegere P, van Domburg R, Boersma E, Franzosi M, Califf R, Schroder R, et al. Individual risk assessment

for intracranial hemorrhage during thrombolytic therapy. Lancet 1993; 342:1523–1528.

69. Grines C, DeMaria A. Optimal utilization of thrombolytic therapy for acute myocardial infarction. J Am Coll Cardiol 1990; 16:223–231.
70. Hillegass W, Jollis J, Granger C, Ohman E, Califf R, Mark D. Intracranial hemorrhage risk and new thrombolytic therapies in acute myocardial infarction. Am J Cardiol 1994; 73:444–449.
71. Anderson H, Willerson J. Thrombolysis in acute myocardial infarction. N Engl J Med 1993; 329:703–709.
72. Aylward P, Wilcox R, Horgan J, White H, Granger C, Califf R, Topol E. Relation of increased arterial blood pressure to mortality and stroke in the context of contemporary thrombolytic therapy for acute myocardial infarction. A randomized trial. GUSTO-I investigators. Ann Intern Med 1996; 125:891–900.
73. Selker H, Beshansky J, Schmid C, Griffith J, Longstreth W, O'Connor C, Caplan L, Massey E, D'Agostino R, Laks M, et al. Presenting pulse pressure predicts thrombolytic therapy-related intracranial hemorrhage. Thrombolytic Predictive Instrument (TPI) Project results. Circulation 1994; 90:1657–1661.
74. Ryan T, Anderson J, Antman E, Braniff B, Brooks N, Califf R, Hillis L, Hiratzka L, Rapaport E, Riegel B, Russell R, Smith E, Weaver W. ACC/AHA guidelines for the management of patients with acute myocardial infarction. A report of the American College of Cardiology/American Heart Association Task Force on Practive Guidelines (Committee on Management of Acute Myocardial Infarction). J Am Coll Cardiol 1996; 28:1328–1498.
75. Tanne D, Gottlieb S, Caspi A, Hod H, Palant A, Reisin L, Rosenfeld T, Peled B, Marmor A, Balkin J, Boyko V, Behar S. Treatment and oucome of patients with acute myocardial infarction and prior cerebrovascular events in the thrombolytic era: the Israeli Thrombolytic National Survey. Arch Intern Med 1998; 158:601–606.
76. Rawles J. Guidelines for general practitioners administering thrombolytics. Drugs 1995; 50:615–625.
77. Ketley D, Woods K. Selection factors for the use of thrombolytic treatment in acute myocardial infarction. Br Heart J 1995; 74:224–228.
78. Cupples A, Gagnon D, Wong N, Ostfeld A, Dannel W. Preexisting cardiovascular conditions and long-term prognosis after initial myocardial infarction: the Farmingham Study. Am Heart J 1993; 125:863–872.
79. Maggioni A, Franzosi M, Santoro E, White H, Vande Werf F, Tognoni G. The risk of stroke in patients with acute myocardial infarction after thrombolytic and antithrombotic treatment. Gruppo Italiano per lo Studio della Sopravvivenza nell'Infarto Miocardico II (GISSI-2), and the International Study Group. N Engl J Med 1992; 327:1–6.
80. Tiefenbrunn A, Sobel B. Thrombolysis and myocardial infarction. Fibrinolysis 1991; 5:1–15.
81. Paoni M, Metz HS, Gillett N, Refino C, Badillo J, Bunting S. An experimental model of intracranial hemorrhage during thrombolytic therapy with t-PA. Thromb Haemost 1996; 75:820–826.
82. Mahaffey K, Granger C, Collins R, O'Connor C, Ohman E, Bleich S, Col J, Califf R. Overview of randomized trials of intravenous heparin in patients with acute

myocardial infarction treated with thrombolytic therapy. Am J Cardiol 1996; 77: 551–556.
83. Neuhaus K, Von Essen R, Tebbe U, Jessel A, Heinrichs H, Maurer W, Doring W, Harmjanz D, Kotter V, Kalhammer E, et al. Safety observations from the pilot phase of the randomized r-Hirudin for Improvement of Thrombolysis (HIT-III) study. A study of the Arbeitsgemeinschaft Leitender Kardiologischer Krankenhausarzte (ALKK). Circulation 1994; 90:1638–1642.
84. Antman E. Hirudin in acute myocardial infarction. Safety report from the Thrombolysis and Thrombin Inhibition in Myocardial Infarction (TIMI) 9A Trial. Circulation 1994; 90:1624–1630.
85. Antman E. Hirudin in acute myocardial infarction. Thrombolysis and Thrombin Inhibition in Myocardial Infarction (TIMI) 9B Trial. Circulation 1996; 94:911–921.
86. Stone G, Grines C, Browne K, Marco J, Rothbaum D, O'Keefe J, Hartzler G, Overlie P, Donohue B, Chelliah N, et al. Comparison of in-hospital outcome in men versus women treated by either thrombolytic therapy or primary coronary angioplasty for acute myocardial infarction. Am J Cardiol 1995; 75:987–992.
87. Gebel J, Sila C, Sloan M, Granger C, Mahaffey K, Weisenberger J, Green C, White H, Gore J, Weaver W, Califf R, Topol E. Thrombolysis-related intracranial hemorrhage: a radiographic analysis of 244 cases from the GUSTO-1 Trial with clinical correlation. Stroke 1998; 29:563–569.
88. Uglietta J, O'Connor C, Boyko O, Aldrich H, Massey E, Heinz E. CT patterns of intracranial hemorrhage complicating thrombolytic therapy for acute myocardial infarction. Radiology 1991; 181:555–559.
89. Caplan L, Stein R. Intracerebral hemorrhage. In: Caplan L, Stein R, eds. Stroke: A Clinical Approach. Boston: Butterworths, 1986:266.
90. LeBlanc R, Haddad G, Robitaille Y. Cerebral hemorrhage from amyloid angiopathy and coronary thrombolysis. Neurosurgery 1992; 31:586–590.
91. Pendlebury W, Iole E, Tracy R, Dill B. Intracerebral hemorrhage related to cerebral amyloid angiopathy and t-PA treatment. Ann Neurol 1991; 29:210–213.
92. Kase C. Cerebral amyloid angiopathy. In: Feldmann E, ed. Current Diagnosis in Neurology. St. Louis: Mosby–Yearbook, 1994:58–62.
93. Masuda J, Tanaka K, Ueda K, Omae T. Autopsy study of incidence and distribution of cerebral amyloid angiopathy in Hisayama, Japan. Stroke 1988; 19:205–210.
94. Schmaier A. Amyloid beta-protein precursor: A new anticoagulant? J Lab Clin Med 1997; 130:5–7.
95. Srinivasan G, Boschman C, Roth S, Hendel R. Unsuspected vasculitis and intracranial hemorrhage following thrombolysis. Clin Cardiol 1997; 20:84–86.
96. Lown B, Perlroth M, Kaidey S, Abe T, Harken D. Cardioversion of atrial fibrillation: a report on the treatment of 65 episodes in 50 patients. N Engl J Med 1963; 269:325–31.
97. Golzari H, Cebul R, Bahler R. Atrial fibrillation: restoration and maintenance of sinus rhythm and indications for anticoagulation therapy. Ann Intern Med 1996; 125:311–323.
98. Burton M. Complications of external cardioversion-defibrillation. In: Lutz J, ed. Complications of Interventional Procedures. New York: Igaku-Shoin, 1995:103–111.

99. Stein B, Halperin J, Fuster V. Should patients with atrial fibrillation be anticoagulated prior to and chronically following cardioversion? Cardiovasc Clin 1990; 21: 231–247.
100. Grimm R, Stewart W, Black I, Thomas J, Klein A. Should all patients undergo transesophageal echocardiography before electrical cardioversion of atrial fibrillation? J Am Coll Cardiol 1994; 23:533–541.
101. Weigner M, Caulfield T, Danias P, Silverman D, Manning W. Risk for clinical thromboembolism associated with conversion to sinus rhythm in patients with atrial fibrillation lasting less than 48 hours. Ann Intern Med 1997; 126:615–620.
102. Harjai K, Mobarek S, Cheirif J, Boulos L, Murgo J, Abi-Samra F. Clinical variables affecting recovery of left atrial mechanical function after cardioversion from atrial fibrillation. J Am Coll Cardiol 1997; 30:481–486.
103. Tabata T, Oki T, Iuchi A, Tamada H, Manabe K, Fukuda K, Abe M, Fukuda N, Ito S. Evaluation of left atrial appendage function by measurement of changes in flow velocity patterns after electrical cardioversion in patients with isolated atrial fibrillation. Am J Cardiol 1997; 79:615–620.
104. Grimm R, Stewart W, Maloney J, Cohen G, Pearce G, Salcedo E, Klein A. Impact of electrical cardioversion for atrial fibrillation on left atrial appendage function and spontaneous echo contrast: characterization by simultaneous transesophageal echocardiography. J Am Coll Cardiol 1993; 22:1359–1366.
105. Laupacis A, Albers G, Dalen J, Dunn M, Weinberg W, Jacobson A. Antithrombotic therapy in atrial fibrillation. From the fourth ACCP Consensus Conference on Antithrombotic Therapy. Chest 1995; 108:352S–359S.
106. Schlicht J, Davis R, Maqi K, Cooper W, Rao B. Physician practices regarding anticoagulation and cardioversion of atrial fibrillation. Arch Intern Med 1996; 156: 290–294.
107. Klein A, Grimm R, Black I, Leung D, Chung M, Vaughn S, Murray R, Miller D, Arheart K. Cardioversion guided by transesophageal echocardiography: the ACUTE pilot study. A randomized, controlled trial. Ann Intern Med 1997; 126: 200–209.
108. Manning W, Silverman D, Gordon S, Drumholz H, Douglas P. Cardioversion from atrial fibrillation without prolonged anticoagulation with use of transesophageal echocardiography to exclude the presence of atrial thrombi. N Engl J Med 1993; 328:750–755.
109. Manning W, Silverman D, Keighley C, Oettgen P, Douglas P. Transesophageal echocardiography facilitated early cardioversion from atrial fibrillation using short-term anticoagulation: final results of a prospective 4.5-year study. J Am Coll Cardiol 1995; 25:1354–1361.
110. Seto T, Taira D, Tsevat J, Manning W. Cost-effectiveness of transesophageal echocardiographic-guided cardioversion: a decision analytic model for patients admitted to the hospital with atrial fibrillation. J Am Coll Cardiol 1997; 29:122–130.
111. Steering and Publications of the ACUTE Study. Design of a clinical trial for the assessment of cardioversion using transesophageal echocardiography (the ACUTE Multicenter Study). Am J Cardiol 1998; 81:877–883.
112. Poole RM, Chimowitz MI. Cardiac imaging for stroke diagnosis. In: Fisher M, Bogousslavsky J, eds. Current Review of Cerebrovascular Disease. Philadelphia: Current Medicine, 1996:197.

6

Asymptomatic Coronary Artery Disease in Patients with Carotid Artery Stenosis: Incidence, Prognosis, and Treatment

INTRODUCTION

Atherosclerosis is a systemic disease that typically involves multiple arterial trees [1]. One implication of the systemic nature of atherosclerosis is that once a patient develops extracranial carotid artery disease (or intracranial arterial stenosis) there is a high likelihood that the patient will have coronary artery disease (CAD). Indeed, several studies have shown that 30% to 45% of patients presenting with carotid stenosis have a history of CAD [2,3] and 25% to 50% of the remaining patients have evidence of asymptomatic CAD on provocative tests for myocardial ischemia (e.g., exercise electrocardiography (ECG) or myocardial perfusion imaging) [4–7]. Therefore, it is not surprising that virtually every population study and stroke therapy trial has shown that CAD is a major cause of death in patients with carotid stenosis.

Recent trials have shown that carotid endarterectomy and medical therapy (aspirin, modification of risk factors) are significantly more effective than medical therapy alone for preventing stroke in patients with carotid stenosis. The benefit is substantial in patients with symptomatic carotid stenosis ≥70% (absolute risk reduction of 17% at 2 years, 13.2% at 5 years) [2] and modest in patients with asymptomatic carotid stenosis ≥60% (absolute risk reduction of 5.9% at 5 years) [8] or symptomatic carotid stenosis 50% to 69% (absolute risk reduction of 6.5% at 5 years) [9]. The results of these trials will lead to a substantial increase in the number of carotid endarterectomies performed worldwide and a concomitant demand on physicians to diagnose and treat coexistent CAD in these patients. While strategies have evolved for evaluating and treating symptomatic CAD in patients with carotid stenosis [10], this is not true for asymptomatic CAD. The focus of this chapter is on the incidence, prognosis, evaluation, and treatment of asymptomatic CAD in patients with carotid stenosis.

INCIDENCE OF ASYMPTOMATIC CAD IN PATIENTS WITH CAROTID DISEASE

The frequency of asymptomatic CAD in patients presenting with TIA or stroke has been evaluated in several studies. Rokey et al. [11] performed exercise thallium-201 scintigraphy and exercise radionuclide ventriculography on 50 consecutive patients presenting with TIA or stroke. Sixteen patients had symptoms suggestive of cardiac ischemia, and the other 34 patients were asymptomatic. Fifteen of 16 symptomatic (94%) patients and 14 of 34 (41%) asymptomatic patients had abnormal myocardial perfusion imaging. Twenty-two patients with abnormal myocardial perfusion imaging underwent coronary angiography, which showed severe CAD (≥70% stenosis of the lumen of at least one coronary artery) in 18 patients (10 of 13 symptomatic patients, 8 of 9 asymptomatic patients). Twelve of these 18 patients had multivessel disease.

Di Pasquale et al. [12] performed exercise ECG on 83 consecutive patients with TIA or minor stroke who had no symptoms of ischemic heart disease. Patients with positive exercise ECG subsequently underwent exercise thallium-201 myocardial scintigraphy. Asymptomatic CAD was detected in 28% of patients studied with these noninvasive techniques. Coronary angiography was performed in only two patients: one had three-vessel CAD and the other had two-vessel CAD. In another study, Di Pasquale et al. [13] performed dipyridamole thallium myocardial imaging in 23 patients without a history of CAD who presented with cerebral ischemia. Sixteen patients (70%) had perfusion defects (reversible in 15 patients, fixed in 1 patient). Love et al. [14] performed thallium-201 myocardial scintigraphy in 27 patients presenting with asymptomatic carotid disease, TIA, or small stroke and without symptoms of CAD. Nine patients (33%) had perfusion defects (reversible in seven patients, fixed in one patient, and both in another).

While these studies show that patients with TIA or stroke have a high frequency of asymptomatic CAD, none of the studies evaluated the frequency of asymptomatic CAD in patients with different vascular causes of TIA or stroke, e.g., carotid artery disease, intracranial atherosclerotic disease, cardioembolism, penetrating artery disease (small-vessel disease). Chimowitz et al. [7] compared the frequency of abnormal cardiac stress tests in 30 patients with atherosclerosis of a major cerebral artery (i.e., cervical carotid artery or a major intracranial artery) versus 39 patients with other causes of cerebral ischemia (penetrating artery disease, cardioembolism, cryptogenic stroke). All 69 patients in the study presented with TIAs or ischemic stroke and no overt CAD. The frequency of risk factors was similar in the two groups except that patients with cervical carotid or intracranial atherosclerosis had a significantly higher frequency of peripheral vascular disease ($P = .04$), and patients with other causes of causes of cerebral ischemia had a significantly higher frequency of hypertension ($P = .03$).

In patients with cervical carotid or intracranial atherosclerosis, the rates of abnormal stress tests were 8 of 16 (50%) in patients with isolated cervical carotid stenosis, 2 of 8 (25%) in patients with isolated intracranial artery stenosis, and 5 of 6 (83%) in patients with coexistent carotid and intracranial stenoses. In patients with other causes of brain ischemia, the rates of abnormal cardiac stress tests were 4 of 20 (20%) in patients with cryptogenic stroke, 3 of 15 (20%) inpatients with penetrating artery disease, and 2 of 4 (50%) in patients with non-valvular atrial fibrillation. Overall, patients with cervical carotid or intracranial atherosclerosis had a significantly higher frequency of abnormal cardiac stress tests than patients with other causes of cerebral ischemia (15 of 30 [50%] vs. 9 of 39 [23%]; $P = .04$). Coronary angiography was performed in seven patients with cervical carotid or intracranial artery stenosis. This showed severe (≥70% stenosis), one-vessel CAD in two patients, severe two-vessel CAD in two patients, and severe three-vessel CAD in three patients. Additionally, two of the seven patients also had left main CAD (50% to 60% stenosis in one patient, 40% to 50% stenosis in the other). Logistic regression analysis showed that smoking (odds ratio 6.5; 95% confidence interval 1.3 to 32.1) and carotid or intracranial atherosclerosis (odds ratio 2.9; 95% confidence interval 1.0 to 8.7) were the only independent risk factors for abnormal stress tests in this study. Another recent study confirms the strong association between carotid artery disease and exercise-induced myocardial ischemia in asymptomatic patients. Okin et al. [15] performed carotid ultrasound and exercise ECG in 204 asymptomatic subjects free of clinical evidence of cardiovascular disease. Exercise-induced myocardial ischemia was detected in 35 patients, 6 of 12 (50%) with carotid atherosclerosis versus 29 of 192 (17%) without carotid disease ($P = .007$). Multivariate analysis showed that carotid artery cross-sectional area ($P = .0007$) and systolic hypertension ($P = .005$) were the only variables that were independently associated with exercise-induced myocardial ischemia.

Other studies have evaluated the frequency of asymptomatic CAD in consecutive patients with carotid artery stenosis. Urbinati et al. [4] performed thallium myocardial perfusion imaging in 106 patients without cardiac symptoms prior to carotid endarterectomy and found that eight of 27 patients (29.6%) had abnormal thallium studies. Sconocchini et al. [5] showed that 21 of 85 (25%) patients with carotid stenosis ≥50% and no history of CAD had abnormal exercise ECG. Only one study has systematically utilized coronary angiography for defining the frequency of asymptomatic CAD in a population presenting with carotid disease. Hertzer et al. [6] performed coronary angiography on 200 patients without symptoms of CAD, most of whom presented with carotid bruits. Eighty patients (40%) had severe CAD defined by >70% stenosis of at least one coronary artery, 93 patients (46%) had mild or moderate CAD, and only 27 patients (14%) had normal coronary arteries. The numbers of patients with single-vessel, multivessel, and left main CAD were not described; however, 22% were considered to have severe, but compensated, CAD; 16% had severe, surgically correctable CAD; and 2% had inoperable CAD.

Overall, these studies suggest that 25% to 50% of patients with carotid disease and no symptoms of CAD have abnormal provocative tests for myocardial ischemia or angiographic evidence of severe CAD. Since provocative tests for myocardial ischemia do not identify patients with atherosclerotic coronary plaques that are not flow-limiting, the true frequency of asymptomatic CAD (i.e., flow-limiting and non-flow-limiting combined) in patients with carotid stenosis is probably substantially greater than 25% to 50%. Patients with non-flow-limiting coronary plaques are at risk of acute MI or sudden death from rupture of an atherosclerotic plaque; however, there are no reliable noninvasive techniques to identify this important subgroup of patients with asymptomatic CAD.

PROGNOSIS OF ASYMPTOMATIC CAD IN PATIENTS WITH CAROTID STENOSIS

Although the risk of myocardial infarction (MI) within 30 days of carotid endarterectomy in patients without a history of CAD is low (1% to 2%) [3], a few studies have established that the long-term cardiac prognosis in these patients is far from benign. Urbinati et al. [4] followed 106 asymptomatic patients who underwent cardiac stress tests prior to carotid endarterectomy and found that 8 of 27 patients (29.6%) with abnormal thallium myocardial perfusion imaging studies had MI or unstable angina during an average of 5.4 years of follow-up, compared with only 1 of 79 patients (1.3%) with normal myocardial studies ($P < .01$).

In another study of 93 patients without overt CAD who underwent carotid endarterectomy, the cumulative incidence of important cardiac events (cardiac death, MI, CABG pulmonary edema, or ventricular tachycardia) at 8 years after endarterectomy was 25% (i.e., approximately 3% per year) [16]. In a large study of 444 male veterans with carotid stenosis, 67 (33%) of 200 patients with a history of CAD and 60 (25%) of 244 patients without a history of CAD had MI or sudden death during a mean follow-up of 47.9 months. This translates into an MI or sudden death rate of approximately 8% per year in patients with a history of CAD and 6% per year in patients without a history of CAD [3]. The higher rate of MI or sudden death in this study [3] may be due to the presence of more severe CAD in veterans who have a higher frequency of vascular risk factors than nonveterans.

These two studies suggest that the rate of MI or sudden death in patients with carotid stenosis and no history of CAD is 3% to 6% per year. However, patients with carotid stenosis and no symptoms of CAD consist of three subgroups: patients without CAD; patients with asymptomatic flow-limiting CAD (approximately 25% to 50% of the entire group); and patients with coronary plaques that are not flow-limiting. Since virtually all of the cardiac events in these two studies would have occurred in the latter two subgroups of patients, the rate of major cardiac events in patients with carotid stenosis and asymptomatic CAD may be as high as 4% to 8% per year [3,16].

TREATMENT OF ASYMPTOMATIC CAD

Although patients with carotid stenosis have a high frequency of asymptomatic CAD and are at high risk of major cardiac events during long-term follow-up, studies have not been performed to evaluate optimal treatment for asymptomatic CAD in these patients. However, there are limited data on the treatment of asymptomatic CAD in noncerebrovascular patients. In a nonrandomized study, Weiner et al. [17] followed 692 patients with asymptomatic ≥70% stenosis of at least one coronary artery who were treated medically (424 patients) or surgically (268 patients). Over a 7-year follow-up period, there were no significant differences in survival rates between the two groups among patients with one-vessel or two-vessel CAD. However, in patients with three-vessel CAD, 58% of medically treated patients survived 7 years, compared with 85% of surgically treated patients ($P < .0001$). Most of the patients who benefited from surgery had impaired left ventricular function. In another nonrandomized study (the CASS registry), 53 patients with asymptomatic ≥ 50% stenosis of the left main CAD were treated medically or surgically. Over a 5-year follow-up, survival rates were 57% in the medical group and 88% in the surgical group ($P = .02$) [18].

A few randomized studies have evaluated different therapies for silent myocardial ischemia in patients with known CAD. These studies focused on patients who were asymptomatic or minimally symptomatic and who had frequent episodes of myocardial ischemia detected by ambulatory ECG. It is well established that patients with silent myocardial ischemia are at high risk of major cardiac events [19,20] but until recently it was unclear how to treat these patients. The Atenolol Silent Ischemia Study (ASIST) randomized asymptomatic or minimally symptomatic patients with known CAD and evidence of silent ischemia to atenolol (100 mg/day) or placebo [21]. The primary outcome was event-free survival at 1 year. Primary events consisted of death, resuscitated ventricular tachycardia/fibrillation, MI, hospitalization for unstable angina, aggravation of angina, or revascularization. Event-free survival improved in patients randomized to atenolol ($P < .007$). These patients had fewer total first events than patients randomized to placebo (relative risk, 0.44; 95% confidence interval, 0.26 to 0.75; $P = .001$). There was a trend for fewer serious events (death, resuscitated ventricular tachycardia/fibrillation, MI, hospitalization for unstable angina) in patients treated with atenolol (relative risk, 0.55; 95% confidence interval, 0.22 to 1.33; $P = .175$). The most powerful correlate of event-free survival was absence of ischemia on ambulatory ECG monitoring at 4 weeks [21]. The results of ASIST have subsequently been supported by another recent trial, which showed that a beta blocker (Bisoprolol) or a calcium channel blocker (Nifedipine) reduced major cardiac events in patients with silent myocardial ischemia [22].

A recent randomized pilot study also suggests that revascularization is more effective than medical therapy for preventing major cardiac events in patients with silent myocardial ischemia detected by ambulatory ECG [23]. In the Asymptomatic Cardiac Ischemia Pilot (ACIP) study, 558 patients with ≥50% stenosis of at least one major coronary artery, at least one episode of asymptomatic ischemia on ambulatory ECG, and a positive exercise stress test were randomized to one of three treatments: (1) medication to suppress angina (angina-guided group); (2) medication to suppress angina and silent ischemia (ischemia-guided group); (3) revascularization (angioplasty or CABG). The medication consisted of a titrated regimen of atenolol followed by sustained-release nifedipine if needed, or a titrated regimen of diltiazem followed by sustained release isosorbide dinitrate if needed. At 1 year, the mortality rate was 4.4% in the angina-guided group, 1.6% in the ischemia-guided group, and 0% in the revascularization group (overall, $P = .004$; angina-guided vs. revascularization, $P = .003$; other pairwise comparisons not significant). The frequency of death, MI, nonprotocol revascularization, or hospital admissions at 1 year was 32% in the angina-guided group, 31% in the ischemia-guided group, and 18% in the revascularization group ($P = .003$). The revascularization group also had less ischemia on serial ambulatory ECG recordings than the medically treated groups [23]. Bypass surgery was superior to angioplasty in suppressing cardiac ischemia despite the fact that patients who underwent CABG had more severe CAD [24].

Longer follow-up data on the ACIP patients has recently been published [25]. The 2-year mortality rate was 6.6% in the angina-guided group, 4.4% in the ischemia-guided group, and 1.1% in the revascularization group ($P < .02$). The rate of death, MI, or recurrent hospitalization at 2 years was 41.8% in the angina-guided group, 38.5% in the ischemia-guided group, and 23.1% in the revascularization group ($P < .001$) [25]. These data clearly show that revascularization (especially CABG) is more effective than medical therapy for preventing major cardiac events in patients with known CAD and silent myocardial ischemia.

SUGGESTED MANAGEMENT OF ASYMPTOMATIC CAD IN PATIENTS WITH CAROTID STENOSIS

In view of the low rate of cardiac complications in the periendarterectomy period in patients without a history of CAD (1% to 2%) [3] the low positive predictive value of provocative tests for myocardial ischemia for predicting perioperative MI [26,27], and the current emphasis on cost containment in medical care, recent guidelines from an American College of Cardiology/American Heart Association (ACC/AHA) task force do not recommend routine cardiac stress testing in patients without a history of CAD who are undergoing carotid endarterectomy [26]. The results of a recent study that used decision analysis to evaluate the role of coronary angiography and coronary revascularization before peripheral vascular surgery or abdominal aortic surgery supports the ACC/AHA recommendations. Since patients undergoing these procedures have a higher rate of MI or cardiac death than patients undergoing carotid endarterectomy [26], the benefit, if any, of coronary angiography and coronary revascularization before vascular surgery should be evident in these patients. In this study, patients who had no angina or mild angina and an abnormal dipyridamole-thallium myocardial study were candidates for three management strategies: (1) to undergo vascular surgery without cardiac intervention; (2) to perform coronary angiography, followed by selective coronary revascularization before vascular surgery or to cancel vascular surgery in patients with inoperable CAD; or (3) to perform coronary angiography, followed by selective coronary revascularization before vascular surgery or proceed directly to vascular surgery in patients with inoperable CAD. The main outcome measures included mortality, nonfatal MI, stroke, and cost within 3 months of surgery. Decision analysis showed that proceeding directly to vascular surgery in patients with an estimated perioperative mortality of $\leq$5% led to better outcomes [28].

The ACC/AHA recommendations [26], which focus on the preoperative management of CAD in patients undergoing vascular surgery, do not address the long-term management of asymptomatic CAD in patients with carotid stenosis. Given the high annual rate of major cardiac events in these patients and mounting evidence that treatment of silent myocardial ischemia improves cardiac outcome, a strong case can be made for performing noninvasive screening for asymptomatic CAD in patients with carotid stenosis after recovery from carotid endarterectomy.

However, noninvasive screening for asymptomatic CAD in all patients with carotid stenosis is unlikely to be cost effective [29]. Efforts have been made to identify subgroups of asymptomatic patients with carotid stenosis who are at highest risk of cardiac events. In one study, factors that were independently associated with cardiac events in patients with carotid stenosis and no history of CAD were coexistent diabetes (relative risk, 2.14; 95% confidence interval, 1.15 to 3.97), intracranial occlusive disease (relative risk, 2.13; 95% confidence interval, 1.13 to 4.02), and peripheral vascular disease (relative risk, 2.04; 95% confidence interval, 1.14 to 3.66). Forty-two percent of patients with two of these factors and 69% of patients with all three factors had cardiac events during a mean follow-up of 4 years [3].

Given these data, what should the cardiac evaluation and treatment of patients with carotid stenosis and no history of CAD entail? A definitive answer is not possible until a randomized study has clearly established the value of screening for CAD and treating asymptomatic CAD in this population. Until such a study is performed, the following approach is suggested based on currently available data: patients with carotid stenosis and no history of CAD who are at high risk of major cardiac events (i.e., diabetics, patients with coexistent intracranial occlusive disease or peripheral vascular disease) [3] should undergo a provocative test for myocardial ischemia. Other patients that should be considered for screening include patients with premature carotid stenosis (i.e., patients younger than 50 years) and patients with a family history of CAD, especially if the CAD occurred at a young age. The most commonly used provocative tests for myocardial ischemia are exercise ECG, myocardial perfusion imaging study, or dobutamine stress echocardiography. A recent meta-analysis has shown that these procedures have similar accuracy rates for detecting underlying CAD [27]. Exercise ECG has the advantage of providing an estimate of the functional capacity of the patient, but is unreliable in patients with an abnormal resting ECG, e.g., left bundle branch block, left ventricular hypertrophy. Dobutamine stress echocardiography is the preferred approach when evaluation of the cardiac chambers and heart valves is necessary.

Patients with abnormal screening studies should be referred to a cardiologist. These patients should be considered for ambulatory ECG monitoring to detect episodes of silent myocardial ischemia. When the noninvasive cardiac studies suggest severe underlying CAD (e.g., patients with a large reversible perfusion defect on a myocardial perfusion imaging study), the patient should undergo coronary angiography, which can be combined safely with carotid angiography [30]. Based on currently available data, patients with severe multivessel or left main disease should be considered for CABG [17,18], especially if they have episodes of silent myocardial ischemic [23–25]. The timing of CABG in patients undergoing carotid endarterectomy is discussed on page 246 of Chapter 4. Patients with less extensive disease (e.g., isolated proximal disease of the left anterior descending artery) should be treated with angioplasty [23–25]. For asymptomatic CAD that is not amenable to revascularization, medical therapy (beta blockers or calcium channel blockers, and antithrombotic therapy) should be instituted, especially in patients with silent myocardial ischemia [21–23,25]. Additionally, management of vascular risk factors (especially hyperlipidemia [31,32], hypertension, diabetes, and smoking) is a critical component of the treatment plan for all patients.

REFERENCES

1. McGill HC Jr, Strong JP. The geographic pathology of atherosclerosis. Ann NY Acad Sci 1968; 149:923–927.
2. North American Symptomatic Carotid Endarterectomy Trial Collaborators. Beneficial effect of carotid endarterectomy in symptomatic patients with high grade carotid stenosis. N Engl J Med 1991; 325:445–453.
3. Chimowitz MI, Weiss DG, Cohen SL, Starling MR, Hobson RW II, Veterans Affairs Cooperative Study Group 167. Cardiac prognosis of patients with carotid stenosis and no history of coronary artery disease. Stroke 1994; 25:759–765.
4. Urbinati S, Di Pasquale G, Andreoli A, Lusa AM, Ruffini M, Lanzino G, Pinelli G. Frequency and prognostic significance of silent coronary artery disease in patients with cerebral ischemia undergoing carotid endarterectomy. Am J Cardiol 1992; 69: 1166–1170.
5. Sconocchini C, Racco F, Pratillo G, Alesi C, Zappelli L. Patients with carotid stenosis and clinical history negative for coronary disease. Usefulness of the ergometric test for the identification of ischemic myocardial disease. Minerva Med 1997; 88: 173–181.
6. Hertzer NR, Young JR, Beven EG, Graor RA, O'Hara PJ, Ruschhaupt WF, de Wolfe G, Maljovec LC. Coronary angiography in 506 patients with extracranial cerebrovascular disease. Arch Intern Med 1985; 145:849–852.
7. Chimowitz MI, Poole RM, Starling MR, Schwaiger M, Gross MD. Frequency and severity of asymptomatic coronary disease in patients with different causes of stroke. Stroke 1997; 28:941–945.
8. Executive Committee for the Asymptomatic Carotid Atherosclerosis Study. Endarterectomy for asymptomatic carotid artery stenosis. JAMA 1995; 273:1421–1428.
9. Barnett HJM, Taylor DW, Eliasziw M, Fox AJ, Ferguson GG, Haynes RB, Rankin RN, Clagett GP, Hachinski VC, Sackett DL, Thorpe KE, Meldrum HE, for the North American Symptomatic Carotid Endarterectomy Trial Collaborators. Benefit of carotid endarterectomy in patients with symptomatic moderate or severe stenosis. N Engl J Med 1998; 339:1415–1425.
10. Graor RA, Hertzer NR. Management of coexistent carotid artery and coronary artery disease. Stroke 1988; 19:1441–1444.
11. Rokey R, Rolak LA, Harati Y, Kutka N, Verani MS. Coronary artery disease in patients with cerebrovascular disease: a prospective study. Ann Neurol 1984; 16: 50–53.
12. Di Pasquale G, Andreoli A, Pinelli G, Grazi P, Manini G, Tognetti F, Testa C. Cerebral ischemia and asymptomatic coronary artery disease: a prospective study of 83 patients. Stroke 1986; 17:1098–1101.

13. Di Pasquale G, Andreoli A, Grazi P, Urbinati S, Corbelli G, Carini G, Pinelli G. Detection of silent myocardial ischemia in cerebrovascular patients by dipyridamole thallium myocardial imaging. Stroke 1989; 20:155. Abstract.
14. Love BB, Grover-McKay M, Biller J, Rezai K, McKay CR. Coronary artery disease and cardiac events with asymptomatic and symptomatic cerebrovascular disease. Stroke 1992; 23:939–945.
15. Okin PM, Roman MJ, Pickering TG, Devereux RB. Relation of exercise-induced myocardial ischemia to cardiac and carotid structure. Hypertension 1997; 30:1382–1388.
16. Rihal CS, Gersh BJ, Whisnant JP, Rooke TW, Sundt TM Jr, Fallon WM, Ballard DJ. Influence of coronary heart disease on morbidity and mortality after carotid endarterectomy: a population-based study in Olmsted County, Minnesota (1970–1988). J Am Coll Cardiol 1992; 19:1254–1260.
17. Weiner DA, Ryan TJ, McCabe CH, Chaitman BR, Sheffield LT, Ng G, Fisher LD, Tristini FE, CASS Investigators. Comparison of coronary artery bypass surgery and medical therapy in patients with exercise-induced silent myocardial ischemia: a report from the Coronary Artery Surgery Study (CASS) registry. J Am Coll Cardiol 1988; 12:595–599.
18. Taylor HA, Deumite NJ, Chaitman BR, Davis KB, Killip T, Roger WJ. Asymptomatic left main coronary artery disease in the Coronary Artery Surgery Study (CASS) registry. Circulation 1989; 79:1171–1179.
19. Gill JB, Cairns JA, Roberts RS, Costantini L, Sealey BJ, Fallen EF, Tomlinson CW, Gent M. Prognostic importance of myocardial ischemia detected by ambulatory monitoring early after acute MI. N Engl J Med 1996; 334:65–70.
20. Gottlieb SO, Weisfeldt ML, Ouyang P, Mellitts ED, Gerstenblith G. Silent ischemia predicts infarction and death during 2 year follow-up of unstable angina. J Am Coll Cardiol 1987; 10:756–760.
21. Pepine CJ, Cohn PF, Deedwania PC, Gibson RS, Handberg E, Hill JA, Miller E, Marks RG, Thadani U, for the ASIST Study Group. Effects of treatment on outcome in mildly symptomatic patients with ischemia during daily life. The Atenolol Silent Ischemia Study (ASIST). Circulation 1994; 90:762–768.
22. von Arnim T, for the TIBBS (Total Ischemic Burden Bisoprolol Study) investigators. Prognostic significance of transient ischemic episodes; response to treatment shows improved prognosis. Results of the TIBBS follow-up. J Am Coll Cardiol 1995; 25(suppl):88A. Abstract.
23. Rogers WJ, Bourassa MG, Andrews TC, Bertolet BD, Blumenthal RS, Chaitman BR, Forman SA, Geller NL, Goldberg AD, Habib, et al. for the ACIP investigators. Asymptomatic Cardiac Ischemia Pilot (ACIP) study: outcome at 1 year for patients with asymptomatic cardiac ischemia randomized to medical therapy or revascularization. J Am Coll Cardiol 1995; 26:594–605.
24. Bourassa MG, Pepine CJ, Forman SA, Rogers WJ, Dyrda I, Stone PH, Chaitman BR, Sharaf B, Mahmarian J, Davies RF, et al. for the ACIP investigators. Asymptomatic Cardiac Ischemia Pilot (ACIP) study: effects of coronary angioplasty and coronary bypass graft surgery on recurrent angina and ischemia. J Am Coll Cardiol 1995; 26: 606–614.
25. Davies RF, Goldberg AD, Forman S, Pepine CJ, Knatterud GL, Geller N, Sopko G, Pratt C, Deanfield J, Conti CR. Asymptomatic cardiac ischemia pilot (ACIP)

study two-year follow-up: outcomes of patients randomized to initial strategies of medical therapy versus revascularization. Circulation 1997; 95:2037–2043.
26. Eagle KA, Brundage BH, Chaitman BR, Ewy GA, Fleisher LA, Hertzer NR, Leppo JA, Ryan T, Schlant RC, Spencer WH III, Spittell JA Jr, Twiss RD, Ritchie JL, Cheitlin MD, Gardner TJ, Garson A Jr, Lewis RP, Givvons RJ, O'Rourke RA, Ryan TJ. Guidelines for perioperative cardiovascular evaluation for noncardiac surgery. Report of the American College of Cardiology/American Heart Association Task Force on Practice Guidelines. Committee on Perioperative Cardiovascular Evaluation for Noncardiac Surgery. Circulation 1996; 93:1278–1317.
27. Mantha S, Roizen MF, Barnard J, Thisted RA, Ellis JE, Foss J. Relative effectiveness of four preoperative tests for predicting adverse cardiac outcomes after vascular surgery: a meta-analysis. Anesth Analg 94; 79:422–433.
28. Mason JJ, Owens DK, Harris RA, Cooke JP, Hlatky MA. The role of coronary angiography and coronary revascularization before noncardiac vascular surgery. JAMA 1995; 273:1919–1925.
29. Goldman L. Cost-effectiveness perspectives in coronary heart disease. Am Heart J 1990; 119:733–740.
30. Chimowitz MI, Lafranchise EF, Furlan AJ, Dorosti K, Paranandi L, Beck GJ. Evaluation of coexistent carotid and coronary disease by combined angiography. J Stroke Cerebrovasc Dis 1991; 1:89–93.
31. Scandinavian Simvastatin Survival Study Group. Randomised trial of cholesterol lowering in 4444 patients with coronary artery disease: the Scandinavian Simvastatin Survival Study (4S). Lancet 1994; 344:1383–1389.
32. Sacks FM, Pfeffer MA, Moye LA, Rouleau JL, Rutherford JD, Cole TG, Brown L, Warnica JW, Arnold JMO, Wun C-C, Davis BR, Braunwald E, for the Cholesterol and Recurrent Events Trial Investigators. The effect of pravastatin on coronary events after myocardial infarction in patients with average cholesterol levels. N Engl J Med 1996; 335:1001–1009.

7

Cardiac and Cardiovascular Findings in Patients with Nervous System Diseases

ANATOMY AND PHYSIOLOGY

Cardiologists and internists will find it useful to think of the cardiac and cardiovascular effects of neurological conditions in terms of nervous system anatomy. (Figs. 1–3). The heart is innervated primarily by the parasympathetic and sympathetic nervous systems. The *parasympathetic innervation* comes from the vagus nerve, whose neurons are located in the medulla in the dorsal motor nucleus of the vagus. The cardiac termination of the vagus nerve is divided into superior, middle, and inferior cardiac rami. The predominant neurotransmitter is acetylcholine. Preganglionic fibers synapse in the cardiac ganglia in which nicotinic cholinergic receptor types predominate. Hexamethonium and other nicotinic receptor blocking agents can inhibit transmission between preganglionic and postganglionic parasympathetic nerve fibers. The short postganglionic fibers then innervate muscarinic cholinergic terminals in the sinoatrial and atrioventricular nodes, and also terminate on cardiac blood vessels, and on heart muscle fibers in all cardiac chambers [1]. Atropine suppresses transmission from postganglionic fibers to cardiac effector cells [2]. Vasoactive intestinal polypeptide is also released from parasympathetic nerve endings and has some effect on cardiac tissues [2]. Parasympathetic fibers innervate the sinoatrial and atrioventricular nodes more than the ventricles and coronary blood vessels [2]. Termination of parasympathetic nerve endings is asymmetrical; the left vagus nerve terminals predominantly in-

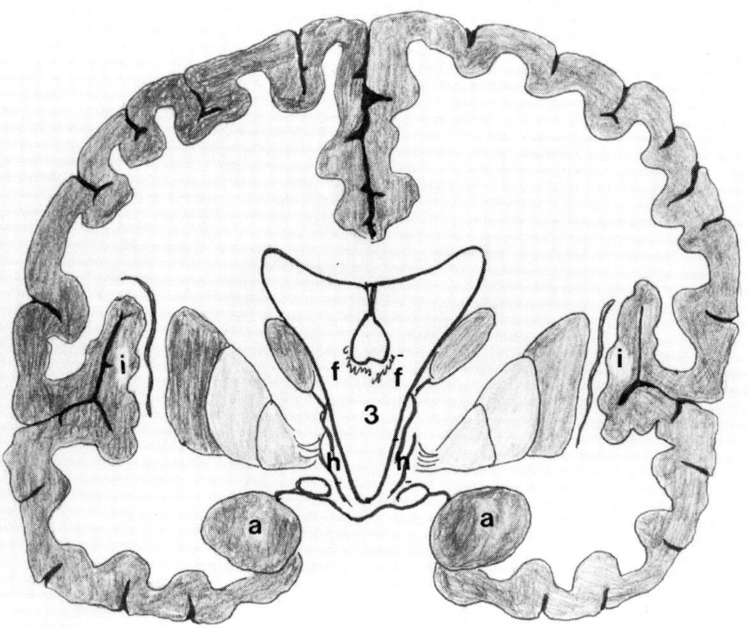

FIG. 1 Artists drawing of the cerebral hemispheres at the level of the foramina of Monro (f) and the third ventricle (3) showing the insular cortex (i), medial temporal lobe limbic system (a for amygdala), and hypothalamic areas (h) posited to be involved in autonomic functions. Drawn by Gloria Wu, M.D.

nervate the atrioventricular node while the right vagus innervates the sinoatrial node [2]. Tonic vagus nerve stimulation prolongs both the length of the cardiac cycle and the refractory period of atrioventricular node fibers [2]. Vagal activity also inhibits atrial contraction and so diminishes the atrial contribution to ventricular filling [2].

The *sympathetic nervous system* originates in the hypothalamus and the medulla. Descending fibers from these regions synapse in the intermediolateral cell columns of the thoracic spinal cord. Fibers from nerve cells in the anterolateral cell columns exit the cord by way of the anterior roots and connect with the sympathetic chain of ganglia which lie outside the spinal cord up and down its length on each side of the vertebral bodies. The bundles that contain preganglionic fibers going from the spinal cord to the sympathetic ganglia are usually called white rami communicates; the white color is related to myelinated visceral afferent fibers, which also travel in these bundles. The upper, middle, and inferior cervical ganglia are the major sympathetic ganglia that innervate the heart and

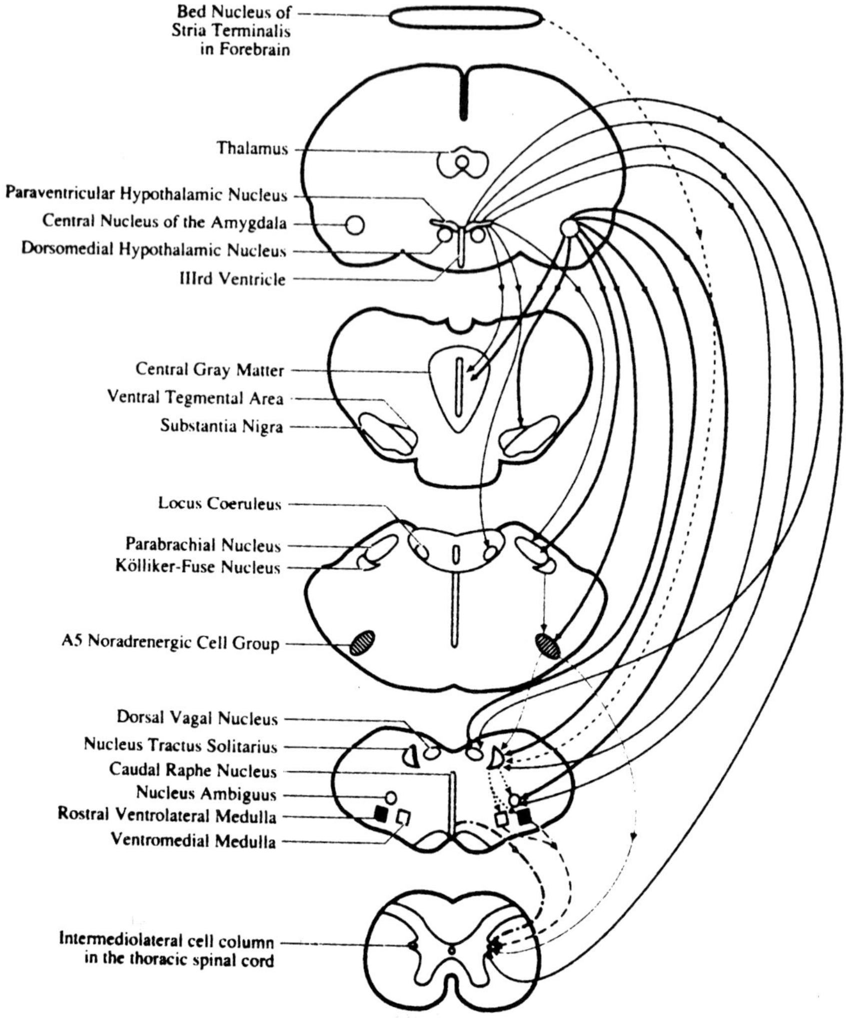

FIG. 2 Descending projections of the central autonomic network (CAN). (From Chokroverty S. Functional anatomy of the autonomic nervous system: autonomic dysfunction and disorders of the central nervous system. Presented in Neurology course No. 144—Correlative Neuroanatomy and Neuropathology for the Clinical Neurologist. Minneapolis: American Academy of Neurology, 1991:77–103. Reproduced with permission.)

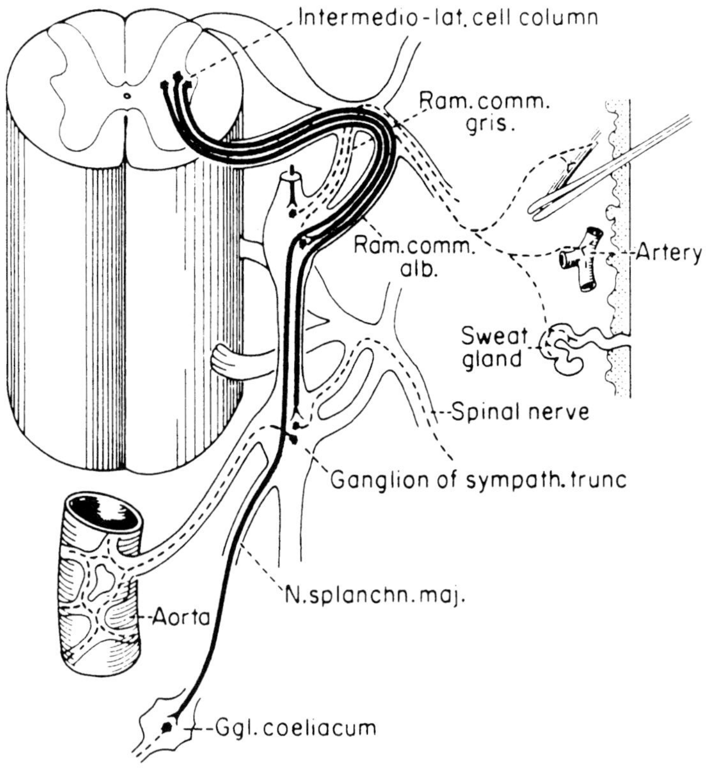

FIG. 3 Cartoon showing the arrangement of the efferent fibers in the sympathetic nervous system. Preganglionic sympathetic fibers (solid lines) from neurons in the intermediolateral cell column leave the spinal cord through the ventral roots and enter the sympathetic trunk via white rami communicant rami to end in one or more sympathetic ganglia. Some preganglionic fibers continue in the splanchnic nerves. Most postganglionic fibers (broken lines) from neurons in the ganglia reenter the spinal nerves via gray communicant rami and follow the nerve peripherally to the skin, supply glands, or to small or major blood vessels. (From Brodal A. Neurological anatomy in relation to clinical medicine, 3rd ed. New York: Oxford University Press, 1981:707. Reproduced with permission.)

each contains fibers from each thoracic segment. The lower cervical and first thoracic ganglia are usually fused to form the *stellate ganglion* on each side. Sympathetic nerve fibers travel from the ganglia to peripheral nerves by unmyelinated gray rami communicantes bundles, and then the sympathetic fibers travel with the peripheral nerves to the end organs [1,3]. Figure 3 shows a thoracic spinal cord segment that contains the sympathetic neurons and their connections with peripheral nerves.

The left and right stellate ganglia have different innervation patterns. The left stellate ganglion fibers terminate in the sinoatrial and atrioventricular nodes and on most of the left ventricle. The right stellate ganglion contains cells whose fibers terminate in the septum, right ventricle, and atria. The postganglionic sympathetic fibers terminate on adrenergic receptors of the alpha or beta types. Stimulation of alpha receptors primarily causes vasoconstriction while stimulation of beta fibers causes more vasodilatation, although there are subtypes of each receptor. Electrical stimulation of the T1 to T5 thoracic anterior roots containing sympathetic nervous system fibers elicits changes in blood pressure, localized changes in cardiac muscle contractile force, and changes in heart rate and electrical impulse conduction [4].

Afferent pathways carry information from the heart and blood vessels mostly derived from chemoreceptors and baroreceptors in the heart, aorta, and carotid arteries that deliver to the nervous system information about cardiac function and blood pressure. This information is carried to the spinal cord via sympathetic afferents that travel in white rami communicantes and to the brainstem through the hypoglossal (cranial nerve IX) and vagus nerves (cranial nerve X). The nucleus of the solitary tract is the major site of fiber termination from cardiopulmonary and arterial baroreceptors and the carotid sinus [5].

A number of brain regions affect the function of these sympathetic and parasympathetic systems. This effect is mediated either by descending fiber tracts that synapse with brainstem and spinal cord neurons of the autonomic nervous system or by the release of chemical neurotransmitters such as epinephrine and norepinephrine, which have profound effects on the heart and blood vessels. Within the cerebral cortex, the insula is the region which probably most relates to cardiac and cardiovascular function. Changes in heart rate and blood pressure occur when various parts of the insula are stimulated [6–9]. Stimulation of limbic system neurons in the frontal and temporal lobes leads to emotional changes and secretion of various neurotransmitter substances which affect cardiovascular functions. The dorsomedial nucleus of the thalamus is an important autonomic nervous system relay station that also influences heart and autonomic functions [9] (Fig. 1 shows the cerebral regions thought to be involved in autonomic functions).

Within the brainstem there is a group of interrelated structures often called the ''central autonomic network'' (CAN) which form an ''internal regulation system through which the brain controls visceromotor, neuroendocrine, pain, and behavioral responses essential for survival'' [10]. Control of autonomic functions such as heart rate, blood pressure, and respirations is closely integrated within the CAN. The principal locations of the CAN are: the medulla (including the ventrolateral medulla, the medullary reticular zone, and the nucleus of the solitary tract (NTS); the parabrachial region in the pons; the periaqueductal grey region of the midbrain; and the preoptic region in the hypothalamus [10,11]. Figure 2 is a cartoon which shows the CAN. These regions within the CAN project to a variety of cerebral regions including the amygdala, insular cortex, and the limbic portions of the striatum. They also project to the spinal cord autonomic neurons and have an important influence on the locus coeruleus and the noradrenergic system [10]. In addition to neural input, circulating neurotransmitter substances such as angiotensin II, atrial naturetic peptide, vasopressin, and endothelin access neural receptors in the midbrain and medulla. Release of chemical transmitters such as epinephrine and norepinephrine from brain structures also can have important effects on the circulation as all of us have experienced after severe stress or fright.

Considering this anatomy and physiology, autonomic dysfunction would be expected in diseases that involve a variety of different areas of the nervous system, including (1) The cerebral cortex, especially the insula and limbic system; (2) the hypothalamus; (3) the brainstem, especially the pons and medulla; (4) the spinal cord; (5) the autonomic ganglia and nerves; and (6) the peripheral nerves.

BRAIN DISEASES

Strokes

Patients with strokes of various types have ECG abnormalities, arrythmias, abnormalities of cardiac enzymes, and pathological abnormalities in the heart at necropsy. Sometimes the strokes in these patients are caused by embolism from the heart. Sometimes the cardiac abnormalities are explained by coexistent coronary artery and other cardiac conditions. However, in many of these patients the cardiac abnormalities are caused by the stroke.

The types of strokes that have been most often associated with secondary cardiac manifestations are subarachnoid hemorrhage, large intracerebral hemorrhages, rapidly developing subdural hematomas, and large cerebral infarcts. Brainstem infarcts and hemorrhages, especially those that involve the medullary and caudal pontine tegmentum, can cause blood pressure, respiratory, and heart rate abnormalities.

The neurological signs depend on the location and size of the stroke. Many patients have some reduction in consciousness.

Cardiovascular Clinical Manifestations

In 1947, Byer, Ashman, and Toth described marked Q-T prolongation with large T and U waves in the electrocardiogram (ECG) of a patient with intracerebral hemorrhage [12]. Levine, in 1953, described a patient with subarachnoid hemorrhage whose ECG seemed to show a myocardial infarct, but the heart was said to be normal at necropsy [13]. Burch and his colleagues, in 1954, first analyzed in detail the *electrocardiographic abnormalities* in patients with strokes, most

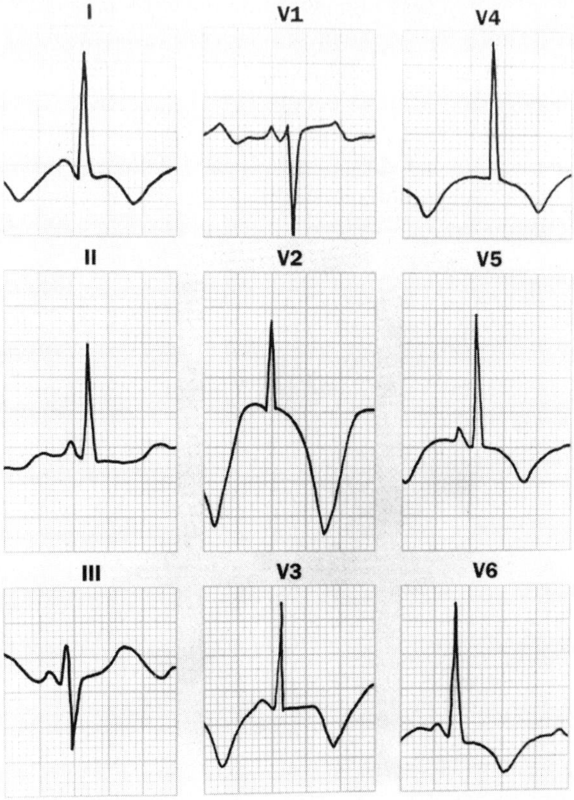

FIG. 4 Abnormal T-waves sometimes associated with strokes (subarachnoid hemorrhage, cerebral hemorrhage, or cerebral thrombosis). (From Burch GE, Meyers R, Abildskov JA. A new electrocardiographic pattern observed in cerebrovascular accidents. Circulation 1954; 9:719. Reproduced with permission.)

often subarachnoid hemorrhages [14]. The ECG abnormalities included deeply inverted T waves, long Q-T intervals, and abnormal U waves. An example of an ECG from their paper is included as Figure 4 [14]. These ECG abnormalities were often referred to as waterfall, or ''cerebral T waves.'' In 1960, Cropp and Manning reported 30 patients with subarachnoid hemorrhage and ECG abnormalities [15]. Prolongation of the Q-T interval was found in 67%; 55% had flat or inverted T waves, and abnormal U waves were also common [15]. The heart, in four patients, was said to be normal at necropsy. Since these early reports, ECG changes have been noted often in patients with subarachnoid hemorrhages and intracerebral hemorrhages, and less often in patients with brain ischemia [16–25].

ECG changes are quite common in stroke patients, but often difficult to interpret because of the concurrence of coronary and other cardiac disease and the frequent absence of prior tracings. In one study, 90 of 100 consecutive acute stroke patients had abnormal ECGs [17]. Compared to controls, the stroke patients had a 7- to 10-fold higher frequency of ST segment depression, prolonged Q-T interval, and atrial fibrillation, and 3.5 times the frequency of T wave inversion [17]. In another study, 138 of 150 (92%) patients with acute stroke had ECG abnormalities [18]. The most common abnormalities also represented changes from prior tracings which were available and included Q-T prolongation (45%), ischemic changes (35%), and abnormal U waves (28%) [18].

Rolak and Rokey summarized the ECG changes found in stroke patients in detail [22]. The characteristic triad includes: (1) a prolonged Q-T interval; (2) T waves that are increased in width and amplitude, either inverted or upright; and (3) abnormal U waves [22]. Prolonged Q-T interval is the most common finding, occurring in up to 66% of acute stroke patients in some series. Since Q-T interval prolongation is otherwise very uncommon (seen in only 46 of every 10,000 [0.46%] hospitalized patients), the presence of this finding should raise high suspicion of stroke or other acute brain lesion [22,23] After Q-T interval widening, T wave inversion is the next most common finding in stroke patients. The T waves after a stroke are usually increased in width and amplitude and are most often inverted although they occasionally remain upright. Large, upright or inverted T waves usually are present soon after stroke onset but can be delayed for as long as a week after subarachnoid hemorrhage [24]. Occasionally, within hours of hospitalization the T wave abnormalities disappear or shift from upright to inverted or from inverted to upright [25]. The abnormal U waves seen after stroke are similar to those found in patients with hypokalemia, and are often hidden in and contribute to the width of the T waves [22]. ST-T changes can also be found after stroke and are often indistinguishable from those found in myocardial infarct patients. If the coronary arteries were normal prior to the stroke, the epicardial ischemia noted in the electrocardiogram is more likely to be limited to the T wave abnormality produced by generalized epicardial ischemia. At times an S-T segment displacement due to generalized epicardial injury may occur when there is prolonged damage to the epicardium. This creates an S-T segment vector directed toward the cardiac apex. The endocardium may not be infarcted, so abnormal initial QRS forces (Q waves) are not produced in such patients.

A variety of *cardiac arrhythmias* have also been noted to develop after strokes [16,18,22,26–30]. In one series arrhythmias were found in 18.5% of stroke patients, compared to 7% of controls [16]. In another study, 41/150 (27%) of consecutive stroke patients had an arrhythmia including 13/53 (25%) in whom comparison with prior available ECG tracings showed that the arrhythmia was new [18]. Atrial fibrillation (21/150; 14%) was the most common arrhythmia in this series; ventricular arrythmias occurred in 5% of patients [18]. Norris and colleagues studied the frequency of cardiac arrhythmias among 312 stroke patients admitted and monitored in an intensive care unit compared to 92 patients admitted to the same unit who were later found not to have strokes [26]. The most common arrythmias in the stroke patients were atrial and ventricular ectopic beats and atrial fibrillation [26].

A particular pattern of changes was observed in patients with brain hemorrhages who had severe increased intracranial pressure related to cerebral herniation. These terminal patients developed progressive bradycardia to a point of nodal escape followed by idioventricular rhythm and finally cardiac arrest [26]. Among 1661 patients with first strokes in the Lausanne Stroke Registry, 24 patients had recent onset atrial fibrillation [27]. A common pattern among these patients was development of atrial fibrillation a few hours to 3 days after stroke and then spontaneous reversion to normal sinus rhythm, a sequence believed to favor a cerebrogenic etiology of the atrial fibrillation by the authors of this study [27].

Two studies of cardiac rhythms in patients with subarachnoid hemorrhage showed a rather high incidence of abnormalities [28,29]. In one study, multifocal ventricular premature beats were found in 54% of 52 patients with subarachnoid hemorrhage [28]. Couplets were present in 40%, and low-frequency unifocal ventricular premature beats in 33% [28]. Unsustained ventricular tachycardia occurred in 28%, sinus bradycardia in 23%, asystolic intervals in 27%, and atrial fibrillation in 4% [28]. Di Pasquale et al. noted that arrhythmias were most often present during the first 48 hours after subarachnoid bleeding [29]. Serious ventricular arrythmias such as bigeminy and multifocal ventricular premature beats were accompanied by a prolonged Q-T interval [29]. Torsade de pointes was found in 4% of patients with subarachnoid hemorrhage and seemed unrelated to the clinical neurological status of the patients [30]. A review of electrocardiographic changes in stroke patients shows that sinus arrhythmia, sinus bradycardia, and sinus tachycardia are the most common rhythm abnormalities found after stroke [22]. Premature ventricular beats are the next most common abnormality, occurring in over 50% of stroke patients. Unifocal and multifocal premature ventricular beats and ventricular tachycardia are reported [22]. Atrial fibrillation, premature atrial beats, supraventricular tachycardia, and paroxysmal atrial tachycardia have also been noted [22].

Elevation of cardiac-origin enzymes may occur in stroke patients, especially those with brain and subarachnoid hemorrhage. Plasma total and MB chain creatine kinase (MB CK) are elevated in a high proportion of patients with subarachnoid hemorrhage, and the magnitude of CK elevation correlates with the prognosis [24,31–34]. Norris and colleagues noted a plasma elevation of MB

CK in 25/230 (11%) of ischemic stroke patients that they studied [34]. In stroke patients peak elevations of cardiac isoenzymes often occur on days 3 and 4 after stroke, a pattern different from most patients with myocardial infarction [31].

After acute myocardial infarction, CK elevations above the normal range are found during the first 8 to 16 hours; there is then a rapid rise in serum enzyme levels with a peak value usually found between 18 and 26 hours and a return to baseline levels by 48 to 72 hours [31]. The brain contains a rich amount of BB CK, so patients with acute brain lesions often have an elevation in serum total CK even when there is no myocardial injury. It is very important to measure cardiac (MB CK) and brain (BB CK) isoenzyme levels, and to monitor these levels during the first week after stroke, in order to attempt to identify patients that have had a myocardial infarct.

Acute pulmonary edema, which is often sudden in onset and sometimes fatal, has been described in patients who have subarachnoid hemorrhage and vertebrobasilar territory ischemia and hemorrhages [35,36]. Pulmonary edema is most likely to develop when there is a sudden onset and severe increase in intracranial pressure. Weir studied the occurrence of pulmonary edema in patients with fatal subarachnoid hemorrhage [37]. Among the 70% of his fatal cases of patients with ruptured aneurysms who developed pulmonary edema, all had the sudden onset of coma. Respiratory symptoms were noted within a short time period after the onset of headache and neurologic symptoms [37]. Weir attributed the occurrence of pulmonary edema to a sudden severe increase in intracranial pressure, which in turn caused massive autonomic stimulation. Experimental data from studies in cats confirm this hypothesis [38].

Centrally mediated sympathetic nervous system discharges can cause intense systemic vasoconstriction [35]. Sympathetic discharges can be triggered by sudden increases in intracranial pressure which cause secondary effects in the hypothalamus and brainstem, and by direct involvement of descending sympathetic fibers traveling in the lateral brainstem tegmentum. Intense vasoconstriction leads to very high resistance in the systemic circulation, which in turn provokes sudden shifts of blood volume into the lower-resistance pulmonary circulation. The sudden increase in volume in the pulmonary vascular bed leads to increased pulmonary capllary pressure, pulmonary hypertension, development of pulmonary edema, rupture of pulmonary capillaries, and lung hemorrhage [36]. The pulmonary edema fluid has a high protein content and can develop despite normal cardiac function and hemodynamics [38].

Cardiac Pathology

The electrocardiographic changes, arrhythmias, and elevation of cardiac enzymes after stroke are explained by morphological changes found in the hearts of stroke patients at necropsy. Although prior authors had not noted changes in the heart, Koskello and colleagues, in 1964, reported three subarachnoid hemorrhage patients who had subendocardial hemorrhages at necropsy [39]. These authors found small petechial, sometimes confluent hemorrhages in the muscle tissue of the left ventricle [39]. Since then, many investigators have described pathologic changes in the heart in stroke patients [1,6,16,17,22,35,36,41–44]. The abnormalities of cardiac muscle cells have usually been referred to as *myocytolysis*. Striations within myocardial muscle cells are lost; the cytoplasm often becomes hyalinized, and measurements show that some enzymes are lost from the muscle cells [22]. The number of muscle cells decrease but the sarcolemma, stroma, and nuclei usually remain. Mononuclear cells are seen infiltrating the myocardium, and connective tissue fibers are increased, producing fibroblastic collagenization and microscopic scars. Lipofuchsin is found within myofibrils. Frequently there is a coagulative type of myocytolysis in which the cardiac muscle cells die in a hypercontracted state with early myofibrillary damage and anomalous irregular cross-band formation [1,45]. This type of pathological change has also been called myofibrillar degeneration and contraction band necrosis. Cells with contraction band necrosis tend to calcify early. These cell lesions, mononuclear infiltrates, and microscopic scars are scatterred throughout the myocardium and are not localized to any particular vascular distribution. Often the most severe myocardial lesions develop near the terminations of intracardiac autonomic nerves [1,22]. Petechial hemorrhages may be found predominantly in the left ventricle, septum, anterior wall, and papillary muscles [22].

Myofibrillar degeneration, the predominant lesion found in the heart in patients dying of subarachnoid hemorrhage and strokes, is similar to the cardiac lesion found in some patients who have sudden unexpected deaths [1]. This lesion is different from coagulation necrosis, the predominant cardiac muscle lesion being found in patients with myocardial infarction due to coronary artery occlusion. In coagulation necrosis, the myocardial muscle cells die in a relaxed state without prominent contraction bands, and the myocardial abnormalities take time to become visible under the microscope. When a cellular infiltrate is present it is usually polymorphonuclear, and calcification occurs quite late after the infarction. In contrast, in myofibrillar degeneration (the lesion found in stroke patients) the muscle cells die in a hypercontracted state with prominent contraction bands; the lesions are visible early, the infiltrate is mononuclear, petechiae are common, and the abnormal cells calcify very quickly [1].

In the brain it has recently become popular to speak of reperfusion injury. Increased release of excitatory neurotransmitters leads to excitotoxic damage to nerve cells [46]. The supply of nutrients does not keep up with the metabolic needs of the hyperactive nerve cells, and they die. Calcium entry into the cells may be the final killing blow. Samuels has likened the myocardial cell injury found in the hearts of patients dying of stroke, contraction band necrosis, to the excitotoxic damage found within the brain [1]. Increased cell activity and early calcification are features common to both excitotoxic nerve cell death and myofibrillar degeneration of myocardial myocytes.

Posited Mechanisms of Myocardial Injury in Stroke Patients

A number of different theories have been proposed to explain the clinical and morphological changes in the heart and heart function that occur after strokes. There are three general ways in which central nervous system lesions, especially strokes cause secondary cardiac, cardiovascular, and respiratory changes:

1. Direct involvement of critical structures such as the cortex of the insula of Reil, the hypothalamus, and brainstem nuclei that make up the central autonomic network (CAN) lead to activation of descending autonomic fiber pathways to the heart, blood vessels, and lungs.
2. Mass effect with compression of the hypothalamus and/or the brainstem also leads to activation of autonomic pathways.
3. The acute brain lesion and its stress effects cause activation of the hypothalamic-pituitary axis, triggering the release of catecholamines and corticosteroids.

Electrical stimulation of the anterior part of the brain, including the frontal pole, premotor and motor cortex, cingulate gyri, orbital frontal gyri, insular cortex, the anterior part of the temporal lobe, amygdala, and hippocampus, has been shown to produce either pressor or depressor effects or atrial and ventricular arrythmias [9,47,48]. Some of the effect may relate to a nonspecific activation of limbic cortex, which has secondary effects on the hypothalamus, autonomic nervous system, and hypothalamic-pituitary endocrine axis. Stimulation of the insula seems to have a more specific relation to cardiac and cardiovascular functions. After showing that stimulation of the posterior portions of the rat insular cortex had reproducible effects on heart rate and rhythm. Oppenheimer and colleagues stimulated the insular cortex of human epileptic patients [7–9]. They found that when they electrically stimulated areas of the left human insular cortex, they produced bradycardia and depressor responses, while stimulation of the right insular cortex elicited tachycardia and pressor effects [7]. Stimulation of the left insula decreases protective parasympathetic effects and increases cardiovascular sympathetic effects on the heart rate and blood pressure. This asymmetry of autonomic function was also shown by Yoon and colleagues, who studied autonomic function in patients given intracarotid amobarbital as part of an evaluation for epilepsy surgery [49]. They found that the right cerebral hemisphere predominantly modulated sympathetic nervous system activity [49]. Hachinski and colleagues showed that rats with experimentally induced right middle cerebral artery

help to localize the origin of the electrical discharge within the brain; these focal discharges then spread to the thalamus and both cerebral hemispheres to cause a frank convulsion. *Partial seizures* (focal epilepsy) are limited to motor (e.g., jerking or twitching of one limb), sensory (paresthesia or visual, olfactory, vestibular, auditory experiences), emotional (e.g., fear, deja vu, pleasure), or cognitive (e.g., feeling outside of oneself, believing one is in another place, feeling that one is in a class) experiences. *Jacksonian seizures* in which twitching or jerking of muscles gradually spreads from one part of the body to another is a form of focal epilepsy. *Partial complex seizures* usually involve similar sensory, emotional, or cognitive experiences followed by some loss of alertness or consciousness without frank generalized convulsive movements. *Petit mal* attacks involve very brief repeated lapses of alertness or posture without sensory or other experiences.

Occasionally a cardiac arrhythmia can accompany epileptic attacks that have focal neurological features (partial or partial complex seizures). It is possible that, in some patients, an arrhythmia could be the only manifestation of an epileptic attack although this occurrence must be quite rare. One of the authors (L.R.C.) consulted on a patient with an intermittent tachycardia that had been very resistant to treatment with the usual cardiac antiarrhythmia drugs. This woman said that sometimes before she developed rapid heart beating she saw a train with several cars coming toward her from the side. When the last car on the short train, the caboose, entered her vision her heart began to beat very rapidly. In some attacks, she saw the train but had no tachycardia. Sometimes she had tachycardia and did not see the train. Most often, however, the vision of the train preceded the tachycardia. She had focal epileptic discharges on her EEG, and prescription of anticonvulsants stopped the train visions and the paroxysmal tachycardias in this patient. A young patient described by Gilchrist had episodes of sudden loss of consciousness that did not respond to phenytoin therapy [77]. Sick sinus syndrome was found after an episode of loss of consciousness but the blackout attacks continued despite insertion of a demand ventricular pacemaker. Combined EEG and ECG monitoring during a seizure showed a left temporal paroxysmal discharge and an ictal cardiac arrythmia [77]. A seizure focus in the frontal or temporal lobes or near the insular cortex could reproduce the same cardiac affects that have been observed during stimulation of these brain regions in animals and humans [6–9].

The frequencies of cardiac and cardiovascular phenomena accompanying focal seizures, including arrhythmias and pulse and blood pressure changes, have only occasionally been well studied. White et al. induced generalized convulsive seizures in paralyzed and ventilated epileptic patients by giving them pentylmetrazol intravenously [78]. All patients had tachycardia at onset of seizures. Frequent atrial and ventricular premature beats occurred and the ECG showed ST segment changes and T wave inversions [78]. Blumhardt and colleagues used ambulatory cassette monitoring to record simultaneously the ECG and ECG during 74 spontaneous seizures among 26 patients who had the diagnosis of temporal lobe epilepsy (partial complex seizures) [79]. In 24 (92%) patients seizures were accompanied by an increase in heart rate; the maximum heart rate was >120 in 67% of seizures, and >160 in 12%. Ictal cardiac arrhythmias occurred in 42% of patients. Most common was an irregular series of abrupt heart rate changes toward the end of the EEG seizure discharge [79]. Sinus arrest can also occur in relation to epileptic seizures. Kiok et al. reported the case of a 23-year-old man with no demonstrable heart disease who had prolonged sinus arrest, lasting up to 9 seconds at the time of clinically observed seizures [80]. The blood pressure may rise during epileptic seizures as much as 50 to 100 mm Hg above the baseline, and catecholamine levels are increased [81].

Sudden death has been described during epileptic attacks, especially during status epilepticus. Patients with epilepsy have a higher frequency of sudden death than the general population [82–85]. The frequency of sudden unexplained death among epileptics has been estimated at 0.05% to 0.2% [84]. Some of these deaths are due to accidents, aspiration, and the primary central nervous system disease that caused the epilepsy. In some patients severe repeated electrical brain discharges could induce the autonomic and neuroendocrine changes described above under strokes and sudden deaths.

Natelson et al. examined the hearts of seven patients with epilepsy who died suddenly [85a]. Five of these seven hearts had foci of myocyte vacuolization, a potentially reversible abnormality. Four of the hearts also showed chronic myocardial damage consisting of perivascular myocardial fibrosis and regions where myocardial fibers had disappeared. Interstitial fibrosis with loss of myocardial fibers was a common finding and was attributed to past episodes of myocytolysis [85a]. Myocytolysis and cardiac arrhythmias are probably important mechanisms of sudden death in epileptic patients. Some epileptic patients may develop chronic myocardial dysfunction and arrythmias caused by myocardial damage during seizures.

Parkinson's Disease and Other "Extrapyramidal" Disorders

The signs of Parkinson's disease are very well known to most practicing physicians. The cardinal manifestations—stooped posture, small-stepped slow gait, masklike facies, lack of arm swing, tremor, and stiffness of the arms and legs—were described by Parkinson in the early years of the 19th century [86]. He noted these manifestations by observing individuals he met on the street without performing formal neurological examinations. Parkinsonian patients also develop drooling, dysarthric low-volume speech, and dysphagia. Parkinson also described altered salivation and sweating as well as dysfunction of the alimentary tract and urinary bladder related to abnormalities of autonomic nervous system function [86]. The predominant pathology found in the brains of Parkinsonian patients is Lewy body inclusions in the substantia nigra of the midbrain and in the locus coeruleus in the pons [87]. These areas are major sites of dopamine synthesis in the brain. The changes in the substantia nigra lead to degenerative changes in the striatum, where the efferent fibers from the substantia nigra synapse. Some patients with Parkinsonism have more extensive Lewy body deposition and degenerative changes that lead to abnormal mental function, hallucinations, and other neurological signs [88]. Neuropathological studies of the autonomic nervous system of patients dying with Parkinsonism also show that Lewy bodies can involve the hypothalamus, intermediolateral cell column of the spinal cord, sympathetic ganglia, and dorsal vagal and other parasympathetic nuclei [89]. Some drugs, e.g., phenothiazines and haloperidol, can cause limb and truncal rigidity, closely mimicking Parkinson's disease.

A number of other neurological degenerative conditions also involve the nigro-striatal dopaminergic regions of the brain, causing some features seen in Parkinsonian patients. These conditions have sometimes been grouped together and called Parkinson's + because they all show other important findings and signs not often found in patients with Parkinson's disease. The most common and important of these Parkinson's + conditions are progressive supranuclear palsy, corticobasal degeneration, and multisystem atrophy.

Progressive supranuclear palsy (PSP) is also often referred to as the Steele-Richardson-Olzewski syndrome, after the neurologists and neuropathologists that first described the disorder [90,91]. It is probably the commonest condition frequently misdiagnosed as Parkinson's disease. Patients with PSP have severe difficulty with truncal balance and often fall when they lean or turn. Frequent falls, often with fractures, remain a problem throughout the course of the disease. Patients with PSP also develop prominent mental changes characterized by apathy, slowness, and decreased speech and cognitive skills. The hallmark of the disease and the sign that gave the disorder its name is the abnormality of voluntary eye movements. Patients most often have difficulty looking up or down spontaneously and when asked to do so. Later, they may also develop difficulty directing their gaze and their eyes horizontally to the sides. This deficiency in conjugate voluntary eye movements makes it difficult for them to direct their gaze at objects that they want to see and makes it difficult to follow lines when reading. Passive movements of the head and neck result in normal or heightened conjugate ocular movements, indicating that the disorder of eye motions is "supranuclear" (that is, involving descending pathways that influence conjugate gaze) and not due to involvement of the oculomotor nuclei or their afferent or efferent nerve fibers. The eye signs may appear as an early manifestation of the disease or occur much later, even after years of other symptoms. Patients with PSP develop loss of facial expression, low-volume dysarthric speech, dysphagia, and limb stiffness. Facial and jaw reflexes are brisk and hyperactive, indicating a supranuclear pseudobulbar mechanism of the dysarthria and dysphagia that invariably accompany the disease. Limb and truncal stiffness resemble that found in Parkinson's disease but the patients do not have tremor. Falls, dementia, Parkinsonian rigidity, pyramidal tract abnormalities, and abnormalities of voluntary gaze are the hallmarks of this progressive disorder [92]. The brain pathology in PSP is neurofibrillary degeneration predominantly in the neurons of the brainstem, thalamus, and basal ganglia. Loss of neurons and gliosis are most prominent in the periaqueductal gray matter of the midbrain, the superior colliculus, subthalamic nucleus, red nucleus, globus pallidus, dentate nucleus of the cerebellum, and the pretectal and vestibular nuclei [91]. The symptoms of PSP usually begin in midlife or older, and the disease insidiously progresses over 5 to 10 years to cause very severe disability and death.

Corticobasal degeneration is a disorder which is also progressive. The neurological abnormalities are asymmetrical, with rigidity, dystonia, and apraxia affecting the limbs on one side of the body [94,95]. The disorder in some ways resembles hemi-Parkinsonism in some patients. Sometimes there is jerking in the affected limbs as well as some sensory loss. Achromatic swollen neurons are often found at necropsy within the cerebral cortex. There are also degenerative changes in the striatum, substantia nigra, thalamus, locus coeruleus, subthalamic nucleus, and the red nucleus.

Multisystem atrophy (MSA) with autonomic failure was formerly called Shy-Drager syndrome [96,97]. It is another degenerative condition that often includes symptoms and findings that mimic Parkinson's disease. In addition to limb stiffness, dysarthria, and dysphagia, patients with MSA often have cerebellar-type limb and gait ataxia and autonomic nervous system abnormalities. Postural hypotension and urinary and sexual dysfunction can be very early symptoms. In the original cases described by Shy and Drager, postural hypotension was the most conspicuous sign of the disease [96,97]. The pathology in patients with MSA is widespread and involves the substantia nigra, striatum, brainstem nuclei, and the intermediolateral columns of the spinal cord. In some patients the disorder begins with ataxia and Parkinsonian-type limb stiffness, and the pathology is similar to that found in patients with sporadic, nonfamilial *olivoponto cerebellar atrophy* (OPCA) [98,99]. Distinctive inclusions of tubular structures are characteristically found within oligodendroglial and neuronal nuclei [98]. In most patients with MSA, dysautonomia, including severe postural hypotension, impotence, and micturition dysfunction, is major and the signs develop early. Hoarseness, dysarthria, and dysphagia are also prominent.

Some patients with multiple lacunar brain infarcts and white matter ischemic changes due to chonic disease of their penetrating brain arteries (*Binswanger's disease*) have Parkinsonian-type extrapyramidal abnormalities as well as altered intellectual functions, weakness, and pyramidal tract signs [100,101]. This disorder was once referred to as ''arteriosclerotic Parkinson's disease. Symptoms do not respond well to L-dopa. A number of other relatively rare conditions affect the extrapyramidal system. *Striatonigral degeneration* is a degenerative condition affecting the basal ganglia and the substantia nigra [102]. Progressive Parkinsonian rigidity, often without tremor, is the cardinal sign of this condition, which does not respond to L-dopa. Many patients with striatonigral degeneration also have *olivoponto cerebellar* atrophy and qualify for the multisystem atrophy syndrome. *Hallevorden-Spatz disease* involves deposition of iron in the basal ganglia, substantia nigra, and the red nucleus [103,104]. Patients have a Parkinsonian gait and trunk and limb rigidity. Response to L-dopa is also poor. MRI scans often can show the iron deposition, thus facilitating recognition of this rare disorder. *Huntington's chorea* is a neurodegenerative disorder involving the caudate nucleus and the frontal lobes. The disorder is characterized predominantly by sudden abnormal limb and facial movements and dementia. Rigidity develops later except in children, in whom stiffness and rigidity may be an early manifestation of this dominantly inherited familial disease. *Machado-Joseph's disease* is a dominantly inherited disease that affects the pons, dentate nucleus, spinocerebellar tracts, and anterior horn cells in the spinal cord. Some patients have prominent Parkinsonian symptoms, often with ataxia. The disease is most prevalent in individuals of Portugese origin.

The major cardiovascular abnormality in patients with these extrapyramidal disorders is *postural hypotension*. The hypotension is most often caused by involvement of the intermediolateral column of sympathetic neurons in the spinal cord in patients with MSA and in some patients with Parkinson's disease, and does not respond to treatment with L-dopa or dopamine agonists. The highest density of dopamine terminals in the spinal cord is found in the intermediolateral cell columns [105]. Degeneration of these cells could follow or coexist with changes in the substantia nigra and striatum. Many of the most effective drugs that are now used to treat Parkinsonian symptoms and signs have hypotension as an important side effect. L-dopa, combinations of carbidopa and L-dopa, dopamine agonists (bromcriptine, pergolide, ropinirole, pramipexole), and newer drugs that increase the availability of L-dopa by inhibiting COMT (catecholamine orthomethyl transferase), including tolcapone and entecapone, all can cause or exacerbate postural hypotension. The decrease in blood pressure is relatively dose dependent; hypotension is most severe at high doses of L-dopa and dopamine agonists. Previously hypertensive patients may gradually require less antihypertensive medication, and in many patients antihypertensive treatment can eventually be discontinued. Postural hypotension is worsened by hypovolemia. Some Parkinsonian patients, because of micturition difficulties and altered gait, which makes it difficult for them to reach the bathroom quickly, reduce their fluid intakes, especially in the evening, and they become relatively volume depleted. In some patients, it is necessary to introduce measures to increase blood pressure such as maximizing fluid intake, using pressure stockings such as Jobst hoses, and/or prescribing pressure-raising drugs such as ephedrine or fludrocortisone (Florinef). Postural hypotension is not a problem in patients with PSP or Hallevorden-Spatz disease, who do not take antiparkinsonian drugs. Huntington's chorea patients do not have postural hypotension.

Other Brain Diseases

Other primary brain diseases have been less thoroughly investigated for their effects on cardiac and cardiovascular functions. The major factors that relate to potential cardiac and cardiovascular effects of brain lesions are their size, location, and whether or not they cause herniation of brain contents and increase intracranial pressure. Focal lesions, such as brain tumors, brain abscesses, focal regions of encephalitis, and focal brain contusions or other traumatic injuries could cause arrhythmias and other cardiovascular abnormalities if they are located in strategic locations known to be potentially arrythmogenic during stimulation, such as the temporal lobes or insula. Electrical stimulation of certain areas within the brain, including the frontal pole, premotor and motor cortex, cingulate gyri, orbital frontal gyri, insular cortex, the anterior part of the temporal lobe, amygdala, and hippocampus, has been known to produce either pressor or depressor effects or atrial and ventricular arrythmias [6–9,47,48]. Slow-growing lesions such as tumors are in general less likely to cause focal disturbances in function including cardiovascular affects than sudden-onset rapidly developing conditions such as strokes and brain injuries.

Degenerative disorders that affect the cerebrum, other than those already discussed under Extrapyramidal Disorders, such as Alzheimer's disease, Pick's disease, motor neuron disease (including amyotrophic lateral sclerosis [ALS]), the slow virus prion protein, diseases Jakob-Creutzfeldt and Gerstmann-Straussler-Scheinker disease, are not known to have important effects on either cardiac or cardiovascular functions. However, in another prion protein disorder called *fatal familial insomnia*, patients often have autonomic nervous system abnormalities [106]. Impotence, micturition abnormalities, constipation, abnormal sweating, and orthoststatic hypotension have been described. The major pathological changes in patients with fatal familial insomnia are found in the thalamus, where there is selective degeneration of some thalamic nuclei, mostly the anterior and dorsomedial nuclei [106]. The dorsomedial thalamic nucleus plays a role in cardiac and cardiovascular functions [9,106]. Chronic neurological degenerative diseases that cause either dementia or bulbar dysfunction and dysphagia may profoundly affect nutrition. Secondary nutritional deficiencies, e.g., of thiamine or niacin, can have important effects on all body systems including the heart, peripheral nervous system, and cardiovascular functions. Patients with *Wernicke's encephalopathy* often have postural hypotension and tachycardia [107,108]. The hypotension may be explained by hypothalamic and brainstem lesions and/or by peripheral neuropathy since both are commonly found in this thiamine deficiency syndrome. The tachycardia could be part of the dysautonomia or be due to the direct effect of thiamine deficiency on the heart. In more severe thiamine deficiency, frank beriberi may occur.

Processes that affect the hypothalamus may affect temperature and blood pressure control. Similarly, disorders that affect the tegmental region of the pons and medulla oblongata within the brainstem can cause lability of blood pressure and have important effects on respiration. Control of autonomic functions such as heart rate, blood pressure, and respiration is closely integrated within the central autonomic network [10,11]. The principal components of the CAN include: (1) the *ventrolateral medulla* and the *medullary reticular zone*; (2) the *nucleus of the solitary tract* (NTS) in the medulla; (3) the *parabrachial region* in the pons; (4) the *periaqueductal gray* in the midbrain; and (5) the *preoptic region* in the hypothalamus. These regions project to a variety of brain regions including the amygdala, insular cortex, and the limbic portions of the striatum. The *parabrachial Kolliker-Fuse* region in the dorsolateral pons relays visceral sensory input to the forebrain and has a very important role in the control of respiration and circulation [10,11].

Reis and colleagues, in a series of experiments, showed that a number of brainstem structures have a very important influence on cerebral blood flow and cerebrovascular autoregulation and metabolism [109,110]. Stimulation of some key structures globally increases cerebral blood flow, affects heart rate and blood pressure, and affects vasodilatation and autoregulation globally and in certain brain regions. The major centers with regulatory function in animal experiments include: the cerebellum—*fastigial nuclei*; the medulla—*NTS, ventrolateral reticular nuclei (RVL)*, and the dorsal medullary reticular formation (DMRF); the pons—*parabrachial nuclei, locus coeruleus*; the midbrain—*dorsal raphe nucleus*; and the thalamus—*centromedian* and *parafascicular complex* [110].

The medulla and pons contain centers that have important effects on respirations. The medulla contains both a dorsal and a ventral respiratory group; lesions below the medulla completely interrupt breathing. The dorsal respiratory group of neurons are located in the ventrolateral portion of the solitary tract and receive visceral sensory afferents through the glossopharyngeral (IX) and vagal (X) cranial nerves. The dorsal medullary respiratory center is mostly inspiratory and drives the phrenic nerve motor neurons and the ventral respiratory group [111,112]. The ventral respiratory group includes neurons in the nucleus ambiguus, supplying the recurrent laryngeal nerve, and the nucleus retroambiguus, which extends from the obex of ventricle IV to the first cervical segment of the spinal cord [112]. The retroambiguus nucleus projects to the spinal cord for control of thoracic and neck muscles involved in breathing. The parabrachial nuclei in the pons have been called the pneumotaxic center because they receive input from the medullary centers to control respiratory patterns and depth [111,112].

Cessation of automatic respiration has long been known to follow high cervical spinal cord injuries and bulbar poliomyelitis [113,114]. High cervical cord lesions disconnect neurons that innervate respiratory muscles from medullary control. The lesions in bulbar poliomyelitis that cause cessation of automatic respirations involve the nerve cells in the lateral medulla. Several reports describe patients with bilateral infarcts in the lateral tegmental regions of the pons and medulla who stopped breathing during sleep [115–118]. The inability to continue to automatically initiate respirations during sleep has often been referred to as *Ondine's curse* after the myth of a water nymph, Ondine, who, in an adaptation by Jean Gradoux of an old German legend, cursed the knight Hans following his marital misconduct by revoking his automatic functions, causing Hans to sleep to death [115]. Unilateral lateral tegmental infarcts have occasionally been reported to also cause Ondine's curse [117,118].

Brainstem tumors, brainstem encephalitis, e.g., caused by *Listeria monocytogenes* [119,120], and strokes are the most common conditions that involve the portions of the brainstem that includes the CAN and are involved in respiratory control. Large, space-taking lesions in the cerebral or cerebellar hemispheres such as hemorrrhages, infarcts, tumors, abscesses, or subdural hematomas can cause secondary pressure effects on the hypothalamus and the brainstem. The Cushing reflex of sudden elevation of systolic blood pressure, lowering of diastolic blood pressure, and slowing of the pulse is probably mediated through brainstem compression of structures within the CAN [121].

SPINAL CORD DISORDERS

Relevant Spinal Cord Anatomy and Physiology

Lesions of the spinal cord can cause cardiac dysfunction and myocardial ischemia, respiratory insufficiency, and various abnormalities of autonomic nervous system functions including lability of pulse and blood pressure, and even cardiac arrest. Descending fiber pathways from the cerebral hemispheres, thalami, and brainstem that relate to the control of respirations and to autonomic nervous system functions travel within the white matter tracts of the spinal cord [122]. Motor pathways, both corticospinal (pyramidal tract) and extrapyramidal, also descend within the white matter tracts of the spinal cord; these fibers subserve voluntary and involuntary control of the muscles of respiration. Within the ventral gray matter of the spinal cord are the neurons that innervate the respiratory muscles including the diaphragm, accessory cervical respiratory muscles, and the intercostal thoracic muscles. Within the intermediolateral columns of the gray matter of the spinal cord are the neurons that are the source of efferent sympathetic nervous system supply to the sympathetic ganglia and to the heart and vascular systems. The predominant afferent input to the spinal cord from visceral afferents carrying information from the heart travels in the second and third thoracic nerves (T2 and T3) [123], while sympathetic nervous system efferents arise from T1 to T5. Electrical stimulation of the rostral five thoracic nerve roots elicits changes in pulse and blood pressure, localized changes in cardiac muscle contractile force, and changes in the pattern of impulse conduction [123].

Effects of Spinal Cord Injuries at Various Levels and Sites

The effects of spinal cord damage most often have been studied clinically in patients with acute spinal cord traumatic injuries. After acute severe injuries, a state of ''spinal shock'' often ensues. Somatic motor and sensory functions are lost below the level of the spinal injury, causing paralysis and loss of pain, temperature, touch, and proprioceptive sensations. There is also a loss of sympathetic nervous system functions. Because the parasympathetic innervation of the heart and vascular system arising from the vagus nerve in the brainstem does not travel within the spinal cord, in patients with cervical, thoracic, and lumbar spinal cord injuries parasympathetic influences are preserved while sympathetic innervation is lost. The skin below the level of the injury becomes hyperemic and warm, blood pools in the veins of the lower extremities, and there is decreased venous return of blood to the heart. Systemic hypotension develops and may be severe. The vagal tone firing action on the heart is unopposed by sympathetic nervous system activity. Tonic stimulation of the vagus nerve prolongs the length of the cardiac cycle and prolongs the refractory period of atrioventricular node fibers. Vagal stimulation also inhibits atrial contraction and thereby attenuates the atrial contribution to ventricular filling [124]. Bradycardia, heart block, and even cardiac arrest can result from the unopposed vagal tone.

Spinal cord injuries have important effects on breathing and respiratory functions. Lesions of the most rostral portions of the cervical spinal cord interrupt descending tracts that control the activity of the muscles of respiration. When spinal cord lesions are near the medullary-spinal junction, as occurs in patients with atlantoaxial dislocations and after hanging, patients stop breathing and all respiratory muscles are paralyzed. When the cervical spinal cord lesion involves the third to the fifth cervical segments (C3–C5), levels that include the neurons that contribute to the phrenic nerves, the diaphragm is paralyzed as well as the thoracic intercostal musculature. Diaphragmatic paralysis can allow the diaphragm on one or both sides to passively move upward during expansion of the upper rib cage by the accessory muscles of respiration (sternocleidomastoid, trapezius, and scalene muscles), causing inward abdominal movement on inspiration. Tidal volume and inspiratory and expiratory reserve volumes are decreased and residual volume is markedly increased [125]. When the spinal cord lesion is below C5, the diaphragms and accessory cervical respiratory muscles are preserved but the thoracic intercostal muscles are paralyzed. Respiratory insufficiency and hypoventilation can also develop in this circumstance [126].

The cardiac and cardiovascular abnormalities accompanying acute spinal cord injuries have been less well studied than the respiratory abnormalities. Lehman et al. monitored 71 consecutive patients with spinal cord injuries using ECG and blood pressure monitoring techniques [127]. Most of the severe cardiac and cardiovascular effects were limited to patients who had severe cervical spinal cord injuries; patients with less severe cervical cord injuries and those with thoracic-lumbar injuries less often had abnormalities and the abnormalities when present were less severe [127]. Hypotension was present in 68% of patients with severe cervical spinal cord injuries but was not present in any of the patients with less severe cervical injuries or those with thoracolumbar lesions. Bradycardia contributed to the hypotension. All of the patients with severe cervical cord lesions had persistent bradycardia (<60 beats/min), and marked bradycardia was present in 71% of these patients. Persistent bradycardia sometimes developed in patients with milder cervical cord lesions (35%) and thoracolumbar lesions (13%) but was less severe. The prevalence of persistent bradycardia peaked at day 4 after injury and gradually declined during the next 10 days. Cardiac arrest occurred in five of the 31 patients with severe cervical cord traumatic injuries and was invariably preceded by persistent bradycardia and hypotension requiring pressor therapy. Repolarizaion changes in the ECG were common in all groups of patients with spinal cord injuries [127]. Four patients with severe cervical cord injuries had new atrioventricular block, including three with first-degree and one with Mobitz type I second-degree block. Supraventricular tachyrhythmias, most commonly atrial fibrillation, developed in 19% of patients with severe cervical spinal cord injuries [127].

The cardiac abnormalities described in patients with spinal cord injuries are mostly explained by the acute autonomic nervous system imbalance that follows disruption of sympathetic nervous system activity leading to unopposed parsympathetic dominance. Baseline and stress-induced catecholamine levels are low, a manifestation of the reduced sympathetic activity [128]. Table 1 lists the evidence supporting the attribution of the cardiovascular effects of spinal injuries to the altered parasympathetic/sympathetic nervous system balance. In recently injured quadriplegic patients, parasympathetic (vagal) activity and reflexes may even be enhanced over the normal situation [129]. For example, tracheal suction can cause bradycardia and even cardiac arrest. This exaggerated response is blocked by premedication with atropine [129].

The decreased sympathetic nervous system activity during the acute stage of spinal cord injury changes after 4 to 6 weeks to increased sympathetic nervous

Patients with *tabes dorsalis*, a syphillitic disorder that involves mostly the thoracic and lumbar spinal nerve roots and the posterior columns of the spinal cord, may also have abnormal circulatory reflexes. Tachycardia is common in patients with tabes dorsalis. Older neurology texts do not mention blood pressure abnormalities as a common finding in tabetics, although blood pressures were not systematically analyzed. In tabetic patients, and likely other individuals who have involvement of their thoracic nerve roots, orthostatic blood pooling could be caused by loss of the afferent input to the baroreflex. Intermittent hypertension could also be a problem.

Patients with intrinsic intramedullary spinal cord tumors (mostly astrocytomas and ependymomas), intradural extramedullary spinal tumors (mostly meningiomas and neurofibromas), and nonneoplastic spinal cord lesions likely also show effects similar to those observed in patients with spinal cord injuries. The major difference between traumatic and nontraumatic spinal cord lesions is the acuteness of onset and the severity of the insults. Since tumors and other nontraumatic spinal cord lesions usually evolve slowly and are most often very incomplete in the extent of spinal cord damage and loss of functions, they probably less often cause cardiac and cardiovascular abnormalities, and the abnormalities are probably less severe than those found in patients with severe spinal cord injuries. Knowing the principles and cardiovascular symptoms and signs found in patients with spinal cord trauma should alert clinicians to the possibility of cardiac and cardiovascular problems in patients with nontraumatic spinal cord disorders. Most important in predicting the likelihood of occurrence of cardiovascular problems are the location (rostrocaudal level, intramedullary vs. extramedullary, and the sites within the cord of involvement of gray and white matter) and the size and rapidity of onset of the spinal cord process. The more acute and severe the process, the more likely are signs of cardiac and cardiovascular dysfunction.

Poliomyelitis is a very unique spinal cord infection. The prevalence of polio during the first half of this century and the seriousness of the disease led to extensive observations of cardiopulmonary and cardiovascular consequences of this dreaded disease. The poliomyelitis syndrome was caused by three enteroviruses: Coxsackie viruses A and B, echovirus, and the poliomyelitis virus. The disease was formerly very common. As late as the mid-1950s summer epidemics occurred during which thousands of children and young adults were paralyzed. Enders, Salk, and Sabin contributed to the development of a vaccine that was highly effective in preventing the disease. Now, poliomyelitis does not occur in the United State except in individuals who do not receive the vaccine, but the disease still occurs in countries that do not have effective vaccination programs.

Poliomyelitis may begin with pharyngitis or gastroenteritis. Fever, headache, sore throat, and diarrhea often ensue. The virus spreads from the intestinal tract to the meninges and to the neurons of the anterior and intermediolateral horns of the spinal cord, and to neurons in the thalamus, hypothalamus, and motor neurons in the brain. Lumbar puncture usually shows signs of a viral meningitis. The first neurologic symptoms are usually headache and muscle aches and pains. A paralytic stage ensues in which paralysis of various muscle groups develops over a period of days. Muscles that were active at the time of infection were most likely to become paralyzed. Bulbar involvement with the poliomyelitis virus leads to respiratory paralysis, vasomotor instability, hypertension, and dysphagia [136]. Death can occur, usually due to respiratory complications.

Cardiovascular abnormalities were common in patients with poliomyelitis [137]. Hypertension was especially common. The virus often directly invaded the heart, causing myocarditis (Fig. 5). Lesions are found at necropsy in all parts of the heart [138]. Myocyte damage was common and there was often widespread focal and perivascular infiltration of polymorphonuclear leukocytes, lymphocytes, plasma cells, and monocytes. Both myocarditis and verrucous endocarditis were found [137]. Hemorrhages were also found within the myocardium [138]. The ECG was often abnormal, showing a long P-R interval, a long Q-T interval, and primary T-wave abnormalities. Pulmonary edema was common during the acute phase. If the patient recovered, the ECG and clinical signs of myocarditis abated and chronic myocardial dysfunction was rarely reported. Lability of blood pressure included episodes of hypotension as well as hypertension, and some patients died in circulatory collapse.

DYSAUTONOMIAS

Some neurological disorders primarily, and sometimes exclusively, affect the autonomic nervous system. These conditions are often referred to in the aggregate as dysautonomias, although different conditions involve different portions of the autonomic nervous system [139]. Although orthostatic, posturally related hypotension is the predominant cardiovascular problem, cardiac abnormalities also occur. Some conditions involve the neurons of the autonomic nervous system within the brain and/or the spinal cord, while others involve the peripheral nervous system which carries information to and from the viscera and the heart and blood vessels. In this section on the dysautonomias, we will discuss the central and peripheral nervous system conditions that have autonomic nervous system dysfunction as the major or only feature. Conditions that affect the peripheral nerves and cause motor, sensory, and autonomic dysfunction will be covered next, in the section on disorders of nerve roots and peripheral nerves. Table 3 lists the most important and commonest symptoms in patients with dysautonomic disorders.

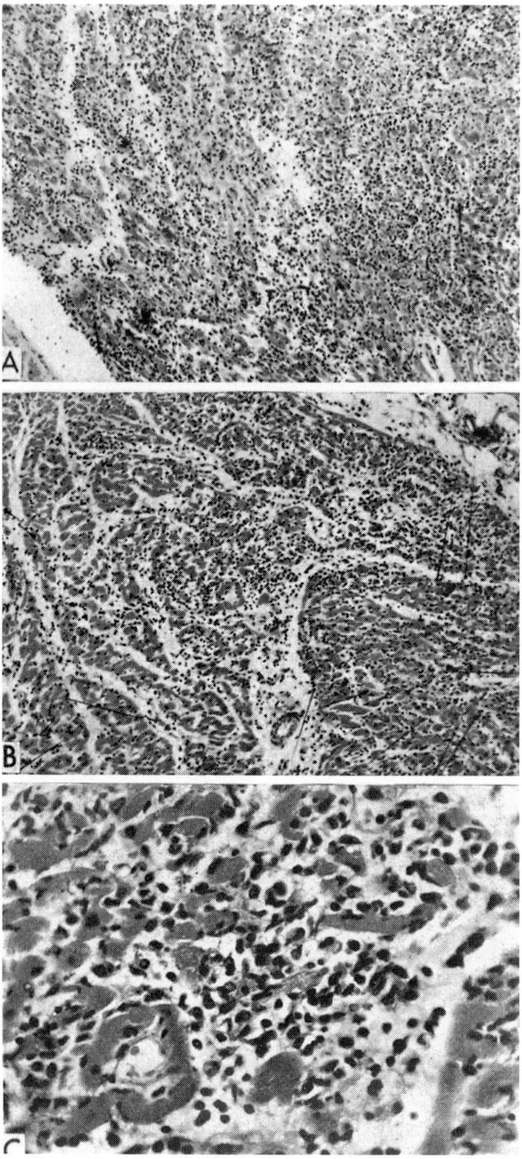

FIG. 5 Myocardial lesions in a patient with poliomyelitis. Myocarditis in poliomyelitis; from a 5-year-old girl with juvenile rheumatoid arthritis (Still's disease). (A) Left ventricle (×75). (B) Right ventricle (×75). (C) Right ventricle (×300). All sections are stained with hematoxylin-eosin. (From Ref. 138. Sections courtesy of Dr. RCB Pugh. Copyright, REB Hudson, 1965. Reproduced with permission.)

TABLE 3 Clinical Findings in Patients with Dysautonomias

System affected	Finding
Cardiovascular	orthostatic hypotension
Sudomotor	anhidrosis, heat intolerance
Gastrointestinal	dysphagia, constipation, fecal incontinence, abdominal distension and pain
Genitourinary	urinary frequency and urgency, urinary incontinence, impotence, failure to ejaculate
Ophthalmic	anisocoria, Horner's syndrome, tonic pupils
Respiratory	stridor, inspiratory gaps, apneic episodes

Source: Modified from Ref. 139, p. 723, with permission.

Pure Autonomic Failure

This disorder was formerly called progressive autonomic failure and idiopathic orthostatic hypotension [139a]. Pure autonomic failure is a primary degenerative condition that affects the peripheral autonomic nervous system. Since the predominant clinical finding and presenting symptoms are usually related to postural hypotension, the condition was initially called idiopathic orthostatic hypotension. The usual age at onset of patients with pure autonomic failure (PAF) is between ages 40 and 60 years, and the condition is more common among men than women [140]. The earliest presenting symptoms are sudden dropping to the ground (syncope), dizziness, or feelings of dizziness, weakness, or visual blurring after standing or walking. Loss of sweating, impotence, urinary urgency and frequency, and later urinary and fecal incontinence are common. The disorder usually gradually progresses and death ensues on average 7 to 10 years after onset of symptoms [140,142]. In some patients, Parkinsonian symptoms and findings, and in other patients, cerebellar, pyramidal, and extrapyramidal signs develop as part of more widespread neural degeneration syndromes which we now classify as Parkinson's disease with dysautonomic features or multisystem atrophy depending on the extent of clinical abnormalities. These more widespread conditions have already been discussed under Extrapyramidal Diseases.

Necropsy studies of patients with PAF show loss of neurons in the intermediolateral column of the spinal cord, loss of neurons in the dorsal vagal nuclei, and degeneration of cells within the sympathetic ganglia [140,143,144]. The extent of the loss of neurons in the intermediolateral columns of the spinal cord closely correlates with the occurrence and severity of autonomic failure. Plasma noradrenaline levels are low and do not rise normally on standing, indicating a failure of release of noradrenaline from postganglionic sympathetic nerve endings [140,145,146]. Recent radioisotope studies of patients with autonomic failure using ^{123}I methyliodobenzylguanidine (MIBG) and single-photon emission tomography (SPECT) scanning of the heart show evidence of sympathetic denervation of the myocardium [147]. The earliest changes are evident in the apical and inferior walls, but later the entire myocardium shows sympathetic denervation [147]. Positron emission tomography (PET) studies and biochemical analyses also confirm that patients with PAF have a progressive loss of sympathetic nerve terminals [148]. The loss of sympathetic innervation can produce an autonomic nervous system imbalance with dominance of the parasympathetic innervation similar to that described in patients with cervical and thoracic spinal cord injuries. Arrythmias and cardiac arrest could result, but extensive or detailed cardiac evaluations have not been reported in patients with PAF.

Familial Dysautonomia (Riley-Day Syndrome)

This hereditofamilial disorder is an autosomal-recessively inherited disorder that begins in very early childhood [140,149–151]. Most affected individuals are Jewish. Difficulty swallowing and recurrent bronchopneumonia are noted during infancy. Later developing symptoms and signs include an absence of tears, poor motor coordination, postural hypotension, vomiting, episodic hypertension, skin blotching, and excessive sweating [151]. Taste perception is often abnormal and there may be loss of somatic sensations, including pain. Temperature control is poor and many patients are quite insensitive to pain. Many children with familial dysautonomia die early in childhood because of recurrent aspiration pneumonia. The recurrent bronchopulmonary infections are explained by dysphagia and recurrent aspiration of food and gastric contents. Necropsy shows decreased numbers of neurons in the sympathetic ganglia and in the intermediolateral column of the spinal cord as well as a decreased number of small myelinated fibers in nerve roots. Sometimes there are also abnormalities within the reticular formation of the brainstem. The posterior columns of the spinal cord may also be demyelinated [152]. Testing shows very abnormal circulatory reflexes [153]. Respiratory control is also abnormal. This familial disorder is probably best understood as a loss of afferent autonomic nervous system input accompanied by a lack of efferent, predominantly sympathetic nervous system output. Most patients with familial dysautonomia do not survive until adulthood.

Holmes-Adie Syndrome

Although this condition is relatively common and is well known to most neurologists, it is not at all familiar to generalists and other nonneurological specialists. The most common manifestations of this condition are tonic, abnormally reactive pupils and loss of deep tendon reflexes [154,155]. This condition is most common among young girls and women. Some patients with the Holmes-Adie syndrome have dry skin, abnormal sweating, and abnormal taste perception. Syncope also occurs and some patients have postural hypotension [156].

The most consistent finding and the abnormality that usually brings patients with the Holmes-Adie syndrome to medical attention is the pupillary abnormalities. Patients may complain of light sensitivity similar to that described by patients who have had mydriatic drops instilled in their eyes for ophthalmoscopy or refraction. In others the pupillary abnormality is noticed by the patient or by a doctor during routine examinations. The pupils are usually asymmetric; often one or both pupils are dilated and irregular. The pupils do not react normally to light. Sometimes long exposure to bright light results in some delayed pupillary constriction. The pupils react better to accommodation than to light, a finding similar to that found in patients with tabes dorsalis. The pupillary response to mecholyl is hyperactive; individuals with the Holmes-Adie syndrome react more vigorously to mecholyl placed in the eye than normals. Dilute pilocarpine (0.125%) constricts the pupil in patients with the Holmes-Adie syndrome but has little effect in normal patients. Later in life the pupils may become small rather than dilated. Cardiovascular reflexes, cardiac autonomic nervous system functions, and sweating responses are often abnormal when tested [157,158]. To date there has been no generally agreed-upon pathological substrate of this syndrome. Abnormalities are often found in the ciliary ganglia which supplies autonomic innervation to the eye. Also posited are abnormalities in the peripheral nerves, which carry both afferent and efferent autonomic nervous system fibers. The loss of deep tendon reflexes, especially knee jerks, is likely due to changes in the peripheral nerves.

TABLE 4 Autonomic Nervous System Tests

1. Response of heart rate and blood pressure to changes in posture; change from supine to standing or using a tilt table [167,169]
2. Response of heart rate, blood pressure, and cardiac output to sustained isometric contraction of a group of muscles [167,170]
3. Heart rate variation during respirations [167,171]
4. Heart rate and blood pressure responses to the Valsalva maneuver [167,172]
5. Tests of sweating after various stimuli [167,168]
6. Changes in blood pressure after application of negative pressure to the lower body while supine [167]
7. Baroreflex sensitivity [167,173]
8. Measurements of peripheral blood flow after radiant heat and after immersion in cold or hot water
9. Tests of pupillary innervation [174,175]
10. Measurements of plasma noradrenaline at rest and after various stimuli [143,167]

TABLE 5 Clinical Tests of Autonomic Function

Test	Normal response	Reflex part tested
1. Noninvasive bedside tests		
BP response to standing or vertical tilt	fall in BP <30/15 mm Hg	afferent and effernet limbs
Heart rate response to standing	Increase 11–29 beats/min; 30:15 ratio > 1.04[a]	afferent and efferent limbs
Isometric exercise	increase 15 mm Hg diastolic BP	sympathetic efferent limb
Heart rate variation with respiration	max-min heart rate >15; expire:inspire ratio >1.2	vagal afferent and efferent limbs
Valsalva ratio	>1.4 depending on age	afferent and efferent limbs
Sweat tests	sweat production, body and limbs	sympathetic efferent limb
Axon reflex	local piloerection, sweating	postganglionic sympathetic efferent
Plasma noradrenaline level	rises on tilt from horizontal to vertical	sympathetic efferent limb
Plasma vasopressin level	rise with induced hypotension	afferent limb
2. Invasive tests using intra-arterial catheter		
Valsalva maneuver	Phase 1—rise in BP Phase 2—gradual decrease BP to plateau; tachycardia Phase 3—fall in BP Phase 4—overshoot of BP, bradycardia	afferent and efferent limbs

Baroreflex sensitivity	1. Slowing of heart rate with induced rise of BP 2. Steady-state repsonses to induced rise and fall of BP	1. Parasympathetic afferent and efferent limbs 2. Afferent and efferent limbs
Pressor drug infusion	1. Rise in BP 2. Heart rate slowing	1. Adrenergic receptors 2. Afferent and efferent parasympathetic limbs
3. Test of vasomotor control		
Radiant heating of trunk	increase hand blood flow	sympathetic efferent limb
Immerse hand in cold water	increase blood flow opposite hand	sympathetic efferent limb
Cold pressor test	reduce blood flow	sympathetic efferent limb
Emotional stress	increase BP	sympathetic efferent limb
Inspiratory gasp	reduce hand blood flow	sympathetic efferent limb

Drug instilled	Normal response	Reflex part tested
4. Tests of pupillary innervation		
4% cocaine	pupil dilates	sympathetic innervation
0.1% adrenaline	no response	postganglionic sympathetic innervation
1% hydroxyamphetamine hydrobromide	pupil dilates	postganglionic sympathetic innervation
2.5% methacholine, 0.125% pilocarpine	no response	parasympathetic innervation

[a] Ratio of R-R intervals corresponding to the 30th and 15th heart beats.
Modified from Ref. 169, p. 520, with permission.

Acute and Subacute Autonomic Neuropathies

Robert Young and his colleagues in 1969, and later in 1975, first described patients who had the acute onset of severe autonomic nervous system abnormalities without other important neurological signs (''pure pandysautonomia''), and then recovered from their illness [159,160]. Patients with acute dysautonomia have the acute or subacute onset of lethargy and fatigue, blurred vision, postural hypotension, decreased tear formation, decreased sweating, dry skin, dry mouth, constipation, urinary retention, impotence, and sometimes urinary and/or fecal incontinence [140,159–162]. Sometimes there are accompanying motor and sensory abnormalities. In most patients the abnormal findings recover during a period of weeks to months, but some patients recover only partially and some do not show any substantial recovery. The cerebrospinal fluid protein content is often elevated. In some patients, especially children, cholinergic abnormalities predominate [140,163,164]. These patients have blurred vision, constipation, dry eyes and mouth, and urinary retention but they do not have postural hypotension. This predominantly cholinergic dysautonomia is often chronic and there is usually less recovery than that found in adults with acute pandysautonomia [140,164].

Most clinicians consider these acute and subacute autonomic neuropathies to be immunologically mediated radiculoneuropathies—a form of Guillain-Barré syndrome that involves predominantly autonomic fibers within the peripheral nervous system. Some patients with the Guillain-Barré syndrome have prominent dysautonomia. Acute pandysautonomia has been described after infectious mononucleosis and other infections [165], and also in patients with various malignancies [166,167]. Lymphocytic infiltrates similar to those found in patients with Guillain-Barré are found in autonomic and sensory ganglia and in nerve roots and peripheral nerves [167].

Testing of Autonomic Nervous System Functions

Recognition that some neurological conditions primarily affect the autonomic nervous system (dysautonomias) and other diseases such as Parkinson's disease and multiple system atrophy, and some peripheral neuropathies such as diabetes mellitus are associated with autonomic nervous system dysfunction amid other signs, has led to the development of sophisticated, objective, quantifiable tests of atonomic nervous system functions [168–177]. Some of these tests are also designed to determine whether the autonomic dysfunction is sympathetic or parasympathetic and whether the abnormalities found relate to preganglionic or postganglionic lesions. Table 4 lists some of the available tests, and Table 5 [169] tabulates in more detail the most common tests, the normal responses to these tests, and the autonomic nervous system components involved.

Space does not permit a lengthy discussion of these tests but references

166, 167, and 168 can be consulted for more details and for other, less commonly used tests. Recently some new treatments for postural hypotension have become available. If patients do not respond to the use of support hose and/or increased salt intake, they can be given flurinef, the artificial amino acid 3,4-dihydroxyphenyl serine (DOPS) [178,179] or midodrine hydrochloride [180].

DISORDERS OF NERVE ROOTS AND PERIPHERAL NERVES

We include in this section diseases whose major manifestation that potentially causes cardiac and/or cardiovascular abnormalities is involvement of peripheral nerves or nerve roots. It would be impossible to include all types and causes of neuropathy in this chapter without rewriting a textbook of neurology. We have selected disorders that are either common or are associated with known cardiac and cardiovascular abnormalities. Although many of the disorders have prominent neurologic manifestations other than neuropathy, it seemed best to include them in this section for the purposes of simplicity and because all have peripheral neuropathy as a very important feature. Autonomic nerve fibers are affected to some degree in many peripheral neuropathies and some radiculopathies, although the clinical manifestations of this involvement are often mild. Segmental demyelination can involve myelinated autonomic nerve fibers in the vagus or sympathetic pathways, e.g., in Guillain-Barré syndrome and some diabetics, and some neuropathies, e.g., amyloid and diabetes, affect small-diameter myelinated and unmyelinated autonomic nervous system fibers within afferent and efferent peripheral nerves [181]. The clinical autonomic dysfunction ranges from slight impairment in sweating to postural hypotension. Orthostatic postural hypotension occurs when damage to small-diameter myelinated and unmyelinated fibers in afferent and efferent peripheral nerves is located within baroreflex pathways and splanchnic outflow [181]. Postural hypotension is especially apt to occur when fibers in the splanchnic vascular bed are pathologically involved, since this innervation has an important influence on blood pressure regulation [181].

Disorders of Cranial Nerves or Nerve Roots

The only disorder of nerve roots that frequently causes cardiac and cardiovascular dysfunction is *glossopharyngeal neuralgia*. This condition is similar to trigeminal neuralgia (tic douleureux) except that the IX nerve (the glossopharyngeal nerve) is involved rather than the V (trigeminal) nerve. Pain is usually felt in the throat, neck, or ear. The pain is sharp and lancinating, and may be precipitated by swallowing or the contact of cold to the pharynx. The glossopharyngeal nerve carries the afferent fibers of the baroreflex. Syncope, bradycardia, and even prolonged sinus arrest can occur during paroxysms of glossopharyngeal neuralgia.

Manipulation of the V cranial nerve, the trigeminal nerve, can cause sudden *increases in blood pressure*, sometimes severe enough to cause hypertensive intracerebral hemorrhages. The trigeminal nerves and their fibers play an important role in the innervation and control of the cerebral blood vessels [182]. Alterations in blood pressure and blood flow follow trigeminal nerve stimulation in animals, and acute rises in blood pressure and tachycardia accompany trigeminal pain and trigeminal stimulation in humans [183]. Elevated blood pressure causing intracerebral hemorrhages has been noted during surgical treatment of patients with *trigeminal neuralgia* [184–186], and dangerous elevations in blood pressure have been noted after heating of trigeminal nerve roots [187] and during percutaneous surgical trigeminal rhizotomies [188]. Elevated blood pressure causing intracerebral hemorrhage has also been described during dental treatments, presumably because of stimulation of the trigeminal nerves [183,186,189].

Infectious and Inflammatory Neuropathies

Acute Inflammatory Polyradiculoneuropathy (Guillain-Barré) [190,191]

The Guillain-Barré syndrome is predominantly a motor neuropathy that often causes severe paralysis. The first symptom is usually weakness of the legs and arms. The lower extremities are often involved before the upper extremities. The weakness is most pronounced in the proximal parts of the limbs (shoulders and thighs). This distribution, which is explained by demyelination of nerve roots and the proximal portions of peripheral nerves, distinguishes the Guillain-Barré syndrome from most peripheral neuropathies, which characteristically cause symptoms first in the distal parts of the limbs. Weakness and paralysis may progress over hours and days, sometimes causing a loss of all limb movements. The weakness is usually symmetrical. The respiratory muscles are often paralyzed so artificial respiration is at times necessary, sometimes for a prolonged period. Paresthesias and occasionally pain are reported in the limbs, especially in the fingers, toes, and feet. Sensory loss is usually minimal, affecting mostly vibration and position sense. The deep tendon reflexes are invariably absent. The cranial nerves are sometimes affected, causing bilateral facial weakness and sometimes hoarseness and dysphagia. The cerebrospinal fluid usually but not always has a high protein content and few or no white blood cells (so-called albuminocytologic dissociation).

This illness usually develops after a respiratory or gastrointestinal infection. Viral illnesses, such as those caused by the human immunodeficiency virus (HIV), the Epstein-Barr virus, cytomegalovirus, and bacterial infections are common. The syndrome can also follow trauma or surgery, and has even been described after myocardial infarction [192]. Necropsy of patients dying early after onset shows a brisk inflammatory response consisting of lymphocytic infiltrates in nerve roots and proximal portions of the peripheral nerves followed by segmental demyelination [193]. The Guillain-Barré syndrome is believed to be an autoimmune disease in which antibodies are directed against elements of peripheral nerves and nerve roots.

In most patients, the weakness is self-limited. Advances in intensive care and respiratory support and excellent nursing care are responsible for the relatively good prognosis despite even severe paralysis. The majority of patients recover completely after paralysis, which lasts weeks to months. In some patients the paralysis is prolonged and recovery very incomplete. In one variant of the Guillain-Barré syndrome (usually called the Miller Fisher variant, after the physician who first described it [194]), the weakness predominantly involves bulbar-innervated muscles and is accompanied by limb incoordination and ataxia. These patients develop ophthalmoplegia and may be unable to move the eyes at all. The facial muscles are often very weak, and the pharynx and larynx may also be involved, causing hoarseness and dysphagia. Deep tendon reflexes are absent and the arms and legs often show severe incoordination. Walking may be impossible because of the gait ataxia.

Cardiac and Cardiovascular Manifestations. Cardiac arrhythmias are common in patients with Guillain-Barré disease and may be related to hypoxia and/or autonomic nervous system involvement [195]. Primary T-wave abnormalities may appear in the electrocardiogram [196]. Bradycardia, atrioventricular block, supraventricular tachycardia, and ventricular tachycardia may be observed during the illness, especially in patients who are treated with mechanical ventilators and who need frequent tracheal aspiration. Tachycardia may be unresponsive to postural change [197]. Sudden death due to arrhythmias or asystole has been described [181]. The systemic blood pressure may fluctuate and can be elevated or abnormally low. Postural hypotension may develop and can be severe [197,198]. Postural hypotension can cause syncope and may be especially hazardous if paralyzed patients are left in a sitting position. The blood pressure and heart rate response to Valsalva maneuvers may be abnormal [181]. The heart rate response to elevated blood pressure induced by intraveous injection of phenylephrine may be abnormal. Tests of sweating are also abnormal, indicating autonomic nervous system dysfunction [181].

Chronic Inflammatory Demyelinative Polyradiculoneuropathy [199]

Austin in 1956 was the first to report a more subacutely developing neuropathy that was characterized by thickened nerves and responsiveness to corticosteroid treatment [200]. Subsequent investigations have shown that the condition is a chronic demyelinative neuropathy probably caused by a hyperimmune response.

The accepted name for this type of neuropathy is chronic inflammatory demyelinative polyradiculoneuropathy (CIDP). It is one of the most common peripheral neuropathies now seen in neurologic practice.

The condition begins subacutely. The course may fluctuate with remissions and periods of worsening, or signs may progress gradually over weeks to months or even years. Both motor and sensory abnormalities may occur. Unlike Guillain-Barré syndrome, with which this condition is often compared (CIDP has often been characterized as a type of "chronic Guillain-Barré"), in CIDP the sensory symptoms and signs may predominate and the findings are quite often asymmetric. The deep tendon reflexes are usually absent or greatly diminished. The spinal fluid protein may be high. The peripheral nerves may be thickened when felt by palpation. Patients often improve with corticosteroid treatment or after being given pooled human immunoglobulin.

Postural hypotension and other signs of autonomic neuropathy occur rarely in CIDP [201]. Ingalls et al. tested autonomic nervous system-mediated responses in 15 patients with CIDP; they studied the ratio of R-R intervals corresponding to the 30th and 15th heart beats, and found it abnormal in three of 14 patients, and they found abnormal sweating responses in five patients [201]. Minor changes were found in unmyelinated nerve fibers in sural nerve biopsy specimens [201].

Motor Neuropathy with Conduction Block

Motor neuropathy with conduction block is another type of chronic demyelinative neuropathy [202,203]. The major and usually only neurological symptom is weakness involving muscles of the limbs. The disease gets its name from the electrophysiological findings. Stimulation of a motor nerve below a block evokes a compound muscle action potential, but stimulation above the block produces a response usually $<10\%$ of that elicited below the block. Weakness develops gradually and is accompanied by muscle cramps and fasciculations. Usually the weakness involves individual peripheral nerves or brachial plexus trunks. The arms are involved much more often than the legs. This condition is often confused with motor neurone disease (amyotrophic lateral sclerosis). Intravenous immunoglobulin therapy is often effective [204]. Cardiac and cardiovascular abnormalities have not been described in this condition.

Diphtheritic Neuropathy

Diphtheria is caused by the organism *Corynebacterium diphtheriae*. The organisms are usually spread by droplets but may enter the body by way of penetrating wounds or skin lesions. The disease is rarely seen now in the United States but is still found in parts of the world where preventive measures are not practiced. The illness usually begins with a sore throat. An inflammatory exudate is visible in the throat and trachea. The bacteria located in the exudate provide the source for a potent exotoxin which is extremely toxic to the nervous system and the heart.

Neurological symptoms usually begin about a week after the onset of sore throat. The palatal muscles become paralyzed [205]. This leads to a change in the voice, regurgitation, and dysphagia. The cranial nerves, including the vagus, facial, trigeminal, and hypoglossal nerves, may become involved at about the same time. Vision may become blurred and accommodation of the pupils becomes abnormal. Later some patients develop symptoms of a peripheral polyneuropathy [206]. The neuropathy is sensorimotor and involves the legs and arms. If the patient does not die of cardiac disease or respiratory failure, the neurologic manifestations gradually subside.

Cardiovascular Findings. Gore reported that the hearts of patients dying of diphtheria were "dilated, pale and flabby" [207]. Among 205 patients who came to necropsy because of fatal outcome of diphtheria, 143 (70%) had myocarditis [207]. Microscopic examination showed frequent hyaline, granular, and fatty changes in the myocytes. Lymphocytes and plasma cells appeared later. Still later there was evidence of scar tissue and occasional calcification [208]. The pathology of diphtheritic myocarditis is shown in Figure 6. The conduction system of the heart is very vulnerable to the toxin. Accordingly, patients may develop complete heart block with its complications [209]. Bundle branch block has also been reported. Most patients die when these complications are observed. Conduction abnormalities have been described in the electrocardiogram years after the disease has abated, and clinical heart block may recur years after the initial diphtheritic infection [210,211].

Acquired Human Immunodeficiency Syndrome

Acquired immunodeficiency syndrome (AIDS) is caused by the human immunodeficiency virus. The virus produces a severe depression of cell-mediated immune function. The decrease in immunity makes individuals susceptible to many types of infections. In the United States the disease affects mostly homosexual and bisexual males and intravenous drug users. The virus can be transmitted by transfusions. Hemophiliacs may become infected when they receive infected blood products, and an infected mother may transmit the disease to her newborn baby.

The initial symptoms may be malaise, diarrhea, and weight loss. Generalized lymphadenopathy commonly develops. The nervous system can be infected directly by the HIV virus or by many of the other opportunistic organisms and neoplasms. The patient may develop meningitis, encephalitis, dementia, neuropathy, and immune inflammatory myopathy.

The nervous system may be involved with opportunistic infections such as toxoplasmosis, cytomegalovirus, herpes simplex or zoster, cryptococcus, and

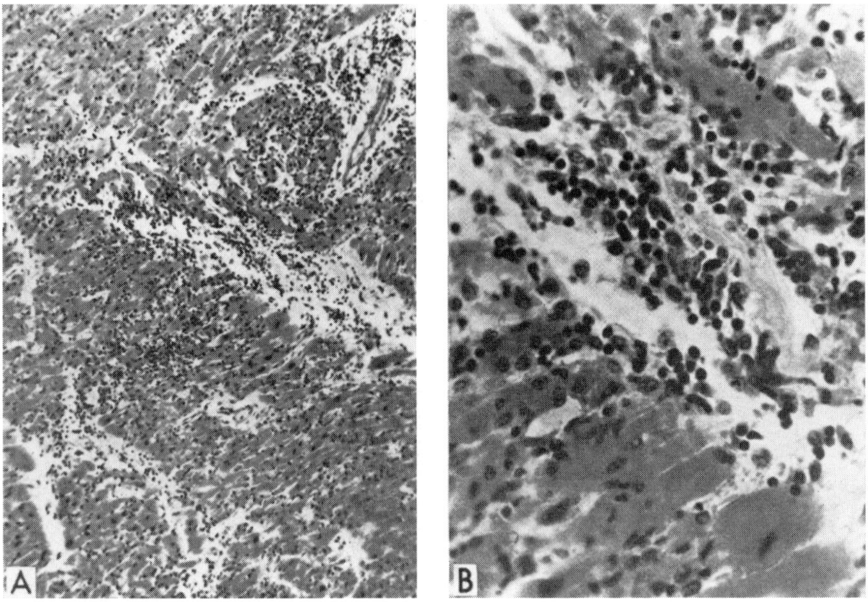

FIG. 6 Diphtheritic myocarditis found in a fatal case in a soldier serving in Egypt. Left ventricle, hematoxylin-eosin. (A) ×85; (B) ×325. (From Ref. 138. Reproduced with permission.)

tuberculosis (several types). Primary lymphoma of the central nervous system may occur. AIDS makes the central nervous system more vulnerable to the spirochete responsible for syphilis. The neuropathy may resemble CIDP. Cytomegalovirus often involves the nerve roots of the cauda equina, causing a painful neuropathy that affects the lower extremities and causes incontinence and impotence.

Patients with AIDS formerly died within 1 to 3 years. The recent use of multiple drug treatment has improved survival considerably and gives hope to affected persons.

Cardiovascular Findings. Patients with AIDS commonly have myocarditis, dilated cardiomyopathy, and pericarditis. These conditions may be caused by the AIDS virus, opportunistic organisms, autoimmune mechanisms, and cardiotoxic drugs used by the patients. An interesting subset of patients are those who have isolated enlargement of the right ventricle [212]. AIDS patients may have marantic endocarditis but infective endocarditis is uncommon except in patients who ‘‘mainline’’ drugs. Lymphoma of the heart may occur in AIDS patients.

Autonomic nervous system function has been described in patients with AIDS [181,213]. Both the sympathetic and parasympathetic nervous systems are involved. Postural hypotension, disorders of sweating, diarrhea, impotence, and abnormal micturition develop in some AIDS patients. In others, although they do not report related symptoms, abnormalities are found on tests of autonomic function. Autonomic dysfunction can be found early in patients with HIV infection although it is more common in patients with established AIDS. Some patients with autonomic nervous system dysfunction do not have a clinically evident peripheral polyneuropathy [214]. The mechanism of the autonomic dysfunction in these patients is not known.

Leprosy

Leprosy is caused by the organism *Mycobacterium leprae*. The clinical picture is produced when the organism invades the cutaneous nerves, subcutaneous nerves, and nerves to the muscles [215,216]. The first sign of leprosy is usually a small, hypopigmented macule or papule on the skin. The disease should be suspected when the lesion has no sensation to painful stimuli. The regions of skin sensory loss may enlarge.

The lack of sensation is produced by invasion of the nerves by the leprosy bacillus. Most sensory loss in leprosy is due to involvement of intracutaneous nerves [216]. The loss of sensation is commonly found in the ears, back of hands, front and side of the thighs, and feet. Sensory loss is most severe in regions of the skin with cooler temperatures, while warm regions such as the palms and soles are characteristically spared [216]. Sweating is decreased in the affected areas. When the organisms invade larger nerves, these nerves may become enlarged. When the nerves of the arms, legs, and face are involved, large areas of sensorimotor abnormalities are produced. When the nerves of the skin are involved the skin becomes simultaneously painful and anesthetic and does not sweat. Trophic changes are quite common in the digits. Chronic longstanding leprosy is sometimes complicated by secondary amyloidosis.

Cardiovascular Findings. Autonomic fibers in the nerves to the limbs are often affected, so insensitive areas often show a loss of sweating and the distal extremities may appear cool and dusky. The autonomic fibers that lie more deeply in the body are much less often affected [216]. Cardiac denervation, postural hypotension, decreased sweating, and impaired response to the cold pressor test have all been described in patients with leprosy but are unusual [181].

Chagas' Disease

Chagas' disease is caused by infestation with the protozoal parasite *Trypanosoma cruzi*. The disease is very common in Brazil and some other parts of South America. Chronic infection causes predominantly cardiac and autonomic nervous system dysfunction. During the acute phase of infection, trypanosomes can be found in the spinal fluid. Schwann cells and satellite cells within parasympathetic ganglia show a predilection for parasitization. Resulting degeneration of host cells and parasites causes an acute inflammatory response which damages the ganglia and surrounding nerve fibers and nerve cells [217]. The autonomic nervous system involvement characteristically causes enlargement of hollow organs (achalasia, megaesophagus, megacolon, and megaureter) [217]. The peripheral nervous system is also damaged but the cardiopathy is mostly related to destruction of the parasympathetic cardiac ganglia [217]. Postural hypotension is common. Autonomic function tests including the response of the blood pressure and heart rate to tilting and the Valsalva maneuver, the sensitivity of the baroreceptor reflex, and measurements of noradrenaline show abnormal responses [181,218].

Cardiac and Cardiovascular Findings. Necropsy studies show abnormalities in the conduction system of the heart as well as in the autonomic ganglia and the myenteric plexus. The heart is usually enlarged and considerably dilated. Focal endomyocardial fibrosis and aneurysmal dilatation are often found in the apex of the left ventricule [217]. Microscopic examination of the heart shows a chronic diffuse myocarditis. Focal regions of myocardial necrosis secondary to an arteriolopathy are common. The cardiac autonomic ganglia, the intracardiac nerves, and the cardiac conduction system, including the bundle of His and its branches, are severely damaged [217]. Impressive parasympathetic devervation has always been found when ganglion cell counts are performed in patients with Chagas' cardiopathy [219]. Multifocal inflammatory lesions and demyelination are found within the peripheral nerves of humans and experimental animals exposed to the parasite [220]. The peripheral neuropathy and autonomic nervous system findings probably have an autoimmune basis [181,217].

The gross cardiac enlargement and dilatation seen in patients with Chagas' disease are mostly the consequence of a loss of autonomic nervous system heart control due to destruction of the cardiac postganglionic vagal neurons. *T. cruzi* selectively destroys these neurons [221]. The severe sympathetic/parasympathetic imbalance can lead to cardiac damage. Studies have also shown blockade of adrenergic receptors in the vascular musculature and partial denervation of the vascular walls of patients with Chagas' disease [222]. This blockade of adrenergic receptors can lead to higher levels of norepinephrine and supersensitivity to the effects of catecholamines on the heart. At the same time, the peripheral nervous system adrenergic blockade can lead to postural hypotension despite the high plasma levels of catecholamines. The cardiomypathy of Chagas' disease is likely multifactoral, with both direct myocardial damage and dysautonomia as important contributors [221].

Lyme Borreliosis

Lyme disease is caused by infection with the spirochete *Borrelia burgdorferi* [223,224]. Because peripheral neuropathy is the most common neurologic manifestation, Lyme disease is considered in this section. Lyme disease is the most common vectorborne disease in the United States, and borreliosis is also common in Europe. The disorder is transmitted by ticks; the type of tick varies according to the region of the United States or Europe where the disease is identified. Small animals are the usual reservoir for the spirochete. *Borrelia* organisms stimulate the production of proteins that are highly antigenic. The spirochetes are also aggressive and invasive. Most cases in the United States have been reported from the northeastern states bordering on the Atlantic Ocean, from the upper midwest, and from northern California. The disorder is also common in Europe, especially in Germany.

Lyme disease is often divided into three clinical stages, but the clinical manifestations vary from patient to patient. The skin, joints, heart, and nervous system bear the brunt of the infection [225,226]. Stage 1 of the illness is limited to the skin and lymph nodes. The patient may notice a localized area of erythema on the skin. The preceding tick bite may not have been noticed or recalled. Systemic influenza like symptoms may occur at the time of the erythema migrans. Regional lymphadenopathy is common. The characteristic skin lesion may precede other manifestations by weeks, months, and even years. Arthritis commonly develops sometime after the skin rash.

Neurological manifestations develop during stages 2 and 3 of the infection. The neurological syndromes and pathogenesis of Lyme borreliosis share many similarities with those caused by the spirochete of syphilis. Neurological syndromes vary; the most common are meningoencephalitis, cranial neuritis, and peripheral radiculoneuropathy [226–228]. The spirochete gains access to the nervous system by first invading the meninges. Patients report headache varying from mild to very severe. The headache is sometimes accompanied by nausea, vomiting, and photophobia. The cerebrospinal fluid at this stage shows a lymphocytic pleocytosis. The meningitic phase is often self-limited as it is in secondary syphylitic infections. In some patients, the *Borrelia* spirochetes spread to the brain, cranial nerves, brain blood vessels, spinal nerve roots, and peripheral nerves.

Brain involvement is most often subtle, causing symptoms of sleepiness, fatigue, difficulty concentrating, slight imprecision in language, and decreased memory [228]. Cranial neuropathies are also common. Isolated involvement of the seventh cranial nerve causing a peripheral Bell's-type facial palsy is most common. Some patients have involvement of multiple cranial nerves, most often nerves V to VIII. Multiple acute cranial neuropathies is a frequent presentation in Europe, where the syndrome is called Bannwarth's syndrome, after the initial describer [229].

The most common symptomatic spread of the spirochete is to the spinal nerve roots and peripheral nerves [230,231]. Lyme disease can cause acute radicular pain and paresthesias that have a root distribution closely mimicking that of

terized by pain in the lower portion of the trunk and lower extremities, usually described as diffuse aching or sharp pain in the thigh and lumbosacral region, accompanied by weakness of the lower-extremity muscles. The weakness is often asymetric and patchy, not following the distribution of any single nerve or nerve root. The knee and ankle reflexes are diminished or lost. Sensory loss is not prominent. The disorder often develops at the onset of diabetes or after its early treatment and very frequently begins after a period of weight loss. Recovery usually occurs after 6 months. Diabetic amyotrophy is caused by infarction of nerve plexi and the proximal portions of peripheral nerves [238,239]. Autonomic nervous system abnormalities are not usually reported.

Diabetic Thoracolumbar Polyradiculopathy [240,241]. This syndrome, although common, is not well known to most clinicians who are not diabetologists. The major symptom is pain in the trunk. The pain is described as burning, sharp, aching, or jabbing [240]. The anterior chest and/or the abdomen are involved but, unlike mechanical root disorders, the pain seldom radiates around the rib cage from the back. The pain and dysesthesias are usually bilateral and cover at least several thoracic nerve root dermatomes. There may be associated weakness and atrophy of intercostal, abdominal, and paraspinal muscles. Fluctuations in pain and dysesthesias are common but the disorder usually remits in 3 to 12 months. The great majority of patients with diabetic thoracolumbar polyradiculopathy also have a diabetic peripheral polyneuropathy. Despite the fact that thoracic nerve roots are involved, cardiac studies have seldom been reported in patients with this syndrome. The pain can mimic angina pectoris and be misdiagnosed as indicating coronary artery disease.

Diabetic Peripheral Polyneuropathy and Accompanying Autonomic Neuropathy [242–252]. Symmetric involvement of the distal portions of peripheral nerves is the most common neuropathic syndrome found in diabetics and often accompanies the other syndromes already mentioned. The most distal ends of the longest peripheral nerves are involved first, so the toes and feet are affected before the fingers. Motor, sensory, and autonomic nerve fibers are all often involved but any one type of involvement can predominate [242]. Sensory symptoms are most common. Numbness, lack of feeling, impaired perception of where the feet are located, "walking on a sponge," are terms often used by patients to describe the sensory abnormality. The ankle reflex is invariably lost and the knee jerk is usually diminished or lost. Significant paralysis of muscles is less common than sensory symptoms and signs, and less common than autonomic dysfunction. At times, especially in insulin-dependent diabetics, the neuropathy can be predominantly autonomic.

Peripheral neuropathy (defined by diminished or absent ankle reflexes and reduced vibration sensation in the feet) is present in about one in every four patients with established diabetes, and about 16% have evidence of an autonomic neuropathy [248]. The frequency of neuropathy increases with the duration of diabetes and both peripheral polyneuropathy and autonomic neuropathy are more common in insulin-dependent diabetics.

Cardiac and Cardiovascular Findings. Coronary atherosclerosis is greatly increased in diabetics and there is a specific type of cardiomyopathy associated with diabetes. Herein we will limit the discussion to the cardiac and cardiovascular findings that relate to the neurological abnormalities found in diabetics. Autonomic nervous system abnormalities often accompany diabetic peripheral polyneuropathy but are usually mild. Occasional patients develop a predominantly autonomic neuropathy. Autonomic nervous system dysfunction includes gastroparesis, diarrhea, resting tachycardia, orthostatic hypotension, abnormal sweating, impotence, and incomplete emptying of the urinary bladder [243–250]. Autonomic dysfunction is due to both axonal loss and segmental demyelination. Small fiber damage is manifested by impaired heart rate variability caused by vagus nerve dysfunction and by diminished peripheral sympathetic tone,which causes increased blood flow in the limbs [249]. Testing of autonomic nervous system function in patients with clinically evident symptomatic diabetic peripheral polyneuropathy very often detects abnormalities even when there are no autonomic nervous system-related symptoms. Diabetics with autonomic neuropathy have a higher than average incidence of ''silent'' myocardial ischemia, myocardial infarction, cardiac arrest, and sudden death [253]. Physicians who attend diabetic patients must be ever mindful of the occurrence of painless ischemia. It is now accepted that diabetic cardiomyopathy is a definite condition.

The prevalence of cardiovascular autonomic dysfunction in diabetics has been estimated to be about 8% in non-insulin-dependent diabetics and 16% in diabetics who are insulin dependent [250,251]. When quantitative cardiovascular autonomic testing is performed, the frequency of abnormalities is higher. Ewing et al. performed heart rate variability testing using the Valsalva maneuver, deep breathing, and standing as stimuli and showed that about 40% of the 543 diabetic patients tested had definite, often severe abnormalities [252]. Only a small proportion of patients with measurable autonomic dysfunction have clinically important cardiovascular symptoms [250].

The maintenance of systemic blood pressure on standing depends on the intactness of afferent impulses from baroreceptors in the carotid sinus and the aortic arch and on efferent sympathetic outflow to the heart and blood vessels. Postural hypotension in diabetics is mostly due to efferent sympathetic vasomotor denervation [249]. Failure to increase heart rate and cardiac output, especially during exercise, can contribute to postural hypotension [249]. Insulin has important direct cardiovascular effects, causing a reduction in plasma volume, increased peripheral blood flow due to vasodilatation, and an increase in heart rate [249]. In patients with autonomic neuropathy and in patients who have had sympathectomies, subcutaneous or intravenous injection of insulin can cause or worsen postural hypotension and lead to fainting. Syncope is also common after eating. Diabetics with autonomic neuropathy are especially apt to faint during a bowel movement after a meal.

Mortality is increased in diabetic patients who have an autonomic neuropathy [250]. In one study, among 506 insulin-dependent diabetic patients, the 5-year mortality was 27% in those who had cardiovascular autonomic neuropathy, compared to 5% in those with normal autonomic function [253]. Deaths in patients with autonomic neuropathy is mostly attributable to renal failure [250]. The nephropathy could be simply a concurrent manifestation related to the severity of the diabetes. Alternatively, the autonomic nervous system dysfunction could contribute to the kidney deterioration because autonomic dysfunction can cause increased urinary albumin excretion and increased renal blood flow. Changes in renal hemodynamics resulting from autonomic dysfunction could contribute to renal failure [250]. Sudden, unexpected cardiorespiratory arrest is the second most common explanation for death in patients with diabetic autonomic neuropathy. Autonomic dysfunction is associated with prolongation of the QT interval on the electrocardiogram. This prolongation may increase the risk of ventricular arrhythmia, especially in the presence of impaired vagus nerve parasympathetic abnormalities. Respiratory abnormalities have also been described in patients with diabetic autonomic neuropathy and could contribute to sudden death [249].

Alcohol-Related Peripheral Neuropathy

The chronic and excessive use of alcohol leads to abnormalities in almost every organ of the body, including the liver, pancreas, brain, peripheral and autonomic nerves, skeletal muscles, and heart. Many alcoholics also suffer from some degree of malnutrition. The cause of the chronic and excessive use of alcohol has been debated for decades. There is increasing evidence that there is a genetic cause of alcoholism. Because peripheral polyneuropathy is the most common neurologic problem in alcoholics, alcoholism is considered in this section.

A number of different neurologic syndromes are related to the excessive use of alcohol [254–258]. Early signs of *alcohol intoxication* are altered mood, impaired intellectual function, and limb and gait incoordination. At blood ethanol concentrations >21.7 mmol/L vestibular and cerebellar dysfunction predominate, causing nystagmus, diplopia, dysarthria, and ataxia [257]. Autonomic involvement due to intoxication can cause hypotension and hypothermia [257]. Alcohol hypoglycemia can also occur. Severe intoxication can cause stupor, then coma, then death.

Alcohol withdrawal seizures (''rum fits'') usually occur between 12 and 48 hours after a sharp decline in alcohol consumption. They can occur while still drinking but the amount of alcohol intake has declined. The seizures are grand mal and are usually one to four in number. They usually stop without treatment. Alchol withdrawal seizures are accompanied by hypomagnesemia and alkalosis [256,259]. Standard anticonvulsants are ineffective, but treatment of the low magnesium and alkalosis prevents or helps stop the seizures. Seizures in alcoholics who have had brain injuries related to head injuries or have other causes of epilepsy, may have precipitation of seizures during alcohol withdrawal; these patients should be treated with anticonvulsants.

Delirium tremens typically begins 1 to 2 days after cessation of alcohol. Patients often stop drinking because they are ill from pneumonia or gastrointestinal problems such as pancreatitis or peptic ulcer disease. The syndrome begins with tremulousness. Later hallucinations, typically visual, occur. In chronic alcoholics with past withdrawal symptoms the delusions can be predominantly auditory and persecutory. Signs of autonomic hyperactivity develop including tachycardia, sweating, hyperactivity, and increased tremulousness. Orthostatic hypotension may occur during alcohol withdrawal, probably due to altered sympathetic activity at times compounded by dehydration.

Wernicke-Korsakoff syndrome consists of four main features: oculomotor abnormalities including opthalmoplegia, vertigo, and nystagmus; short-term memory loss often with confusion; cerebellar gait ataxia; and a peripheral polyneuropathy [260]. The memory loss is often severe. Some patients with Korsakoff's psychosis never regain the ability to make new memories. The pathology of Wernicke's encephalopathy involves acute neuronal and vascular changes in the mammillary bodies and structures surrounding the cerebral aqueduct and the third and fourth ventricles of the brain. Hemorrhages are sometimes found in these regions due to capillary leakage. Deficiency of thiamine causes a diffuse decrease in the metabolism of glucose in the brain [257]. Thiamine deficiency is associated with abnormalities of cocarboxylase and transketolase, two enzymes active in the metabolism of pyruvic acid. Abnormalities in the metabolism of sugars in relation to thiamine deficiency are thought to be important in the pathogenesis of the brain lesions [260]. The onset of Wernicke's encephalopathy is sometimes precipitated by intravenous administration of glucose. Some patients with Wernicke's encephalopathy have postural hypotension [108].

Although some alcoholics show evidence of poor cognition and intellectual deterioration, the issue of whether or not there is a specific alcohol dementia is controversial. Wernicke's disease, head injury, and nutritional deprivation can all cause brain lesions that affect cognition and behavior. CT scans of chronic alcoholics often show a pattern of enlarged ventricles and dilated cerebral sulci, changes that often reverse after abstinence and improved nutritional intake [261,262]. The increased CSF fluid content found in alcoholics and its later correction is most likely due to changes in spinal fluid production and absorption and is not explained by true brain atrophy.

Some alcoholics develop a syndrome of ataxia and dysarthria due to degeneration of Purkinje cells, predominantly in the anterior and superior regions of the cerebellar vermis [263]. The gait ataxia of *alcoholic cerebellar degeneration* may develop acutely and sometimes improves after nutritional supplementation. The lower extremities and gait are involved more than the upper limbs. Speech is often dysrhythmic, poorly modulated in volume, and scanning in character.

Marchiafava-Bignami disease is a rare disorder first described in Italian red wine drinkers [264]. In this condition there is acute necrosis of the corpus callosum and adjacent cerebral white matter. The clinical picture is that of a confusional state with frontal lobe-type behavioral dysfunction and an abnormal gait. CT and MRI scans now can show the focal abnormalities in the corpus callosum and cerebral white matter [258,265].

Central pontine myelinolysis is another disorder sometimes found in alcoholics [261]. The white matter in the central portion of the pons is acutely damaged, causing weakness of all limbs, with ataxia and dysarthria. This condition is often associated with correction of hyponatremia [267,268].

Acute loss of vision has also been described in alcoholics. These patients have poor central vision and scotomas involving macular vision including the area of central vision up to and including the blind spot. This condition has sometimes been referred to as the *tobacco-alcohol amblyopia* syndrome [269,270]. The syndrome represents an acute retrobulbar optic neuropathy presumably due to nutritional deficiency.

Myopathy is also an important and underrecognized sequela of alcohol abuse. The injury to muscle cells probably represents a direct toxic effect of alcohol [257]. Both skeletal muscle and cardiac muscle are vulnerable to the toxic effects of alcohol [271]. Associated electrolyte imbalances can also exacerbate or cause muscle weakness and necrosis. Myopathy can present acutely, often in relation to a binge of alcohol drinking, and causes muscle weakness and pain, tenderness, and swelling in affected muscles [272]. Proximal limb muscles are most severely involved. Levels of muscle enzymes such as creatine kinase are strikingly elevated and there may be myoglobinuria. Chronic myopathy is also very common in alcoholics and is characterized by proximal muscle weakness and atrophy and muscle cramps [273]. The hip and shoulder girdle muscles are most severely involved. A peripheral neuropathy often coexists with the neuropathy.

Peripheral neuropathy is almost ubiquitous among chronic alcoholics. Controversy still surrounds the issue of whether the neuropathy represents a direct toxic effect of alcohol or instead is due to accompanying nutritional deficiencies. Neuropathy is often a minor clinical feature found on examination in patients admitted to the hospital with alcohol withdrawal syndrome or Wernicke's encephalopathy. In other patients, peripheral neuropathy is the major neurologic manifestation of their alcoholism.

The most common early symptom of alcohol-related neuropathy is unpleasant dysesthetic feelings in the toes and feet. Burning and stabbing feelings are described, and the feet may be extremely sensitive to stimulation. Patients often withdraw from sensory testing of the involved regions because of the unpleasant character of the burning pain induced by touching and manipulating the hyperesthetic regions. These symptoms are often referred to as the ''burning feet syndrome.'' Examination when possible shows diminished appreciation of pain, touch, and temperature in the distal portions of the lower extremities and fingers. The sensory loss is invariably distal and roughly symetrical, and fits a so-called glove-and-stocking distribution [274]. Ankle reflexes are invariably lost. The knee jerks may also be reduced. Weakness occurs only when the neuropathy is severe, but occasional patients develop a paralyzing neuropathy with severe weakness of all limb muscles. Gait ataxia is a frequent accompaniment and is probably due to a combination of loss of proprioception and degeneration of the cerebellar vermis. The neuropathy may temporarily progress even after patients stop drinking and despite nutritional and vitamin supplementation. However, the prognosis for recovery is good with prolonged abstinence from alcohol [275].

Cardiovascular Manifestations. The acute ingestion of alcohol may cause dilatation of the arterioles in the skin, tachycardia, and a drop in systemic blood pressure. Alcohol can also cause a slight decrease in cardiac ejection fraction in individuals who have normal hearts. This change in the ejection fraction does not cause any difficulty in patients with normal hearts but can contribute to left ventricular dysfunction in patients with heart disease [276].

Alcohol has the potential to produce cardiac arrhythmias in patients with heart disease and even in those with normal hearts. Atrial premature depolarizations and atrial fibrillation are the usual arrhythmias related to alcohol use. The catchy name ''holiday heart'' is often given to alcohol-related arrhythmias because the situation often involves busy individuals who overindulge in alcohol during holidays from work.

Chronic alcohol use can cause a dilated cardiomyopathy [277]. It is not always possible to blame alcohol alone for the dilated cardiomyopathy because it is not possible to eliminate myocarditis or other causes of cardiomyopathy in patients who may also consume alcohol. The fact that cardiomyopathy does not develop in all or even most heavy alcohol consumers indicates that other factors may make affected individuals susceptible to the toxic cardiac effects of alcohol. Dilated cardiomyopathy is common and is recognized more now than in the past. The condition leads to chronic congestive heart failure and all of its complications.

Patients who use alcohol and eat very poorly may develop thiamine deficiency. This may lead to beriberi, which not only causes peripheral neuropathy but also causes high-output cardiac failure in which the extremities are warmer than normal. Clinical beriberi is rarely seen today, even in patients who consume excessive alcohol and eat poorly.

Most patients with alcohol-related peripheral neuropathy do not show autonomic dysfunction. Some patients have orthostatic hypotension during alcohol withdrawal [108]. Occasional alcoholic patients with a chronic peripheral polyneuropathy have chronic postural hypotension due to sympathetic nervous system dysfunction [278]. Although sympathetic autonomic nervous system involvement in the peripheral neuropathy found in alcoholics is relatively uncommon, studies show that abnormalities of parasympathetic function are relatively common [279]. Vagus nerve involvement can affect cardiac function and contributes to hoarseness and dysphagia [279,280]. Necropsy examination of patients with alcohol-related neuropathy has shown degeneration of the vagus nerves [281]. Vagal abnormalities that occur as a result of alcoholism can reverse after several months of abstinence from alcohol [282].

Whereas small amounts of regular alcohol consumption may help prevent atherosclerosis by altering the lipid profile, the chronic use of excess alcohol increases the likelihood of developing hypertension [283]. Heavy alcohol intake probably increases the likelihood of strokes both ischemic and hemorrhagic [284,285].

Uremic Neuropathy

Peripheral neuropathy develops in the great majority of patients who have chronic uremia. Patients with acute renal failure show segmental damage to the Schwann cell–myelin sheith of peripheral nerves, and the axis cylinders and myelin sheiths of nerves are damaged in patients with chronic uremia [286–288]. The neuropathy is probably caused by toxic substances that accumulate because of the renal failure. The symptoms of uremic polyneuropathy begin in the lower extremities long before symptoms are noted in the arms [286,289]. Patients describe burning feelings in the toes and feet, itching of the legs, and the sensation of ''something crawling on the skin.'' Patients soon learn that moving the legs tends to temporarily relieve the unpleasant sensations. Sensory symptoms and signs usually predominate over motor. Position sense and vibration sense are lost in the feet and diminished at the knees and fingers. Deep tendon reflexes are lost. If untreated, uremic patients often develop a bilateral foot drop. The combination of position sense loss and foot drop creates a rather characteristic high-steppage, ataxic gait. Dialysis may stabilize the neuropathy but usually does not lead to important improvement in symptoms or signs. The neuropathy usually improves considerably after renal transplantation. An acute or subacutely developing neuropathy characterized by generalized limb weakness worsening over days or weeks, severe gait imbalance, diminished reflexes, and limb sensory loss is occasionally found in patients with severe or end-stage renal failure [290]. Seizures and a toximetabolic encephalopathy are common in chronic severe uremia if patients are not dialyzed. The encephalopathy is characterized by drowsiness, lack of interest and spontaneity, tremulousness, asterixis, and slow intellectual functioning.

Cardiovascular Findings. Pericarditis is common in patients with uremia who have signs of a polyneuropathy. It is always wise to look for other causes of pericarditis in uremic patients because nonuremic causes also occur in such patients. Unlike the symptoms of polyneuropathy, the signs and symptoms of uremic pericarditis are relieved by renal dialysis.

The chest pain of pericarditis is located in the precordial area and is made worse by inspiration. The pain may be felt on top of the left shoulder; this is attributed to involvement of the phrenic nerve. It should be emphasized, however: all patients with uremic pericarditis do not have chest pain. A loud pericardial friction rub may be heard. The rub tends to be louder when it is due to uremia than when it is due to other causes. Sometimes three components to the rub can be defined. A pericardial rub is heard when the heart moves with atrial systole, ventricular systole, and ventricular diastole. Cardiac tamponade is more likely to occur during dialysis if the patient's blood volume becomes decreased. Then, too, the use of heparin may produce abrupt pericardial bleeding and subsequent cardiac tamponade.

The electrocardiographic signs of acute pericarditis due to viral infection, collagen disease, or neoplasia are well known. The changes in the electrocardiogram can be dividied into four stages:

1. An S-T vector due to generalized epicardial injury develops. It is directed toward the anatomic cardiac apex. The T-wave vector remains normally directed. The P-R segment may be displaced.
2. The mean S-T vector may decrease in size, and the mean T vector may tend to point away from the anatomic cardiac apex.
3. The mean S-T vector may continue to decrease in size until it almost vanishes and the T wave vector becomes large.
4. The electrocardiogram may return to normal or the T-waves may remain abnormal.

The electrocardiographic signs of acute pericarditis are illustrated in Figures 8 and 9. The electrocardiographic signs of pericarditis related to uremia are seen less often than when the pericarditis is due to viral infections, collagen disease, or neoplasia.

Spodick wrote the following paragraph on uremic pericarditis in his book on the pericardium [291]. It is reproduced here with permission.

> Uremic exudates tend to be abundant, with considerable fibrin and inflammatory cells. Despite destruction of the pericardial mesothelium and gross hemorrhage, pure—that is, uninfected—uremic pericarditis is

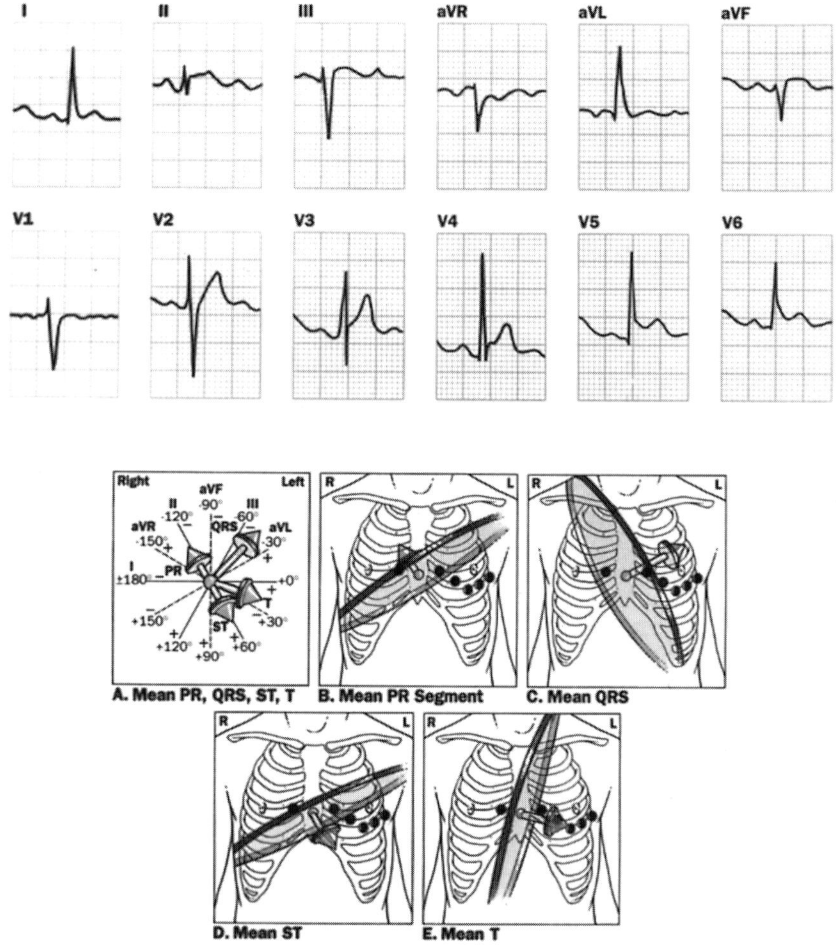

FIG. 8 Electrocardiogram in early-stage pericarditis. This electrocardiogram shows the abnormalities of stage 1 pericarditis as most often occurs with viral pericarditis. Note that the P-Q segment is displaced. The mean S-T vector is directed toward the cardiac apex. The mean T vector has not as yet changed in direction. The mean QRS vector is directed about −45° to the left and about 20° posteriorly; it is abnormal because of left anterior-superior division block that is unrelated to the pericarditis. ([*Top*] Modified from Shabetai R. The Pericardium. New York: Grune & Stratton, 1981:359. Reproduced with permission. [*Bottom*] From Hurst JW. Ventricular electrocardiography. New York: Gower Medical Publishing, 1991:10.3. Copyright, JW Hurst.)

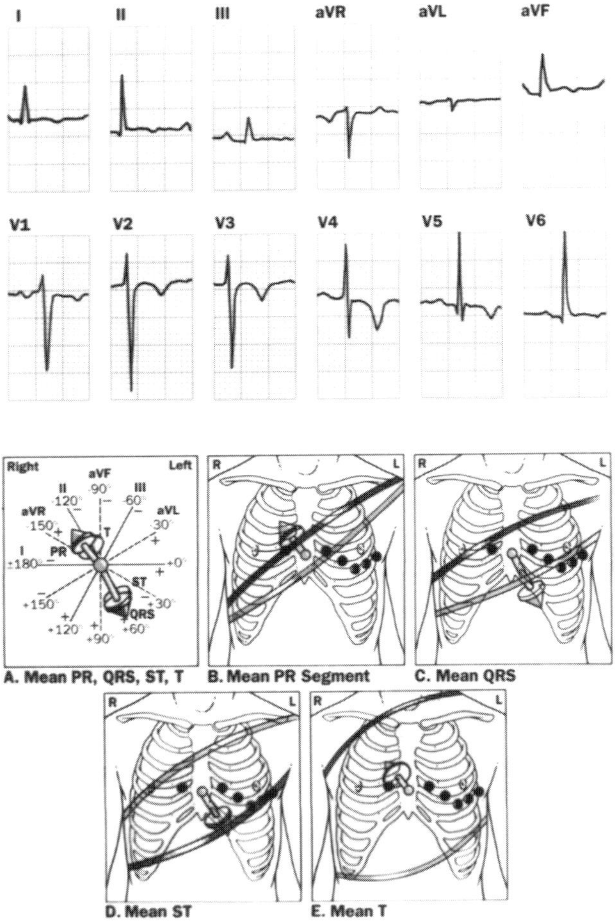

FIG. 9 Electrocardiogram of late-stage pericarditis. This electrocardiogram shows the abnormalities associated with a later stage of acute pericarditis than was illustrated in Figure 8. Note that the mean S-T segment vector is not as prominent but that the mean T-vector tends to point away from the cardiac apex. These changes are typical of those found in patients with acute viral pericarditis. (From Hurst JW, Woodson GC Jr. Atlas of Spatial Vector Electrocardiography. New York: Blakiston Company, 1952:199. Reproduced with permission. Hurst JW. Ventricular electrocardiography. New York: Gower Medical Publishing, 1991:10.4. Copyright, JW Hurst.)

gene. The most common form is caused by mutant transthyretin [292]. Transthyretin is a transport protein for thyroxin and retinol-binding protein that is synthesized in the liver and in the choroid plexus [292]. Amyloid may be found in the arteries, heart, liver, kidneys, skin, gastrointestinal system, tongue, gums, rectum, peripheral nerves, autonomic nerves, and ganglia. The anterior horn cells become abnormal and the posterior columns of the cord degenerate.

In patients with primary amyloidosis, neuropathic symptoms usually begin in the lower extrremities, and sensory symptoms are more prominent than motor. Altered feeling, loss of feeling, prickling numbness, and pain are commonly reported. Both small and large fiber sensory fibers are involved. Muscle weakness may develop later. Autonomic dysfunction is often prominent and may be responsible for the presenting complaints. Decreased sweating, postural hypotension, syncope, and impotence are common [295]. In some patients pain and temperature sensation and autonomic nervous system functions are selectively involved, and biopsies of nerves show predominant loss of unmyelinated nerve fibers. Some patients present with symptoms of carpal tunnel syndrome. Occasionally masses of amyloid involve skeletal muscles, causing muscle weakness and atrophy. Muscle biopsy in these patients shows deposition of amyloid material between muscle fibers with compression of the fibrils and loss of fibril detail.

In some familial forms of amyloidosis the peripheral nerves are involved early and neuropathy is the predominant feature. Familial amyloidotic peripheral neuropathy was first reported by Andrade, who studied a Portuguese family who developed progressive sensory loss in their limbs [296]. The disorder is often called Andrade's syndrome. The signs of polyneuropathy begin in the second and third decades of life. Death usually occurs one to two decades later. The patient notices numbness, parathesias, and pain in the legs and feet. The tendon reflexes are commonly diminished. Autonomic dysfunction leads to a loss of pupillary reflexes, decreased sweating, and postural hypotension. Vibration sense may be diminished and the patient may have difficulty walking. Late in the course of the disease, cranial nerve neuropathy may become apparent. Patients may lose their sense of taste and develop weakness of the facial muscles. Visual complaints are due to opacites in the vitreous, and deafness may develop. Transthyretin is the protein most often involved. Transthyretin (also often referred to as prealbumin) is a 127-amino acid residue single-chain polypeptide [297,298]. Liver transplantation is probably effective in halting and even reversing the disease [297,298].

There is a subset of patients with familial amyloidosis that have the carpal tunnel syndrome. These patients, often of Swiss descent, develop paresthesias of the fingertips due to nerve compression secondary to amyloid deposits in the ligaments located in the carpal tunnel. The muscles of the hands that are innervated by the median nerve become atrophic and sensation may be markedly diminished.

Another subset of familial amyloidosis was originally observed in Finland. The patients have predominately cranial neuropathy and corneal lattice dystrophy. All organs are involved in patients with this variant of the disease.

Cardiovascular Findings. Amyloidosis produces very serious cardiovascular problems. Amyloid deposits occur in all parts of the heart and may occur in the coronary arteries (Fig. 11).

Restrictive cardiomyopathy may develop in patients with cardiac amyloidosis. The ventricles are stiff and resist filling. This restrictive form of cardiomyopathy produces a clinical picture of diastolic myocardial dysfunction similar to that seen in patients with constrictive cardiomyopathy. The heart may not be enlarged or may be slightly enlarged. The external jugular veins become distended and peripheral edema develops. Orthopnea is uncommon in such patients. The right ventricular pressure curve reveals a ''square-root sign'' which is similar to the abnormality found in patients with constrictive pericarditis.

Patients with amyloidosis of the heart may also have dilated cardiomyopathy. Such patients have systolic myocardial dysfunction. These patients may also have atrial amyloidosis that limits atrial contractility. This could be referred to

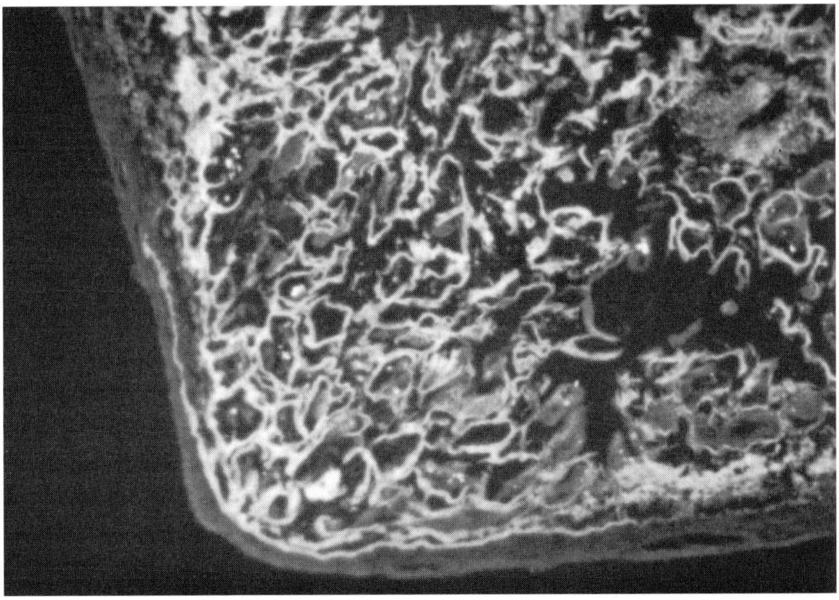

FIG. 11 Amyloid deposits in the myocardium. Thioflavine T stain examined under ultraviolent light shows interstitial amyloid deposits around individual myocytes. (Photograph courtesy of Michael B. Gravanis M.D., Emory University Hospital, Atlanta, GA.)

as atrial cardiomyopathy. Atrial thrombi may be present even when patients are in sinus rhythm; the onset of atrial fibrillation is associated with a high risk of thromboembolism [292]. The heart is larger than normal and congestive heart failure is progressive. Death commonly occurs a few months after the development of severe heart failure.

Patients with all forms of amyloidosis have postural hypotension due to autonomic dysfunction that results from amyloid deposits in autonomic nervous system fibers. Autonomic control of cardiac function as shown by radiolabeled meta-iodobenzylguanidine (MIBG) is often abnormal [299]. Patients with familial amyloid polyneuropathy show a high incidence of myocardial adrenergic denervation on MIBG radionuclide scans even before they show significant wall thickening or have abnormal technetium myocardial scanning [299].

The physical examination may show hypotension, a left ventricular diastolic gallop sound, pulsus alternans, distended external neck veins, a large V-wave in the internal jugular vein, an enlarged liver, and peripheral edema.

Cardiac arrhythmias, including atrial fibrillation and serious ventricular arrhythmias, and cardiac conduction abnormalities may be seen in the electrocardiogram. The QRS amplitude is almost always diminished and primary T-wave abnormalities are commonly found. Abnormal initial QRS forces (Q-waves) may be seen. This abnormality, which suggests a myocardial infarction due to coronary atherosclerosis, is usually due to a large area of electrically inert amyloid deposits. The intact cardiac muscle located opposite to the inert area creates the abnormal initial force. On rare occasions amyloid deposits in the coronary arteries can produce myocardial ischemia and infarction. Angina pectoris can occur in patients with amyloid cardiomyopathy, as it does in other types of cardiomyopathy, even when the coronary arteriogram is normal. The electrocardiogram of a patient with cardiomyopathy due to amyloidosis is shown in Figure 12.

The echocardiogram shows diastolic dysfunction when there is restrictive cardiomyopathy. Systolic function may be preserved in such cases, and left ventricular dilatation is rare. Left atrial enlargement may be present because of the elevated atrial-filling pressure. In a small percent of patients the chambers are dilated and systolic dysfunction is evident. The ventricles are echogenic; that is, they appear brighter than usual on the echocardiogram. A nuclear scan using technetium 99m pyrophyosphate is often positive.

Although the diagnosis is commonly made on clinical grounds, a biopsy may be needed in some patients. Biopsy of a skin lesion, gums, rectum, kidney, liver, bone marrow, abdominal fat, or the right and left ventricular endocardium may be needed.

Porphyrias and Neuropathy

The porphyrias are caused by genetically related deficiencies in enzymes related to heme synthesis. Acute intermittent porphyria (AIP) is the disorder most linked

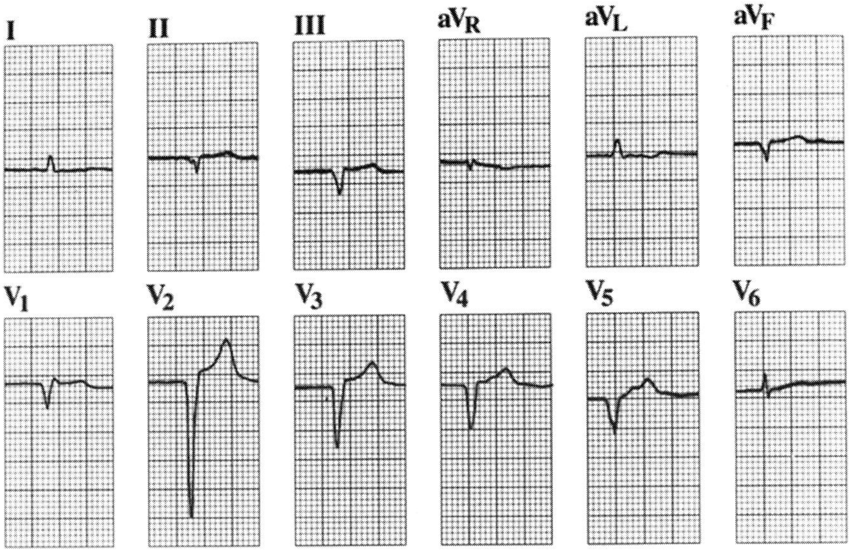

FIG. 12 Amyloid cardiomyopathy. Low voltage (amplitude) of the QRS complexes is noted. This electrocardiogram was recorded from a 69-year-old woman with restrictive cardiomyopathy due to amyloid disease. Amyloid cardiomyopathy commonly produces low amplitude of the QRS complexes, and the abnormally directed initial 0.04-second QRS vector may suggest a dead zone simulating myocardial infarction due to atherosclerotic coronary heart disease. (From Hurst JW. Cardiovascular Diagnosis: The Initial Examination. St. Louis: Mosby, 1993:300–301. Reproduced with permission.)

to neurologic dysfunction. This condition is inherited as an autosomal-dominant trait. There is an increase in production and urinary excretion of porphobilinogen related to a deficiency in the enzyme porphobilinogen deaminase; this inborn error of metabolism can be present in a latent form for long periods of time. Patients have attacks that most often include neurologic abnormalities, abdominal pain, and autonomic nervous system dysfunction.

Patients with intermittent porphyria are commonly women who have otherwise unexplained episodes of abdominal pain, severe constipation, and peripheral neuropathy. Attacks can be precipitated by starvation, infection, and certain drugs. Virtually all drugs that induce the hepatic microsomal cytochrome P450 system have the potential to precipitate attacks of AIP [300]. A history of barbiturate ingestion should increase one's suspicion because this drug, as well as sulfonamides, female sex hormones, and antiepileptic drugs commonly precipitate's attacks. The condition is diagnosed by detecting excess excretion of the porphyrin precursors porphobilinogen and alpha-aminolevulinic acid in the urine. The Watson-Schwartz test is a useful screening test for the presence of porphobilinogenin the urine. Definitive diagnosis of AIP depends on showing a decrease in porphobilinogen deaminase levels in red blood cells.

The most common features of attacks are related to autonomic nervous system dysfunction. In patients dying of AIP, acute demyelination is found in the vagus nerve and chromatolysis is found in the dorsal nucleus of the vagus in the medulla oblongata; the hypothalamus and the sympathetic chain are also involved [301–304]. Abdominal pain, often severe, is a central feature of attacks. The abdominal pain is probably caused by the autonomic neuropathy which results in an imbalance in the innervation of the gastrointestinal tract with resultant areas of spasm and dilatation. The abdominal pain is usually accompanied by constipation, and vomiting may occur. A small number of patients have diarrhea [301,304]. Other manifestations of autonomic dysfunction such as labile hypertension, postural hypotension, tachycardia, sweating, and urinary retention are often found during attacks [301,302]. Hyponatremia is common and may relate to the hypothalamic pathology [300,305].

Abdominal pain is the first symptom of an attack in about 85% of patients [301]. Abdominal pain almost always precedes the development of neuropathy. Mental symptoms including confusion and psychosis may also precede the neuropathy [306]. Some patients have severe hypertension, and may develop edema in the posterior portions of the cerebral hemispheres associated with transient cortical blindness—a posterior leukoencephalopathy syndrome [307]. Convulsive seizures may also occur [308].

The neuropathy in a full, severe attack of AIP usually develops within 2 to 3 days of the onset of abdominal pain and neuropsychiatric symptoms [300]. Back or limb pain may precede paralysis. Motor weakness is often severe and outweighs sensory abnormalities. The disease closely resembles Guillain-Barré syndrome. The weakness may be asymmetric and often begins in the upper limbs or in muscles innervated by the cranial nerves. Swallowing difficulty, facial weakness, and weakness of the tongue are common. Proximal limb muscles are affected along with distal muscles. Unpleasant migratory paresthesias are sometimes reported by patients. Progression to maximal weakness usually occurs within a few days, but the disorder can progress over weeks [300].

Patients with other hereditary porphyrin disorders (hereditary coproporphyria, variegate porphyria, and hereditary tyrosinemia) can also develop attacks with neuropathy but usually less severe than in AIP [300].

Cardiovascular Findings. AIP and the other porphyrias have not been reported to cause direct effects on the heart. The autonomic nervous system dysfunction can cause tachycardia and abnormal cardiac autonomic responses. Labile hypertension and postural hypotension are also common and are related to the autonomic neuropathy.

Lipoprotein Deficiency Disorders

Abetaliproproteinemia (Bassen-Kornsweig disease [309]). This disorder is transmitted as an autosomal-recessive trait. The serum cholesterol, triglycerides, fatty acids, and triglycerides are low, and all plasma lipoproteins containing apolipoprotein B are absent [310]. Macular degeneration and retinitis pigmentosa are common, as is acanthocytosis of the red blood cells. Malabsorption occurs because of an abnormality in the intestinal epithelium. Steatorrhea in infancy and slowness of growth are characteristic features of this disease. Children are usually small and show slow psychomotor development. The brain abnormalities are probably related to nutritional factors. The neuromuscular manifestations are the most disabling feature of the disorder. Large sensory neurons in the dorsal root ganglia and their central pathways are most heavily involved.

The tendon reflexes often disappear in early childhood, and vibratory and position sense may be absent in the lower extremities. Cerebellar abnormalities including gait, trunk, and extremity ataxia develop later [311]. Temperature and pain sensation may be lost and Babinski's sign may be present. Eye movements are also often abnormal [311]. Kyphoscoliosis and pes cavus foot deformity may develop secondary to the extensive neuropathy. The kyphoscoliosis, foot deformity, can lead to an erroneus diagnosis of Friedreich's ataxia, which shares many clinical features with abetalipoproteinemia.

Cardiovascular Manifestations. Cardiac enlargement and heart failure are serious and late manifestations in patients with abetalipoproteinemia. Malabsorption, fat-soluble vitamin deficiencies, and the lipoprotein disorders may play a role in the development of cardiovascular disease. The autonomic nervous system is usually not involved [311].

Tangier Disease. Tangier disease is inherited as an autosomal recessive condition. The patients have low serum cholesterol, low serum high-density lipoprotein, elevated triglycerides, absent or low high-density lipoprotein, and decreased phospholipids [310,311]. Cholesterol esters accumulate in the tonsils, spleen, liver, thymus, intestinal mucosa, peripheral nerves, and cornea. The presence of enlarged, yellow-orange cholesterol-laden tonsils is the most conspicuous diagnostic feature of patients with Tangier disease. Splenomegaly is common. The condition is caused by the increased catabolism of the lipids rather than a decrease in production. The disorder was named after Tangier Island, Virginia, home of the first two reported patients [312].

Peripheral neuropathy is common in patients with Tangier disease; it is sensorimotor in type and tends to fluctuate in severity. Tendon reflexes are usually lost or diminished. The sensory and motor abnormalities may be quite asymmetric. Although in some patients abnormalities can be shown on neurologic examination, patients may not have prominent symptoms [310]. The neuropathy may

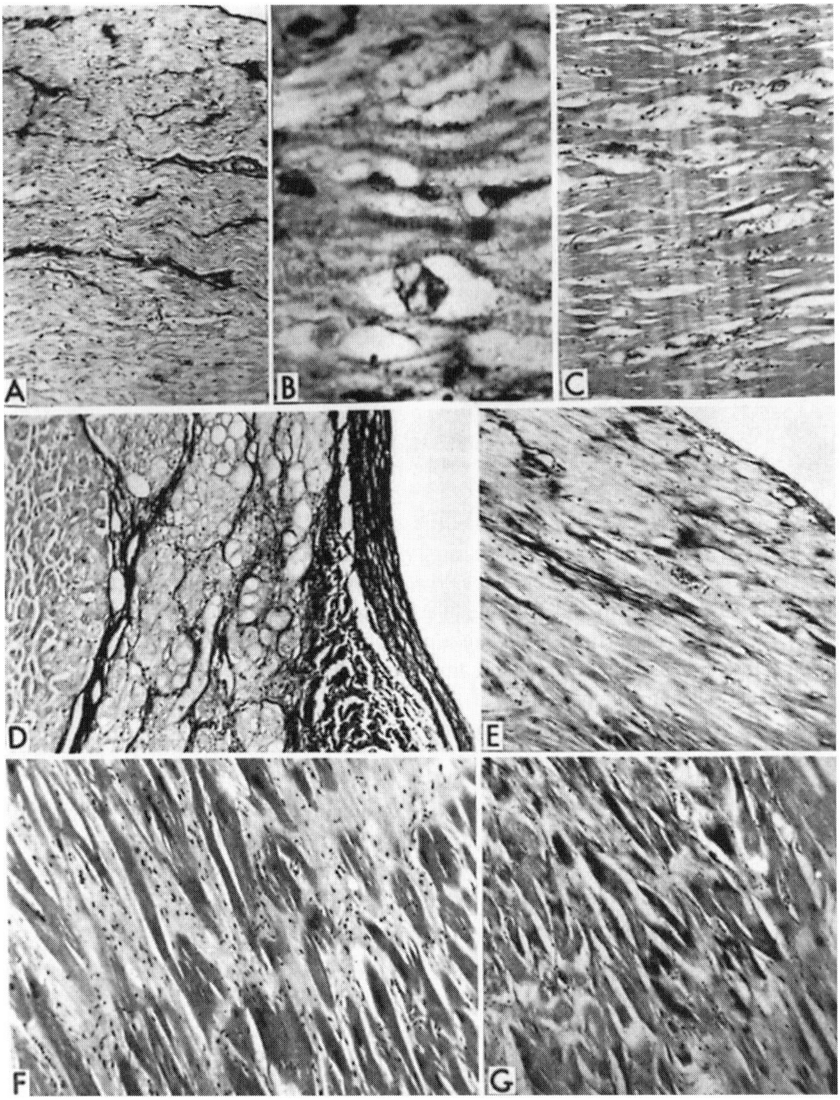

FIG. 14 Abnormalities of the atrium and ventricles in Refsum's disease. (A) and (B) Right atrial myocardium showing marked loss of structure. Transverse striations are still visible in B, but the fibers appear to be in a state of dissolution (A, ×75; B, ×565). (C) Right ventricular myocardium showing similar degenerative change (×75). (D) Left ventricle showing endocardial fibroelastosis and marked vacuolation of the subendocardial myocardium (×75). (E) Left ventricle showing replacement fibrosis and hypertrophy of surviving myocardial fibers (×75). (G) Left ventricle showing degenerative myocardium and replacement fibrosis (×75). (F) Stained by haematoxylin-eosin; all the remainder stained by elastic—van Gieson. No glycogen or excess of fat was demonstrated in the spaces which are conspicuous in several of the pictures. (From Ref. 138. Copyright, REB Hudson, 1965. Reproduced with permission.)

legs [320]. There is often a reddish-purple maculopapular skin rash concentrated near the umbilicus and in the scrotal, inguinal, and gluteal regions. Telangiectases may be prominent under the nail beds and in the oral mucosa and conjunctiva. The most important cause of disability and death is kidney disease that is caused by the gradual accumulation of glycolipid in the renal glomeruli and tubules. Strokes, hypertension, and premature myocardial infarcts are also common. Some patients have decreased sweating, corneal opacities, and peripheral edema. The peripheral edema may appear before any signs of kidney disease or hypertension and may represent lymphedema [320,321]. The major manifestation of the peripheral neuropathy is painful paresthesias.

Cardiac and Cardiovascular Findings. Lipid infiltration of the myocardium leads to a hypertrophic cardiomyopathy. There is also deposition of glycolipid in the cardiac conduction system. Occasional patients who are shown to have very low plasma levels of alpha-galactosidase activity have only heart disease manifested mainly by left ventricular hypertrophy [321a]. These patients have no other manifestations of Fabry disease. Myocardial biopsies in these patients show lysosomal inclusions in the sarcoplasma of cardiac myocytes [321a]. Mitral valve prolapse is found in more than half of patients studied by echocardiography [321,322]. The ECG often shows a shortened PR interval, and ventricular irritability is also common [323]. Arrhythmias and heart block may develop, requiring placement of pacemakers [321]. Premature myocardial infarctions occur because of the vascular disease and because of enhanced platelet aggregation [324]. The myocardial and rhythm abnormalities predispose to the formation of mural thrombi in the heart, which can be the cause of brain embolism [321].

Strokes are also very common in patients with Fabry disease [322a]. Strokes occur in relatively young patients and are predominantly ischemic. The strokes are often caused by small penetrating artery occlusive disease. The media of penetrating arteries is thickened by the deposition of glycolipid. Some patients have had dolichoectatic changes in intracranial arteries, especially involving the intracranial vertebral and basilar arteries [322a]. Deposition of glycolipid in endothelial, perithelial, and smooth muscle cells of large arteries probably leads to dilatation and tortuosity of these vessels. Blood flow in dilated ectatic arteries is often inefficient, leading to thrombus formation and poor perfusion of branches of the dolichoectatic arteries.

Other Hereditary and Familial Neuropathies

Familial neuropathic disorders are quite common. Experienced neurologists have opined often that the most important single test in patients with undiagnosed neuropathy is to examine relatives of the affected patient [325–327]. Advances in genetics and clinical and pathological studies have recently led to almost constant revision in the classification of these hereditofamilial neuropathies so that even experts in the field cannot keep pace with the complicated classification system and nomenclature. Drs. Peter Dyck and Anita Harding have been leaders in this complex field. These disorders are now customarily described as ''hereditary and sensory neuropathies'' (HMSN), and as of 1993 there were at least HMSN I–HMSN XII [325].

The first reported hereditary neuropathy and the best-known and most common disorder was described during the late 19th century and named after two very well known French neurologists—Jean Martin Charcot and Pierre Marie—and an English neurologist named Tooth. This condition is usually called peroneal muscular atrophy or Charcot-Marie-Tooth (CMT) disease. The disorder is now known to be somewhat heterogeneous and is composed of both a neuronal and a peripheral form. The conditions are inherited as an autosomal-dominant trait, but in some families the disorder is inherited as an autosomal-recessive trait. Historically, early observers sometimes linked the disease to Friedreich's ataxia because of somewhat similar clinical and pathological findings. Later, students of the disease established that Charcot-Marie-Tooth syndrome is predominantly a neuropathy and distinguishable clinically and pathologically from the disease described by Freidreich, which was a form of spinocerebellar degeneration. One variety of disease begins in late childhood and another variety begins later in life. The disease is characterized by atrophy of the muscles of the feet and legs. The muscles of the hands may become involved as time passes. Deformity of the feet and hands is characteristic of the disease; the feet develop an equinovarus deformity and the hands become clawlike. Sensation is diminished and paresthesias may be noted. The tendon reflexes are diminished. Walking eventually becomes difficult or impossible. Some patients have a very mild form of the disorder characterized by slight atrophy of peroneal innervated muscles. The condition has been divided into several types depending on the results of nerve conduction velocity studies [325].

Cardiovascular Findings. Most patients with the Charcot-Marie-Tooth forms of hereditary motor and sensory neuropathies do not have autonomic nervous system involvement. In one study, the authors found no abnormalities of cardiovascular reflexes in patients with this disorder when compared to controls [328]. Occasional patients have been reported to have paroxysmal atrial flutter [329], cardiac conduction abnormalities [330], and congestive heart failure due to cardiomyopathy [331]. However, cardiomyopathy and arrhythmias are rare in patients with this neurologic abnormality, and it may not be possible to exclude an unrelated cause.

Dejerine Sotas Disease

This is another form of hereditary neuropathy which is inherited as an autosomal-recessive trait but may also be inherited as autosomal-dominant trait [325,332].

Neuropathy begins in childhood or earlier. The first symptoms are paresthesias and pain in the feet, and then weakness of the forearms and lower legs develops. The feet and hands begin to appear clawlike. Sensation of the arms and legs may be decreased and tendon reflexes become diminished. The peroneal, ulnar, median, radial, and other superficial nerves may become sufficiently large to be felt by the examiner. The nerves, however, are not tender to the touch. The spinal cord may become compressed because the spinal roots of the nerves become larger than normal. The enlargement is due, as in other diseases in which demyelination of the nerves occurs, to the repair of demyelinated segments of nerves with connective tissue and collagen. Cardiovascular abnormalities have not been reported in patients with this form of hereditary neuropathy.

DISEASES OF MUSCLE AND THE NEUROMUSCULAR JUNCTION

Many of the conditions that affect skeletal muscle fibers also involve cardiac muscle.

Muscle Dystrophies

Duchenne Muscular Dystrophy

''Dystrophinopathy'' is now the term often used to describe allelic disorders ranging from Duchenne muscular dystrophy to patients who have only an elevation of serum creatine kinase [333,334]. Duchenne dystrophy is the second most common hereditary disease of muscle, behind only myotonic dystrophy in frequency. Until recently Duchenne dystrophy was thought to be due to a mutation of the responsible gene. Now it is known that 20% of cases may be familial and are inherited as an X-linked autosomal-dominant or -recessive trait. Males have the disease and females are carriers. The gene that is responsible for the production of dystrophin is located on the short arm of the X chromosome situated at the xp21 locus [335]. Simply stated, dystrophin is needed for the normal development of muscle cells. This type of dystrophinopathy, which occurs in one of 4000 male births, may be associated with abnormalities of neurons, skeletal muscle, cardiac muscle, and smooth muscle [336]. Some patients with Duchenne dystrophy show mild forms of mental retardation.

Although the condition is present at birth, it is usually not recognized until the male child is about 2 years old. Gowers' sign is useful in making the diagnosis; the child learns to move from the sitting position to the standing position by using his arms to climb up his legs. There is pseudohypertrophy of the calves of the legs, but the strength in the muscles is decreased (Fig. 15). Lumbar lordosis is evident and the Achilles' tendons are shorter than normal. Kyphoscoliosis may

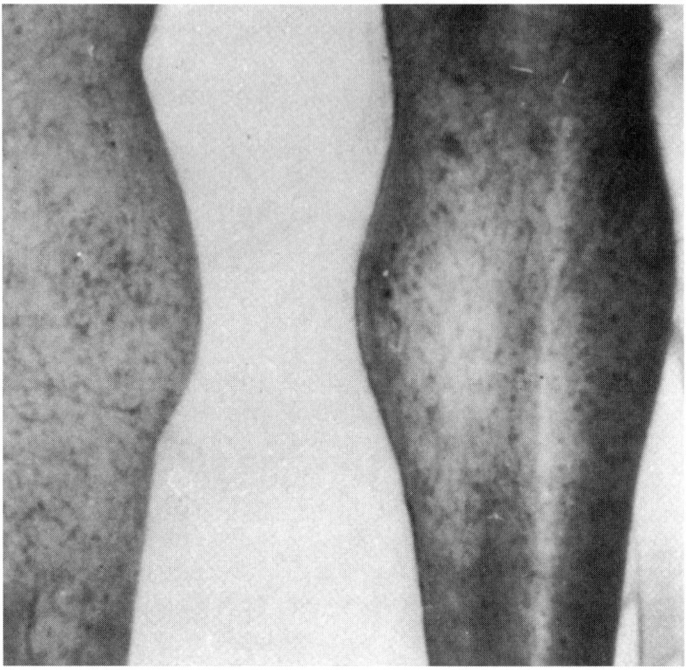

FIG. 15 Duchenne's muscular dystrophy showing pseudohypertrophy of the calves. (From Silverman ME, Hurst JW. Inspection of the patient. In: Hurst JW, Logue RB, eds. The Heart, 2nd ed. New York: McGraw-Hill, Inc. 1970:152. Reproduced with permission.)

be present. The diaphragm may be involved and this makes coughing difficult. The limbs are usually initially loose and flaccid, but later fibrosis and contractures develop. The last years of life are spent in a wheelchair, and terminally affected patients become bedridden. Patients with Duchenne dystrophy usually die in late adolescence or their early 20s, most often due to pulmonary infections, respiratory failure, and cardiac decompensation. The serum level of creatine kinase (CK) is markedly elevated in patients with Duchenne muscular dystrophy. The enzyme is elevated at birth before other signs of the disease are evident. The muscle cells obtained by skeletal muscle biopsy contain very little if any dystrophin. If any is found, it has normal molecular weight.

Cardiovascular Findings. Duchenne muscular dystrophy is commonly associated with a rather specific type of dilated cardiomyopathy (Fig. 16) [336,337]. Abnormalities of cardiac myocytes can be detected by examining biopsy material obtained from the right ventricle using an electron microscope. Presumably such abnormalities can be identified throughout the heart. Although

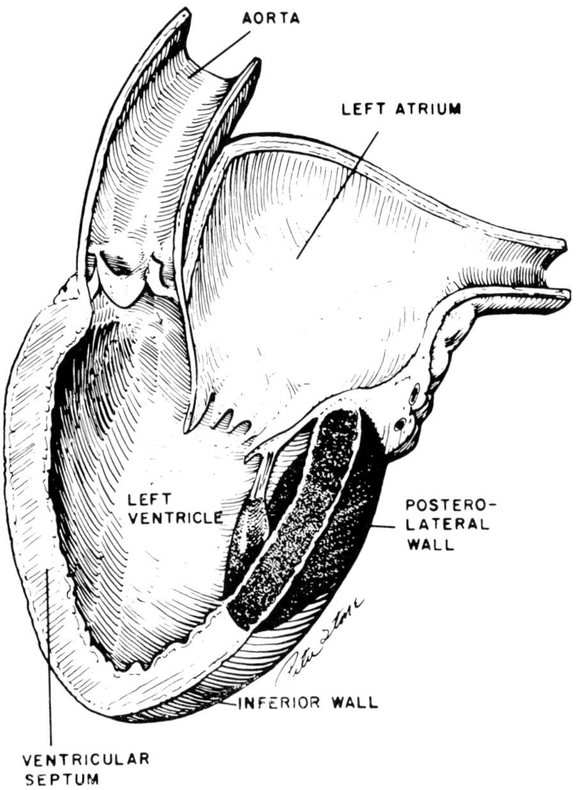

FIG. 16 Cardiomyopathy due to Duchenne dystrophy. Cartoon of the left side of the heart illustrating the distribution of fibrous scarring. The scarring was focal and limited to the posterolateral free wall of the left ventricle. No scarring was observed in the diaphragmatic or inferior free wall or in the ventricular septum, but the papillary muscle was involved. (From Ref. 337. Reproduced with permission of Dr. Joseph Perloff and the publisher.)

fibrosis may be found throughout the heart, it is located predominantly in the posterior-basilar and posterior-lateral portion of the left ventricle [337]. The posterior-lateral papillary muscle to the mitral valve may be involved. Many of the clinical manifestations of the disease are produced by the unique location of the fibrosis found in the heart [337]. Patients may complain of dyspnea on effort due to heart failure and palpitation. The physical examination is distinctive. The chest of patients with Duchenne muscular dystrophy may be distorted and the diaphragm may be located higher in the chest than usual. These two abnormalities alter the location of the heart and its normal relationship to the chest wall; the pulmonary artery and right ventricle may be adjacent to the anterior chest wall.

years of age. Severe congestive heart failure may develop late in the course of the disease [339]. Reports are now appearing that indicate that the cardiomyopathy may occur before there are obvious signs of abnormalities of the skeletal muscle [340]. Pulmonary emboli may occur, as they do in other patients who are bedridden. Cerebral emboli and emboli to the extremities and other organs may occur, as they do in other patients who have dilated cardiomyopathy and atrial fibrillation. Verapamil may produce respiratory arrest [341], and drugs used in cardiovascular medicine, such as procainamide and phenytoin, may aggravate the skeletal muscle weakness. Halothane, suxamethonium isofluron, and succinylcholine, given for anesthesia, have been reported to produce cardiac arrest [342].

Facioscapulohumeral Muscular Dystrophy

Facioscapulohumeral dystrophy (Landouzy-Dejerine dystrophy) is usually inherited as an autosomal-dominant. It is the third most common hereditary disease of muscle, superseded in frequency only by Duchenne dystrophy and myotonic dystrophy. The abnormal gene is located on chromosome 4 [343]. Virtually all patients with facioscapulohumeral dystrophy have deletions of variable size on the distal portion of chromosome 4q35 [344]. The patient, who is usually an older child or adolescent, commonly notices difficulty in raising the arms above the head [333]. The scapulae project prominently; this is referred to as ''winging'' of the scapulae. The zygomaticus muscles, obicularis oculi, and orbicularis oris muscles become weak and atrophic. The patient has difficulty closing the eyes or using the lips to whistle. The trapezius and pectoral muscles are usually involved. The upper muscles of the arms become smaller than the muscles of the lower arms. As time passes the sternocleoidmastoid and back muscles may become involved. The muscles of the pelvis may eventually become involved. Finally, the pretibial muscles may become atrophic and foot drop may develop. The condition may progress, but for unexplained reasons may cease progressing. The disease may be so mild that it is unnoticed by the patient. Mental functions are normal. The only common nonmuscular manifestations of the condition are high-frequency hearing loss and tortuosity of retinal vessels [344]. The level of serum CK is slightly elevated above normal. Although many patients do not recognize that they have the condition and the great majority of patients live a normal life span, on rare occasions the disease may occur in infants, in whom it may progress to an early death.

Cardiac and Cardiovascular Findings [345]. Labile hypertension of unknown pathogenesis may occur. Cardiac conduction abnormalities are also described. Abnormalities have been observed in the atria, atrioventricular node, and the infranodal area. Accordingly, patients may have sinus node dysfunction, atrial fibrillation or flutter, atrioventricular node dysfunction, slow junctional rhythm, all varieties of bundle branch block, and complete heart block. The cardiac rhythm disturbances are similar to, but more benign than, those seen in patients with the Emery-Dreifuss syndrome. In fact, a few patients with the Emery-Dreifuss syndrome were erroneously initially reported to have facioscapulohumeral dystrophy.

Becker's Muscular Dystrophy

Becker's muscular dystrophy occurs less often than Duchenne's muscular dystrophy and can be viewed as a milder form of Duchenne dystrophy [346]. It is an X-linked recessive condition that is carried by females and transmitted to one-half of the male offspring. An even milder form of the condition may be seen in females [346]. The condition is due to a mutation of the same gene that causes Duchenne muscular dystrophy. The Duchenne and Becker types of dystrophy can be separated by analyzing the material obtained by skeletal muscle biopsy [347]. There is very little or no dystrophin found in the skeletal muscle of patients with Duchenne muscular dystrophy. If any is found, it has a normal molecular weight. The biopsy of skeletal muscle from a patient with Becker's muscular dystrophy reveals dystrophin with an abnormal molecular weight.

The condition is characterized by weakness and pseudohypertrophy of the same muscles that are affected in Duchenne muscular dystrophy. However, the condition is much milder than Duchenne muscular dystrophy. The patient may not detect any difficulty until early adulthood, and death may not occur until after midlife. Serum creatine kinase levels are commonly 25 to 200 times normal.

Cardiac and Cardiovascular Findings. Cardiac abnormalities may occur early in life and do not correlate with the extent of skeletal muscle dystrophy [348]. Dilated cardiomyopathy due to fibrosis commonly occurs in both ventricles [349]. This leads to severe congestive heart failure [350]. Ventricular dysrhythmia may cause death. Conduction defects identified in the electrocardiogram include right or left bundle branch block, left bundle branch block with left anterior superior division block, right bundle branch block with left anterior-superior block, and complete heart block [341,352]. These conduction defects are not specific for Becker cardiomyopathy because they also occur in patients with other types of dilated cardiomyopathy. The diagnosis of cardiomyopathy related to Becker's muscular dystrophy can be made by showing abnormal immunohistochemical staining for dystrophin in endomyocardial biopsy specimens of patients with cardiomyopathy [352a].

Emery-Dreifuss Muscular Dystrophy Syndrome

The Emery-Dreifuss type of muscular dystrophy is an X-linked recessive condition [353,354]. The disease is caused by deletion of the gene encoding emerin, which is located on the X chromosome [355]. Muscle weakness is noted initially in the upper arms and pectoral girdle. The abnormality may be detected in childhood or later. Weakness may then develop in the muscles of the pelvic girdle and lower extremities. The muscles are not ''hypertrophic.'' Contractures of the flexor muscles of the elbows, Achilles' tendons, and posterior muscles of the neck may occur. The serum level of CK is moderately elevated. Several variants of the disease occur. These are clinically similar to the Emery-Dreifuss syndrome but are genetically different.

Cardiac and Cardiovascular Findings [356–358]. Myocardial fibrosis is commonly observed in patients with this condition. The most remarkable cardiac abnormality that may be found in the Emery-Dreifuss syndrome is that of atrial paralysis. Patients may also have sinus bradycardia, atrial fibrillation or flutter, slow junctional rhythm (Fig. 18), partial atrioventricular block, and complete heart block. In addition, the electrocardiogram may show conduction defects such as left anterior-superior division block and left bundle branch block. Sudden death may occur in these patients because of complete heart block and other arrhythmias.

Myocardial fibrosis may be seen in the heart on myocardial biopsy, but heart failure is not usually a major problem. Patients die of cardiac arrhythmias. As occurs with the Duchenne and Becker types of muscular dystrophy, female carriers of Emery-Dreifuss syndrome may have the cardiac rhythm abnormalities without obvious muscular dystrophy. Sudden death is also a threat to such patients.

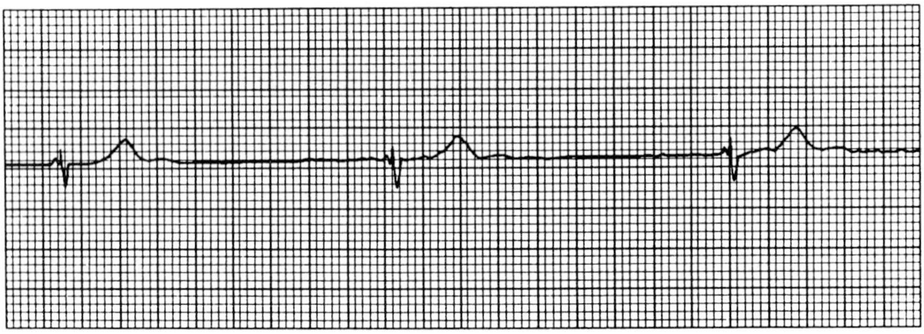

FIG. 18 This electrocardiogram was recorded from a 37-year-old man with Emery-Dreifuss syndrome. No P-waves are seen, and the ventricular rate is about 30 depolarizations per minute. Despite the installation of a pacemaker, this patient died suddenly while mowing the lawn. (Electrocardiogram courtesy of Linton Hopkins, M.D., Emory University School of Medicine, Atlanta, GA. Reproduced with permission.)

Oculopharyngeal Dystrophy

Oculopharyageal dystrophy is inherited as an autosomal-dominant trait [359]. This dystrophy involves the muscles that lift the eyelids. The other external muscles of the eyes may be affected to a minor degree. Accompanying the gradually progressive ptosis are difficulty swallowing and a change in the voice. The muscles of the pharynx and upper part of the esophagus may become weak. The condition begins in adulthood and, as times passes, the proximal muscles of the extremities may become weak. The level of serum creatine kinase is usually normal, and cardiac and cardiovascular abnormalities have not been described in this disorder.

Limb Girdle Muscular Dystrophies

There are a variety of conditions that are currently designated as belonging to the limb girdle muscular dystrophy syndromes [333,360]. They are inherited and the recessive form of the condition is the most common. Some of the patients have an X-linked inheritance. As time passes, the genetics of these conditions will undoubtedly be clarified further. The condition may be noted in childhood or early adulthood. The muscles around the hips or shoulders become weak and atrophic. The muscle weakness often is not progressive or only slowly worsens. The serum level of CK may be normal or moderately elevated.

Cardiac and Cardiovascular Findings [361,362]. The limb-girdle group of muscular dystrophies is so diverse that specific cardiac abnormalities cannot be assigned to them. Cardiac conduction defects have been described in patients diagnosed as having limb-girdle syndromes. Right and left bundle branch block, left anterior-superior division block, and left posterior-inferior division block have been reported.

Myotonic Dystrophy

This disorder is the most common adult form of muscle dystrophy and it is very distinct from all of the other conditions that are called dystrophic. The abnormal gene is located on chromosome 19g13.3 [363]. At this site there is an unstable trinucleotide sequence (cytosine, thymine, guanidine; CTG) that is larger in those affected with the disorder than in unaffected control individuals [363]. Myotonic dystrophy is one of the so-called trinucleotide repeat disorders. Inheritance is autosomal dominant with variable penetrance.

The condition is seen in adults and is known as Steinert disease. The muscles of the hands, forearms, and pretibial area may be affected as may the facial, masseter, sternocleidomastoid, and levator palpebrae muscles [364,365]. Myotonia may be apparent before the muscles become weak and atrophied. Patients report that they have difficulty letting go of objects that they have grasped. Myotonia is recognized when the relaxation phase following muscle contraction is delayed. This may be elicited by percussion of the proximal muscles of the limbs and of the tongue. A firm handshake by the patient may be sustained because of the failure of the muscles of the hand to relax. Gentle movement of the muscles, however, does not evoke the prolonged contraction. Later in the course of the disease, the muscles of the hands and forearms become weak and atrophic [364,365]. A characteristic facial expression is created when the masseter muscles become atrophic, producing a thinness to the lower portion of the face. At the same time, the neck may become smaller because of the atrophy of the sternocleidomastoid muscles. The voice begins to have a nasal tone because of the atrophy of the laryngeal and pharyngeal muscles. Myotonic dystrophy is often accompanied by several additional abnormalities, including weak uterine muscle, dilated esophagus, megacalon, weak diaphragm, cataracts, frontal baldness, testicular atrophy with its associated sequalae, ovarian deficiency, and low levels of intelligence. Diabetes mellitus is also often present. The serum level of creatine kinase may be normal or slightly elevated. Low intelligence and cognitive and behavioral abnormalities and seizures are common in patients with myotonic dystrophy, and anatomical, brain imaging, and magnetic resonance spectrosopy studies have shown a very high frequency of brain abnormalities in patients with myotonic dystrophy [366,367]. Patients with the highest number of CTG repeats have the most severe brain abnormalities [366].

The abnormalities of children of mothers with myotonic dystrophy deserve special comment. The newborn has facial paralysis. There is no myotonia. The eyelids droop and the mouth has a characteristic appearance. The infants often die a respiratory death because of weak intercostal muscles and a weak diaphragm. Those who survive to an older age are very often mentally retarded. Myotonia becomes evident and the clinical course is then similar to that for the adult form of the disease. The reasons for the different clinical manifestations in the newborn are not clear.

Cardiac and Cardiovascular Findings. The cardiac conduction system is involved more than the functional myocytes [368–370]. There may be fibrosis, fatty infiltration, and atrophy of the conduction system of the heart. The electrocardiogram may reveal partial or complete atrioventricular block, right bundle branch block, left anterior-superior division block, left bundle branch block, or right bundle branch block plus left anterior-superior division block. All types of atrial and ventricular arrhythmias may occur. The patient may die of complete heart block or ventricular arrhythmia. Dilated cardiomyopathy due to myocardial fibrosis is not as common as cardiac arrhythmias and conduction abnormalities. Therefore, heart failure is uncommon. Conduction defects are sometimes observed in the electrocardiogram of the children of mothers who have myotonic dystrophy.

Congenital and Metabolic Myopathies

Nemaline Myopathy

This is inherited as an autosomal-dominant or -recessive trait. Areas of minute rodlike structures can be seen in the striated muscles of these patients. Children with this disease have weakness of the muscles of the extremities and trunk, and the muscles are small [371,372]. In most children muscle weakness is diffuse, symetric, and nonprogressive. The facies of the children are distinctive; the face is narrow and there is a high arched palate reminiscent of the abnormality seen in patients with Marfan syndrome. Tendon reflexes are diminished or absent. Older patients sometimes develop scapuloperoneal weakness and foot drop [373]. Patients may die of pneumonia.

Cardiac and Cardiovascular Findings. There are few data regarding the cardiac involvement in patients with nemaline myopathy. The same rodlike structures may be seen in the cardiac myocytes and conduction tissue that are seen in striated muscle. Meier et al. reported that cardiomyopathy may be seen in patients with nemaline myopathy; in fact, in one report they emphasized that cardiomyopathy may be the presenting problem [374,375].

Centronuclear Myopathies

These are a group of hereditofamilial diseases having in common the central placement of cell nuclei of skeletal muscles [372]. The disease usually becomes apparent at a young age, sometimes with hypotonia and respiratory distress noted in the neonatal period. Children look frail and the skeletal muscles are diffusely weak and atrophic. Tendon reflexes are absent. Some patients have seizures, mental retardation, or psychosis. Ptosis of the eyelids is common.

Cardiovascular Findings. This disease is rare among the myopathies, and few facts are available regarding the cardiovascular system. The few data available suggest that dilated cardiomyopathy due to myocardial fibrosis and cardiac arrhythmias may occur [376,377].

Central Core Myopathy

This is another type of congenital myopathy characterized by the presence in the central portion of each muscle fiber of a dense, amorphous condensation of myofibril or myofibrillar material. Infants are usually floppy and muscles are weak from birth, especially proximal muscles. Patients with this disorder have a predilection to develop malignant hyperthermia when anesthetized. The gene for central core disease has been localized to chromosome 19q13.1, where it is tightly linked to the ryanodine receptor gene—a mutation also linked to malignant hyperthermia [378]. There is an unusual predominance of type 1 muscle fibers in this disorder [372,378]. Electrocardiograms are described as normal, and cardiomyopathy has not been common in patients with this disorder.

Desmin Storage Myopathies

In this disorder abundant electron-dense material identified biochemically as desmin accumulates under the sarcolemma and between myofibrils. The disorder is familial and both skeletal and cardiac muscle are involved. The onset can be during childhood or middle life. The muscle weakness is usually diffuse and symmetrical; proximal and distal limb muscles and muscles of the neck, trunk, and pharynx may be involved [372,379,380]. Some patients present with a nonobstructive hypertrophic cardiomyopathy as the most important clinical feature [381–383].

Glycogen Storage Disease (Acid Maltase Deficiency)

The synthesis and degradation of glycogen are controlled by different enzymes. The first such disorder described was Von Gierke's disease, a hepatic form of glycogen storage disease which was found to be caused by a deficiency of glucose-6-phosphatase. To date, seven different enzymes have been identified. This has created seven different syndromes that are classified as glycogenoses I through VII. The names of the syndromes are Von Gierke, Pompe, Illingsworth-Cori-Farber, Anderson, McArdle, Herr, and Tauri. Each of these syndromes is inherited as an autosomal-recessive trait. The McArdle and Tauri syndromes may, on rare occasions, be inherited as an autosomal-dominant trait.

An increased amount of glycogen is stored in the skeletal muscles, liver, and heart of patients with type II glycogen storage disease (Pompe's disease). This disorder has been called cardiomegalic glycogenosis to capture the prominent feature of cardiac involvement. There is a deficiency of alpha-1,4-glucosidase (acid maltase) in such patients [384,385]. The abnormal gene has been located in the distal portion of the long arm of human chromosome 17 (17q23). The heart is much less often involved in the other glycogen storage diseases, but cardiomyopathy may occur rarely in patients with type III, IV, and VI glycogen storage disease [386].

Pompe's disease (type II glycogen storage disease), in which the heart is always involved, can be subdivided into infantile, childhood, and adult syndromes. The heart, skeletal muscles, and liver may be affected in the infant with type II glycogen storage disease (Fig. 19). The skeletal muscles are weak and hypotonic and the tongue is often larger than normal. The enlarged liver may be palpated. The childhood form is associated with weakness of the proximal skeletal muscles. The large calves may suggest Duchenne muscular dystrophy, and patients may develop respiratory difficulty and death.

The adult form of the disease is characterized by an increasing degree of skeletal myopathy, including the diaphragm, and respiratory difficulty. In adults, the disorder can mimic polymyositis or limb girdle dystrophy. Skeletal muscle biopsy is diagnostic in that the enzyme, acid maltase, is absent and there is a great increase in the amount of glycogen. In addition, the location of the glycogen particles in the lysosomes is abnormal. Acid maltase is not identified in liver biopsy or in lymphocytes.

Cardiac and Cardiovascular Findings. The amount of glycogen located in the cardiac myocytes is greatly increased in the infantile type of Pompe's disease. The heart becomes hypertrophic and may become greatly enlarged (see Figure 19a and 19b). The heart has many of the features of hypertrophic cardiomyopathy [386,387]. There may be abnormal murmurs due to subaortic obstruction as well as mitral regurgitation [387].

The electrocardiogram is striking in that the QRS voltage is so large it often goes off the paper used to record it. The x-ray film of the chest may reveal a large heart. The findings on the echocardiogram as well as those found on angiography resemble the abnormalities found in obstructive hypertrophic cardiomyopathy. Heart failure and rhythm disturbances occur. These may lead to death, which invariably occurs within a year or two.

McArdle's Disease and Tauri Disease

McArdle's disease (glycogenosis type V) is inherited as an autosomal-recessive trait [388,389]. It may rarely be inherited as an autosomal-dominant trait. There is a defect in myophosphorylase. It is this defect that prevents the conversion of glucogen to glucose-6-phosphate that causes McArdle's disease. The gene for muscle phosphorylase has been localized to chromosome 11 [389]. Phosphofructokinase deficiency prevents the conversion of glucose-6-phosphate to glucose-1-phosphate. This abnormality produces Tauri disease (glycogenosis type VII), which is clinically similar to McArdle's disease.

The patient, who is most often a boy under age 15, complains of pain, stiffness, and weakness of the muscles of the extremities during exercise. The muscles contract during vigorous exercise, and the pain may last for hours after the exercise is discontinued. The symptoms do not occur when the patient is resting. During mild exercise the patient may feel fatigue and weakness, but these symptoms subside even if the mild exercise is continued. This is possible because the muscles utilize fatty acids and glucose which are provided by the increase in cardiac output [388].

During an episode the patient's urine may be dark red because of myoglo-

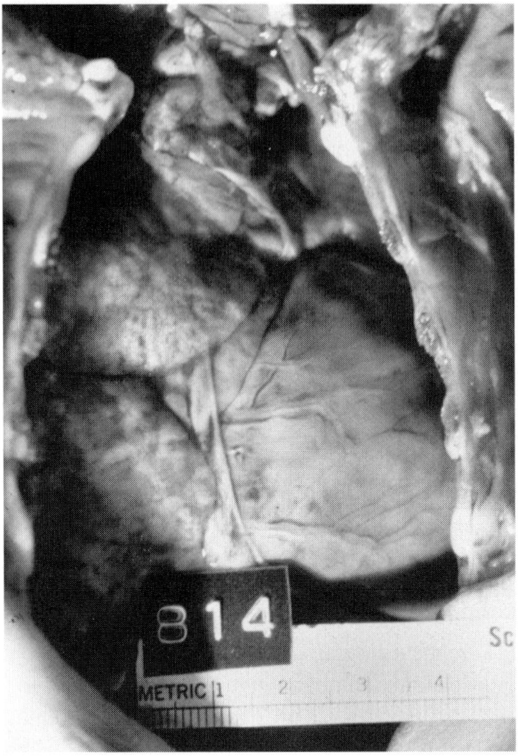

(A)

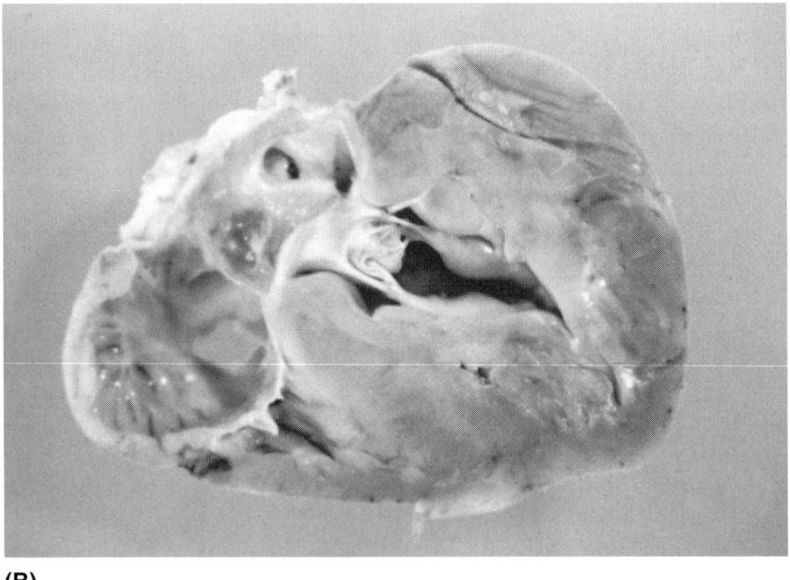

(B)

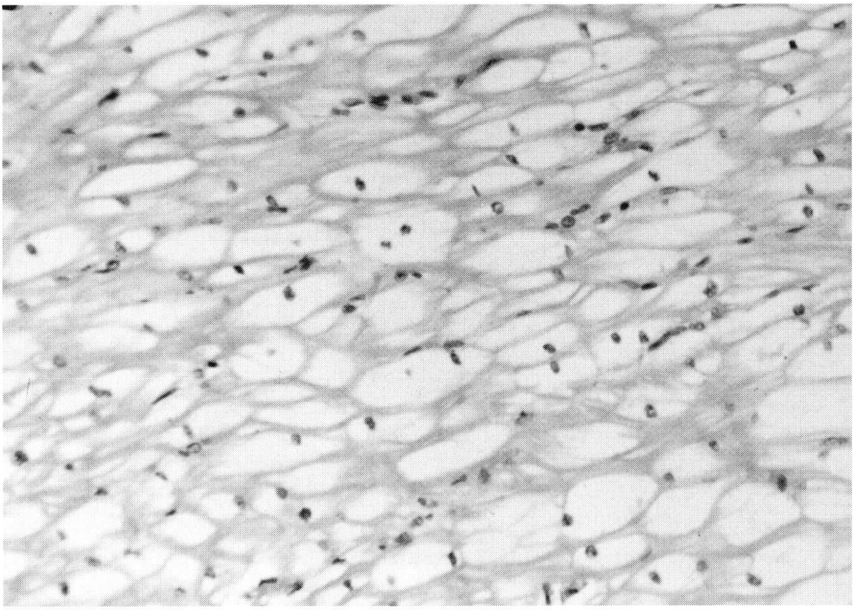

(C)

FIG. 19 Glycogen storage disease. Pompe's disease of the heart (type II glocogen storage disease). The 6-month-old patient died of progressive heart failure. (A) The heart is shown in situ. Note how large it is compared to the chest. (B) Transverse section of the heart showing a great increase in the thickness of the ventricles. (C). Microscopic section showing the lacework appearance of the myocardium. (Illustration courtesy of Dr. Carlos R. Abramowsky, M.D. Emory University School of Medicine, Atlanta, GA.)

binuria produced by the muscles during the time they are painful. The muscles of patients who have this condition do not produce lactic acid. This fact is the basis of the most commonly used diagnostic test. A blood pressure cuff is placed on the arm. The pressure in the cuff is elevated until it is higher than the systolic blood pressure. The patient then exercises the hand until the palm of the hand is white. A blood sample is obtained from the anticubical vein and analyzed for lactic acid. There is no rise in the level of lactic acid in patients with McArdle's or Tauri disease, as occurs normally. Some affected patients have a very mild form of McArdle's disease and have neither muscle cramps or myoglobinuria but merely report tiredness and lack of stamina. About one-third of patients with McArdle's disease develop some persistent proximal muscle weakness as they age. Hemolysis and severe muscle weakness have occasionally been reported in patients with Tauri disease [389]. Muscle biopsy is used to separate the two diseases. Analysis of the tissue reveals the absence of phosphorylase in McArdle disease and the absence of phosphofructokinase in Tauri disease.

Cardiac and Cardiovascular Findings. The cardiac abnormalities are commonly limited to first-degree atrioventricular block (a long P-R interval), large QRS voltage, and sinus tachycardia soon after beginning exercise [390]. An inordinate increase in respiratory rate and depth may also be apparent. Electrocardiographic abnormalities may resemble those found in other glycogen storage diseases. The amplitude of the QRS complex may be greatly increased [390].

Carnitine Deficiency Myopathies and Systemic Disorders

About 75% of carnitine (beta-hydroxy-gamma-N-trimethylamino-butyrate) comes from dietary sources, especially red meats and dairy products, and the rest is synthesized in the liver and kidneys from methionine and lysine [391,392]. After being formed, carnitine enters the bloodstream and is used to assist in the oxidation of fatty acids located in the mitochondria of muscle cells. The primary carnitine deficiency syndromes are inherited as autosomal-recessive traits. Engel and associates were the first to describe muscle carnitine deficiency associated with a progressive lipid storage myopathy [393,394]. This condition is characterized by weakness of the proximal limb muscles as well as the muscles of the trunk. The condition can appear at any age. Muscle biopsy reveals an excess in fat and a decrease in muscle carnitine. Levels of carnitine are variable in plasma and are normal in the liver and heart.

Karpati and associates described a second syndrome, characterized by systemic carnitine deficiency associated with hepatic encephalopathy and myopathy [395]. This syndrome consisted of weakness of the proximal muscles plus episodes of vomiting, stupor, and coma. Metabolic crises in these patients with systemic carnitine deficiency were associated with hepatomegaly, hyperammonemia, hypoglycemia, and elevation of liver enzymes in the blood [392].

A third syndrome of carnitine deficiency, first described by Tripp et al., was characterized by systemic carnitine deficiency associated with a progressive cardiomyopathy [396].

A fourth syndrome occurs when there is deficiency of carnitine palmitoyltransferase. This deficiency leads to an infantile form of the condition, characterized by attacks of hepatic failure with nonketotic hypoglycemia and coma.

There is another, later-onset disorder that begins in the second decade of life or later and is characterized by recurrent attacks of muscle pain often with myoglobinuria [392].

A number of diverse metabolic disorders can cause a secondary deficiency of carnitine. These conditions include: organic acidurias, which are genetic disorders of mitochondrial metabolism that cause an accumulation of nonmetabolizable organic acids in tissues and fluids; defects of the mitochondrial respiratory chain; renal Fanconi syndrome; and treatment with some drugs, for example, valproate and pivampicillin, that increase excretion of carnitine [392].

Cardiac and Cardiovascular Findings. Cardiomyopathy is often associated with hypoglycemic attacks and systemic carnitine deficiency [392,397]. Progressive dilatative cardiomyopathy can develop and progress to death [398]. Endocardial fibroelastosis may also be observed [396]. Patients with carnitine deficiency syndromes may develop congestive heart failure and die. Some students of cardiomyopathy suggest that the level of carnitine should be measured in children with cardiomyopathy because carnitine supplementation in the diet may be helpful [399]. The clinical response to carnitine dietary supplementation (2 to 6 g oral l-carnitine each day) can be dramatic in some patients. Heart function and muscle strength improve and patients stop having episodes of hypoglycemia [392].

Mitochondrial Encephalomyopathies

The abnormalities in mitochondrial diseases derive from deficiencies in the energy-producing systems of many organs [400,401]. The syndromes are diverse but have in common expression in skeletal muscle. Even when myopathy is not evident clinically, muscle biopsy specimens usually indicate the presence of a mitochondrial disorder [400]. The hallmark of mitochondrial myopathy is the so-called ragged-red muscle fiber, which contains large collections of mitochondria immediately beneath the plasmalemma and between myofibrils. These fibers are readily visible as red-staining granular deposits when Gomori trichome stains are used [400,402].

The mildest form of *mitochondrial myopathy* may cause only slight proximal muscle weakness most notable in the arms associated with exercise intolerance. At the other end of the spectrum of mitochondrial myopathies is an infantile form characterized by a fatal myopathy in which muscle weakness and lactic acidosis are found shortly after birth and prove fatal during the first year of life [401].

Other conditions now known to be due to abnormalities of mitochondrial function include: progressive external opthalmoplegia; Kearns-Sayre syndrome; subacute necrotizing encephalomyelopahty (Leigh disease); MELAS syndrome (mitochondrial myopathy, encephalopathy, lactic acidosis, and strokelike episodes) [403–406]; MERRF (myoclonic epilepsy with ragged-red fiber myopathy); NARP (neuropathy, ataxia, retinitis pigmentosa syndrome); MNGIE (myoneurogastrointestinal encephalopathy); LHON (Leber's hereditary optic neuropathy); and Alper's progressive infantile poliodystrophy [400,401]. Different disorders of molecular genetics, pathology, and respiratory chain function underlie the different clinical conditions. Undoubtedly, as advances in molecular biology and genetics occur, other neurological disorders will be identified as being related to various diverse abnormalities of mitochondrial energy production.

Space limitations prevent full discussion of each of the known mitochondrial disorders, so only brief descriptions are included herein. Patients with *progressive external ophthalmoplegia* develop progressive ptosis and weakness of their extrocular muscles usually without diplopia [400–402]. Some patients also have limb weakness. A closely related disorder is the *Kearns-Sayre syndrome*, which consists of retinitis pigmentosa with visual loss beginning before age 20, ataxia, heart block, short stature, and increased cerebrospinal fluid protein content [400,401,406]. Some patients also have sensorineural deafness seizures, and pyramidal tract signs.

Leigh's subacute necrotizing encephalomyelopathy [407] is a clinically diverse disorder characterized mainly by its distictive neuropathology. The brain shows bilaterally symmetyrical regions of spongy necrosis with myelin degeneration, vascular proliferation, and gliosis in the spinal cord, medulla, pons, midbrain, thalami, and bilateral basal ganglia. The lesions in many ways resemble those found in Wernicke's encephalopathy. Lesions in these areas are characteristically seen on MRI imaging [408,409]. Failure to thrive in infants, myoclonic jerks, seizures, respiratory difficulties, ataxia, dysarthria, gaze abnormalities, and abnormal limb movements have all been reported. This is a serious, often fatal disorder of infancy and childhood.

The *MELAS syndrome* is relatively common and distinctive [403-406]. Seizures and migrainelike headaches are common symptoms. Patients develop attacks characterized by focal neurological signs, especially visual loss accompanied by lactic acidosis. Brain imaging usually shows focal lesions in the posterior portions of the brain in the parietal and occipital lobes [404,405,408]. The lesions resemble brain infarcts. In most cases there is some resolution of the imaging abnormalities. The brain lesions are probably caused by energy failure within the brain regions, producing regions of ischemia and edema. There are no occlusions within the supplying blood vessels, so these lesions are not true brain infarcts. Loss of intellectual and visual functions often develops over years.

Leber's hereditary optic neuropathy [410–412] is becoming increasingly more commonly recognized since genetic testing of patients with visual loss has become more available. Vision is usually lost between ages 18 and 25, but the visual loss can also develop in the 30- and 40-year-old age group. Men are predominantly but not exclusively affected. The visual loss is usually gradual over weeks to months but can evolve rapidly, mimicking optic neuritis. Usually both eyes are involved together, but visual loss may begin in one eye and then later affect the other eye. The optic nerves show axonal degeneration and demyelination of the central portion of the optic nerves, optic chiasm, and optic tracts. The disorder is maternally inherited and is caused by missense mutations in mitochondrial DNA. Occasional patients also have other abnormalities, including ataxia, dystonia, peripheral neuropathy, and cardiac conduction abnormalities.

Patients with *MERRF* (myoclonus, epilepsy, and ragged red fibers) [413–415] usually first develop myoclonic jerking in childhood or early adulthood. Seizures also develop. A gradually worsening ataxia is common. Myopathy is usually mild or inapparent. Lactate levels are increased in the serum and cerebrospinal fluid. The most common genetic defect (80% of MERRF patients) is a point mutation of the mitochondrial genome at locus 8344 which codes for a transfer RNA [401,415]. MRI may show some cerebral and cerebellar atrophy [408].

The *NARP syndrome* of sensory neuropathy, ataxia, and retinitis pigmentosa is apparently due to a single mitochondrial gene mutation—the substitution of one amino acid in the mitochondrial DNA at position 8993 [401]. Patients with this syndrome may have developmental delays, seizures, and proximal muscle weakness in addition to the other findings.

The *MNGIE syndrome* is characterized by intestinal malabsorption, progressive external opthalmoplegia, generalized muscle wasting and weakness, and peripheral neuropathy [400,416]. CT may show hypointensity of the cerebral white matter. The disorder is probably due to a partial deficiency of cytochrome c oxidase (COX) activity.

Alper's disease (progressive cerebral poliodystrophy) is a disorder of infancy and early childhood characterized by seizures, failure to thrive, and developmental delays [417,418]. The disorder is progressive and usually fatal. There is spongy atrophy of the cerebral cortex and the basal ganglia and thalamus. Liver abnormalities also occur. Cortical thinning, delayed myelination, and diminished white matter are shown by MRI scans [408]. Patients with Alper's syndrome have deficiencies of cytochrome c oxidase, pyruvate cocarboxylase, and mytochondrial electron transport chain complex 1 activity [408,419].

Menkes disease (trichopoliodystrophy, or kinky-hair disease) is an X-linked recessive condition in which mitochondrial dysfunction is due to impaired intestinal absorption of copper [420]. Low copper levels lead to cytochrome oxidase deficiency. The hair is very abnormal and is coarse, stiff, and easily broken. Hypotonia, hypothermia, seizures, and failure to thrive are common. Ragged red fibers may be seen on muscle biopsy [421], and electron microscopic studies of the brain can show abnormal mitochondria. MRI studies of the brain show rapidly developing cerebral atrophy [408].

Cardiac and Cardiovascular Findings. The heart and cardiovascular system have not been investigated thoroughly in most patients with mitochondrial encephalomyopathies, so there are insufficient data at present. Because muscle and peripheral nerves are so prominently affected, cardiac muscle and conduction system pathology is likely to occur more often than has been reported. Cardiac

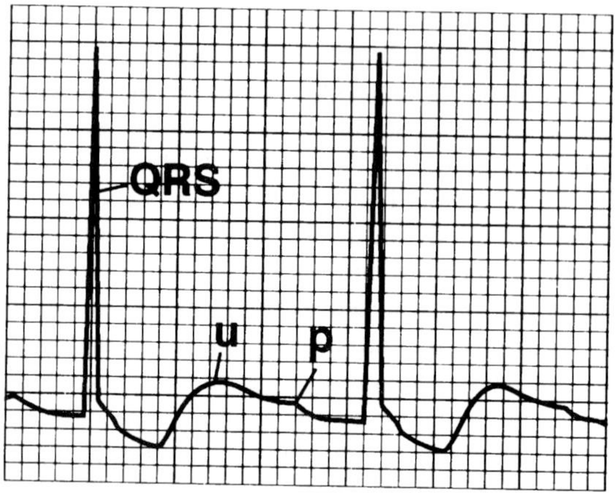

Fig. 20 This electrocardiogram was recorded from a 33-year-old male with hypokalemic periodic paralysis. There was total paralysis of his arms and legs at the time of admission. His serum potassium at the time this electrocardiogram was recorded was 1.9 mEq/L. The electrocardiogram shows a prominent wave that was considered to be a large U wave. He gave a history of previous episodes, including one in which respiratory function was markedly diminished. Episodes were sometimes precipitated by a large, high-carbohydrate meal, such as the ingestion of pizza dough. (Tracing courtesy of Dr. David Propp, Emory University. Reproduced with permission.)

malities of the sodium channel gene that underlies hypokalemic periodic paralysis. In past years, before genetic analysis of patients with the periodic paralyses became available, some of the cases reported as arrhythmias associated with hypokalemic paralysis probably had Andersen's syndrome.

Potassium-Sensitive Periodic Paralysis (Hyperkalemic Periodic Paralysis)

This disorder has been linked to a mutation in the alpha subunit of the sodium ion channel as an autosomal-dominant trait. The gene for this subunit is located on the long arm of chromosome 17 [428–430]. It is interesting to note that a small increase in serum potassium as well as a decrease in serum potassium may provoke periodic paralysis in some patients. Actually these rare patients should be referred to as being exquisitely sensitive to the level of serum potassium because periodic paralysis can occur when the serum potassium is within the normal range, elevated, or lower than normal.

Sometimes the illness is noted during infancy or early childhood. Attacks during the teens are often provoked by rest after a period of exercise. Weakness develops quickly, but attacks are milder than those seen in patients with hypokalemic periodic paralysis. The affected muscles may be painful during an attack. Other provocative factors include exposure to cold, anesthesia, sleep, and ingestion of fruit juices.

Patients with hyperkalemic periodic paralysis also often have myotonia that can be demonstrated in the muscles of the face, tongue, eyelids, and hands. One bedside test for the myotonia is to place a small towel soaked in ice water over the patient's eyes for several minutes. Eyelid myotonia is then demonstrated by asking the patient to sustain upward gaze for a few seconds and then look down. The eyelids remain up, baring the sclera above the iris in patients with eyelid myotonia [427].

Very high levels of serum potassium can also precipitate weakness in patients without the familial form of the disease. High levels are most often found in patients with renal failure and in patients who take both potassium supplements and potassium-retaining diuretics.

Cardiac and Cardiovascular Findings. The electrocardiogram may reveal a long Q-T interval. The prolongation may be due to prolongation of the T-waves and prolongation of the QRS complexes because the S-T segment duration is usually normal. The T-waves are "tent shaped." This appearance is created by the steep and equal slant of the ascending and descending limbs of the T-wave. All types of QRS conduction abnormalities can occur with hyperkalemia. P-waves may not be seen in the electrocardiogram, and serious atrial and ventricular arrhythmias may occur. Arrhythmias are not an intrinsic part of the syndrome. Previously reported cases of arrhythmias in patients with hyperkalemic periodic paralysis likely had Andersen's syndrome.

Andersen's Syndrome

Since the availability of genetic analysis of patients with the periodic paralyses, clinicians have identified a syndrome that is distinct and unique from the hypokalemic and hyperkalemic syndromes discussed above. The syndrome has been named after its initial description by Andersen [431]. A triad of findings distinguish this entity: episodic muscle weakness; distinctive facial features, often associated with abnormal fingers and toes; and prolonged QT interval on the electrocardiogram, associated with frequent arrythmias [432]. Genetic studies show that these patients do not have abnormalities of the sodium channel and do not have the chromosomal abnormalities found in the patients with hyperkalemic paralysis. The syndrome is also distinct from the other congenital long QT syndromes (Jervell and Lange-Nielsen, and Romano-Ward syndromes), which will be discussed later [432].

Patients with this syndrome have periodic episodes of weakness, usually lasting hours. Attacks can be precipitated by low potassium or high potassium; in many attacks the potassium levels are normal. Patients may have high potassium in one attack and either low or normal potassium in other attacks [432]. Dysmorphic facial appearances and limb abnormalities are a consistent part of the syndrome but vary among families. Low-set ears, broad nose, and small jaw are common characteristics of the facies. Some patients have short fingers, and clinodactyly of fingers and syndactyly of toes are common but vary among families. Hepatomegaly and cirrhosis may be detected early in infancy.

Cardiac and Cardiovascular Findings. A long QT interval is an integral part of the syndrome. Some patients have only this abnormality, but most patients have arrhythmias. Some of the patients with a long QT interval and syndactyly do not have periodic attacks of weakness [433,434]. The commonest serious arrhythmia is ventricular tachycardia. Cardiac arrest has also been described. Premature ventricular contractions and bidirectional tachycardias also occur [432].

Paramyotonia Congenita

This rare, autosomal-dominant disorder is associated with a slightly different mutation in the gene for the sodium channel alpha subunit [427]. In this condition muscle stiffness is provoked by cold. Paramyotonia is similar to myotonia in that muscles do not relax following voluntary contraction. However, in paramyotonia repetitive use of the muscles causes an increased delay in relaxation. This can be shown clinically by asking the patient to repeatedly shut the eyelids. After repeated attempts, patients with paramyotonia can no longer open the eyelids. The facial, tongue, and forearm muscles are mostly involved. Exposure to cold provokes muscle weakness, which may take time to recover even when the temperature warms. Electromyography of resting muscles at room temperature shows myotonia on percussion of the muscle or movement of the recording needle. As the muscle is cooled, low-amplitude fibrillation develops but disappears with further cooling [427]. Cardiac and cardiovascular findings have not been mentioned in this disorder.

Myotonia Congenita

This myopathy was first described by Thomsen in his own family and has often been referred to as Thomsen's disease. The disorder has been associated with an abnormality in the gene for the chloride channel, which is on the long arm of chromosome 7 [429]. Muscle stiffness is the predominant problem in patients with Thomsen's disease. After resting, muscles are stiff and may appear weak because muscles that are myotonic cannot be used with full power. With repetitive use, muscles relax and regain power. Most typically, gait appears stiff when patients first arise from a chair but with continued walking the muscles loosen up and gait normalizes. Percussion myotonia can be demonstrated and patients' muscles may hypertrophy. Electromyography confirms the presence of myotonia. Mexilitine may improve symptoms in patients with paramyotonia and myotonia congenita [427]. Cardiac and cardiovascular dysfunction has not been prominent in patients with Thomsen's disease though cardiac muscle function has not been extensively studied.

Inflammatory Myopathies

Polymyositis and dermatomyositis are now known to be conditions that share an autoimmune pathogenesis. They are each associated with an inflammatory process that is characterized by the heavy infiltration of lymphocytes. The two disorders are, however, quite different in their basic mechanisms. Dermatomyositis is mostly a disease of blood vessels, which are attacked by humoral mechanisms; in the inflammatory infiltrate around blood vessels there is a higher proportion of B cells and CD4 (helper) cells than CD8 (cytotoxic) cells [427]. In polymyositis, the inflammatory reaction is related mostly to muscle fibers which may become necrotic. In this condition there is a high proportion of CD8 cells among the T-cells found among the necrotic muscle fibers during the early phase of the disease [427]. In polymyositis the disorder is most often limited to muscle while dermatomyositis involves the skin, muscles, and often other organs. Each condition is sometimes accompanied by findings that suggest the presence of other collagen vascular diseases.

Polymyositis [427,435]

Females are more commonly affected than males. In most instances the disease develops gradually and progresses over a number of months and years, but it may begin abruptly and progress rapidly. The major symptom is muscle weakness. Muscles of the shoulder, girdle, thighs, and legs are often involved. Weakness is noted by the patient when he or she has trouble climbing stairs or performing other simple physical tasks. Pain in the muscles is sometimes noted but may be absent or minor. Sometimes the muscles are tender to palpation and may have a slightly nodular, grainy feeling. The patient may complain of difficulty swallowing; the muscles of the pharynx and upper part of the esophagus are involved in such cases. Usually the eye muscles and other bulbar innervated muscles are not affected. The deep tendon reflexes are usually reduced or absent in patients with severe weakness. The serum creatine kinase concentrations are usually elevated, sometimes to several thousand mU/mL. Diagnosis is usually established by muscle biopsy which demonstrates necrotic muscle fibers and an inflammatory response. Cardiac involvement is frequent.

Dermatomyositis [427,435]

This disorder is common in childhood but also occurs in adults. The skin lesions may appear before or after the myositis. The skin lesions consist of a heliotrope, which is a lilac-colored rash on the eyelids, nose, or some other part of the face, or on the chest, knees, or elbows. Periorbital edema may also occur. Other skin lesions include erythema, a maculopapular rash, and eczematoid dermatitis. The rash on the cheeks and elsewhere often blanches on compression. Small hemorrhages and erythema are often found in the nail beds and over the knuckles. On rare occasions calcification of the subcutaneous tissue may develop. The muscle weakness may be widespread but varies in severity. Other organs are often involved. Raynaud's phenomenon is common, and gastric and esophageal emptying are often delayed. Cardiac involvement is relatively frequent. The creatine kinase level is raised. Biopsy shows perivascular infiltrates and involvement of the connective tissue within muscles.

Neoplasms are found in more than the expected frequency in adult patients with dermatomyositis [436]. This interesting association must always be on the clinician's mind. The neoplasm may be apparent before or after the skin and muscle disease. The association of the skin and muscle disease is more often seen in older patients, those beyond the sixth decade of life. It is proper to search for commonly occurring neoplasms in the lung, gastrointestinal tract, breast, ovary, and lymphoid tissue.

Polymyositis or dermatomyositis may be associated with progressive systemic sclerosis, lupus erythematosis, polyarteritis nodosa, rheumatoid arthritis, and rheumatic fever. When more than one syndrome is present, the term "overlap syndrome" or "mixed connective tissue disorder" is often used.

Cardiac and Cardiovascular Findings in Patients with Polymyositis/Dermatomyositis

Cardiac lesions commonly occur in patients with primary idiopathic polymyositis [437]. Cardiac myocytes are destroyed, but the inflammatory response is minimal. The electrocardiogram may show conduction defects [438] and abnormalities suggesting myocardial infarcts, which may be due to myocardial fibrosis or actual infarction, and repolarization abnormalities. In one series one-third of the patients with polymyositis had ECG abnormalities. The most frequent abnormalities were left anterior superior division block and right bundle branch block [438]. The myocardial damage may be so severe that heart failure, including pulmonary edema, may occur. Pericarditis, including cardiac tamponade, has been reported [439]. When other collagen disease is associated with the skin and muscle disease, other cardiac abnormalities may occur. For example, the patient with systemic sclerosis may have progressive pulmonary arteriolar disease and pulmonary hypertension, Reynaud's phenomenon, pericarditis, and cardiomyopathy due to cardiac myocyte damage. The patient with lupus erythematosus may have pericarditis, myocardial disease, aortic valve regurgitation, and mitral valve disease.

INCLUSION BODY MYOSITIS

This disorder takes its name from abnormal structures seen within the muscle in muscle biopsy specimens. The inclusions resemble autophagic vacuoles or rimmed vacuoles [427]. Although this disease may be inherited as an autosomal-recessive or autosomal-dominant trait, it usually occurs sporadically. Inclusion body myositis occurs more often in men than women. The patient is usually a middle-aged individual who develops weakness of the lower extremities [440–442]. The hips are most often involved, but the shoulders and forearms are also affected. In some patients distal muscles are involved more than proximal muscles, an unusual pattern for a myopathy. Especially common are finger flexor and wrist extensor weakness [443]. The muscles are not painful. The knee jerk reflex is markedly diminished. Facial weakness and dysphagia sometimes occur.

The serum creatine phosphate level may be very high (>12 times normal), but in some patients the levels are normal or only slightly elevated [442]. Skeletal muscle biopsy is needed to separate the condition from polymyositis. Rimmed vacuoles and abnormal intracellular accumulation of proteins are seen in the muscle fibers, as well as mononuclear cell infiltrates [443]. Cardiac abnormalities have not been prominent, but most patients have not had thorough cardiac evaluations.

TRICHINOSIS

Trichinosis may develop after eating pork that is not thoroughly cooked. It is caused by the pork tapeworm *Trichinella spiralis*. Larvae are produced when gastric juice acts on the ingested cysts and the worms develop in the small bowel. The fertilized female enters the intestinal mucosa and produces larvae. The larvae enter the lymphatic system and bloodstream. The larvae invade all tissue but prefer to reside in the skeletal and heart muscle, where they become encysted.

The patient may have gastroenteritis beginning 1 or 2 days after eating undercooked pork. Other symptoms may begin 1 week to several weeks later. The patient may develop fever, headache, edema of the eyelids, and painful, tender muscles. Symptoms are related to the invasion of the larvae in the tongue; extraocular muscles; muscles of the neck and back; and other muscles including the diaphragm [444]. Occasional patients develop hemiplegia, aphasia, delirium, stiff neck, or coma [445]. Bilateral facial paralysis has been reported [446]. The eosinophil count may be markedly increased and the spinal fluid may reveal lymphocytosis. The skin test may become positive and a skeletal muscle biopsy may reveal the larvae. Later, the patient may develop seizures and encephalitis. These conditions are thought to be caused by larvae in the capillaries of the brain or from emboli from the heart.

Cardiac and Cardiovascular Findings. Myocarditis occurs commonly in patients with trichinosis [447]. The heart may become enlarged and pericardial effusion may be present. There may be an abundance of eosinophils and lymphocytes noted in the myocardium, but larvae are rarely seen. The myocytes appear to be degenerated and areas of necrosis may be seen. Some students of the

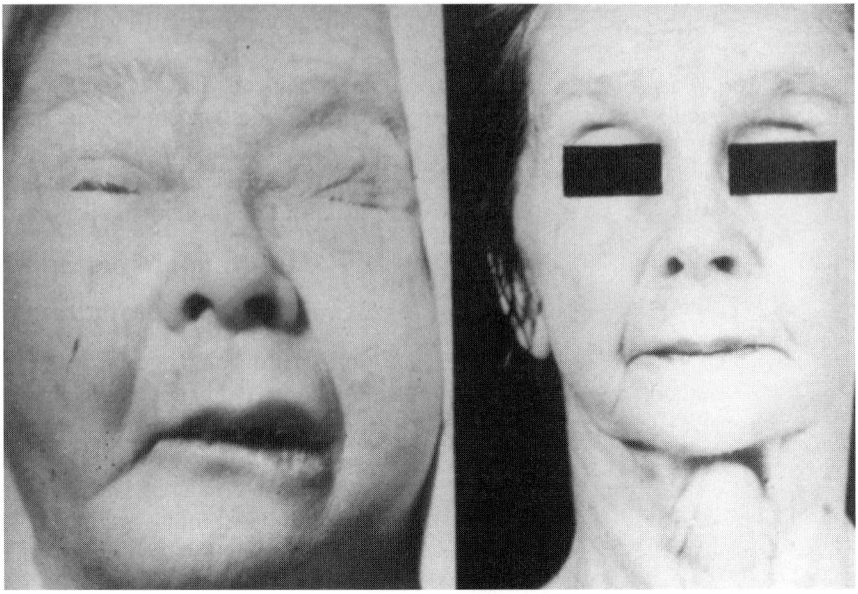

(A) (B)

FIG. 22 Facies of a patient with myxedema before and after treatment. (A) Patient in near-coma shows typical facies. (B) Some months after thyroid therapy. Pericardial effusion is common in myxedema and is the major cause of the large cardiac silhouette seen on the x-ray. (From Logue RB, Hurst JW. General inspection of the patient with cardiovascular disease. In: Hurst JW, Logue RB, eds. The Heart, 1st ed. New York: McGraw-Hill, Inc., 1966:61. Reproduced with permission.)

thetic defects, iodine deficiency, panhypopituitarism, and deficiency of thyroid-stimulating hormone [448]. The serum level of thyroid hormones is low and the level of TSH is increased. Hyperlipidemia is common in patients with hypothyroidism.

The clinical abnormalities associated with myxedema include slow speech, slow movements, a husky voice, a large tongue, dry and thickened skin, loss of the lateral aspect of the eyebrows, and slow contraction and relaxation of the muscles produced by tapping the tendon reflexes (Fig. 22). The speed of muscle contraction is thought to be related to the quantity of myosin ATPase available. The amount of this enzyme is increased in hyperthyroidism and decreased in hypothyroidism [449]. The rate of release and reaccumulation of calcium in the endoplasmic reticulum is also decreased in hypothyroidism, contributing to the slowness of muscle relaxation [449]. Hypothyroid patients often report muscle aching and muscle stiffness, and the muscles may appear larger than normal. The serum level of creatine kinase may be markedly increased.

Peripheral neuropathy and evidence of spinal cord dysfunction can also be prominent in patients with myxedema. Position sense and vibration sense are reduced in the lower extremities, and the gait may become quite ataxic. The carpal tunnel syndrome is more common in patients with hypothyroidism than in euthyroid patients. Mental functions are occasionally severely reduced in patients with frank myxedema. These patients are extremely slow and inert and apathetic. They often show poor judgment and poor memory.

Cardiac and Cardiovascular Findings. Patients with myxedema may develop an excess of pericardial fluid but cardiac tamponade does not occur. Bradycardia is commonly present and myocardial dysfunction is rare. Congestive heart failure is rare and when present should lead the physician to look for other cardiac disease. The electrocardiogram is highly suggestive of hypothyroidism when there are bradycardia and low amplitude of the P-waves and QRS complexes, a long Q-T interval, and primary T-wave changes. The low voltage may be due to pericardial effusion, a marked increase in skin resistance, or myocardial damage [450].

Hyperparathyroidism and Hypercalcemia

Hypercalcemia is usually defined as a serum calcium level >10.6 mg/dL. The most common cause for an elevation of serum calcium is hyperparathyroidism. The next most common cause is malignancy. Other causes are acute renal failure with rhabdomyolysis, thyrotoxicosis, vitamin D intoxication, milk alkali syndrome, carcinomatosis, sarcoidosis, multiple myeloma, vitamin A intoxication, Addison disease, and thiazide and lithium medication [451,452]. Determination of the blood level of parathyroid hormone is very helpful; a high serum calcium accompanied by a low blood level of parathyroid hormone rules out hyperparathyroidism. A high serum level of calcium accompanied by a high blood level of parathyroid hormone is almost diagnostic of hyperparathyroidism.

Common symptoms of hypercalcemia include fatigue, generalized weakness, constipation, polyuria, and depression. Peptic ulcer, renal stones, renal colic, and kidney failure may also develop. Dysphagia, constipation, and muscle weakness are caused by hypercalcemia-related hypotonia of smooth and skeletal muscles. Tongue tremor, hoarseness, and dysphagia are sometimes noted [453]. Hyperactive deep tendon reflexes, paresthesias and sensory loss in the pattern of a peripheral polyneuropathy, and unsteadiness of gait are other signs found in patients with hyperparathyroidism [453]. When the serum calcium level exceeds 15 mg/dL, patients often become drowsy and may even become stuporous or comatose at very high calcium levels. Hypophosphatemia, sometimes associated with bone cysts, can cause important muscle weakness. Muscle strength improves when the serum phosphate returns toward normal [449]. Removal of bone cysts may help increase serum phosphate levels and improve the myopathy [449]. Strokes and intracranial vessel vasoconstriction occasionally develop in patients with hypercalcemia [450,451].

Cardiac and Cardiovascular Findings. Hypercalcemia due to hyperparathyroidism causes the Q-T interval to shorten. The electrocardiographic signs of hypercalcemia may resemble those due to digitalis—a short Q-T interval and S-T and T-wave abnormalities. The S-T segment displacement may be so marked in some patients that myocardial infarction is suspected. The J-point in the electrocardiogram may be displaced in patients with hypercalcemia; such a J-wave may be somewhat similar to an Osborn wave [456].

There is antecdotal evidence indicating that serious digitalis intoxication occurs when digitalis is given to a patient with hypercalcemia due to any cause; life-threatening cardiac arrhythmias may occur. The anecdotal evidence is so powerful and the cardiac complications are so serious that no clinical trials have been conducted to study the problem.

Hypoparathyroidism and Hypocalcemia

Hypocalcemia is usually defined as a serum calcium level <8.5 mg/dL. Hypocalcemia may be caused by hypoparathyoidism which may be idiopathic, postsurgical, or due to acute renal failure, vitamin D deficiency, or hypomagnesemia; it also might occur in some patients with acute pancreatitis [450]. Parathyroid hormone may be deficient or it may fail in its direct action on certain body tissues. The most common symptoms are muscle cramps, carpopedal spasm, and tingling of the lips, hands, and feet. Decreased intellectual function choreic movements, seizures, psychosis, and dementia may occur.

The patient may have carpopedal spasm and a positive Chvostek's sign (tapping the facial nerve). Trousseau's sign (adduction of the thumb followed by flexion of the wrist and metacarpophalangeal joints) may be illicited by inflating a blood pressure cuff on the patient's arm above systolic pressure for 3 minutes.

Cardiac and Cardiovascular Findings. The QT interval in the electrocardiogram is commonly prolonged in patients with hypocalcemia due to hypoparathyroidism. It is the ST segment that is prolonged rather than the QRS complex or T-wave. Atrial fibrillation and ventricular arrhythmias, including torsades de pointes, may occur in patients with hypocalcemia [457]. Cardiomyopathy and heart failure have been reported in patients with hypocalcemia [458–460].

Cushing's Syndrome and Myopathy

Cushing's disease is caused by an increase in adrenocorticophic hormone (ACTH) production by a pituitary tumor. Excess adrenocortical hormones are also caused

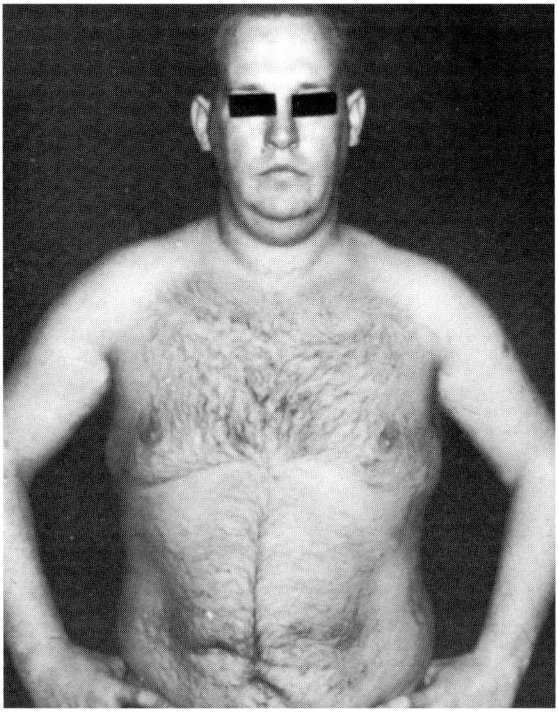

FIG. 23 Cushing's syndrome. Note the absence of typical ''moon facies.'' The striae on the lateral aspects of the upper portion of the abdomen suggest the diagnosis. (From Logue RB, Hurst JW. General inspection of the patient with cardiovascular disease. In: Hurst JW, Logue RB, eds. The Heart, 1st ed. New York: McGraw-Hill, Inc., 1966:59. Reproduced with permission.)

by cortisone-producing tumors of the adrenal gland, the ectopic production of adrenocorticotrophic hormone or corticopropin-releasing hormone, or the administration of glucocorticoids or adrenocorticotrophic hormone. Patients with Cushing's disease have hypertension, central obesity, diabetes mellitus, mental depression, loss of hair on the head, an increase in facial and body hair in women, red-purple striae, easy bruising, weakness of proximal muscles, and osteoporosis (Fig. 23). Enlargement of the pituitary gland may cause bitemporal visual-field defects and headache.

The diagnosis is usually confirmed by an elevated level of ACTH or a high level of cortisol in the blood. The morning cortisol blood level is usually >35 μg/dL. Further investigation usually includes CT and/or MRI scans of the adrenal and pituitary glands. A cortisol suppression test may be indicated. When high doses of dexamethasone suppress the level of cortisol in the blood, it suggests the presence of a primary pituitary disease.

Cardiac and Cardiovascular Findings. About 80% of patients with Cushing's disease have arterial hypertension. The P-R interval in the electrocardiogram may be shorter than average [461]. The serum potassium may be lower than normal, and this may be reflected as T-wave abnormalities in the electrocardiogram. The electrocardiogram and chest x-ray film may show left ventricular hypertrophy. Left ventricular hypertrophy and asymmetric septal hypertrophy are probably more prominent in patients with Cushing's syndrome than in patients with comparable hypertension who do not have excess adrenocortical hormone levels [461]. Carnay et al. reported the association of myxoma of the heart in patients with Cushing's syndrome. The patients also have subcutaneous myxomas and pigmented areas of the skin [462].

Adrenal Insufficiency (Addison's Disease)

Adrenal insufficiency is caused by a decrease in function of the adrenal cortex or failure of the pituitary gland to secrete an adequate amount of adrenal corticotrophic hormone (ACTH). Primary adrenocortical insufficiency (Addison's disease) is an autoimmune disease. Other causes of primary adrenocortical insufficiency include involvement of the adrenal glands with tuberculous, metastatic lesions; fungi; hemorrhage; surgical removal; acute sepsis; heparin therapy; neoplastic disease; AIDS; and drugs such as mitotane and warfarin. Adrenoleukodystrophy is a type of familial primary adrenal insufficiency in which there is demyelination of the brain, spinal cord, and peripheral nerves (see pp. 419–422).

The causes of secondary adrenal insufficiency include pituitary tumors, pituitary gland infarction, and surgical removal of the pituitary gland. The chronic use of glucocorticoid medication may cause suppression of the function of the pituitary gland and its secretion of ACTH. Other rare causes include hypoaldosteronism associated with diabetes and renal disease [463] and congenital absence of ACTH.

Patients with primary adrenal insufficiency report weakness, weight loss, fatigue, nausea, and vomiting. Encephalopathy may be responsible for coma in such patients. There is an increase in the skin pigmentation. The same symptoms develop in patients with secondary adrenal insufficiency but because of the suppression of ACTH, the skin is not hyperpigmented. Patients with secondary adrenal insufficiency due to pituitary tumor also have the neurologic and endocrine abnormalities produced by the tumor. The proximal muscles of the arms and legs, as well as the muscles of the pelvic girdle, may show considerable muscle weakness in patients who have used a large amount of corticosteroids for a long period of time.

The serum sodium may be lower than normal and the serum potassium level may be elevated above normal [464,465]. The diagnosis of primary adrenal insufficiency can be made by identifying an elevation of the serum level of ACTH and a decrease in the serum level of cortisol plus a poor adrenocortical response to the injection of corticotropin. The diagnosis of secondary adrenal insufficiency can be made when the serum levels of ACTH and cortisol are low and there is no response to ACTH secretagogs, such as insulin-induced hypoglycemia and corticotropin-releasing hormone.

Cardiac and Cardiovascular Findings [466]. The heart is smaller than usual in patients with chronic adrenal insufficiency. Patients with Addison's disease have systemic arterial hypotension. The systemic blood pressure usually decreases to even lower levels when the patient stands. The P-R interval and QT interval in the electrocardiogram may be longer than normal. Low amplitude of the QRS complexes and T-waves are common, and primary T-wave abnormalities may occur. The electrocardiogram rarely shows T-waves that are characteristic of hyperkalemia. Heart failure rarely occurs in patients with Addison's disease [466].

Acromegaly

Acromegaly is caused by an increase in the production of growth hormone by a pituitary adenoma [467]. The most common symptoms are headache, poor vision, muscle weakness, symptoms of hypertrophic arthritis, and overgrowth of bones including the mandible, hands, and feet. The facial features gradually change from almost handsome to coarse (Fig. 24). The tongue becomes large as do the parotid glands. There may be signs of kyphoscoliosis and spinal stenosis, and galactorrhea may be troublesome. The liver, kidneys, and heart are often larger than normal. There is an increase in likelihood that patients with acromegaly will develop colon polyps and cancer of the colon [468].

Diabetes mellitus may be present because of insulin resistance, and renal stones occur more often than in the general population. The serum calcium and prolactin may be elevated. The level of growth hormone in the blood should be measured 1 to 2 hours after the oral ingestion of 100 g glucose. Acromegaly is likely to be present when the growth hormone level is >10 pg/L. The insulinlike growth factor–somatomedin C is also increased in patients with acromegaly.

Common neurological manifestations include headache, spinal cord compression due to overgrowth of vertebral bones, proximal muscle weakness, and the carpal tunnel syndrome.

Cardiac and Cardiovascular Findings [468]. Many patients with acromegaly develop hypertension, and the level of renin and aldosterone are suppressed. Although the liver and kidneys may become larger than normal they continue to function normally, but not the heart. The heart is commonly enlarged

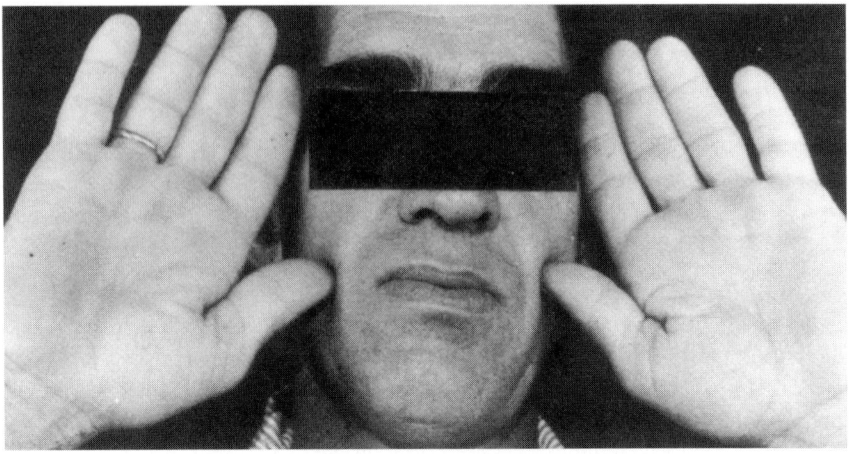

FIG. 24 Acromegaly. Note the coarse features, protruding forehead and mandible, and spadelike hands associated with hypertension. (From Silverman ME, Hurst JW. Inspection of the patient. In: Hurst JW, ed. The Heart, 3rd ed. New York: McGraw-Hill, 1974:154. Reproduced with permission.)

even when the blood pressure is normal. The excess of growth hormone affects the myocytes of the entire heart, and cardiac failure may ensue [469]. Patients with acromegaly often have left ventricular hypertrophy, increased left ventricular mass, and abnormal left ventricular diastolic function [469]. Patients with acromegaly develop coronary atherosclerosis more often than normal subjects.

Disorders That Affect the Neuromuscular Junction and Neuromuscular Transmission

Myasthenia Gravis

Myasthenia gravis is caused by an acquired immunological abnormality. Antibodies are developed against acetylcholine receptors at the motor end plate [470,471]. There is a decrease in the number of acetylcholine receptors at the neuromuscular junctions in patients with myasthenia gravis [472]. The skeletal muscles become weak with usage but their strength is restored quickly by resting. The condition is associated with thymoma in 10% of patients and with thyrotoxicosis in 5% of patients [470]. About 75% of patients with myasthenia gravis have thymic abnormalities; among these, 85% have thymic hyperplasia and 15% have thymomas [472]. Other conditions thought to be due to autoimmune disease, such as rheumatoid arthritis, lupus erythematosus, and polymyositis, seem to be associated with myasthenia gravis more often than would be predicted by chance alone [470]. This fact is used to support the contention that myasthenia gravis is an autoimmune disease.

The disease can begin at any age but most often symptoms begin between the ages of 20 and 30 years in women and at 60 to 70 years in men. The extraocular muscles and the muscles of the face, jaws, throat, and neck are the first to be involved. Weakness remains localized to the eyelids and eye muscles in about 15% of patients [472]. As time passes, the other muscles of the body become affected. This causes the patient to be unable to ''lift'' their eyelids, speak as usual, or swallow. Double vision is a very common symptom. The muscles that are used most often are generally the most often involved. When the facial and bulbar muscles are involved, a characteristic flattened smile (''snarl'') develops and patients develop a ''mushy'' or nasal speech and have difficulty chewing and swallowing [472]. The voice may become softer and more dysarthric as patients continue to speak or count. Chewing and swallowing may become more difficult toward the end of a large meal. The respiratory muscles are often weak. The muscles of the shoulder girdle, hips, and spine may be involved.

The condition may remain localized to the extraocular muscles and the bulbar muscles. The spread of weakness to other muscles usually occurs within 1 to 3 years. Remissions and relapses characterize the disease. Death occurs due to respiratory complications including aspiration pneumonia and pulmonary hypertension.

The diagnosis can often be established by the clinical findings. The eyelids are usually drooped, especially if the patient is asked to continuously look at the examiner's finger which is held slightly above the patient's gaze. The orbicularis oculi are weak and so the patient has some weakness of eye closure. (The pupils are normal.) The facial muscles and neck flexors are also weak. Intravenous administration of edrophonium often quickly but temporarily improves muscle strength. Electromyography usually documents a decremental response to repetitive nerve stimulation. Single-fiber electromyography is the most sensitive test for disorders of the neuromuscular junction [471]. This test shows an increased ''jitter'' in almost all patients with myasthenia gravis. Jitter refers to the variability in relationships of two motor units to each other. Anticholinesterase receptor antibodies are usually elevated.

A number of drugs can cause defective neuromuscular transmission and increase muscle weakness in patients with established myasthenia gravis [473]. These include antibiotics (aminoglycosides and some tetracyclines, polymyxins), d-penicillamine used to treat Wilson's disease, quinidine, procainamide, trimethaphan, propanolol, oxprenolol, practolol, phenytoin, and lithium carbonate [473].

Cardiac and Cardiovascular Findings. In 1975 Gibson reviewed the literature provoked by the controversy regarding the cardiac abnormalities seen in some patients with myasthenia gravis [474]. Some patients, especially those in whom the myasthenia is associated with thymomas, have abnormalities in the myocardium. Pathological specimens may reveal myofibrillar necrosis, inflammatory changes, hemorrhage, and lymphocytic infiltration [475]. The electrocardiogram may show conduction abnormalities. Myocardial abnormalities definitely occur but controversy centers around their cause. Gibson points out that these lesions may not be due to myasthenia because many patients have other conditions that may produce myocardial lesions including coronary atherosclerosis, electrolyte abnormalities, and iatrogenic causes [474]. However, Gibson does not deny the possibility that some of the lesions may be directly associated with myasthenia.

Pulmonary hypertension may develop as part of cor pulmonale in patients with myasthenia gravis [476]. Hypoventilation, poor diaphragmatic function, and aspiration conspire to produce lung disease and cor pulmonale.

Although the heart disease that is found in a myasthenic patient may not be directly related to myasthenia gravis, the disease should be discussed here because drugs used to treat cardiac disease and infections can worsen myasthenic weakness. Cardiac drugs such as quinidine and procainamide are anticholinergic. Accordingly, these drugs may unmask myasthenia gravis or aggravate the signs of the disease when it is known to be present. Chapter 3 contains information on drugs used to treat cardiac patients that have been known to exacerbate myasthenia.

Lambert-Eaton Syndrome

The Lambert-Eaton myasthenic syndrome (LEMS) is commonly related to neoplasia. The most common associated neoplasm is small-cell carcinoma of the lung, but the condition has been observed in patients with carcinoma of the prostate, breast, stomach, rectum, sarcoma, and lymphoma. The cancer may be known before or discovered only years after the symptoms of LEMS begin [471]. Although the condition may occur before there are signs of neoplasia, it may also occur in the complete absence of neoplastic disease. The disease is now thought to be related to an immune-mediated process directed against the voltage-gated calcium channels of muscle [477,478]. Antibodies to the voltage-gated calcium channel are found in the serum of about 75% of patients with LEMS and small-cell lung cancers. Patient with LEMS who do not have cancer more often have antibodies than patients with small-cell lung cancer. Some of the chemical markers of an autoimmune disease are commonly present.

Men are more commonly affected than women. Unlike myasthenia gravis, it is the muscles of the lower extremities, pelvic girdle, trunk, and shoulder girdle that are most affected. Weakness of the proximal muscles especially in the lower extremities is the most important finding and it usually develops gradually. In contrast to myasthenia gravis, ocular and oropharyngeal muscles are usually spared or involved to only a minor extent in LEMS.

Autonomic dysfunction also occurs [479]. The dysautonomia is mostly cholinergic [479]. Patients often report paresthesias, dry mouth, and impotence. Postural hypotension can also occur. Abnormally reacting pupils, constipation, and bladder dysfunction are occasionally reported [479]. Tendon reflexes may be diminished. Muscle strength may be increased after the first few contractions. Patients often say that they feel stronger after warming up.

The diagnosis is usually made by electromyography. Low-frequency repetitive stimulation produces a decremental response in amplitude and the area of compound muscle action potential while high-frequency repetitive stimulation causes an incremental response [480]. The response to neostigmine and pyridostigmine is not consistent. Should d-tubocurarine be injected during anesthesia, it may produce severe muscle weakness and precipitate respiratory paralysis. A muscle biopsy may show an increase in postsynaptic folds in which there are large ''clefts.'' Succinylcholine, beta-adrenergic blockers, and some antiarrhythmics such as quinidine and procainamide may worsen muscle weakness in patients with LEMS.

Cardiac and Cardiovascular Findings. There is little literature concerning cardiac abnormalities in patients with LEMS. Postural hypotension may be present. The presence of cholinergic dysautonomia predicts that there might be abnormalities of autonomic control of the heart, but such abnormalities have not be systematically sought among patients with LEMS.

Botulism

Botulism is a potentially very serious, usually foodborne illness characterized by neuroparalytic abnormalities. Foodborne botulism results from eating food containing neurotoxin produced by *Clostridium botulinum*. The disease may also result from toxin produced by the bacterium in vivo in infected wounds [481] or by colonization of the gastrointestinal tract [482]. The great majority of cases are food related. Food that is preserved at home is more likely to cause the disease than food purchased at the grocery store. There are different toxins which are usually designated as types A to F. Botulism toxins prevent the release of acetylcholine from cholinergic nerve terminal at the neuromuscular junctions of skeletal muscle and at peripheral synapses of autonomic nerves [483]. Spontaneous release of acetylcholine and release after nerve stimulation are both affected in patients with botulism [483].

Constipation, anorexia, nausea, and vomiting develop in some patients a day or two after eating contaminated food. Symptoms usually begin between 24 and 48 hours after ingestion. The first neurological symptoms usually relate to weakness of muscles innervated by the cranial nerves. The first signs of the disease are often diplopia, ptosis, strabismus, and blurred vision [484]. Symptoms and signs of cholinergic autonomic nervous system dysfunction are also prominent [484,485]. Dry mouth, blurred vision, constipation, urinary retention, and postural hypotension may occur. The pupils often do not react normally to light and may be dilated. The condition may simulate myasthenia gravis except that the pupils are reactive in the latter disease. The patient may have dysphagia, hoarseness, dysarthria, and weakness of the muscles of the trunk, limbs, and neck. After bulbar abnormalities persist, patients may develop progressive descending weakness or paralysis. Respiration may become increasingly difficult. The tendon reflexes become hypoactive or absent. The condition may be mistaken as Guillian-Barré syndrome, but muscle pain and paresthesias do not occur in patients with botulism. Sensation is retained in botulism. The spinal fluid reveals no abnormalities.

The diagnosis of botulism is confirmed by detection of toxin in the serum or stool or in food ingested before the illness began. Electromyography can also be very helpful. There is a decrease in the amplitude of the muscle action potential [483]. Maximal exercise or tetanic stimulation of nerves leads to an abnormal facilitation of the muscle action potential [483]. Most patients died prior to the development of intensive care units and antitoxin. Now, with such treatment available, the majority of the patients survive, but it remains a very serious disease.

Cardiac and Cardiovascular Findings. Cholinergic autonomic dysfunction is often present. The most common manifestation is postural orthostatic hypotension. Botulinus toxin has a direct toxic effect on the heart when given to experimental animals [486]. Abnormal T-waves and incomplete right bundle branch block have been observed in patients with botulism [486]. These changes can be related to hypokalemia but have also been noted in patients with normal electrolytes. Sudden unexpected death from cardiac arrest or ventricular fibrillation have also been described in patients with botulism [486].

SELECTED GENETIC AND HEREDITOFAMILIAL SYSTEM DISEASES THAT HAVE CARDIAC AND/OR CARDIOVASCULAR ABNORMALITIES

Friedreich's Ataxia

Friedreich's ataxia is the most common type of ataxia inherited as an autosomal recessive and accounts for at least 50% of hereditary ataxias in most large American and European series [487]. The disease is caused by a gene mutation that maps to the pericentromeric long arm of chromosome 9 [487]. The mutation consists of an unstable expansion of GAA repeats in the first intron of the frataxin gene on chromosome 9 [488]. The size of the GAA expansions determines the

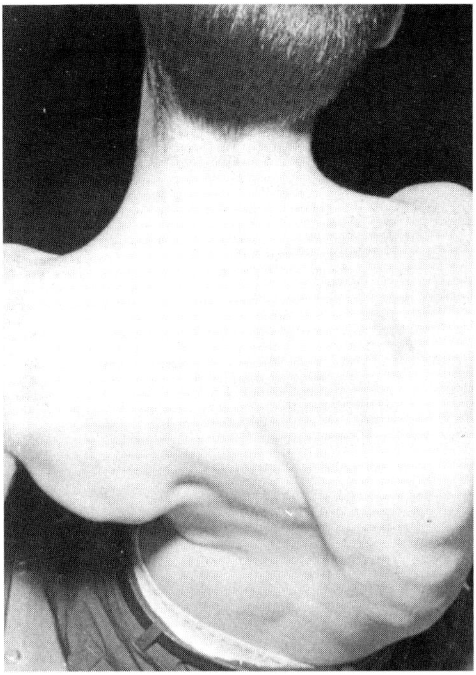

FIG. 25 Kyphoscoliosis secondary to Friedreich's ataxia. This young boy developed marked cardiac enlargement of the type seen in Friedreich's ataxia before kyphoscoliosis developed. (From Hurst JW, Logue RB, eds. The Heart: Arteries and Veins, 1st ed. New York: McGraw-Hill, Inc., 1966:69. Reproduced with permission.)

frequency of cardiomyopathy and the severity of the clinical neurological findings [488]. Necropsy examination of patients with Friedreich's ataxia shows that the myelinated fibers of the posterior columns and the corticospinal and spinocerebellar tracts of the spinal cord are greatly diminished and are incompletely replaced with gliosis [489]. The large cells in the dorsal root ganglia are often lost [487].

The age of onset of symptoms is most often between 8 and 15 years but can vary from 18 months to 25 years [487]. The first sign of the disease is ataxia. Neurologic signs gradually progress and include dysarthria, limb and gait ataxia, areflexia, pyramidal tract distribution weakness in the lower limbs, extensor plantar reflexes, and loss of joint position sense and vibration sense in the feet. About 50% of patients have distal wasting, especially in the upper limbs [487]. Unfortunately, the ataxia progresses rapidly and most patients are unable to ambulate a few years after the onset of symptoms. Kyphoscoliosis (Fig. 25) and pes cavus

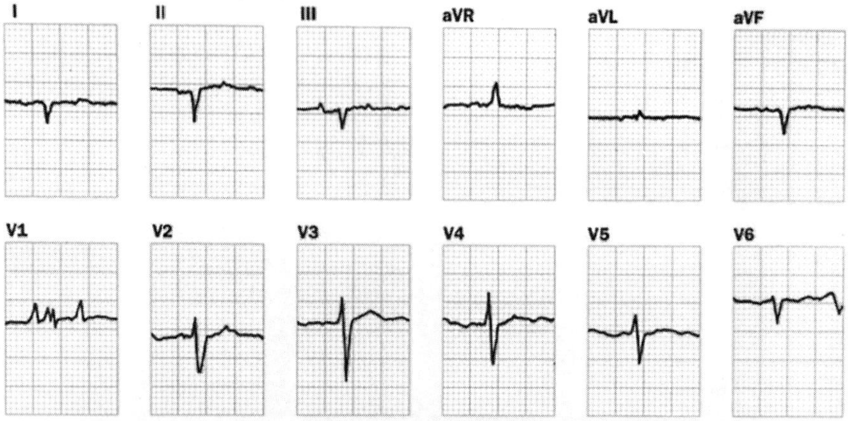

FIG. 26 Electrocardiographic abnormalities in a patient with Friedreich's ataxia. This electrocardiogram, illustrating an example of pseudoinfarction, was recorded from a 31-year-old man with Friedreich's ataxia. An atrial ectopic rhythm is present; the atrial rate is about 210 depolarizations per minute. (From Hurst JW. Ventricular Electrocardiography. New York: Gower Medical Publishing, 1991:11.33. Copyright, JW Hurst. Reproduced with permission.)

deformity of the feet may be noted before or after the neurologic abnormalities are detected.

The abnormality of gait has been characterized as both cerebellar and tabetic in type. Patients may spread their legs apart in an effort to stand but will fall if the eyes are closed. Tendon reflexes disappear but the ability to think and reason remains intact. There is a loss of proprioception in the arms and legs. Nystagmus and deafness are occasionally found. At the end of life patients are totally bedridden. On average, patients become unable to walk about 15 years after the onset of symptoms [487]. Age at death is variable but now averages in the mid-30s. Occasional patients survive into the sixth or seventh decade.

Cardiac and Cardiovascular Findings. The heart is diseased in most patients with Friedreich's ataxia. However, the severity of the heart disease does not parallel the severity of the neurologic abnormalities [490]. As a rule, the neurologic abnormalities appear long before symptoms of heart disease are apparent. Electrocardiographic (Fig. 26) and echocardiographic abnormalities are detected in almost all patients. The abnormalities noted on physical examination, electrocardiogram, and chest x-ray can be difficult to interpret when there is kyphoscoliosis.

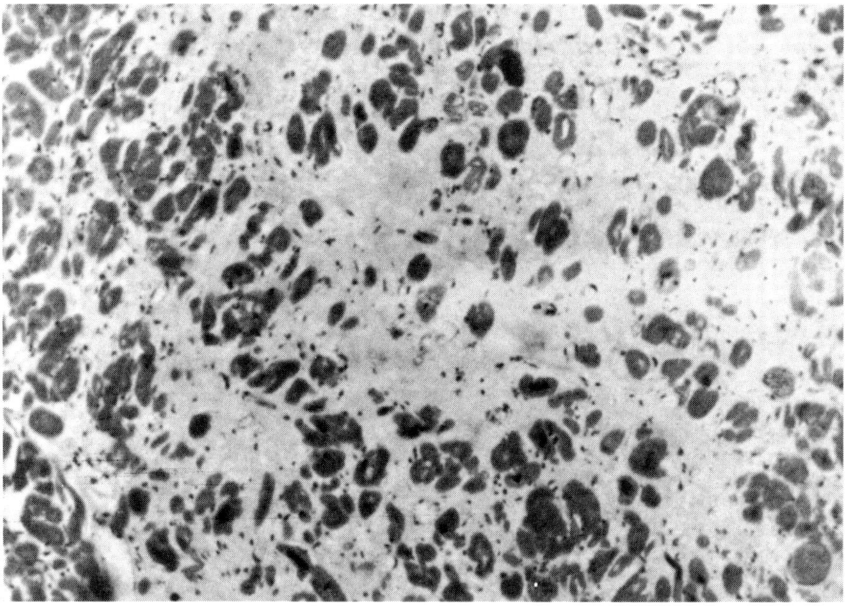

FIG. 27 Myocardial abnormalities in Friedreich's ataxia. Area of myocardium showing replacement fibrosis. Hematoxylin-eosin (×80). (From Ref. 138. Copyright, REB Hudson, 1965. Reproduced with permission.)

Two types of cardiomyopathy are found in patients with Friedreich's ataxia [491]. *Hypertrophic* cardiomyopathy can be identified by echocardiography. Asymmetric septal hypertrophy and left ventricular tract obstruction may or may not be apparent. Cardiac myocyte disarray is not usually present and ventricular arrhythmias do not usually occur [492]. These findings differ markedly from those found in isolated hypertrophic cardiomyopathy, which is also genetically predestined [491]. Cardiac function may be maintained, which is also unlike isolated hypertrophic cardiomyopathy [492]. In one study hypertrophic cardiomyopathy, most commonly concentric, was thought to be specific for Friedreich's ataxia and was found in all patients studied by echocardiography [493].

Dilated cardiomyopathy may also occur in patients with Friedreich's ataxia [491]. The functioning myocytes degenerate, as do the components of the conduction system. These cells are replaced with connective tissue and macrophages (Fig. 27). Initially, there may be generalized hypocontractility of the heart muscle even when the heart size is normal. Later, there is generalized cardiac enlargement with very poor systolic wall motion [492]. The ejection fraction becomes markedly diminished. Whereas this type of cardiomyopathy is less common in patients with Friedreich's ataxia, it is far more serious than the hypertrophic cardiomyopathy that is commonly found. The electrocardiogram is usually abnormal [494,495]. Atrial flutter and fibrillation may occur, and ventricular dysrhythmias may lead to death. The electrocardiogram may reveal conduction system abnormalities in which the terminal portion of the QRS complex is abnormally directed. Any type of conduction abnormality can occur, including uncomplicated and complicated right and left bundle branch block. The initial portion of the QRS complex can also become abnormal. Such an abnormality can be caused by a localized area of fibrosis. The vector representing the abnormal electrical force will be directed away from the inert area of myocardium. Such an abnormality is caused by the intact cardiac muscle that is located in the region of the myocardium that is opposite to the localized area of disease. Such an abnormal Q-wave may lead the clinician to misdiagnose the patient as having a myocardial infarction (see Fig. 26). Patients often die of severe congestive heart failure, cardiac arrhythmia, or pulmonary dysfunction.

Ataxia Telangiectasia

Ataxia telangiectasia is often referred to as the Louis-Bar syndrome, after Madame Louis-Bar, who described the first cases. The condition is an autosomal-recessively inherited disorder in which the gene locus maps to chromosome 11q [487]. The initial descriptions were those of an early-life ataxic syndrome in children who were usually mentally retarded. It is now recognized that this disorder is a multisystem disease that includes variable immunodeficiency of both the cellular and humoral immune systems [496]. Patients have a markedly increased frequency of developing various neoplasms.

Motor development is usually delayed, and ataxia is usually noted when the children first begin walking. Growth and sexual development are delayed and most patients have mild mental retardation [487]. The patients have difficulty moving their eyes conjugately at will. The face is described as having an impassive appearance, and drooling and a slow slurred voice are common findings. Motor abnormalities include dystonic postures, choreic movements, and limb and gait ataxia. Telangiectases are found on the skin and conjunctiva [487]. Necropsy shows a severe loss of Purkinje cells in the cerebellum, and degeneration of the posterior columns in the spinal cord.

Patients are quite sensitive to ionized radiation and some drugs [496]. Recurrent infections are a major clinical feature of the disease. Bronchiectasis and recurrent pulmonary infections are common and are due to the immunodeficiency. About 10% of patients with ataxia telangiectasia develop neoplasms, which occur in 80% before the age of 15 [496]. The commonest neoplasms are non-Hodgkin's lymphoma and lymphocytic leukemia [496].

Cardiac and Cardiovascular Findings. Cor pulmonale can develop in relation to the chronic bronchopulmonary infections. Cardiac neoplasms have not been described. Cardiac and cardiovascular abnormalities have not been reported in patients with ataxia telangiectasia, but these have not been sought or studied systematically.

Neurofibromatosis

The term neurofibromatous is now applied to two genetically different disorders. Neurofibromatosis I (NF-I) (von Recklinghausen's disease) is inherited as an autosomal-dominant trait and is the most common genetically transmitted disorder affecting the nervous system [497]. The gene locus for NF-I is chromosomal region 17q11.2 [497].

NF-I is characterized by café-au-lait spots on the skin, neurofibromas, schwannomas, and optic nerve tumors [497,498]. The café-au-lait skin spots are noted after infancy and gradually increase in number during the first decade of life. Axillary and inguinal freckles, usually about 2 to 3 mm in diameter, are also important markers of the disease. Neurofibromas of the peripheral nerves are detected as pedunculated subcutaneous nodules (Fig. 28). Vascular nevi and an excess of hair in the sacral area may be present. Lisch nodules are pigmented hamartomas of the iris that are characteristic of NF-I. All adult patients with NF-I have these nodules by age 65, and half have them by age 29 [497]. Neurofibromas may also involve the central nervous system, and meningiomas, schwannomas, and gliomas, as well as other brain tumors, may occur. Patients with NF-I may have decreased hearing but do not develop acoustic nerve tumors [498]. Optic nerve tumors are the most common of the intracranial tumors. Neurofibromas may also involve the viscera and autonomic ganglia. Pheochromocytomas develop in about 1% of patients with NF-I. Neurofibromas secrete norepinephrine, which must be kept in mind when searching for a pheochromocytoma in such patients [499]. Ganglioneuromas, carotid glomus tumors, Wilms' tumors, leukemia, and rhabdomyosarcomas are more common in patients with NF-I than in the general population. Gastrointestinal neurofibromas are especially common and occur most often in the jejunum and stomach but may be multiple [500]. Mental retardation, congenital absence of the greater wing of the sphenoid bone, and pseudoarthrosis of the tibia and radius are other features of NF-I. Nerve growth factor activity is increased in patients with NF-I [501], and the genetic disorder is linked to the nerve growth factor receptor on the distal long arm of chromosome 17 [498].

Neurofibromatosis-2 (NF-2) has also been called bilateral acoustic neuromas neurofibromatosis, or central neurofibromatosis [497,498,502]. The genetic locus for the disease is near the center of the long arm of chromosome 22 [502]. The inheritance is of an autosomal-dominant pattern with high penetrance [502].

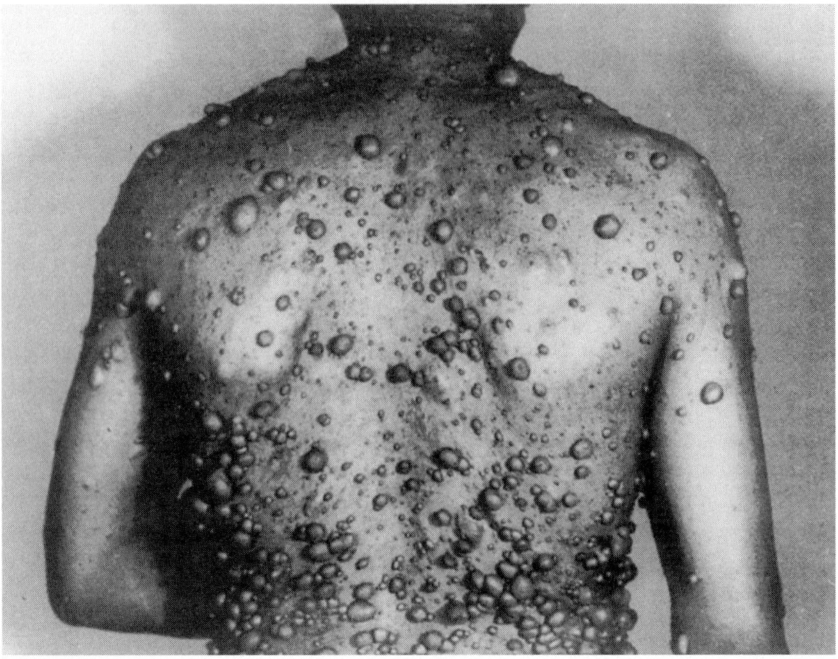

FIG. 28 Neurofibromatosis in a patient without pheochromocytoma. These lesions, which probably arise from the neurilemma of peripheral nerves, are subcutaneous, freely mobile, and may be tender. They seldom interfere with nerve function. Rarely, a sarcomatous degeneration occurs. (Courtesy of the late Dr. A. Domonkos. From Manger WM, Gifford RW Jr. Pheochromocytoma. New York: Springer-Verlag, 1977. Reproduced with permission.)

The main signature of this disorder is the presence of bilateral acoustic nerve tumors. Other central nervous system neurofibromas and other tumors, especially meningiomas and ependymomas, are also very common and most patients with NF-2 have multiple tumors. Café-au-lait spots and subcutaneous neurofibromas also occur but are not as numerous as in NF-I [497].

Cardiac and Cardiovascular Findings. Pheochromocytomas may be present in patients with neurofibromatosis. The finding of labile hypertension in a patient with pheochromocytoma suggests the existence of an excess of catecholamines. However, hypertension in patients with NF-I can also be related to renal vascular occlusive disease or to an incidental association with essential hyperten-

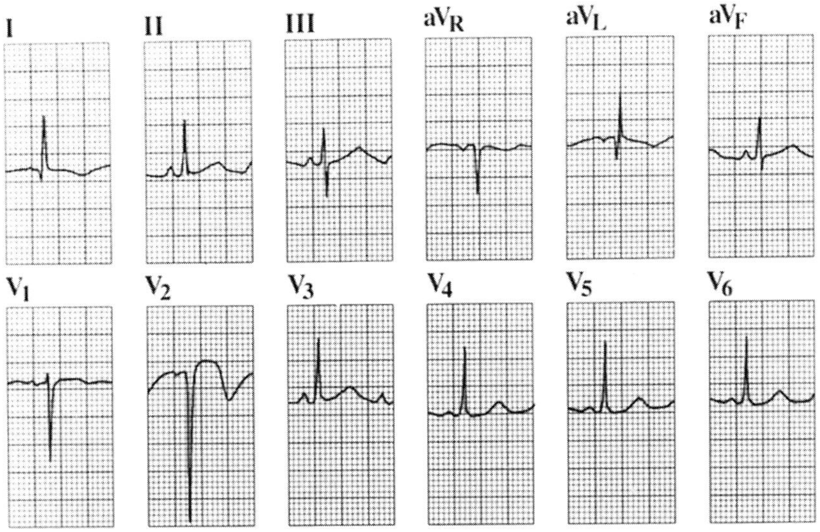

FIG. 29 ECG in a patient with myocardial infarction due to pheochromocytoma. This patient did not have neurofibromatosis. This electrocardiogram was recorded from a 23-year-old woman with pheochromocytoma who had episodes of hypertension. She developed pulmonary edema and a systolic blood pressure of 320 mm Hg and a diastolic blood pressure of 140 mm Hg. The serum creatine phosphokinase rose to 600 with 10% MB band. This patient undoubtedly had myocardial damage and infarction due to severe catecholenemia. (Electrocardiogram courtesy of Dallas Hall, M.D., Emory University School of Medicine, Atlanta, GA. From Hurst JW. Cardiovascular Diagnosis: The Initial Examination. St. Louis: Mosby-Year Book, Inc., 1993:388–389. Reproduced with permission.)

sion [497]. The patient with pheochromocytoma may have episodes of headache, sweating, palpitations, anxiety, tremulousness, chest pain, nausea, vomiting, and weakness. A patient with pheochromocytoma may have a myocardial infarction. Whereas the usual amount of catecholamines may dilate the coronary arteries, an excess amount of catecholamines, as occurs with a catecholamine storm, may overwhelm the receptors in the coronary arteries and cause them to constrict. Figure 29 shows an ECG from a patient with myocardial infarction related to a pheochromocytoma. Some patients may have a stroke due to brain hemorrhage, and sudden death has occurred.

The measurement of plasma catecholamines in the fasting, resting state is the most reliable test. Most patients with a tumor have a plasma level combination of epinephrine and norepinephrine of 2000 ng/L. The physician must be certain

to migrate normally during early life. Gliomas also often develop in patients with tuberous sclerosis. Renal cysts and angiomyolipomas are often found in the kidneys. Renal angiomyolipomas are found in nearly 50% of patients with tuberous sclerosis who are studied using renal ultrasound, CT scans, or both [497,505].

Cardiac and Cardiovascular Findings. Webb and colleagues reported that 80% of patients with rhabdomyomas of the heart have tuberous sclerosis and that 60% of patients, under 18 years of age with tuberous sclerosis have rhabdomyomas [506]. The tumors of the myocardium may or may not obstruct or obliterate the ventricular cavity. The larger tumors may cause death within a few hours of birth. The cardiac abnormalities of a 36-week-old infant are shown in Figure 31. The myocardial tumors are not encapsulated and are considered by many pathologists to be hamartomas. Biopsy of the lesions is often possible and the cells are characteristic of rhabdomyoma. The lesions most often involve the left ventricle and the interventricular septum. Large obstructing lesions and those that interfere with cardiac function have a poor prognosis [506]. Cardiac failure and arrhythmias can develop in patients with rhabdomyomas. Some patients with tuberous sclerosis have fibromuscular dysplasia of the renal arteries and may develop hypertension [497]. Renal failure due to severe hypertension is rare.

Von Hippel–Lindau Disease

The condition known as von Hippel–Lindau syndrome is inherited as an autosomal-dominant disorder. The tumor suppressor gene on chromosome 3 is involved in this syndrome. Positional cloning has localized the gene responsible to chromosome 3p25–26 [497,507]. The most common features are retinal and cerebellar hemangiomas and hemangioblastomas. Other cysts, angiomas, and tumors are also common. These include: renal cysts and carcinomas; pheochromocytomas; hepatic cysts, adenomas, and hemangiomas; pancreatic cysts, hemangiomas, hemangioblastomas, and carcinomas; epidydimal cysts, adenomas, and hemagiomas; adrenal cysts and adenomas; lung cysts and adenomas; and bone cysts [497,508]. Within the central nervous system, hemangioblastomas are most often located in the cerebellum, spinal cord (especially at the craniocervical junction and the conus medullaris), and brainstem [509]. The hemangioblastomas are composed of vascular elements that may organize into channels or caverns. They do not contain nerve cells but do contain a great deal of reticulin and swollen, lipid-filled endothelial cells [510].

Careful examination of the retina almost invariably shows retinal hemangiomatous lesions. At first these hemagiomas are flat and resemble aneurysmal dilatations of a single vessel. Later the lesions become globular and orange. An afferent arteriole and efferent veinule can sometimes be seen entering and leaving

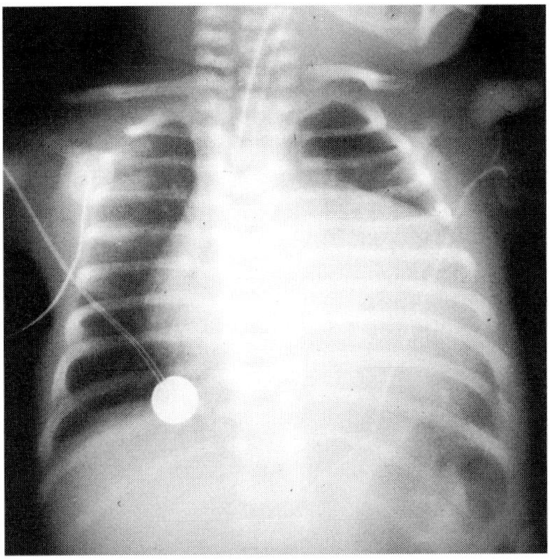

(A)

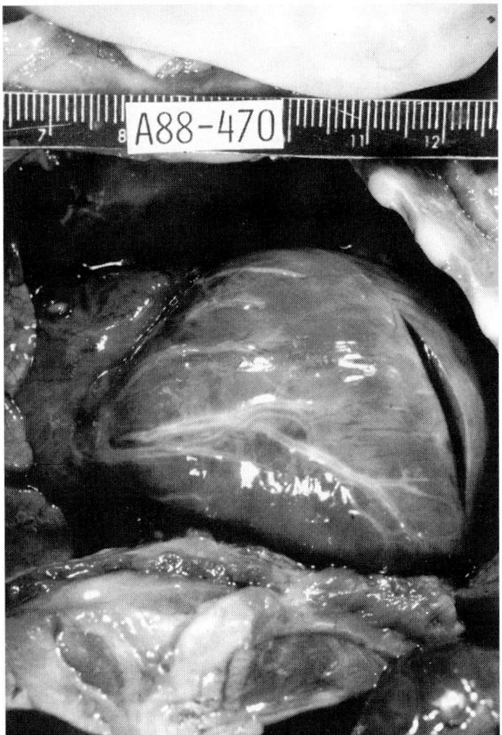

(B)

Fig. 31 (See legend on following page.)

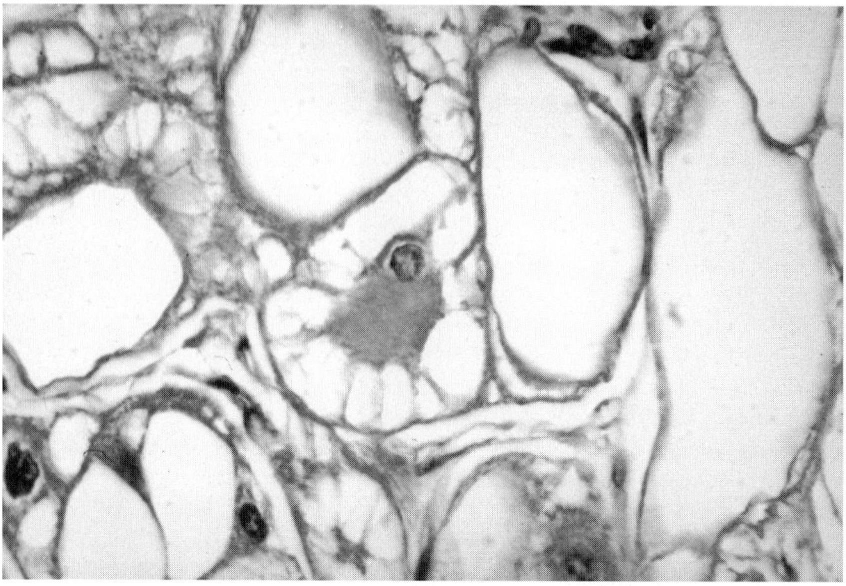

(C)

FIG. 31 Rhabdomyoma of the heart. The patient was a 36-month-old female who died as the result of congenital rhabdomyoma of the heart. (A) X-ray film of the chest showing enormous cardiac enlargement. (B) Heart shown at autopsy. (C) Microscopic section of rhabdomyoma. The infant had seizures and a cardiac mass was noted on the echocardiogram. There was evidence of heart failure. The rhabdomyoma involved the septum as well as the left and right ventricles. The outflow tracts of the left and right ventricles were obstructed and there was possible compression of the AV node and main bundle branches. (Illustration courtesy of Carlos H. Abramowsky, M.D., Egleston Hospital for Children, Emory University, Atlanta, GA.)

the retinal hemangiomas. Exudate and gliosis can obscure the lesions, which often grow slowly.

Hypernephroma are found in 45% to 70% of affected patients and are the cause of death in over one-fourth of patients [497,511].

Cardiac and Cardiovascular Findings. Pheochromocytomas develop in 7% to 20% of patients with von Hippel–Lindau disease, and can be bilateral and malignant [511]. Hypertension may occur in these patients, either in relation to renal disease, pheochromocytoma, or the polycythemia that often accompanies cerebellar hemangioblastomas. The cystic fluid within cerebellar hemangioblastomas contain erythropoietic activity.

Adrenoleukodystrophy

Adrenoleukodystrophy and adrenomyeloneuropathy are X-linked recessive disorders characterized by demyelination within the central and peripheral nervous systems and adrenal insufficiency. Men are almost exclusively affected, but 10% to 15% of women who are heterozygous for adrenoleukodystrophy will develop neurological signs. In this condition [512] the defective gene maps to Xq28, the terminal segment of the long arm of the X chromosome, and codes for a peroxisomal membrane protein [513]. Adrenal cortical cells and Schwann cells of patients with these disorders contain lamellar cytoplasmic inclusions that consist of cholesterol esterified with abnormally long-chain saturated fatty acids [514]. Saturated very long chain fatty acids accumulate in body fluids and tissues because of defective peroxisomal oxidation of these very long chain fatty acids [512,514].

Often the first symptoms of patients who have adrenoleukodystrophy are neurologic. The onset is often during early childhood or adolescence. Hemianopia and other visual-field defects are due to demyelination in the posterior portions of the cerebral hemispheres. Motor signs and loss of interest and intellectual functions may occur and are secondary to more widespread cerebral demyelination. MRI usually shows widespread bilateral white matter demyelination, most severe in the parieto-occipital regions and often asymmetric [515]. The childhood-onset form is the most severe and can be fatal during the first decade of life.

Symptoms in patients with adrenomyeloneuropathy usually develop during adolescence. A progressive spastic paralysis occurs usually with abnormal urinary and sexual function. Electrophysiological studies usually show slowing of motor and sensory nerve velocities. MRI in these patients shows hyperintensity within the corticospinal tracts and spinal cord atrophy [515]. Women who are heterozygous for X-linked adrenoleukodystrophy often develop a spastic paraparesis that begins in their 20s or 30s [514].

Clinical and biochemical evidence of adrenal cortical insufficiency develops in most patients with these syndromes. Hypogonadism is also common. Dietary restriction of very long chain fatty acids may lower the plasma levels of these substances but does not reverse the neruological abnormalities.

Cardiac and Cardiovascular Findings. Patients with adrenal insufficiency have the same cardiovascular abnormalities seen in other patients with Addison's disease. No other specific cardiac or cardiovascular abnormalities have been related to adrenoleukodystrophy or adrenomyeloneuropathy.

Zellweger's disease

This disorder is a multisystem, autosomal-recessive condition characterized by an absence of perioxisomal function [512]. Perioxisomes cannot be found in the liver or kidneys of patients with Zellweger's syndrome [516,517]. Perioxisomes are round, cytoplasmic organelles that are found abundantly in all eukaryotic cells. These structures play an important role in fatty acid and phytanic acid metabolism. Infants with Zellweger's syndrome are hypotonic and underactive at birth. Seizures are common. Deep tendon reflexes are absent. Ocular and retinal abnormalities are common. Biochemical tests usually show adrenal insufficiency. Most infants die within the first year of life.

Cardiac and Cardiovascular Findings. Cardiac defects are very common. The most frequent defects are ventricular septal defects and abnormalities of the aortic valve region [512].

Hereditary Hemorrhagic Telangiectasia (Osler-Weber-Rendu Syndrome)

This disorder is transmitted as an autosomal-dominant trait. Genetic linkages have been shown to chromosome 9q33–q34 in some families and to chromosome 12q in others [518]. The gene for this disorder at chromosome 9q3 has been shown to be endoglin, which encodes an integral membrane protein most abundant on endothelial cells [518]. Angiomas and telangiectasias are found in the skin, nasal membranes, pharynx, urinary bladder, and the gastrointestinal tract. The vascular lesions range from pinhead to 3 mm in size. Nosebleeds, hematuria, and gastrointestinal bleeding are all common. Angiomas and arteriovenous malformations are also found in the brain and spinal cord of these patients [518,519]. About 33% of patients have brain or spinal cord arteriovenous or venous malformations [518,519]. The brain malformations cause intracerebral or subarachnoid hemorrhages or seizures. Patients with spinal malformations may develop a paraparesis. Angiomas in the liver can be accompanied by shunting of blood around the liver and develpment of a portosystemic encephalopathy.

About 15% of patients with hereditary hemorrhagic telangiectasia have pulmonary arteriovenous malformations, and about 40% to 60% of patients with pulmonary arteriovenous fistulas have hereditary hemorrhagic telangiectasia [520–522]. The right-to-left shunting of blood often causes polycythemia. Brain abscesses are common in children and young adults who have pulmonary arteriovenous fistulas. Transient ischemic attacks and ischemic strokes can result from paradoxical embolism through the pulmonary shunts; air embolism has also been postulated [523].

Cardiac and Cardiovascular Findings. Pulmonary arteriovenous fistulae are common and are often associated with polycythemia. The lung fistulas often grow, increasing the right-to-left shunting of blood. Polycythemia often causes hypertension. The increased blood viscosity decreases blood flow to the brain and heart. These factors can exacerbate coronary and cerebrovascular disease. Severe anemia can develop in patients, with severe recurrent epistaxis and/or gastrointestinal bleeding when transfusions are not given. Transfusions can lead to an iron overload and clinical features of hemachromatosis.

Mental Retardation and Congenital Heart Disease

Down Syndrome

Down syndrome is present in about 1 in every 600 to 700 births and accounts for about 10% of cases of mental retardation [524–526]. The majority of patients with Down syndrome have a trisomy of chromosome 21 but some have a translocation. The children are mentally retarded. Intelligence quotients (IQs) range from 20 to 70 (mean, 40 to 50) but most children aquire some speech by the age of 5. Epicanthic folds, slant eyes, and Brushfield's spots on the iris are common physical features (Fig. 32). The palms of the hands commonly have a single crease rather than the several which are normally present. The young infant has a characteristic cry, and the tongue protrudes more than usual. Adults with Down

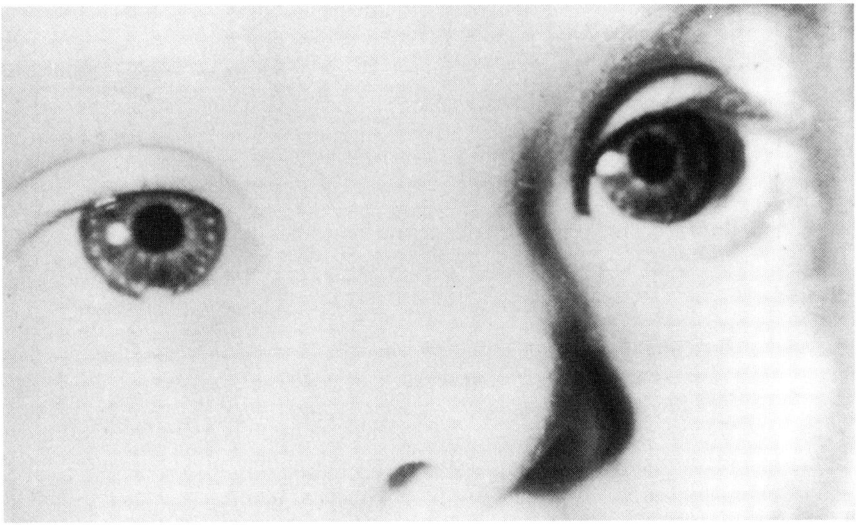

FIG. 32 Face of a patient with Down syndrome. Brushfield's spots in the iris and epicanthal folds are apparent. Atrial septal defect and endocardial cushion defects may be present in such patients. (From Logue RB, Hurst JW. General inspection of the patient with cardiovascular disease. In: Hurst JW, Logue RB, eds. The Heart, 1st ed. New York: McGraw-Hill, Inc., 1966:57. Reproduced with permission.)

syndrome often become progressively demented after age 40, and their brains show prominent Alzheimer's disease changes at necropsy. They develop Alzheimer's changes 10 to 20 years before individuals in the general population, and men develop Alzheimer's changes earlier than women with Down syndrome [527,528]. There is an increased frequency of myelocytic and lymphocytic leukemia among patients with Down syndrome.

Cardiac and Cardiovascular Findings. Fifty percent of patients with Down syndrome have congenital heart disease, and 50% of those with congenital heart disease have an endocardial cushion defect [529]. The patient may have an ostium primum atrial defect or a complete atrioventricular canal. Some patients have only a secundum atrial septal defect.

The patient with an ostium primum atrial septal defect may have a large heart. There is commonly a prominent anterior movement of the chest, and the pulsation of the pulmonary artery may be felt. There is a loud systolic murmur at the apex because of a cleft mitral valve, and the murmur of tricuspid regurgitation may be heard. There is fixed splitting of the second heart sound, and the pulmonary valve closure sound may be louder than normal.

Chest x-rays show a large heart, large left and right atria, a large pulmonary artery, and right and left ventricular enlargement. Electrocardiograms almost always show right bundle branch block (or right ventricular conduction delay) plus left anterior-superior division block. Heart failure is common and atrial fibrillation is likely to occur. The cardiac examination of a patient with a complete atrioventricular canal reveals many of the same features described for an ostium primum defect. There is, in effect, an atrial septal defect plus a ventricular septal defect in such patients. The heart functions as a two-chambered structure with the connecting atria above and the connecting ventricles below. This severe defect leads to heart failure, and respiratory infections are common. Embolic strokes also develop as a result of the congenital heart lesions.

Other Trisomies

The *trisomy of chromosome 18 syndrome* is the second most common multiple congenital malformation syndrome [530]. This condition is found in about three births in every thousand [530]. There is a strong female preponderance; three out of every four affected infants are girls. Affected babies are usually small at birth and are quite feeble. Infants often require resuscitation at birth and may later have apneic periods. Half of affected infants die during the first week, and many of the early survivers die within the first year [530,531]. About 5% to 10% survive as severely mentally retarded adults [531].

The most common congenital anomalies involve the face (low-set, malformed ears; small oral openings; small jaws), hands and feet (second and fourth fingers overlie the third finger and the fifth finger overlies the fourth [Fig. 33],

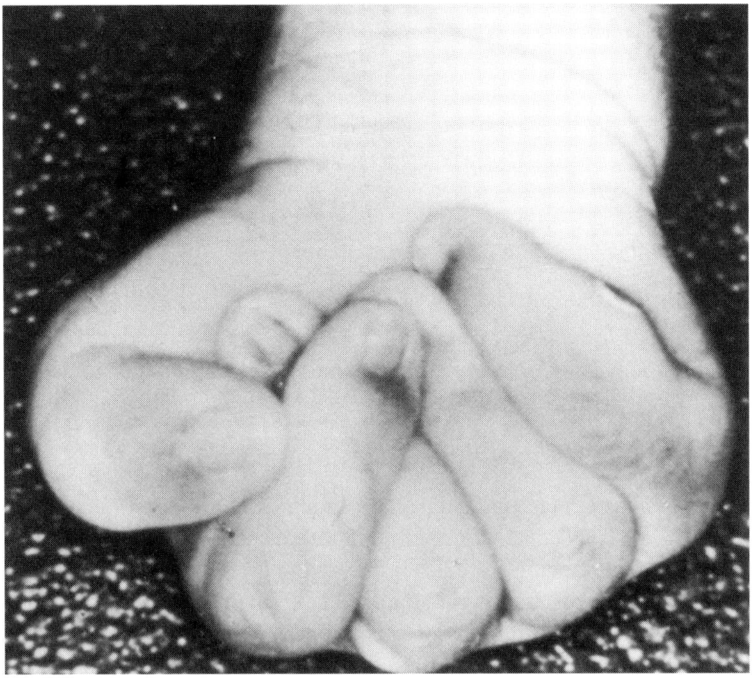

FIG. 33 Hand of a patient with trisomy 18 syndrome. Typical posturing of the hands occurs in these patients. A variety of cardiac abnormalities has been reported with this syndrome. (From Logue RB, Hurst JW. General inspection of the patient with cardiovascular disease. In: Hurst JW, Logue RB, eds. The Heart, 1st ed. New York: McGraw-Hill, Inc., 1966:58. Reproduced with permission.)

retroflexed thumbs and short dorsiflexed big toes), inguinal and umbilical hernias, and small pelvis [524,530,532]. Some patients have partial trisomies of either the short or long arm of chromosome 18; these patients have partial syndromes. Decreased muscle tone, seizures, and severe mental retardation are common features.

Cardiac and Cardiovascular Findings. Congenital heart lesions are an integral part of the clinical findings. The most frequently found defects are ventricular septal defects, atrial septal defects, patent ductus arteriosus, and pulmonary valve stenosis [529,530].

Trisomy of Chromosome 13

Patients with trisomy of chromosome 13 (Patau syndrome) are usually also small at birth and are most often girls. Congenital abnormalities involve mostly the middle of the face, the brain, hand, visceral organs, and heart [533,534]. The craniofacial anomalies are characteristic and include microcephaly, sloping forehead, agenesis of the olfactory apparatus, cleft lip and/or cleft palate, large capillary angiomas of the brow and occipital region, and small and abnormal eyes and ears [533]. They also often have polydactyly. Urogenital defects are also common. Most patients are severely mentally retarded. The brains of these patients are often severely malformed [535]. These patients rarely survive beyond the neonatal period because of their extensive malformations. Partial trisomy 13 cases are also well known.

Cardiac and Cardiovascular Findings. Patients may have dextrocardia, ventricular septal defects, double-outlet right ventricle, patent ductus arteriosus, or atrial septal defects [529].

Congenital Rubella (Gregg-Swan) Syndrome

Gregg was the first to relate congenital malformations to rubella infection acquired in utero [536]. The congenital rubella syndrome occurs in >80% of infants when the rubella infection with rash occurs during the first 3 months of gestation [537,538]. The brains of patients with congenital rubella show a chronic leptomeningitis and multiple focal regions of infarction and gliosis [537]. Deafness, cataracts, chorioretinitis, mental retardation, and congenital heart disease are the commonest findings. The newborn most often has the triad of eighth-nerve deafness, mental retardation, and cataracts (Fig. 34).

Cardiac and Cardiovascular Findings. Patients with the congenital rubella syndrome have been reported to have patent ductus arteriosus, pulmonary valve stenosis, and coarctation of a pulmonary artery [529].

Noonan Syndrome

This syndrome has often been referred to as the Turner-like syndrome because the morphological features closely resemble those found in girls who have Turner's syndrome [530]. Both boys and girls are affected. Noonan syndrome can be transmitted as an autosomal-dominant condition or be sporadic in occurrence. Affected individuals are short and have distintive facial appearances with hypertelorism, epicanthal folds, low-set ears, and a webbed neck. Myopia, keratoconus, and strabismus are common [530]. Some also have café-au-lait spots and lentigines. The gene for this disorder has been mapped to chromosome 12q22 [539]. Patients may be mentally retarded but the degree of retardation is usually not severe [540].

Cardiac and Cardiovascular Findings. Children with the Noonan syndrome have a high frequency of congenital cardiac defects, especially dysplasia of the pulmonary valve.

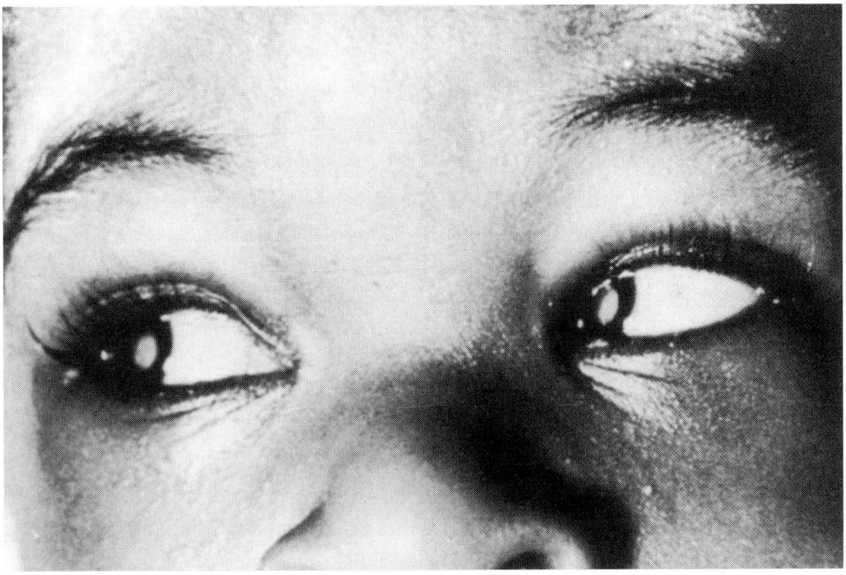

FIG. 34 Face of a patient with Gregg-Swan, or congenital rubella syndrome. Note cataracts. Patent ductus arteriosus with or without pulmonary stenosis is common in these patients. Coarctation of the pulmonary artery may occur. (From Logue RB, Hurst JW. General inspection of the patient with cardiovascular disease. In: Hurst JW, Logue RB, eds. The Heart, 1st ed. New York: McGraw-Hill, Inc., 1966:57. Reproduced with permission.)

Williams Syndrome

This syndrome is due to a microdeletion in the region that encodes elastin on chromosome 7q11.23 [512,530]. Patients may have mild microcephaly and may be mildly mentally retarded but are usually talkative and friendly. They have difficulty with visual-spatial functions and hypersensitivity to sound. Periods of autistic behavior are described. Some patients have hyperactive reflexes and slight spasticity in the legs. Some patients during adulthood develop hypertension, progressive joint disease, hypercalcemia, and recurrent urinary tract infections [530].

Cardiac and Cardiovascular Findings. These patients often have supravalvular aortic stenosis, supravalvular pulmonary stenosis, and mitral valve regurgitation [529,530]. Hypoplasia of the aorta and other arterial anomalies may be present. Some patients develop renal artery stenosis with hypertension [530].

Cornelia de Lange Syndrome

Patients with this syndrome have a characteristic physiognomy. They have bushy confluent eyebrows, downward-slanting eyes, small mandibles, low-set ears, hirsutism, growth retardation, and a peculiar "chicken wing" appearing arm with a single, thumblike digit [541,542]. They are often severely mentally retarded and have hearing loss and speech delay. Most cases have had sporadic occurrence but there may also be autosomal-dominant inheritance [530].

Cardiac and Cardiovascular Findings. Associated congenital cardiac lesions are very common and include ventricular and atrial septal defects, patent ductus arteriosis, pulmonic stenosis, anaomalous venous return, and an atrioventricular canal.

Rubenstein-Taybi's Syndrome

This syndrome is characterized by postnatal onset of growth deficiency with short stature, mental retardation, speech difficulties, and a stiff, unsteady gait [530]. Rubenstein and Taybi, who described the syndrome in 1963, emphasized the association of facial dysmorphic features and broad thumbs and toes with mental retardation [543]. The maxilla is hypoplastic with a narrow palate; the nose is prominent and often beaked, and the palpebral fissures often slant downward [530]. Most cases are of sporadic occurrence. The gene locus for this condition is at chromosome 16p13.3, a region that encodes the human cAMP-regulated, enhancer-binding protein [530,544].

Cardiac and Cardiovascular Findings. About 25% of patients with the Rubinstein-Taybi syndrome have ventricular septal defects, atrial septal defects, or patent ductus arteriosus.

Velocardiofacial Syndrome

This syndrome was first described by Shprintzen and colleagues and is sometimes also called the Shprintzen syndrome [545,546]. The major features of this syndrome are: mental retardation; learning disabilities; cleft palate; conductive hearing loss; prominent, square-shaped nose; retruded small mandible; and slender and hypotonic limbs with hyperextendable hands and fingers [530]. The condition is inherited as an autosomal-dominant disorder. Affected individuals have an interstitial deletion of chromosome 22q11.21–q11.23 [530].

Cardiac and Cardiovascular Findings. Cardiac defects are an integral part of the syndrome, being present in 85% of affected individuals [530]. The most common abnormalities are ventricular septal defect, right-sided aortic arch, tetralogy of Fallot, and aberrant left subclavian artery [530,547].

DiGeorge Sequence Abnormalities

This developmental disorder was first described by DiGeorge and includes defects of development of the thymus, parathyroid glands, and the great vessels. Affected individuals sometimes have lateral displacement of the inner canthi of the eyes, short palpebral fissures, small jaw, and ear anomalies. The children are usually mildly mentally retarded. The thymus and parathyroid glands may be absent or hypoplastic. Hypocalcemia with seizures may occur in young infants and provide a clue to the presence of this syndrome. Most individuals are a result of a partial monosomy of the proximal long arm of chromosome 22 due to a microdeletion of 22q11.2 [530,548,549]. The velocardiofacial syndrome and the DiGeorge sequence may represent different clinical manifestations of the same genetic defect [530].

Cardiac and Cardiovascular Findings. The aortic arch is often malformed. The arch may be right-sided or the aorta may be interupted [530,550]. Truncus arteriosis, ventricular septal defects, and tetralogy of Fallot also occur [530,550].

Syndromes Associated with Prematurely Accelerated Aging

There are two well-recognized but rare syndromes in which aging processes are accelerated. *Progeria*, also called the Hutchinson-Gilford syndrome after the physicians who reported the initial cases [551,552], is a condition evident at or soon after birth. In patients who have *Werner's syndrome*, accelerated aging usually begins when affected individuals reach their third decade [553].

Progeria

Infants with progeria are noted at birth to have abnormal, scerodermalike skin, especially over the abdomen [530,554,555]. By the time they reach their first birthday, decreased weight gain and retarded growth are apparent. The craniofacial features are quite characteristic and allow instant recognition of the disorder by physicians who are familiar with the syndrome and have seen other patients with progeria. The face seems relatively small for the head; hair is lost early and alopecia persists throughout life. The mandible is small and the teeth are crowded. The face has a triangular appearance because of the absence of subcutaneous fat [554]. Eyelashes and eyebrows are often absent. The voice is unusual and has a high, squeaky sound. The muscles are atrophic and poorly developed, and subcutaneous fat is virtually absent throughout the body. Intelligence is usually normal [554–556].

The incidence of progeria is about one in every 8 million births. Most cases are sporadic but there are reports of occurrence in siblings and in consanguineous offspring, suggesting an autosomal-recessive inheritance.

Accelerated aging begins during the first years of life. Degenerative arthritis and osteoporosis develop. The average age of death among 13 patients was 14.2 years (range, 7 to 27) [530]. By the teens, progeric patients look like very sick, feeble, and aged.

Cardiac and Cardiovascular Findings. Hypertension, coronary atherosclerosis with angina pectoris, and myocardial infarction are quite common. Cardiomegaly and congestive heart failure often develop in the early teens. Occlusive cerebrovascular disease is also quite common. One of the authors (L.R.C.) has cared for a patient who had multiple brain infarcts related to extensive extracranial vascular occlusive disease that developed before age 6.

Werner's Syndrome

In 1904, Otto Werner in his doctoral thesis described the findings in four siblings who had premature aging [553,557]. Little has been added since this original description of the findings. Werner's original patients were short and had a senile appearance. Their hair started to become gray during their 20s. They had cataracts that appeared during the third decade of life, and had atrophic, hyperkeratotic, ulcerated skin, mostly over the hands and feet, and their skeletal limb muscles showed marked atrophy [553,557]. With time, physicians have learned that diabetes, hypogonadism, and retinitis pigmentosa are additional associated features. Cataracts are described as posterior cortical and subcapsular and are always bilateral [553]. Liver dysfunction, hyperuricemia, and hyperlipidemia are usually present. Some patients have subnormal intelligence. Seizures and hyperreflexia are also common.

The facies are usually quite characteristic. Affected individuals look 20 to 30 years older than their actual age. The face is thin and the sharp angle of the bridge of the nose gives it a beaked appearance. Most patients have a high-pitched voice due to a variety of different vocal cord abnormalities. The muscles of the extremities usually show severe atrophy. Electromyographic studies show a myopathic pattern of abnormality.

Patients with Werner's syndrome have a striking predilection for developing noncarcinomatous tumors. Meningiomas and neural sheath sarcomas are found within the central nervous system. Age at death averages about 48 (range, 30 to 63) [553]. Death is often from malignancies, diabetic coma, or liver failure [553].

Cardiac and Cardiovascular Findings. Patients develop accelerated atherosclerosis. The aorta and great vessels are often calcified. The atherosclerosis in patients with Werner's syndrome has the typical distribution and involves the coronary and craniocervical arteries [553,558]. Myocardial infarcts are common. Often there is heavy calcification of the mitral and/or aortic valves [558].

Homocystinuria and Homocysteinemia

Severe hyperhomocysteinemia and homocystinuria is a genetic disorder first described in children and known to be associated with premature strokes, mental retardation, and a Marfan-like syndrome. In more recent years, it has become clear that lesser degrees of hyperhomocysteinemia are associated with premature atherosclerosis.

Classic homocystinuria is caused by a hereditary deficiency of the enzyme cystathione-beta-synthase; this enzyme is necessary for the conversion of methionine-derived homocysteine to cystathione. In humans, about 15 to 20 mmol of homocysteine is formed each day by demethylation of the amino acid methionine [559]. Homocysteine is then metabolized by one of two pathways, either remethylation or transulfuration [560]. In the remethylation process, homocysteine is remethylated to methionine in a reaction catalyzed by methionine synthase [561]. Vitamin B_{12} is an essential cofactor for methionine synthase. N^5-methyl-tetrahydrofolate is the methyl donor in this reaction, and N^5, N^{10}-methylene-tetrahydrofolate reductase functions as the catalyst in this remethylation reaction [560]. Homocysteine can also be transulfurated. In this process homocysteine condenses with serine to form cystathione, a reaction that is catalyzed by the vitamin B_6-dependent enzyme cystathione beta-synthase [560,561]. Cystathione is then hydrolyzed to cysteine which in turn can be incorporated into glutathione or further metabolized to sulfate and excreted in the urine [560,562].

Cystathione-beta-synthase deficiency is the most common genetic cause of severe hyperhomocysteinemia. The homozygous form of this disorder is called congenital homocystinuria and is associated with plasma homocystine concentrations of up to 400 μmol/L during the fasting state [560]. This clinical disorder is rare (five in 1 million births). Affected individuals have lens ectopias, skeletal deformities, a Marfan-like habitus, and severe premature atherosclerosis. Typically a clinical thromboembolic event would occur before age 30 in these individuals; this would typically be a stroke rather than a myocardial infarct [563]. A homozygous deficiency of N^5, N^{10}-methylene-tetrahydrofolate reductase, the enzyme involved in the B_{12}-dependent remethylation of homocysteine can also cause severe hyperhomocysteinemia. Patients with this metabolic defect have an even worse prognosis than those with cystathione-beta-synthase deficiency [560].

Milder forms of hyperhomocysteinemia occur in heterozygotes with these enzyme deficiencies. Deficiencies in the cofactors, folate, vitamin B_{12}, and vitamin B_6, which are required for homocysteine metabolism, can also cause an elevated homocysteine level. In patients with nutritional deficiencies in these vitamin cofactors, prescribing these substances can reduce homocysteine levels. Increased levels of homocysteine also occur in patients with: renal insufficiency;

hyperthyroidism; breast, pancreatic, and ovarian cancers; lymphatic leukemia; treatment with methotrexate, theophylline, and phenytoin; and pernicious anemia [560]. Cigarette smoking has also been associated with elevated homocysteine levels presumably because of interference with the synthesis of pyridoxal phosphate [564].

Elevated levels of homocysteine have now been unequivocably related to strokes, premature atherosclerosis, myocardial infarction, and venous thromboembolism [560,565,566]. Evidence from more than 20 case-controlled studies that included over 2000 individuals has validated the relationship between elevated homocysteine levels and accelerated atherosclerosis [560]. Experimental evidence shows that increased homocysteine level injures the vascular endothelium and that this injury leads to platelet activation and the formation of thrombi [567,568]. Homocysteine also stimulates vascular smooth muscle cells to proliferate [569].

Cardiac and Cardiovascular Findings. Increased homocysteine levels are associated with an increase in occlusive atherosclerotic disease [560,570,573]. This leads to an increased frequency of myocardial infarction, increased frequency of carotid artery disease [571], and increased severity of coronary artery occlusive disease [560,572,573].

Neurocutaneous Diseases and the Heart

Lentigenosis-Deafness-Cardiomyopathy Syndrome

Lentigenosis is a neurocutaneous disease that is inherited as an autosomal-dominant trait with variable expression [574]. Sporadic cases due to mutation of the gene also occur. Polani and Moynahan postulated that the condition is due to a defect of the neuroectoderm [575]. The patient has multiple lentigenes (Fig. 35), deafness, hypertelorism, short stature, psychomotor retardation, poor muscle development, and genital abnormalities. Biopsy of the skin lesions reveals an increase in pigment in the dermis.

Cardiac and Cardiovascular Findings. Hypertrophic cardiomyopathy is commonly found in patients with lentigenosis [576,577]. The cardiac abnormalities include a pulsus bisferiens which can be noted by palpating the pulsation of the carotid artery and hearing a systolic murmur along the left sternal border. The murmur is intensified by the Valsalva maneuver [578]. These abnormalities are caused by dynamic subaortic valve stenosis. The murmur of subpulmonic valve stenosis may also be heard. An atrial gallop sound is commonly audible. Mitral valve regurgitation may develop.

The electrocardiogram is usually abnormal. It may show a left atrial abnormality, left ventricular hypertrophy, left anterior-superior division block, right

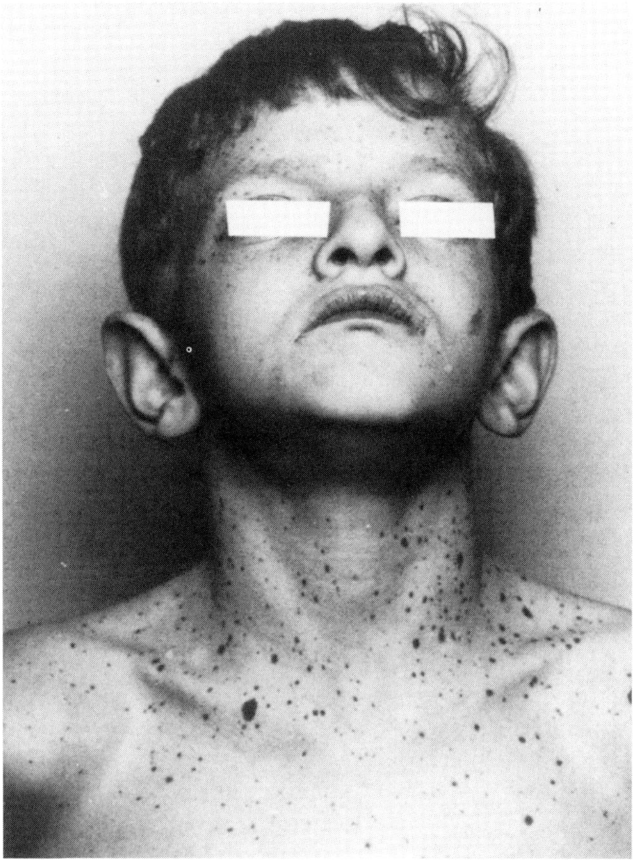

FIG. 35 Face and trunk of a patient with lentigenosis-deafness-cardiomyopathy syndrome. Nine-year-old boy with multiple lentigenes, mental retardation, growth retardation, and hypertrophic cardiomyopathy. He did not have genital abnormalities or sensorineural deafness. (From Ref. 574. Reproduced with permission.)

ventricular hypertrophy, a persistent abnormal ST vector due to persistent epicardial injury, a persistent T-wave vector due to epicardial ischemia, and, at times, a deeply inverted T-wave due to a vector directed away from the epicardium of the cardiac apex. The initial electrical forces of the QRS complex may be directed away from a segment of the endocardium, producing an abnormality suggesting a myocardial infarction.

Atrial fibrillation and ventricular arrhythmias may develop. Heart failure may develop late in the course of the disease if the patient does not succumb earlier to the arrhythmias mentioned above.

Long QT—Deafness Syndromes

The *Jervell and Lange-Nielsen's syndrome* consists of a prolonged QT interval and congenital deafness [579]. In childhood the children are diagnosed as having bilateral high-tone deafness, and they develop fainting spells, often precipitated by exertion, rage, or fear. Such individuals are subject to sudden death. The *Romano-Ward syndrome* consists of a long QT interval and sudden death, but patients are not deaf [580,581]. They also often have exertionally related syncope.

The Jervell and Lange-Nielsen's syndrome is an inherited autosomal-recessive condition. The Romano-Ward syndrome is inherited as an autosomal-dominant condition. Three or more genetic markers have been identified in patients with the long QT sudden death syndrome [582]. Some investigators believe that they have a decrease in right cardiac sympathetic activity and an increase in left cardiac sympathetic activity.

Patients with the Jervell, and Lange-Nielsen's syndrome are deaf and are more likely to be female. The patients may have syncope due to ventricular tachycardia. Syncopal attacks may be misdiagnosed as epilepsy.

Cardiac and Cardiovascular Findings. The electrocardiogram reveals a long QT interval (Figs. 36,37). The syncope and sudden death in these patients is usually due to ventricular arrhythmia which may be ventricular tachycardia or ventricular fibrillation. Torsades de pointes is common [583]. Patients with this syndrome may develop a lethal arrhythmia as the result of a sudden sympathetic discharge, such as may come from fright, anger, and startle. The serious arrhythmia may also occur with physical exercise or upon awakening.

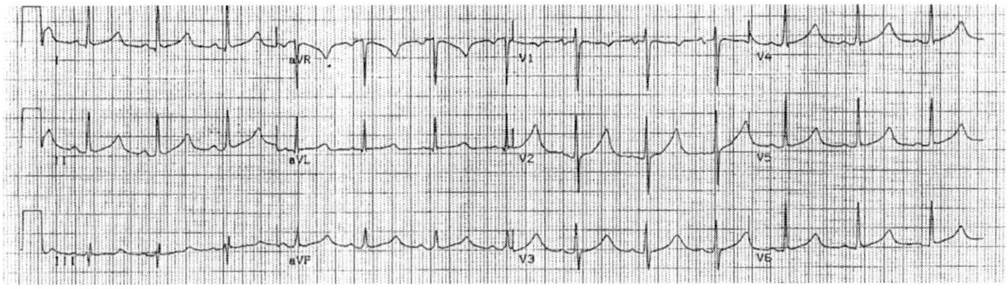

FIG. 36 This electrocardiogram was recorded from a 10-year-old boy with the Jervell-Lange-Nielsen syndrome. Note the long Q-T interval. (Electrocardiogram courtesy of Arthur J. Moss, M.D., University of Rochester Medical Center, Rochester, NY.)

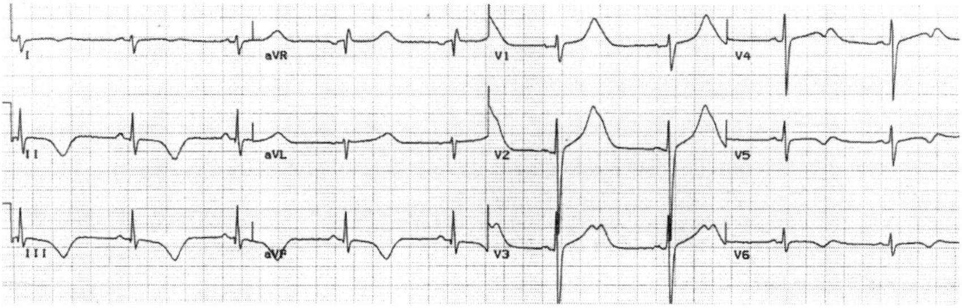

FIG. 37 This electrocardiogram was recorded from a 22-year-old male with the Jervell-Lange-Nielsen syndrome. Note the long Q-T interval and large T waves. In addition, the mean T vector is directed at $-90°$ in the frontal plane and about 70° anteriorly, while the mean QRS vector is directed at about $+110°$ in the frontal plane and about 70° posteriorly. Note the difference in the T wave shown in this tracing compared to the T wave shown in Figure 36. (Electrocardiogram courtesy of Arthur J. Moss, M.D., University of Rochester Medical Center, Rochester, NY.)

Prolongation of the QT interval is a common finding among neonates who subsequently have the sudden infant death syndrome (SIDS). This finding could be explained by a variant of the Romano-Ward or Jervell and Lange-Nielsen syndromes in these infants [584,585].

REFERENCES

1. Samuels M. ''Voodoo'' death revisited: the modern lessons of neurocardiology. Neurologist 1997; 3:293–304.
2. Levy MN, Warner MR. Parasympathetic effects on cardiac function. In: Armour JA, Ardell JL, eds. Neurocardiology. New York: Oxford University Press, 1994: 53–76.
3. Appenzeller O. The Autonomic Nervous System 2d ed. Amsterdam: North-Holland Publishing Company, 1976.
4. Randall WC, McNally L, Caliguiri L, Rohse WG. Functional analyses of the cardiac augmentor and cardioaccelerator pathways in the dog. Am J Physiol 1957; 91:213–217.
5. Barnes KL, Ferrario CM. Role of the central nervous system in cardiovascular regulation. In: Furlan A, ed. The Heart and Stroke. London: Springer-Verlag, 1987: 155–169.
6. Ali AS, Levine SR. Heart and brain relationships. In: Brain Ischemia, Basic Concepts and Clinical Relevance. London: Springer-Verlag, 1995:317–328.
7. Oppenheimer SM, Cechetto DF, Hachinski VC. Cerebrogenic cardiac arrythmias: cerebral ECG influences and their role in sudden death. Arch Neurol 1990; 47: 513–519.

8. Oppenheimer SM, Wilson JX, Guiraudon C, Cechetto DF. Insular cortex stimulation produces lethal cardiac arrythmias: a mechanism of sudden death. Brain Res 1991; 550:115–121.
9. Oppenheimer SM, Hopkins DA. Suprabulbar neural regulation of the heart. In: Armour JA, Ardell JL, eds. Neurocardiology. New York: Oxford Press, 1994:309–341.
10. Benarroch EE. The central autonomic network: functional organization, dysfunction, and perspective. Mayo Clin Proc 1993; 68:988–1001.
11. Loewy AD. Central autonomic pathways. In: Loewy AD, Spyer KM, eds. Central Regulation of Autonomic Functions. New York: Oxford University Press, 1990: 88–103.
12. Byer E, Ashman R, Toth LA. Electrocardiogram with large upright T waves and long Q-T intervals. Am Heart J 1947; 33:796–806.
13. Levine HD. Non-specificity of the electrocardiogram associated with coronary heart disease. Am J Med 1953; 15:344–354.
14. Burch GE, Myers R, Abildskov JA. A new electrocardiographic pattern observed in cerebrovascular accidents. Circulation 1954; 9:719–723.
15. Cropp GJ, Manning GW. Electrocardiographic changes simulating myocardial ischemia and infarction associated with spontaneous intracranial hemorrhage. Circulation 1960; 22:25–38.
16. Lavy S, Stern S, Herishianu Y, et al. Electrocardiographic changes in ischemic stroke. J Neurol Sci 1968; 7:409–415.
17. Dimant J, Grob D. Electrocardiographic changes and myocardial damage in patients with acute cerebrovascular accidents. Stroke 1977; 8:448–455.
18. Goldstein DS. The electrocardiogram in stroke: relationship to pathophysiological type and comparison with prior tracings. Stroke 1979; 10:253–258.
19. Samuels MA. Electrocardiographic manifestations of neurologic disease. Sem Neurol 1984; 4:453–459.
20. Oppenheimer SM, Cechetto DF, Hachinski VC. Cerebrogenic cardiac arrythmias. Cerebral electrocardiographic influences and their role in sudden death. Arch Neurol 1990; 47:513–519.
21. Brouwers PJ, Wijdicks EF, Hasan D, et al. Serial electrocardiographic recording in aneurysmal subarachnoid hemorrhage. Stroke 1989; 20:1162–1167.
22. Rolak LA, Rokey R. Electrocardiographic features. In: Rolak LA, Rokey R, eds. Coronary and Cerebral Vascular Disease. A Practical Guide. Mount Kisco, NY; Futura, 1990:139–197.
23. Hansson L, Larsson O. The incidence of ECG abnormalities in acute cerebrovascular accidents. Acta Med Scand 1974; 195:45–47.
24. Hunt D, McRae C, Zapf P. Electrocardiographic and serum enzyme changes in subarachnoid hemorrhage. Am Heart J 1969; 77:479–488.
25. Kreus KE, Kemila SJ, Takala JK. Electrocardiographic changes in cerebral vascular accidents. Acta Med Scand 1969; 185:327–334.
26. Norris JW, Frogatt GM, Hachinski VC. Cardiac arrhythmias in acute stroke. Stroke 1978; 9:392–396.
27. Vingerhoets F, Bogousslavsky J, Regli F, Van Melle G. Atrial fibrillation after acute stroke. Stroke 1993; 24:26–30.

28. Stober T, Anstatt T, Sen S, Schimrigk K, Jager H. Cardiac arrhythmias in subarachnoid hemorrhage. Acta Neurochir (Wien) 1988; 93:37–44.
29. Di Pasquale G, Pinelli G, Andreoli A, Manini G, Grazi P, Togneyyi F. Holter detection of cardiac arrhythmias in intracranial subarachnoid hemorrhage. Am J Cardiol 1987; 59:596–600.
30. Di Pasquale G, Pinelli G, Andreoli A, Manini GL, Grazi P, Tognetti F. Torsade de pointes and ventricular flutter-fibrillation following spontaneous cerebral subarachnoid hemorrhage. Int J Cardiol 1988; 18:163–172.
31. Puleo P. Cardiac enzyme assessment. In: Rolak LA, Rokey R, eds. Coronary and Cerebral Vascular Disease. A Practical Guide. Mount Kisco, NY: Futura, 1990: 199–216.
32. Fabinyi G, Hunt D, McKinley L. Myocardial creatine kinase isoenzyme in serum after subarachnoid hemorrhage. J Neurol Neurosurg Psychiatry 1977; 40:818–820.
33. Neil-Dwyer G, Cruikshank J, Stratton C. Beta blockers, plasma total creatine kinase and creatine kinase myocardial isoenzyme, and the prognosis of subarachnoid hemorrhage. Surg Neurol 1986; 25:163–168.
34. Norris JW, Hachinski VC, Myers MG, et al. Serum cardiac enzymes in stroke. Stroke 1979; 10:548–553.
35. Norris JW, Hachinski V. Cardiac dysfunction following stroke. In: Furlan A, ed. The Heart and Stroke. London: Springer-Verlag, 1987:171–183.
36. Caplan LR. The heart: concluding comments. In: Brain Ischemia, Basic Concepts and Clinical Relevance. London: Springer-Verlag, 1995:329–334.
37. Weir BK. Pulmonary edema following fatal aneurysmal rupture. J Neurosurg 1978; 49:502–507.
38. Hoff JT, Nishimura M. Experimental neurogenic pulmonary edema in cats. J Neurosurg 1978; 18:383–389.
39. Theodore J, Robin ED. Pathogenesis of neurogenic pulmonary edema. Lancet 1975; 2:749–751.
40. Koskello P, Punsar S, Sipila W. Subendocardial hemorrhages and electrocardiographic changes in intracranial bleeding. Br Med J 1964; 1:1479–1480.
41. Duren DR, Becker AE. Focal myocytolysis mimicking the electrocardiographic pattern of transmural anteroseptal myocardial infarction. Chest 1976; 69:506–511.
42. Connor RCR. Heart damage associated with intracranial lesions. Br Med J 1968; 3:29–31.
43. Greenhoot JH, Reichenbach DD. Cardiac injury and subarachnoid hemorrhage. J Neurosurg 1969; 30:521–531.
44. Kolin A, Norris JW. Myocardial damage from acute cerebral lesions. Stroke 1984; 15:990–993.
45. Baroldi G. Different morphological types of myocardial cell death in man. In: Fleckstein A, Rona G, eds. Recent Advances in Studies in Cardiac Structure and Metabolism. Pathophysiology and Morphology of Myocardial Cell Alteration. Vol. 6. Baltimore: University Park Press, 1975:385–397.
46. Choi DW. Excitotoxicity and stroke. In: Brain Ischemia, Basic Concepts and Clinical Relevance. London: Springer-Verlag, 1995:29–36.
47. Levine SR, Patel VM, Welch KMA, Skinner JE. Are heart attacks really brain

attacks? In: Furlan A, ed. The Heart and Stroke. London: Springer-Verlag, 1987: 185–216.
48. Talman WT. Cardiovascular regulation and lesions of the central nervous system. Ann Neurol 1985; 18:1–12.
49. Yoon R-W, Morillo CA, Cechetto DF, Hachinski V. Cerebral hemispheric lateralization in cardiac autonomic control. Arch Neurol 1997; 54:741–744.
50. Hachinski VC, Oppenheimer SM, Wilson JX, Guiraudon C, Cechetto DF. Asymmetry of sympathetic consequences of experimental stroke. Arch Neurol 1992; 49: 697–702.
51. Giubilei F, Strano S, Lino S, et al. Autonomic nervous system activity during sleep in middle cerebral artery infarction. Cerebrovasc Dis 1998; 8:118–123.
52. Schenk EA, Moss AJ. Cardiovascular affects of sustained norepinephrine infusions. II. Morphology. Circ Res 1966; 605–615.
53. Szakacs JE, Mehlman B. Pathological changes induced by norepinephrine. Am J Cardiol 1960; 5:619–627.
54. Myers MG, Norris JW, Hachinski VC, Sole MJ. Plasma norepinephrine in stroke. Stroke 1981; 12:200–204.
55. Benedict CR, Loach AB. Sympathetic nervous system activity in patients with subarachnoid hemorrhage. Stroke 1978; 9:237–244.
56. McNair JL, Clower BR, Sanford RA. Effect of reserpine pretreatment on myocardial damage associated with simulated intracranial hemorrhage in mice. Eur J Pharmacol 1970; 9:1–6.
57. Hawkins WE, Clower BR. Myocardial damage after head trauma and simulated intracranial hemorrhage in mice: the role of the autonomic nervous system. Cardiovasc Res 1971; 5:524–529.
58. Offerhaus I, Van Gool J. Electrocardiographic changes and tissue catecholamines in experimental subarachnoid hemorrhage. Cardiovasc Res 1969; 3:433–440.
59. Jacob WA, Van Bogaert A, DeGroot-Lasseel MHA. Myocardial ultrastructural and hemodynamic reactions during experimental subarachnoid hemorrhage. J Moll Cell Cardiol 1972; 4:287–298.
60. Hunt D, Gore I. Myocardial lesions following experimental intracranial hemorrhage: prevention with propanolol. Am Heart J 1972; 83:232–236.
61. Natelson BH. Neurocardiology. Arch Neurol 1985; 42:178–184.
62. Selye H. The Chemical Prevention of Cardiac Necrosis. New York: Ronald Press, 1958.
63. Pine DS, Tierney L Jr. A stressful interaction. N Engl J Med 1996; 334:1530–1534.
64. Cebelin M, Hirsch CS. Human stress cardiomyopathy. Hum Pathol 1980; 11:123–132.
64a. Weiner N. Atropine, scopolamine, and related antimuscarinic drugs. In: Gilman AG, Goodman LS, Gilman A, eds. Goodman and Gilman's The Pharmacologic Basis of Therapeutics. 6th ed. New York: Macmillan, 1980:146–167.
65. Cannon W. ''Voodoo'' death. Am Anthropol 1942; 4:1–10.
66. Engel G. Sudden and rapid death during psychological stress. Ann Intern Med 1971; 4:771–782.

67. Pavlov I. The Complete Collection of Works. Vol. 1. Moscow: ANSSR, 1951:419–457.
68. Zavodskaya IS, Moreua EV, Novikova NA. Neurogenic Heart Lesions. Oxford: Pergamon Press, 1980.
69. West TC, Falk G, Cervoni P. Drug alteration of transmembrane potentials in atrial pacemaker cells. J Pharmacol Exp Ther 1956; 117:245–252.
70. Kralios FA, Millar CK. Sympathetic neural effects on regional atrial recovery properties and cardiac rhythm. Am J Physiol 1981; 240:H590–H596.
71. Scher AM, Ohm WW, Bumgarner K et al. Sympathetic and parasympathetic control of heart rate in the dog, baboon, and man. Fed Proc 1972; 31:1219–1225.
72. Lown B. Sudden cardiac death: the major challenge confronting contemporary cardiology. Am J Cardiol 1979; 43:313–328.
73. Schwartz PJ, Stome HL, Brown AM. Effects of unilateral stellate ganglion blockade on the arrhythmia associated with coronary occlusion. Am Heart J 1976; 92:588–599.
74. Verrier RL, Thompson P, Lown B. Ventricular vulnerability during sympathetic stimulation: role of heart rate and blood pressure. Cardiovasc Res 1974; 8:602–610.
75. Richter CP. On the phenomenon of sudden death in animals and man. Psychosom Med 1957; 19:191–198.
76. McEwen BS. Protecting and damaging effects of stress mediators. N Eng J Med 1998; 338:171–179.
77. Gilchrist JM. Arrhythmogenic seizures: diagnosis by simultaneous EEG/ECG recording. Neurology 1985; 35:1503–1506.
78. White PT, Grant P, Mosier J, Gray A. Changes in cerebral dynamics associated with seizures. Neurology 1961; 11:354–361.
79. Blumhardt LD, Smith PE, Owen L. Electrocardiographic accompaniments of temporal lobe seizures. Lancet 1986; 1:1051–1056.
80. Kiok MC, Terrence CF, Fromm GH, Lavine S. Sinus arrest in epilepsy. Neurology 1986; 36:115–116.
81. Johnson RH, Lambie DG, Spalding JMK. Autonomic nervous system. In: Joynt RJ, ed. Clinical Neurology. Philadelphia: Lippincott, 1993(Chap. 57):1–94.
82. Jay GW. Leitsma JE. Sudden death in epilepsy. Acta Neurol Scand 1981; 63(suppl): 1–66.
83. Lathers CM, Schraeder PR. Epilepsy and Sudden Death. New York: Marcel Dekker, 1990.
84. Nashef L, Garner S, Sander WAS, Fish DR, Shorvon SD. Circumstances of death in sudden death in epilepsy: interviews of bereaved relatives. J Neurol Neurosurg Psychiatry 1998; 64:349–352.
85. Leetsma JE, Kalelkar MB, Teas SS, Jay GW, Hughes JR. Sudden unexpected death associated with seizures. analysis of 66 cases. Epilepsia 1984; 25:84–88.
85a. Natelson BH, Suarez R, Terrence CF, Turizo R. Patients with epilepsy who die suddenly have cardiac disease. Arch Neurol 1998; 55:857–860.
86. Parkinson J. An Essay on the Shaking Palsy. London: Whittingham and Rowland, 1817.
87. Jellinger K. Overview of morphological changes in Parkinson's disease. In: Yahr MD, Bergmann KJ, eds. Advances in Neurology. Vol. 45. New York: Raven Press, 1986: 1–18.

88. Burkhardt CR, Filley CM, Kleinschmidt-Demasters BK, et al. Diffuse Lewy body disease and progressive dementia. Neurology 1988; 38:1520–1528.
89. Wakabayashi K, Takahashi H. Neuropathology of autonomic nervous system in Parkinson's disease. Eur Neurol 1997; 38(suppl 2):2–7.
90. Steele JC, Richardson JC, Olszewski J. Progressive supranuclear palsy. Arch Neurol 1964; 10:333–359.
91. Steele JC. Progressive supranuclear palsy. Brain 1972; 95:693–704.
92. Litvan I, Agid Y, Calne D, et al. Clinical research criteria for the diagnosis of progressive supranuclear palsy (Steele-Richardson-Olszewski syndrome): report of the NINDS-SPSP international workshop. Neurology 1996; 47:1–8.
93. Daniel SE, de Bruin VMS, Lees AJ. The clinical and pathological spectrum of Steele-Richardson-Olszewski syndrome (progressive supranuclear palsy): a reappraisal. Brain 1995; 118:759–770.
94. Riley DE, Lang AE, Lewis A, et al. Cortical-basal ganglionic degeneration. Neurology 1990; 40:1203–1212.
95. Rinne JO, Lee MS, Thompson PD, Marsden CD. Corticobasal degeneration. A clinical study of 36 cases. Brain 1994; 117:1183–1196.
96. Shy GM, Drager GA. Neurological syndrome associated with orthostatic hypotension. Arch Neurol 1960; 2:511–527.
97. Schwarz GA. The orthostatic hypotension syndrome of Shy-Drager. Arch Neurol 1967; 16:123–139.
98. Gilman S, Quinn NP. The relationship of multiple system atrophy to sporadic olivopontocerebellar atrophy and other forms of idiopathic late-onset cerebellar atrophy. Neurology 1996; 46:1197–1199.
99. Penney JB. Multiple systems atrophy and nonfamilial olivopontocerebellar atrophy are the same disease. Ann Neurol 1995; 37:553–554.
100. Caplan LR, Schoene W. Clinical features of subcortical arteriosclerotic encephalopathy (Binswanger disease). Neurology 1978; 28: 1206–1215.
101. Caplan LR. Binswanger disease revisited. Neurology 1995; 45:626–633.
102. Adams RD, van Bogaert L, Vander Eecken H. Striato-nigral degeneration. J Neuropathol Exp Neurol 1964; 23:584–608.
103. Vakili S, Drew AL, von Schuching S, Becker D, Zeman W. Hallevorden-Spatz syndrome. Arch Neurol 1977; 34:729–738.
104. Dooling EC, Schoene WC, Richardson EP Jr. Hallevorden-Spatz syndrome. Arch Neurol 1974; 30:70–83.
105. Lindvall O, Bjorklund A, Skagerberg G. Dopamine-containing neurons in the spinal cord: anatomy and some functional aspects. Ann Neurol 1983; 14:255–260.
106. Lugaresi E, Medori R, Montagna P, et al. Fatal familial insomnia and dysautonomia with selective degeneration of thalamic nuclei. N Engl J Med 1986; 315:997–1003.
107. Gravellese MA, Victor M. Circulatory studies in Wernicke's encephalopathy. Circ Res 1957; 15: 836–844.
108. Birchfield RI. Postural hypotension in Wernicke's disease. Am J Med 1964; 36: 404–414.
109. Reis DJ, Iadecola C, Nakai M. Control of cerebral blood flow and metabolism by intrinsic neural systems in brain. In: Cerebrovascular Diseases. Proceedings of the 14th Princeton Conference. New York: Raven Press, 1985:1–22.

110. Reis DJ, Golanov EV. Central neurogenic regulation of regional blood flow (rCBF) and relationship to neuroprotection. In: Caplan LR, ed. Brain Ischemia: Basic Concepts and Clinical Relevance. London: Springer-Verlag, 1994: 273–288.
111. Vingerhoets F, Bogousslavsky J, Caplan LR. Respiratory dysfunction. In: Bogousslavsky J, Caplan LR, eds. Stroke Syndromes. London: Cambridge University Press, 1995: 223–231.
112. Berger AJ, Mitchell RA, Severinghaus JW. Regulation of respiration. N Engl J Med 1977; 297:138–143.
113. Plum F, Swanson AG. Abnormalities in central regulation of respiration in acute and convalescent poliomyelitis. Arch Neurol Psychiatry 1958; 80:267–285.
114. Brown JR, Baker AB. Poliomyelitis: 1. Bulbar poliomyelitis: a neurophysiological interpretation of the clinico-pathological findings. J Nerv Ment Dis 1949; 109:54–78.
115. Caplan LR. Posterior Circulation Vascular Disease. Boston: Blackwell Science, 1996
116. Devereaux MW, Keane JR, Davis RL. Automatic respiratory failure associated with infarction of the medulla. Arch Neurol 1973; 29:46–52.
117. Levin BE, Margolis G. Acute failure of automatic respirations secondary to a unilateral brainstem infarct. Ann Neurol 1977; 1:583–586.
118. Bogousslavsky J, Khurana R. Deruaz JP, et al. Respiratory failure and unilateral caudal brainstem infarction. Ann Neurol 1990; 28:668–673.
119. Brown RH, Sobel RA. Case records of the Massachusetts General Hospital. N Engl J Med 1989; 321:739–750.
120. Frayner J, Gates P. *Listeria* rhombencephalitis. Clin Exp Neurol 1987; 24:175–179.
121. Cushing H. Concerning a definite regulatory mechanism of the vaso-motor centre which controls blood pressure during cerebral compression. Bull Johns Hopkins Hosp 1901; 12:290–292.
122. Fox JL. Localization of the respiratory motor pathway in the upper cervical spinal cord following percutaneous cordotomy. Neurology 1969; 19:1115–1118.
123. Randall WC, McNally L, Caliguiri L. Rohse WG. Functional analysis of the cardio-augmentor and cardio-accellerator pathways in the dog. Am J Physiol 1957; 191: 213–217.
124. Levy MN, Warner MR. Parasympathetic effects on cardiac function. In: Armour JA, Ardell JL, eds. Neurocardiology. New York: Oxford University Press, 1994: 53–76.
125. Rodts GE, Haid RW. Intensive care management of spinal cord injury. In: Narayan RK, Wilberger JE, Povlishock JT, eds. Neurotrauma. New York: McGraw-Hill, 1995:1201–1212.
126. Bergofsky EH. Mechanism for respiratory insufficiency after cervical cord injury. Ann Intern Med 1964; 61:435–446.
127. Lehman KG, Lane JG, Piepmeier J, Batsford WP. Cardiovascular abnormalities accompanying acute spinal cord injury in humans: incidence, time course, and severity. J Am Coll Cardiol 1987; 10:46–52.
128. Mathias CJ, Christensen NJ, Frankel HL, Spalding JMK. Cardiovascular control in recently injured tetraplegics in spinal shock. Q J Med 1979; 48:273–287.

129. Mathias CJ. Bradycardia and cardiac arrest during tracheal suction—mechanisms in tetraplegic patients. Eur J Intens Care Med 1976; 2:147–156.
130. Mathias CJ, Frankel HL. Autonomic disturbances in spinal cord lesions. In: Bannister R, Mathias CJ, eds. Autonomic Failure, a Textbook of Clinical Disorders of the Autonomic Nervous System. Oxford: Oxford University Press, 1992 (Chap. 43):839–881.
131. Mathias CJ, Christensen NJ, Frankel HL, Spalding JMK. Enhanced pressor response to noradrenaline in patients with cervical spinal cord transection. Brain 1976; 99:757–770.
132. Curt A, Nitsche B, Rodic B, Schurch B, Dietz V. Assessment of sutonomic dysreflexia in patients with spinal cord injury. J Neurol Neurosurg Psychiatry 1997; 62:473–477.
133. Lalouschek W, Muller C, Gamper G, Weissel M, Turetscheli K. Myocardial ischemia with normal coronary arteries associated with thoracic myelitis. N Engl J Med 1997; 337:1920.
134. Aminoff MJ, Wilcox CS. Autonomic dysfunction in syringomyelia. Postgrad Med J 1972; 48:113–115.
135. Nogues MA, Newman PK, Male VJ, Foster JB. Cardiovascular reflexes in syringomyelia. Brain 1982; 105:835–849.
136. Adams RD, Victor M, Ropper AH. Principles of Neurology. 6th Ed. New York: McGraw-Hill, 1997:764–767.
137. Weinstein L, Shelovok A. Cardiovascular manifestations of acute poliomyelitis. N Engl J Med 1951; 244:281–285.
138. Hudson REB. Cardiovascular Pathology. Vol. 1. London: Edward Arnold, 1965: 735, 787–790.
139. Mathias CJ. Autonomic disorders and their recognition. N Engl J Med 1997; 336: 721–724.
139a. Schatz IJ, Bannister R, Freeman RL, et al. Consensus statement. The definition of orthostatic hypotension, pure autonomic failure, and multiple system atrophy. J Auton Nerv Syst 1996; 58:123–124.
140. McLeod JG, Tuck RR. Disorders of the autonomic nervous system. Part 1. Pathophysiology and clinical features. Ann Neurol 1987; 21:419–430.
141. Thomas JE, Schirger A. Idiopathic orthostatic hypotension. Arch Neurol 1970; 22: 289–293.
142. Bannister R. Clinical features of progressive autonomic failure. In: Bannister R, ed. Autonomic Failure. Oxford: Oxford University Press, 1983:67–73.
143. Terrao Y, Takeda K, Sakuta M, et al. Pure progressive autonomic failure: a clinicopathological study. Eur Neurol 1993; 33:409–415.
144. Oppenheimer DR. Lateral horn cells in progressive autonomic failure. J Neurol Sci 1980; 46:393–404.
145. Sever PS. Plasma noradrenaline in autonomic failure. In: Bannister R, ed. Autonomic Failure. Oxford: Oxford University Press, 1983:155–173.
146. Goldstein DS, Polinsky RJ, Garty M, et al. Patterns of plasma levels of catechols in neurogenic orthostatic hypotension. Ann Neurol 1989; 26:558–563.
147. Yoshida M, Fukumoto Y, Kuroda Y, Ohkoshi N. Sympathetic denervation of myocardium demonstrated by ^{123}I-MIBG scinigraphy in pure progressive autonomic failure. Eur Neurol 1997; 38:291–296.

148. Goldstein DS, Holmes C, Cannon RO III, Eisenhofer G, Kopin IJ. Sympathetic cardioneuropathy in dysautonomias. Nietzsche English 331—19th century. N Engl J Med 1997; 336:696–702.
149. Riley CM, Day RL, Greeley DM, Langford WS. Central autonomic dysfunction with defective lacrimation. 1. Report of 5 cases. Pediatrics 1949; 3:468–478.
150. Riley CM. Familial dysautonomia. Adv Pediatr 1957; 9:157–190.
151. Dancis J, Smith AA. Current concepts. Familial dysautonomia. N Engl J Med 1966; 274:207–209.
152. Fogelson MH, Rorke LB, Kaye R. Spinal cord changes in familial dysautonomia. Arch Neurol 1967; 17:103–108.
153. Mason DT, Kopin IJ, Braunwald E. Abnormalities in reflex control of the circulation in familial dysautonomia. Am J Med 1966; 41:898–909.
154. Adie WJ. Tonic pupils and absent tendon reflexes: a benign disorder sui generis: its complete and incomplete forms. Brain 1932; 55:98–113.
155. Holmes G. Partial iridoplegia associated with symptoms of other diseases of the nervous system. Trans Ophthal Soc UK 1931; 51:209–224.
156. Johnson RH, McLellan DL, Love DR. Orthostatic hypotension and the Holmes-Adie syndrome: a study of two patients with afferent baroreceptor block. J Neurol Neurosurg Psychiatry 1971; 34:562–570.
157. Lucy DD, Van Allen MW, Thompson HS. Holmes-Adie syndrome with segmental hypohydrosis. Neurology 1967; 17:763–770.
158. Berkowitz JS, Zweifach PH. Evidence for cardiac autonomic dysfunction in patients with tonic pupils. Neurology 1970; 20:1096–1102.
159. Young RR, Asbury AK, Adams RD, Corbett JL. Pure pandysautonomia with recovery. Trans Am Neurol Assoc 1969; 94:355–357.
160. Young RR, Asbury AK, Adams RD, Corbett JL. Pure pandysautonomia with recovery. Description and discussion of diagnostic criteria. Brain 1975; 98:613–635.
161. Low PA, Dyck PJ, Lambert EH, et al. Acute pandysautonomic neuropathy. Ann Neurol 1983; 13:412–417.
162. Appenzeller O, Kornfeld M. Acute pandysautonomia. Clinical and morphological study. Arch Neurol 1973; 29:334–349.
163. Harik SI, Ghandour MH, Farah FS, Afifi AK. Postganglionic cholinergic dysautonomia. Ann Neurol 1977; 1:393–396.
164. Hopkins IJ, Shield LK, Harris M. Subacute cholinergic dysautonomia in childhood. Clin Exp Neurol 1980; 17:147–151.
165. Yahr MD, Frontera AT. Acute autonomic neuropathy. Arch Neurol 1975; 32:132–133.
166. Lieshout JJV, Wieling W, Montfrans GV, et al. Acute dysautonomia associated with Hodgkin's disease. J Neurol Neurosurg Psychiatry 1986; 49:830–832.
167. Stoll G, Thomas C, Reiners K, Schober R, Hartung H-P. Encephalo-myelo-radiculo-ganglionitis presenting as pandysautonomia. Neurology 1991; 41:723–726.
168. Low PA. Non-invasive evaluation of autonomic function. Neurol Chron 1992; 2(5)1–8.
169. McLeod JG, Tuck RR. Disorders of the autonomic nervous system: Part 2. Investigation and treatment. Ann Neurol 1987; 21:519–529.
170. Mathias CJ, Bannister R. Investigation of autonomic disorders. In: Bannister R,

Mathias CJ, eds. Autonomic Failure: A Textbook of Clinical Disorders of the Autonomic Nervous System. 3d ed. Oxford: Oxford University Press, 1992:334–358.
171. Low PA. Quantitation of autonomic function. In: Dyck PJ, Thomas PK, eds. Peripheral Neuropathy. 3d ed. Philadelphia: WB Saunders 1993:729–745.
172. Lind AR, Taylor SH, Humphreys PW, et al. The circulatory effects of sustained voluntary muscle contraction. Clin Sci 1964; 27:229–244.
173. Sundqvist G, Almer L-O, Lilja B. Respiratory influences on heart rate in diabetes mellitus. Br Med J 1979; 1:924–925.
174. Levin AB. A simple test of cardiac function based upon the heart-rate change during the Valsalva maneuver. Am J Cardiol 1966; 18:90–99.
175. Kirchheim HR. Systemic arterial baroreceptor reflexes. Physiol Rev 1976; 56:100–176.
176. Lepore FE. Diagnostic pharmacology of the pupil. Clin Neuropharmacol 1985; 8: 23–37.
177. Ponsford JR, Bannister R, Paul EA. Methacholine pupillary responses in third nerve palsy and Adie's syndrome. Brain 1983; 106:503–511.
178. Freeman R, Young J, Landsberg L, Lipsitz L. The treatment of postprandial hypotension in autonomic failure with 3,4-DL-threodihydroxyphenylserine. Neurology 1996; 47:1414–1420.
179. Kaufman H. Could treatment with DOPS do for autonomic failure what DOPA did for Parkinson's disease. Neurology 1996; 47:1370–1371.
180. McTavish D, Goa KL. Midodrine. A review of its pharmacological properties and therapeutic use in orthostatic hypotension and secondary hypotensive disorders. Drugs 1989; 38:757–777.
181. McLeod JG. Autonomic dysfunction in peripheral nerve disease. In: Bannister R, Mathias CJ eds. Autonomic Failure. A Textbook of Clinical Disorders of the Autonomic Nervous System. 3d ed Oxford: Oxford University Press, 1992:659–681.
182. Moskowitz MA. The neurobiology of vascular head pain. Ann Neurol 1984; 16: 157–168.
183. Barbas N, Caplan LR, Baquis, G, et al. Dental chair intracerebral hemorrhage. Neurology 1987; 37:511–512.
184. Haines SJ, Maroon JC, Janetta PJ. Supratentorial intracerebral hemorrhage following posterior fossa surgery. J Neurosurg 1978; 49:881–886.
185. Waga S, Shimosaka S, Sakakura M. Intracerebral hemorrhage remote from the site of the initial neurosurgical procedure. Neurosurgery 1983; 13:662–665.
186. Caplan LR. Hypertensive intracerebral hemorrhage. In: Kase CS, Caplan LR, eds. Intracerebral Hemorrhage. Boston: Butterworth-Heinemann, 1994:99–116.
187. Sweet WH, Poletti CE, Roberts JT. Dangerous rises in blood pressure upon heating of trigeminal rootlets: increased bleeding times in patients with trigeminal neuralgia. Neurosurgery 1985; 17:843–844.
188. Kehler CH, Brodsky JB, Samuels SL, et al. Blood pressure during percutaneous rhizotomy for trigeminal neuralgia. Neurosurgery 1982; 10:200–202.
189. Cawley CM,Rigamonti D, Trommer B. Dental chair apoplexy. South Med J 1991; 84:907–909.
190. Ropper A. Current concepts: the Guillain-Barré syndrome. N Engl J Med 1992; 326:1130–1136.

191. Ropper AH, Wijdicks EFM, Truax BT. Guillain-Barré Syndrome. Philadelphia: FA Davis, 1991.
192. McDonagh AJG, Dawson J. Guillain-Barré syndrome after myocardial infarction. Br Med J 1987; 294:613–614.
193. Asbury AK, Arnason BG, Adams RD. The inflammatory lesion in idiopathic polyneuritis. Medicine 1969; 48:173–215.
194. Fisher CM. An unusual variant of acute idiopathic polyneuritis (syndrome of opthalmoplegia, ataxia, and areflexia). N Engl J Med 1956; 255:57–65.
195. Greenland P, Griggs RC. Arrhythmic complications in the Guillain-Barré syndrome. Arch Intern Med 1980; 140:1053–1055.
196. Palferman TG, Wright I, Doyle DV, Amiel S. Electrocardiographic abnormalities and autonomic dysfunction in Gullain-Barré syndrome. Br Med J 1982; 284:1231–1232.
197. Tuck RR, McLeod JG. Autonomic dysfunction in Guillain-Barré syndrome. J Neurol Neurosurg Psychiatry 1982; 44:983–990.
198. Fagius J, Wallin G. Microneurographic evidence of excessive sympathetic outflow in the Guillain-Barré syndrome. Brain 1983; 106:589–600.
199. Dyck PJ, Lais AC, Ohta M, Bastron JA, Okazaki H, Groover R. Chronic inflammatory polyradiculoneuropathy. Mayo Clin Proc 1975; 50:621–640.
200. Austin JH. Recurrent polyneuropathies and their corticosteroid treatment. With five-year observations of a placebo-controlled case treated with corticotrophin, cortisone, and prednisone. Brain 1958; 81:157–192.
201. Ingall TJ, McLeod JG, Tamura N. Autonomic function and unmyelinated fibers in chronic inflammatory demyelinating polyradiculoneuropathy. Muscle Nerve 1990; 13:70–76.
202. Lewis RA, Summer AJ, Brown MJ, et al. Multifocal demyelinative neuropathy with persistent conduction block. Neurology 1982; 32:958–964.
203. Kornberg AJ, Pestronk A. Chronic motor neuropathies. In: Serratrice G, Munsat T, eds. Pathogenesis and Therapy of Amyotrophic Lateral Sclerosis. Advances in Neurology. Philadelphia: Lippincott-Raven, 1995:113–119.
204. Azulay J-P, Ribet P, Pouget J, et al. Long term follow up of multifocal motor neuropathy with conduction block under treatment. J Neurol Neurosurg Psychiatry 1997; 62:391–394.
205. Fisher CM, Adams RD. Diphtheritic polyneuritis: a pathological study. J Neuropathol Exp Neurol 1956: 15:243–268.
206. McDonald WI, Kocen RS. Diphtheritic neuropathy. In: Dyck PJ, Thomas PK, eds. Peripheral Neuropathy. 3d ed. Philadelphia: WB Saunders, 1993:1412–1423.
207. Gore I. Myocardial changes in fatal diphtheria. A summary of observations in 221 cases. Am J Med Sci 1948; 215:257–266.
208. Hudson REB. Diptheria in Cardiovascular Pathology. Vol. 1. London: Edward Arnold, 1965:805–806.
209. Leys DG. Heart block following diphtheria. Br Heart J 1945; 7:57–58.
210. Perry CB. Persistent conduction defects following diphtheria. Br Heart J 1939; 1: 117–122.
211. Hoel J. Reappearance of complete heart block years after diphtheritic myocardial disease. Acta Med Scand 1958; 160:237–244.

212. McNulty CM. Aids and the heart. In: Hurst JW, ed. New types of Cardiovascular Diseases. New York: Igaku-Shoin, 1994:46–62.
213. Freeman R, Roberts MS, Friedman LS, Broadbridge C. Autonomic function and human immunodeficiency virus infection. Neurology 1990; 40:575–580.
214. Cohen JA, Laudenslager M. Autonomic nervous system involvement in patients with human immunodeficiency virus infection. Neurology 1989; 39:1111–1112.
215. Adams RD, Victor M, eds. Principles of Neurology. 5th ed. New York: McGraw-Hill, 1993:1145–1146.
216. Sabin TD, Swift TR, Jacobson RR. Leprosy. In: Dyck PJ, Thomas PK, Griffin JW, et al., eds. Peripheral Neuropathy. Philadelphia: WB Saunders, 1993:1354–1379.
217. Connor DH, Manz HJ. Parasitic infections of the peripheral nervous system. In: Dyck PJ, Thomas PK, Griffin JW, et al., eds. Peripheral Neuropathy. Philadelphia, WB Saunders, 1993:1380–1383.
218. Iosa D, Dequattro V, Lee D, et al. Pathogenesis of cardiac neuromyopathy in Chagas' disease and the role of the autonomic nervous system. J Auton Nerv Syst 1990; 30:583–588.
219. Oliveira JSM, Preta R. A natural human model of intrinsic heart nervous system degeneration: Chagas' cardiopathy. Am Heart J 1985; 110:1092–1098.
220. Said G, Joskowicz M, Barreira AA, Eisea H. Neuropathy associated with experimental Chagas' disease. Ann Neurol 1985; 18:676–683.
221. Davila DF, Rossell RO, Donis JH. Cardiac parasympathetic abnormalities: cause or consequence of Chagas' heart disease. Parasitol Today 1989; 5:327–329.
222. Iosa D, Dequattro V, Lee DD, et al. Pathogenesis of cardiac neuro-myopathy in Chagas' disease and the role of the autonomic nervous system. J Auton Nerv Syst 1990; 30:583–588.
223. Burgdorfer W, Barbour AG, Hayes SF, et al. Lyme disease—a tick-borne spirochetosis? Science 1982; 216:1317–1319.
224. Steere AC, Grodzicke RL, Kornblatt AN, et al. The spirochetal etiology of Lyme disease. N Engl J Med 1983; 308:733–740.
225. Steere AC, Schoen RT, Taylor E. The clinical evolution of Lyme arthritis. Ann Intern Med 1987; 107:725–731.
226. Pachner AR, Steere AC. The triad of neurologic manifestations of Lyme disease: meningitis, cranial neuritis, and radiculoneuritis. Neurology 1985; 35:47–53.
227. Pachner AR, Duray P, Steere AC. Central nervous system manifestations of Lyme disease. Arch Neurol 1989; 46:790–795.
228. Logigian EL, Kaplan R, Steere AC. Chronic neurologic manifestations of Lyme disease. N Engl J Med 1990; 323:1438–1444.
229. Bannwarth A. Zur klinik und pathogenese der ''chronischen lymphocytaren meningitis.'' Arch Psychiatr Nervenkr 1944; 117:161–185.
230. Halperin JJ, Little BW, Coyle PK, Dattwyler RJ. Lyme disease: cause of a treatable peripheral neuropathy. Neurology 1987; 37:1700–1706.
231. Logigian EL, Steere AC. Clinical and electrophysiologic findings in chronic neuropathy of Lyme disease. Neurology 1992; 42:303–311.
232. Duffy J, Rodeheffer RJ. The heart and Lyme disease. In: Hurst JW, ed. New Types of Cardiovascular Diseases. New York: Igaku-Shoin, 1994:164–174.

233. Steere AC, Batsford WP, Weinberg M, et al. Lyme carditis: cardiac abnormalities of Lyme disease. Ann Intern Med 1980; 93:8–16.
234. McAlister HF, Klementowicz PT, Andrews C, et al. Lyme carditis: an important cause of reversible heart block. Ann Intern Med 1989; 110:339–345.
235. Nagi KS, Joshi R, Thakur RK. Cardiac manifestations of Lyme disease: a review. Can J Cardiol 1996; 12:503–506.
236. Garland H. Diabetic amyotrophy. Br Med J 1955; 2:1287–1290.
237. Locke S, Lawrence DG, Legg MA. Diabetic amyotrophy. Am J Med 1963; 34: 775–785.
238. Chokroverty S, Reyes MG, Rubino FA, Tunaki H. The syndrome of diabetic amyotrophy. Ann Neurol 1977; 2:181–194.
239. Raff MC, Sangalang V, Asbury AK. Ischemic mononeuropathy multiplex associated with diabetes mellitus. Arch Neurol 1968; 18:487–499.
240. Bastron JA, Thomas JE. Diabetic polyradiculopathy. Mayo Clin Proc 1981; 56: 725–732.
241. Kikta DG, Breuer AC, Wilbourn AJ. Thoracic root pain in diabetes; the spectrum of clinical and electrographic findings. Ann Neurol 1982; 11:80–85.
242. Brown MJ, Asbury AK. Diabetic neuropathy. Ann Neurol 1984; 15:2–12.
243. Clarke BF, Ewing DJ, Campbell IW. Diabetic autonomic neuropathy. Diabetologia 1979; 17:195–212.
244. Faerman I, Glacer L, Celemer D, et al. Autonomic nervous system and diabetes: histological and histochemical study of the autonomic nerve fibers of the urinary bladder in diabetic patients. Diabetes 1973; 22:225–237.
245. Low PA, Walsh JC, Huang CY, McLeod JG. The sympathetic nervous system in diabetic neuropathy: a clinical and pathological study. Brain 1975; 98:341–356.
246. Page MM, Watkins PJ. Cardiorespiratory arrest and diabetic autonomic neuropathy. Lancet 1978; 1:14–16.
247. Hilsted J. Pathophysiology in diabetic autonomic neuropathy: cardiovascular, hormonal, and metabolic studies. Diabetes 1982; 31:730–737.
248. O'Brien IAD, Corrall RJM. Epidemiology of diabetes and its complications. N Engl J Med 1988; 318:1619–1620.
249. Edmonds ME, Watkins PJ. Clinical presentation of diabetic autonomic failure. In: Bannister R, Mathias CJ, eds. Autonomic Failure. A Textbook of Clinical Disorders of the Autonomic Nervous System. 3d ed. Oxford: Oxford Med. Publ., 1992:698–720.
250. Neil HAW. Epidemiology of diabetic autonomic neuropathy. In: Bannister R, Mathias CJ, eds. Autonomic Failure. A Textbook of Clinical Disorders of the Autonomic Nervous System. 3d ed. Oxford: Oxford Med. Publ. 1992:682–697.
251. Bilious RW. Diabetic autonomic neuropathy. Br Med J 1990; 301:565–566.
252. Ewing DJ, Martyn CN, Young RJ, Clarke BF. The value of cardiovascular autonomic function tests: 10 years experience in diabetes. Diabetes Care 1985; 8:491–498.
253. O'Brien IA, McFadden JP, Corrall RJM. The influence of autonomic neuropathy on mortality in insulin-dependent diabetes. Q J Med 1991; 79:495–502.
254. McMicken DB. Alcohol: tolerance, addiction, and withdrawal. In: Hurst JW, ed.

Medicine for the Practising Physician. 4th ed. Stamford, CT: Appleton & Lange, 1996:1975–1980.
255. Victor M, Adams RD. The effect of alcohol on the nervous system. Res Publ Assoc Res Nerv Ment Dis 1953; 32:526–573.
256. Adams RD, Victor M, Ropper A. Principles of Neurology. 6th ed. New York: McGraw-Hill, 1997:1166–1185.
257. Charness ME, Simon RP, Greenberg DA. Ethanol and the nervous system. N Engl J Med 1989; 321:442–454.
258. Charness ME. Neurologic complications of alcoholism In: Samuels MA, Feske S, eds. Office Practice of Neurology. New York: Churchill-Livingstone, 1996:1047–1055.
259. Wolfe SM, Victor M. The relationship of hypomagnesemia and alkalosis to alcohol withdrawal symptoms. Ann NY Acad Sci 1969; 162:973–998.
260. Victor M, Adams RD, Collins GH. The Wernicke-Korsakoff Syndrome. Philadelphia: FA Davis, 1971.
261. Carlen PL, Wortzman G, Holgate RC, Wilkinson DA, Rankin JC. Reversible cerebral atrophy in recently abstinent alcoholics measured by computed tomography scans. Science 1978; 200:1076–1078.
262. Carlen PL, Wilkinson DA, Wortzman G, Holgate R. Partially reversible cerebral atrophy and functional improvement in recently abstinent alcoholics. Can J Neurol Sci 1984; 11:441–446.
263. Victor M, Adams RD, Mancall EL. A restricted form of cerebellar degeneration occurring in alcoholic patients. Arch Neurol 1959; 1:579–688.
264. Marchiafava E, Bignami A. Sopra un'alterazione del corpo calloso osservaba in sogetti alcooliste. Riv Patol Nerv Ment 1903; 8:544–549.
265. Kawamura M, Shiota J, Yagashita T, Hirayama K. Marchiafava-Bignami disease: computed tomographic scan and magnetic resonance imaging. Ann Neurol 1985; 18:103–104.
266. Adams RD, Victor M, Mancall EL. Central pontine myelinolysis: a hitherto undescribed disease occurring in alcoholic and malnourished patients. Arch Neurol Psychiatry 1959; 81:154–172.
267. Norenberg MD, Leslie KO, Robertson AS. Association between rise in serum sodium and central pontine myelinolysis. Ann Neurol 1982; 11:128–135.
268. Laureno R. Central pontine myelinolysis following rapid correction of hyponatremia. Ann Neurol 1983; 13:232–242.
269. Carroll FD. The etiology and treatment of tobacco-alcohol amblyopia. Amer J Ophthalmol 1944; 27:713–725, 847–863.
270. Victor M. Tobacco-alcohol amblyopia. A critique of current concepts of this disorder, with special reference to the role of nutritional deficiency and its causation. Arch Ophthalmol 1963; 70:313–318.
271. Rubin E. Alcohol myopathy in heart and skeletal muscle. N Engl J Med 1979; 301: 28–33.
272. Haller RG, Knochel JP. Skeletal muscle disease in alcoholism. Med Clin North Am 1984; 68:91–103.
273. Martin F, Ward K, Slavin G, Levi J, Peters TJ. Alcoholic skeletal myopathy, a clinical and pathological study. Q J Med 1985; 55:233–251.

274. Behse S, Buchtal F. Alcoholic neuropathy: clinical, electrophysiological, and biopsy findings. Ann Neurol 1977; 2:95–110.
275. Hillbom M, Wennberg A. Prognosis of alcoholic peripheral neuropathy. J Neurol Neurosurg Psychiatry 1984; 47:699–703.
276. Segel LD, Klausner SC, Gnadt JTH, Amsterdam EA. Alcohol and the heart. Med Clin North Am 1984; 68:147–161.
277. Piano MR, Schwertz DW. Alcoholic heart disease: a review. Heart Lung 1994; 23: 3–17.
278. Eisenhofer GE, Whiteside EA, Johnson RH. Plasma catecholamine responses to change of posture in alcoholics during withdrawal and after continued abstinence from alcohol. Clin Sci 1985; 68:71–78.
279. Novak DJ, Victor M. The vagus and sympathetic nerves in alcohol neuropathy. Arch Neurol 1974; 30:273–284.
280. Duncan G, Johnson RH, Lambie DG, et al. Evidence of vagal neuropathy in chronic alcoholics. Lancet 1980; 2:1053–1057.
281. Johnson RH, Lambie DG. Autonomic function and dysfunction. In: Asbury A, McKann GM, McDonald WI, eds. Diseases of the Nervous System. Clinical Neurobiology. Philadelphia: WB Saunders, 1986:665–678.
282. Tan ETH, Johnson RH, Lambie DG, et al. Alcoholic vagal neuropathy: recovery following prolonged abstinence. J Neurol Neurosurg Psychiatry 1984; 47:1335–1337.
283. Saunders JB. Alcohol: an important cause of hypertension. Br Med J 1987; 294: 1045.
284. Gill JS, Shipley MJ, Tsementzis SA, et al. Alcohol consumption: a risk factor for hemorrhagic and nonhemorrhagic stroke. Am J Med 1991; 90:489–497.
285. Gorelick PB. Alcohol and stroke. Stroke 1987; 18:268–271.
286. Asbury A, Victor M, Adams RD. Uremic polyneuropathy. Arch Neurol 1963; 8: 413–428.
287. Dayan AD, Gardner-Thorpe C, Down PF, Gleadle RI. Peripheral neuropathy in uremia. Neurology 1970; 20:649–658.
288. Dyck PJ, Johnson WJ, Lambert EH, O'Brien PC. Segmental demyelination secondary to axonal degeneration in uremic neuropathy. Mayo Clin Proc 1971; 46:400–430.
289. Tyler HR. Neurologic disorders in renal failure. Am J Med 1968; 44:734–748.
290. Ropper AH. Accelerated neuropathy of renal failure. Arch Neurol 1993; 50:536–539.
291. Spodick DH. The Pericardium: A Comprehensive Textbook. New York: Marcel Dekker, 1997:293–296.
292. Falk RH, Comenzo RL, Skinner M. The systemic amyloidoses. N Engl J Med 1997; 337:898–909.
293. WHO-IUIS Nomenclature Sub-Committee. Nomenclature of amyloid and amyloidosis. Bull World Health Organ 1993; 71:105–112.
294. Kyle RA, Gertz MA. Primary systemic amyloidosis: clinical and laboratory features in 474 cases. Semin Hematol 1995; 32:45–59.
295. Kyle RA, Dyck PJ. Amyloidosis and neuropathy. In: Dyck PJ, Thomas PK, Griffin JW, et al., eds. Peripheral Neuropathy. Vol. 2. Philadelphia: WB Saunders, 1993: 1294–1309.

296. Andrade C. A peculiar form of peripheral neuropathy: atypical generalized amyloidosis with special involvement of the peripheral nerves. Brain 1952; 75:408.
297. Coelho T. Familial amyloid polyneuropathy: new developments in genetics and treatment. Curr Opin Neurol 1996; 9:355–359.
298. Bergethon PR, Sabin TD, Lewis D, et al. Improvement in the polyneuropathy associated with familial amyloid polyneuropathy after liver transplantation. Neurology 1996; 47:944–951.
299. Ando Y, Obayashi K, Tanaka Y, et al. A new and sensitive tool for autonomic dysfunction: analysis by radiolabelled meta-iodobenzylguanidine (MIBG) in patients with familial amyloidotic polyneuropathy (PAL). Int J Exp Clin Invest 1995; 2:183–187.
300. Windebank AJ, Bankovsky H. Porphyric Neuropathy. In: Dyck PJ, Thomas PK, Griffin JW, et al., eds. Peripheral Neuropathy. Vol. 2. Philadelphia: WB Saunders, 1993:1161–1168.
301. Tschudy DP, Valsamis M, Magnussen CR. Acute intermittent porphyria: clinical and selected research aspects. Ann Intern Med 1975; 83:851–864.
302. Kushner JP. The porphyrias. In: Hurst JW, ed. Medicine for the Practicing Physician. 4th ed. Stamford, CT: Appleton & Lange, 1996:917–923.
303. Perloth MG, Tschudy DP, Marver HS, et al. Acute intermittent porphyria: new morphologic and biochemical findings. Am J Med 1966; 41:149–162.
304. Gibson JB, Goldberg A. The neuropathy of acute porphyria. J Pathol Bacteriol 1965; 71:495–509.
305. Suarez JI, Cohen ML, Larkin J, et al. Acute intermittent porphyria: clinicopathological correlation. Report of a case and review of the literature. Neurology 1997; 48: 1678–1683.
306. Bonkovsky HL, Schady W. Neurologic manifestations of acute porphyria. Semin Liv Dis 1982; 2:108–124.
307. Kupferschmidt H, Bont A, Schnorf H, et al. Transient cortical blindness and bioccipital brain lesions in two patients with acute intermittent porphyria. Ann Intern Med 1995; 123:598–600.
308. Magnussen CR, Doherty JM, Hess RA, Tschudy DP. Grand mal seizures and acute intermittent porphyria. Neurology 1975; 25:1121–1125.
309. Bassen FA, Kornzweig AL. Malformation of the erythrocytes in a case of atypical retinitis pigmentosa. Blood 1950; 5:381–387.
310. Yao JK, Herbert PN. Lipoprotein deficiency and neuromuscular manifestations. In: Dyck PJ, Thomas PK, Griffin JW, et al., eds. Peripheral Neuropathy. Vol. 2. Philadelphia: WB Saunders, 1993:1179–1193.
311. Adams RD, Victor M, Ropper A. Principles of Neurology. 6th ed. New York: McGraw-Hill, 1997:1347–1348.
312. Fredrickson DS, Altrocchi PH, Avioli LV, Goodman DS, Goodman HC. Tangier disease—combined clinical staff conference at the National Institute of Health. Ann Intern Med 1961; 55:1016–1031.
313. Assmann G, von Eckardstein A, Brewer HB Jr. Familial high density lipoprotein deficiency: Tangier disease. In: Scriver CR, Beaudet AL, Sly WM, et al., eds. The Metabolic and Molecular Bases of Inherited Disease. Vol. II. New York: McGraw-Hill, 1995:2053–2072.

314. Schaefer EJ, Zech LA, Schwartz DE, Brewer HB Jr. Coronary heart disease prevalence and other clinical features in familial high-density lipoprotein deficiency (Tangier disease). Ann Intern Med 1980; 93:261–266.
315. Refsum S. Heredopathia atactica polyneuritiformis: phytanic acid storage disease (Refsum disease). In: Vinken PJ, Bruyn GW, eds. Vol 21. Handbook of Clinical Neurology. System Disorders and Atrophies. Amsterdam: North-Holland, 1975: 181–229.
316. Skjeldal OH, Stokke O, Refsum S. Phytanic acid storage disease. In: Dyck PJ, Thomas PK, Griffin JW, et al., eds. Peripheral Neuropathy. Vol. 2. Philadelphia: WB Saunders, 1993:1149–1160.
317. Cammermeyer J. Neuropathological changes in hereditary neuropathies: manifestation of the syndrome heredopathia atactica polyneuritiformis in the presence of interstitial hypertrophic polyneuropathy. J Neuropathol Exp Neurol 1956; 15:340–361.
318. Gordon N, Hudson REB. Refsum's syndrome—heredopathia atactica polyneuritiformis. Brain 1959; 82:41–55.
319. Hudson REB. Cardiovascular Pathology. Vol. 1. London: Edward Arnold, 1965: 736–737.
320. Brady RO. Fabry disease. In: Dyck PJ, Thomas PK, Griffin JW, et al., eds. Peripheral Neuropathy. Vol 2. Philadelphia: WB Saunders, 1993:1169–1178.
321. Kolodny EH. Fabry disease. In: Bogousslavsky J, Caplan LR, eds. Stroke Syndromes. New York: Cambridge University Press, 1995:453–459.
321a. Nakao S, Takenaka T, Maeda M, et al. An atypical variant of Fabry's disease in men with left ventricular hypertrophy. N Engl J Med 1995; 333:288–293.
322. Goldman ME, Cantor R, Schwartz MF, Baker M, Desnick RJ. Echocardiographic abnormalities and disease severity in Fabry's disease. J Am Coll Cardiol 1986; 7: 1157–1161.
322a. Mitsias P, Levine SR. Cerebrovascular complications of Fabry's disease. Ann Neurol 1996; 40:8–17.
323. Efthimiou J, Mclelland J, Betteridge DJ. Short PR intervals and tachyarrhythmias in Fabry's disease. Postgrad Med J 1986; 62:285–287.
324. Sakuraba H, Igarashi T, Shibata T, Suzuki Y. Effect of vitamin E and ticlopidine on platelet aggregation in Fabry's disease. Clin Genet 1987; 31:349–354.
325. Dyck PJ, Chance P, Lebo R, Carney JA. Hereditary motor and sensory neuropathies. In: Dyck PJ, Thomas PK, Griffin JW, et al., eds. Peripheral Neuropathy. Vol. 2. Philadelphia: WB Saunders, 1993:1094–1136.
326. Dyck PJ, Dyck JB, Chalk CH. The 10 P's: a mnemonic helpful in characterization and differential diagnosis of peripheral neuropathy. Neurology 1992; 42:14–18.
327. Dyck PJ, Dyck JB, Grant IA, Fealey RD. Ten steps in characterizing and diagnosing patients with peripheral neuropathy. Neurology 1996; 47:10–17.
328. Ingall TJ, McLeod JG. Autonomic function in hereditary motor and sensory neuropathy (Charcot-Marie-Tooth disease). Muscle Nerve 1991; 14:1080–1083.
329. Leak D. Paroxysmal atrial flutter in peroneal muscular atrophy. Br Heart J 1961; 23:326–328.
330. Lowry PJ, Littler WA. Peroneal muscular atrophy associated with cardiac conduction tissue disease. Postgrad Med J 1983; 59:530–532.

331. Martin–Du Pan RC, Juge C, Perrenoud JJ. Cardiomyopathie congestive et augmentation du pyruvate dans un case de maladie du Charcot-Marie-Tooth. Schweiz Med Wochenschr 1984; 114:625–629.
332. Adams RD, Victor M, Ropper AH. Principles of Neurology. 6th ed. New York: McGraw-Hill, 1997:1345.
333. Banker BQ. The congenital muscular dystrophies. In: Engel AG, Franzini-Armstrong, eds. Myology. 2d ed. New York: McGraw-Hill, 1994:1275–1289.
334. Beggs AH. Dystrophinopathy, the expanding phenotype: dystrophin abnormalities in X-linked dilated cardiomyopathy. (Editorial.) Circulation 1997; 95:2344–2347.
335. Politano L, Nigro V, Nigro G, Petretta VR, Passamano L, Papparella S, Di Somma S, Comi LI. Development of cardiomyopathy in female carriers of Duchenne and Becker muscular dystrophies. JAMA 1975; 275:1335–1338.
336. Emery AEH. Duchenne Mucular Dystrophy. 2d ed. Oxford: Oxford University Press, 1993.
337. Perloff JK, Roberts, WC, de Leon A, O'Doherty D. The distinctive electrocardiogram of Duchenne's progressive muscular dystrophy. Am J Med 1967; 42:179–188.
338. Perloff JK. Cardiac rhythm and conduction in Duchenne's muscular dystrophy. A prospective study of 20 patients. J Am Coll Cardiol 1984; 3:1263–1268.
339. Nigro G, Comi LI, Politano L, Bain RJ. The incidence and evolution of cardiomyopathy in Duchenne muscular dystrophy. Int J Cardiol 1990; 26:271–277.
340. Angelini C, Fanin M, Pegoraro E, Freda MP, Cadaldini M, Martinello F. Clinical-molecular correlation in 104 mild X-linked muscular dystrophy patients: characterization of subclinical phenotypes. Neuromuscul Disord 1994; 4:349–358.
341. Zalman F, Perloff JK, Durant NN, Campion DS. Acute respiratory failure following intravenous verapamil in Duchenne's muscular dystrophy. Am Heart J 1983; 105: 510–511.
342. Chalkiadis GA, Branch KG. Cardiac arrest after isofluraneanaesthesia in a patient with Duchenne's muscular dystrophy. Anaesthesia 1990; 45:22–25.
343. Wijmenga C, Sandkuijl LA, Moerer P, et al. Genetic linkage map of facioscapulohumeral muscular dystrophy and five polymorphic loci on chromosome 4q35-qter. Am J Hum Genet 1992; 51:411–415.
344. Tawil R, Figlewicz DA, Griggs RC, Weiffenbach, B, FSH Consortium. Facioscapulohumeral dystrophy: a distinct regional myopathy with a novel molecular pathogenesis. Ann Neurol 1998; 43:279–282.
345. Stevenson WG, Perloff JK, Weiss JN, Anderson TL. Facioscapulohumeral muscular dystrophy: evidence for selective, genetic electrophysiologic cardiac involvement. J Am Coll Cardiol 1990; 15:292–299.
346. Politano L, Nigro V, Nigro G, Petretta VR, Passamano L, Papparella S, Di Somma S, Comi LI. Development of cardiomyopathy in female carriers of Duchenne and Becker muscular dystrophies. JAMA 1975; 275:1335–1338.
347. Hoffman EP, Kunkel LM. Dystrophin abnormalities in Duchenne/Becker muscular dystrophy. Neuron 1989; 2:1019–1029.
348. Comi GT, Prelle A, Bresolin N, et al. Clinical variability in Becker muscular dystrophy: genetic, biochemical and immunohistochemical correlates. Brain 1994; 117: 1–14.

349. de Visser M, de Voogt WG, la Riviere GV. The heart in Becker muscular dystrophy, facioscapulohumeral dystrophy, and Bethlem myopathy. Muscle Nerve 1992; 15:591–596.
350. Yazawa M, Ikeda S, Owa M, et al. A family of Becker's progressive muscular dystrophy with severe cardiomyopathy. Eur Neurol 1987; 27:13–19.
351. Levin RN, Narahara KA. Right-axis deviation and anterior wall thallium-201 defect in Becker's muscular dystrophy. Am J Cardiol 1985; 56:203–207.
352. Melacini P, Fanin M, Danieli GA, et al. Cardiac involvement in Becker muscular dystrophy. J Am Coll Cardiol 1993; 22:1927–1934.
352a. Jones HR, de la Monte SM. Case records of the Massachusetts General Hospital—case 22-1998. N Engl J Med 1998; 339:182–190.
353. Emery AEH, Dreifuss FE. Unusual type of benign X-linked muscular dystrophy. J Neurol Neurosurg Psychiatry 1966; 29:338–342.
354. Hopkins LC, Jackson JA, Elias LJ. Emery-Dreifuss humeroperoneal muscular dystrophy: an X-linked myopathy with unusual contractures and bradycardia. Ann Neurol 1981; 10:230–237.
355. Small K, Iber J, Warren ST. Emerin deletion reveals a common x-chromosome inversion mediated by inverted repeats. (Letter.) Nature Genet 1997; 16:96–99.
356. Wooliscroft J, Tuna N. Permanent atrial standstill: the clinical spectrum. Am J Cardiol 1982; 49:2037–2041.
357. Dickey RP, Ziter FA, Smith RA. Emery-Dreifuss muscular dystrophy. J Pediatr 1984; 104:555–559.
358. Emery AEH. X-linked muscular dystrophy with early contractures and cardiomyopathy (Emery-Dreifuss type). Clin Genet 1987; 32:360–367.
359. Adams RD, Victor M, Ropper AH. Principles of Neurology. 6th ed. New York: McGraw-Hill, 1997:1423.
360. Adams RD, Victor M, Ropper AH. Principles of Neurology. 6th ed. New York: McGraw-Hill, 1997:1421–1422.
361. Stubgen J-P. Limb girdle muscular dystrophy: a non-invasive cardiac evaluation. Cardiology 1993; 83:324–330.
362. Hoshio A, Kotake H, Saitoh M, et al. Cardiac involvement in a patient with limb-girdle muscular dystrophy. Heart Lung 1987; 16:439–441.
363. Mahadevan M, Tsilfidis C, Sabourin L, et al. Myotonic dystrophy mutation: an unstable CTG repeat in the 3′ untranslated region of the gene. Science 1992; 255: 1253–1255.
364. Harper PS. Myotonic Dystrophy. 2d ed. Philadelphia: WB Saunders, 1989.
365. Adams RD, Victor M, Ropper AH. Principles of Neurology. 6th ed. New York: McGraw-Hill, 1997:1423–1425.
366. Chang L, Ernst T, Osborn D, et al. Proton spectroscopy in myotonic dystrophy. Correlation with CTG repeats. Arch Neurol 1998; 55:305–311.
367. Ashizawa T. Myotonic dystrophy as a brain disorder. Arch Neurol 1998; 55:291–292.
368. Bharati S, Bump FT, Bauernfeind R, Lev M. Dystrophica myotonia: correlative electrocardiographic, electrophysiologic and conduction system study. Chest 1984; 86:444–450.
369. Fragola PV, Luzi M, Calo L, et al. Cardiac involvement in myotonic dystrophy. Am J Cardiol 1994; 74:1070–1072.

370. Nguyen HH, Wolfe JT III, Holmes DR Jr, Edwards WD. Pathology of the cardiac conduction system in myotonic dystrophy: a study of 12 cases. J Am Coll Cardiol 1988; 11:662–671.
371. Adams RD, Victor M, Ropper AH. Principles of Neurology. 6th ed. New York: McGraw-Hill, 1997:1453.
372. Fardeau M, Tome FMS. Congenital myopathies. In: Engel AG, Franzini-Armstrong, eds. Myology. 2d ed. Vol. 2. New York: McGraw-Hill, 1994:1487–1532.
373. Kinoshita M, Satoyoshi E. Type I fiber atrophy and nemaline bodies. Arch Neurol 1974; 31:423–425.
374. Meier C, Gertsch M, Zimmerman A, Voellmy W, Geissbuhler W. Nemaline myopathy presenting as cardiomyopathy. N Engl J Med 1983; 308:1536–1537.
375. Meier C, Voellmy W, Gertsch M, et al. Nemaline myopathy appearing in adults as cardiomyopathy: a clinicopathologic study. Arch Neurol 1984; 41:443–445.
376. Shafiq SA, Sande MA, Carruthers RR, Killip T, Milhorat AT. Skeletal muscle in idiopathic cardiomyopathy. J Neurol Sci 1972; 15:303–320.
377. Verhiest W, Brucher JM, Goddeeris P, Lauweryns J, De Geest H. Familial centronuclear myopathy associated with cardiomyopathy. Br Heart J 1976; 38:504–509.
378. Adams RD, Victor M, Ropper AH. Principles of Neurology. 6th ed. New York: McGraw-Hill, 1997:1452–1453.
379. Fardeau M, Godet-Guillain J, Tome FMS, et al. Une nouvelle affection musculaire familiale: definie par l'accumulation intra-sarcoplasmique d'un materiel granulofilamentaire dense en microscopie electronique. Rev Neurol 1978; 134:411–425.
380. Edstrom L, Thornell LE, Eriksson A. A new type of hereditary distal myopathy with characteristic sarcoplasmic bodies and intermediate (skeleton) filaments. J Neurol Sci 1980; 47:171–190.
381. Sabatelli M, Bertini E, Ricci E, et al. Peripheral neuropathy with giant axons and cardiomyopathy associated with desmin type intermediate filaments in skeletal muscle. J Neurol Sci 1992; 109:1–10.
382. Takatsu T, Kawai C, Tsutsumi J, Inoue K. A case of idiopathic myocardiopathy with deposits of a peculiar substance in the myocardium. Diagnosis by endomyocardial biopsy. Am Heart J 1968; 76:93–104.
383. Porte A, Stoeckel ME, Sacrez A, Batzensclager A. Unusual familial cardiomyopathy with storage of intermediate filaments in the cardiac muscle cells. Virchows Arch 1980; 386:43–58.
384. Bordiuk JM, Legato MJ, Lovelace RE, Blumenthal S. Pompe's disease: electron myographic, electron microscopic and cardiovascular aspects. Arch Neurol 1970; 23:113–119.
385. Engel AG, Hirschhorn R. Acid maltase deficiency. In: Engel AG, Franzini-Armstrong, eds. Myology. 2d ed. Vol. 2. New York, McGraw-Hill, 1994:1533–1553.
386. Labrune P, Huguet P, Odievre M. Cardiomyopathy in glycogen-storage disease type II: clinical and echographic study of 18 patients. Pediatr Cardiol 1991; 12: 161–163.
387. Hwang G, Meng CC, Lin C-Y, Hsu H-C. Clinical analysis of five infants with glycogen storage diseae of the heart—Pompe's disease. Jpn Heart J 1986; 27:25–34.

388. Adams RD, Victor M, Ropper AH. Principles of Neurology. 6th ed. New York: McGraw-Hill, 1997:1433–1436.
389. DiMauro S, Tsujino S. Nonlysosomal glycogenoses. In: Engel AG, Franzini-Armstrong, eds. Myology. 2d ed. Vol. 2. New York: McGraw-Hill, 1994:1554–1576.
390. Ratinov G, Baker WP, Swaiman KF. McArdle's syndrome with previously unreported electrocardiographic and serum enzyme abnormalities. Ann Intern Med 1965; 62:328–335.
391. Adams RD, Victor M, Ropper AH. Principles of Neurology. 6th ed. New York: McGraw-Hill, 1997:1437–1439.
392. Di Donato S. Disorders of lipid metabolism affecting skeletal muscle: carnitine deficiency syndromes, defects in the catabolic pathway, and Chanarin disease. In: Engel AG, Franzini-Armstrong, eds. Myology. 2d ed. Vol. 2. New York: McGraw-Hill, 1994:1587–1609.
393. Engel AE, Angelini C. Carnitine deficiency of human skeletal muscle with associated lipid storage myopathy: a new syndrome. Science 1973; 179:899–902.
394. Engel AG, Banker BQ, Eiben RM. Carnitine deficiency: clinical morphological and biochemical observations in a fatal case. J Neurol Neurosurg Psychiatry 1977; 40:313–322.
395. Karpati G, Carpenter S, Engel AG, et al. The syndrome of systemic carnitine deficiency: clinical, morphological, biochemical, and pathophysiological features. Neurology 1975; 25:16–24.
396. Tripp ME, Katcher ML, Peters HA, et al. Systemic carnitine deficiency presenting as familial endocardial fibroelastosis: a treatable cardiomyopathy. N Engl J Med 1981; 305:385–390.
397. Bakker HD, Scholte HR, Luyt-Houwen IE, et al. Neonatal cardiomyopathy and lactic acidosis responsive to thiamine. J Inherit Metab Dis 1991; 14:75–79.
398. Bautista J, Rafel E, Martinez A, et al. Familial hypertrophic cardiomyopathy and muscle carnitine deficiency. Muscle Nerve 1990; 13:192–194.
399. Bratton SL, Garden AL, Bohan TP, French JW, Clarke WR. A child with valproic acid-associated carnitine deficiency and carnitine-responsive cardiac dysfunction. J Child Neurol 1992; 7:413–416.
400. Morgan-Hughes JA. Mitochondrial diseases. In: Engel AG, Franzini-Armstrong, eds. Myology. 2d ed. Vol. 2. New York: McGraw-Hill, 1994:1610–1660.
401. Adams RD, Victor M, Ropper AH. Principles of Neurology. 6th ed. New York: McGraw-Hill, 1997:982–987.
402. Olson W, Engel WK, Walsh GO, Einaugler R. Oculocraniosomatic neuromuscular disease with ''ragged-red'' fibers: histochemical and ultrastructural changes in limb muscles in a group of patients with idiopathic progressive external ophthalmoplegia. Arch Neurol 1972; 26:193–211.
403. Goto Y, Horai S, Matsuoka T, et al. Mitochondrial myopathy, encephalopathy, lactic acidosis, and stroke-like episodes (MELAS): a correlative study of the clinical features and mitochondrial DNA mutation. Neurology 1992; 42:545–550.
404. Koo B, Becker LE, Chuang S, et al. Mitochondrial encephalomyopathy, lactic acidosis, stroke-like episodes (MELAS): clinical, radiological, pathological, and genetic observations. Ann Neurol 1993; 34:25–32.
405. Clark JM, Marks MP, Adalsteinsson E, et al. MELAS: clinical and pathologic corre-

lations with MRI, xenon/CT, and MR spectroscopy. Neurology 1996; 46:223–227.

406. Lowes M. Chronic progressive external ophthalmoplegia, pigmentary retinopathy and heart block (Kearns-Sayre syndrome). Acta Ophthalmol 1975; 53:610–619.
407. Leigh D. Subacute necrotizing encephalomyelopathy in an infant. J Neurol Neurosurg Psychiatry 1951; 14:216–221.
408. Barkovich AJ, Good WV, Koch T, Berg BO. Mitochondrial disorders: analysis of their clinical and imaging characteristics. AJNR 1993; 14:1119–1137.
409. Medina L, Chi TL, DeVivo DC, Hilal SK. MR findings in patients with subacute necrotizing encephalomyelopathy (Leigh syndrome). AJNR 1990; 11:379–384.
410. Adams J, Blackwood W, Wilson J. Further clinical and pathological observations on Leber's optic atrophy. Brain 1966; 89:15–26.
411. Newman N, Wallace D. Mitochondria and Leber's hereditary optic neuropathy. Am J Ophthalmol 1990; 109:726–730.
412. Newman N, Lott M, Wallace D. The clinical characteristics of pedigrees of Leber's hereditary optic neuropathy with the 11778 mutation. Am J Ophthalmol 1991; 111: 750–762.
413. DiMauro S, Bonilla E, Lombes A, et al. Mitochondrial encephalomyopathies. Neurol Clin 1990; 8:483–506.
414. Rowland L, Blake D, Hirano M, et al. Clinical syndromes associated with ragged red fibers. Rev Neurol 1991; 147:467–473.
415. Shoffner J, Lott M, Wallace D. MERRF: a model disease for understanding the principles of mitochondrial genetics. Rev Neurol 1991; 147:431–435.
416. Bardosi A, Creutzfeldt W, DiMauro S, et al. Myo-, neuro-, gastrointestinal encephalopathie (MNGIE syndrome) due to partial deficiency of cytochrome c oxidase. Acta Neuropathol 1987; 74:248–258.
417. Alpers B. Progressive cerebral degeneration in infancy. J Nerv Ment Dis 1960; 130:442–448.
418. Harding BN. Progressive neuronal degeneration of childhood with liver disease (Alpers-Huttenlocher syndrome): a personal review. J Child Neurol 1990; 5:273–287.
419. Tulinius MH, Holme E, Kristiansson B, et al. Mitochondrial encephalomyopathies in childhood. 1. Biochemical and morphological investigations. J Pediatr 1991; 119: 242–250.
420. Menkes J, Alter M, Steigleder G, Weakley D, Sung J. A sex-linked recessive disorder with retardation of growth, peculiar hair and focal cerebral and cerebellar degeneration. Pediatrics 1962; 29:764–779.
421. Morgello S, Peterson HD, Kahn LJ, Laufer H. Menkes kinky hair disease with 'ragged red fibers.' Dev Med Child Neurol 1988; 30:812–816.
422. Channer KS, Channer JL, Campbell MJ, Rees JR. Cardiomyopathy in the Kearnes-Sayre syndrome. Br Heart J 1988; 59:486–490.
423. Clark DS, Myerberg RJ, Morales RR, et al. Heart block and Kearnes-Sayre syndrome: electrophysiologic-pathologic correlation. Chest 1975; 68:727–730.
424. Petty RKH, Harding AE, Morgan-Hughes JA. The clinical features of mitochondrial myopathy. Brain 1986; 109:915–938.
425. Mastaglia F, Thompson PL, Papadimitriou JM. Mitochondrial myopathy with car-

diomyopathy, lactic acidosis, and response to prednisone and thiamine. Aust NZ J Med 1980; 10:660–664.

426. Sato W, Tanaka M, Sugiyama S, et al. Cardiomyopathy and angiopathy in patients with mitochondrial myopathy, encephalopathy, lactic acidosis, and stroke-like episodes. Am Heart J 1994; 128:733–741.
427. Brooke MH, Cwik VE. Disorders of skeletal muscle. In: Bradley WG, Daroff RB, Fenichel GM, Marsden CD, eds. Neurology in Clinical Practice. Vol. 2. The Neurological Disorders. 2d ed. Boston: Butterworth-Heinemann, 1996:2003–2047.
428. Ptacek LJ, Gouw L, Kwiecinski H, et al. Sodium channel mutations in paramyotonia congenita and hyperkalemic periodic paralysis. Ann Neurol 1993; 33:300–307
429. Ptacek LJ, Johnson KJ, Griggs RC. Mechanisms of disease: genetics and physiology of the myotonic muscle disorders. N Engl J Med 1993; 328:482–489.
430. Fontaine B, Khurana TS, Hoffman EP, et al. Hyperkalemic periodic paralysis and the adult muscle sodium channel alpha-subunit gene. Science 1990; 250:1000–1002.
431. Andersen ED, Krasilnikoff PA, Overvad H. Intermittent muscular weakness, extrasystoles, and multiple developmental anomalies: a new syndrome? Acta Pediatr Scand 1971; 60:559–564.
432. Sansone V, Griggs RC, Meola G, et al. Andersen's syndrome: a distinct periodic paralysis. Ann Neurol 1997; 42:305–312.
433. Marks ML, Trippel DL, Keating M. Long QT syndrome associated with syndactyly in females. Am J Cardiol 1995; 76:744–745.
434. Marks ML, Whisler SL, Clericuzio C, Keating M. A new form of long QT syndrome associated with syndactyly. J Am Coll Cardiol 1995; 25:59–64.
435. Banker BQ, Engel AG. The polymyositis and dermatomyositis syndromes. In: Engel AG, Banker BQ, eds. Myology. New York: McGraw-Hill, 1986:1385–1422.
436. Sigurgeirsson B, Lindelof B, Edhag O, Allander E. Risk of cancer in patients with dermatomyositis or polymyositis. A population-based study. N Engl J Med 1992; 326:363–367.
437. Denbow CE, Lie JJ, Robert TL, Tancredi RG, Bunch JW. Cardiac involvement in polymyositis: a clinicopathologic study of 20 autopsied patients. Arthritis Rheum 1979; 27:1088–1092.
438. Stern R, Godbold JH, Chess Q, Kagen L. ECG abnormalities in polymyositis. Arch Intern Med 1984; 144:2185–2189.
439. Yale SH, Adlakha A, Stanton MS. Dermatomyositis with pericardial tamponade and polymyositis with pericardial effusion. Am Heart J 1993; 126:997–999.
440. Lotz BP, Engel AG, Nishino H, Stevens JC, Litchy WJ. Inclusion body myositis: observations in 40 patients. Brain 1989; 112:727–747.
441. Dalakas MC. Polymyositis, dermatomyositis, and inclusion-body myositis. N Engl J Med 1991; 325:1487–1498.
442. Griggs RC, Askanas V, DiMauro S. Inclusion body myositis and myopathies. Ann Neurol 1995; 38:705–713.
443. Van der Meulen MFG, Hoogendijk JE, Jansen GH, Veldman H, Wokke JHJ. Absence of characteristic features in two patients with inclusion body myositis. J Neurol Neurosurg Psychiatry 1998; 64:396–398.

444. Adams RD, Victor M, Ropper AH. Principles of Neurology. 6th ed. New York: McGraw-Hill, 1997:634–635.
445. Fourestie V, Douceron H, Brugieres P, et al. Neurotrichinosis. A cerebrovascular disease associated with myocardial injury and hypereosinophilia. Brain 1993; 116: 603–616.
446. Lopez-Lozano JJ, Garcia Merino JA, Liano H. Bilateral facial paralysis secondary to trichinosis. Acta Neurol Scand 1988; 78:194–197.
447. Ursell PC, Habib A, Babchick O, et al. Myocarditis caused by *Trichinella spiralis*. Arch Pathol Lab Med 1984; 108:4–5.
448. Wartofsky L. Diseases of the thyroid. In: Isselbacher KJ, Braunwald E, Wilson JD, et al., eds. Harrison's Principles of Internal Medicine. 13th ed. New York: McGraw-Hill, 1994:1941–1946.
449. Adams RD, Victor M, Ropper AH, The endocrine myopathies. In: Principles of Neurology. 6th ed. New York: McGraw-Hill, 1997:1440–1443.
450. Zonszein J, Fein FS, Sonnenblick EH. The heart and endocrine disease. In: Schlant RC, Alexander RC, eds. Hurst's The Heart. 8th ed. New York: McGraw-Hill, 1994: 1908–1911.
451. Potts JT Jr. Diseases of the parathyroid gland and other hyper- and hypocalcemic disorders. In: Fauci AS, Braunwald E, Isselbacher KJ, Wilson JD, Martin JB, Kasper DL, Hauser SL, eds. Harrison's Principles of Internal Medicine. 13th ed. New York: McGraw-Hill, 1998:2227–2247.
452. Bilezikian JP. Management of acute hypercalcemia. N Engl J Med 1992; 326: 1196–1203.
453. Patten BM, Bilezikian JP, Mallette LE, et al. Neuromuscular disease in primary hyperparathyroidism. Ann Intern Med 1974; 80:182–193.
454. Gorelick PB, Caplan LR. Calcium, hypercalcemia, and stroke. Curr Concepts Cerebrovasc Dis (Stroke) 1985; 20:13–17.
455. Yarnell PR, Caplan LR. Basilar artery narrowing and hyperparathyroidism. Illustrative case. Stroke 1986; 17:1022–1024.
456. Lind L, Ljunghall S. Serum calcium and the ECG in patients with primary hyperparathyroidism. J Electrocardiol 1994; 27:99–103.
457. Lavis VR, Mueller SD, Willerson JT. Endocrine disorders and the heart. In: Willerson JT, Cohn JN, eds. Cardiovascular Medicine. New York: Churchill Livingstone, 1995:1617–1618.
458. Giles TD, Iteld BJ, Rives KL. The cardiomyopathy of hypoparathyroidism. Another reversible form of heart muscle disease. Chest 1981; 79:225–228.
459. Rimailho A, Bouchard P, Schaison G, Richard C, Auzepy P. Improvement of hypocalcemic cardiomyopathy by correction of serum calcium level. Am Heart J 1985; 109:611–613.
460. Levine SN, Rheams CN. Hypocalcemic heart failure. Am J Med 1985; 78:1033–1035.
461. Sugihara N, Shimizu M, Kita Y, et al. Cardiac characteristics and postoperative courses in Cushing's syndrome. Am J Cardiol 1992; 69:1475–1480.
462. Carney JA, Gordon H. Carpenter PC, Shenoy BV, Go VLW. The complex of myxomas, spotty pigmentation, and endocrine overactivity. Medicine 1985; 64:270–283.
463. Schambelan M, Sebastian A, Biglieri KG, et al. Prevalance, pathogenesis and func-

tional significance of aldosterone deficiency in hyperkalemic patients with chronic renal insufficiency. Kidney Int 1980; 17:89–101.
464. Williams GH, Dlahy RG. Diseases of the adrenal cortex. In: Isselbacher KJ, Braunwald E, Wilson JD, Martin JB, Fauci AS, Kasper DL, eds. Harrison's Principles of Internal Medicine. New York: McGraw-Hill, 1994:1970–1973.
465. Schteingart DE. Adrenal failure. In: Hurst JW, ed. Medicine for the Practicing Physician. Stamford, CT: Appleton & Lange, 1996:570–574.
466. Knowlton AI, Baer L. Cardiac failure in Addison's disease. Am J Med 1983; 74: 829–836.
467. Daniels GH, Martin JB. Neuroendocrine regulation and diseases of the anterior pituitary and hypothalamus. In: Isselbacher KJ, Braunwald E, Wilson JD, et al., eds. Harrison's Principles of Internal Medicine. 13th ed. New York: McGraw-Hill, 1994:1899–1904.
468. Ezzat S, Melmed S. Clinical review 18: are patients with acromegaly at increased risk for neoplasia? J Clin Endocrinol Metab 1991; 72:245–249.
469. Rodrigues EA, Caruana MP, Lahiri A, et al. Subclinical cardiac dysfunction in acromegaly: evidence for a specific disease of heart muscle. Br Heart J 1989; 62: 185–194.
470. Adams RD, Victor M, Ropper AH. Principles of Neurology. 6th ed. New York: McGraw-Hill, 1997:1459–1475.
471. Sanders DB, Howard JF. Disorders of Neuromuscular transmission. In: Bradley WG, Daroff RB, Fenichel GM, Marsden CD, eds. Neurology in Clinical Practice. Vol. 2. The Neurological Disorders. 2d ed. Boston: Butterworth-Heinemann, 1996: 1983–2001.
472. Drachman DB. Myasthenia gravis. N Engl J Med 1994; 330:1797–1810.
473. Argov Z, Mastaglia FL. Disorders of neuromuscular transmission caused by drugs. N Engl J Med 1979; 301:409–413.
474. Gibson TC. The heart in myasthenia gravis. Am Heart J 1975; 90(3):389–396.
475. Rottino A, Poppiti R, Rao J. Myocardial lesions in myasthenia gravis. Review and report of a case. Arch Pathol 1942; 34:557–561.
476. Naeye RL. Alveolar hypoventilation and cor pulmonale secondary to damage to the respiratory center. Am J Cardiol 1961; 8:416–419.
477. Leys K, Lang B, Johnston I, Newsome-Davis J. Calcium channel autoantibodies in the Lambert-Eaton myasthenic syndrome. Ann Neurol 1991; 29:307–314.
478. Lennon VA, Kryzer T, Griesmann GE, et al. Calcium-channel antibodies in the Lambert-Eaton syndrome and other paraneoplastic syndromes. N Engl J Med 1995; 332:1467–1474.
479. Rubinstein AE, Horowitz SH, Bender AN. Cholinergic dysautonomia and Eaton-Lambert syndrome. Neurology 1979; 29:720–723.
480. Weinberg D, Cros D. Case records of the Massachusetts General Hospital. Case 32-1994. N Engl J Med 1994; 331:528–535.
481. Merson MH, Dowell VR. Epidemiologic, clinical and laboratory aspects of wound botulism. N Engl J Med 1973; 289:1005–1010.
482. McCroskey LM, Hatheway CL. Laboratory findings in four cases of adult botulism suggest colonization of the intestinal tract. J Clin Microbiol 1988; 26:1052–1054.

483. Gutmann L, Pratt L. Pathophysiologic aspects of human botulism. Arch Neurol 1976; 33:175–179.
484. Adams RD, Victor M, Ropper AH. Principles of Neurology. 6th ed. New York: McGraw-Hill, 1997:1208–1209.
485. Jenzer G, Mumenthaler M, Ludin HP, Robert F. Autonomic dysfunction in botulism B: a clinical report. Neurology 1975; 25:150–153.
486. Koenig MG, Drutz DJ, Mushlin A, Schaffner W, Rogers DE. Type B botulism in man. Am J Med 1967; 42:208–219.
487. Harding AE. Cerebellar and spinocerebellar disorders. In: Bradley WG, Daroff RB, Fenichel GM, Marsden CD, eds. Neurology in Clinical Practice. 2d ed. Vol. 2. Boston: Butterworth-Heinemann, 1996:1773–1792.
488. Durr A, Cossee M, Agid Y, et al. Clinical and genetic abnormalities in patients with Friedreich's ataxia. N Engl J Med 1996; 335:1169–1175.
489. Adams RD, Victor M, Ropper AH. Principles of Neurology. 6th ed. New York: McGraw-Hill, 1997:1081–1084.
490. James TN, Cobbs BW, Coghlan HC, NcCoy WC, Fisch C. Coronary disease, cardioneuropathy, and conduction system abnormalities in the cardiomyopathy of Friedreich's ataxia. Br Heart J 1987; 57:446–457.
491. Gottdiener JS, Hawley RJ, Maron BJ, Bertorini TF, Engle WK. Characteristics of the cardiac hypertrophy in Friedreich's ataxia. Am Heart J 1982; 103:525–531.
492. Giunta A, Maione S, Biagini R, et al. Noninvasive assessment of systolic and diastolic function in 50 patients with Friedreich's ataxia. Cardiology 1988; 75:321–327.
493. Morvan D, Komajda M, Doan LD, et al. Cardiomyopathy in Friedreich's ataxia: a Doppler-echocardiographic study. Eur Heart J 1992; 13:1393–1398.
494. Alboliras ET, Shub C, Gomez MR, et al. Spectrum of cardiac involvement in Friedreich's ataxia: clinical, electrocardiographic and echocardiographic observations. Am J Cardiol 1986; 58:518–524.
495. Harding AE, Herver RL. The heart disease of Freidreich's ataxia: a clinical and electrocardiographic study of 115 patients, with an analysis of electrocardiographic changes in 30 cases. Q J Med 1983; 28:489–502.
496. Waldmann TA, Misiti J, Nelson DL, Kraemer KH. NIH conference. Ataxia telangiectasia: a multisystem hereditary disease with immunodeficiency, impaired organ maturation, x-ray hypersensitivity, and a high incidence of neoplasia. Ann Intern Med 1983; 99:367–379.
497. Gomez MR. Neurocutaneous diseases. In: Bradley WG, Daroff RB, Fenichel GM, Marsden CD, eds. Neurology in Clinical Practice. 2d ed. Vol. 2. Boston: Butterworth-Heinemann, 1996:1561–1581.
498. Mulvihill JJ, Parry DM, Sherman JL, Pikus A, Kaiser-Kupfer MI, Eldridge R. NIH conference. Neurofibromatosis I (Recklinghausen disease) and neurofibromatosis 2 (bilateral acoustic neurofibromatosis). An update. Ann Intern Med 1990; 113: 39–52.
499. Manger WM, Gifford RW Jr. Clinical and Experimental Pheochromocytoma. Cambridge: Blackwell Science, 1996.
500. Hochberg FH, Dasilva AB, Galdabini J, Richardson EP. Gastrointestinal involvement in von Recklinghausen's neurofibromatosis. Neurology 1974; 24:1144–1151.

501. Fabricant RN, Todaro GJ. Increased serum levels of nerve growth factor in von Recklinghausen's disease. Arch Neurol 1981; 38:401–405.
502. Wertelecki W, Rouleau GA, Superneau D, et al. Neurofibromatosis 2: clinical and DNA linkage studies of a large kindred. N Engl J Med 1988; 319:278–283.
503. Hilal SK, Solomon GE, Gold AP, Carter S. Primary cerebral arterial occlusive disease in children. II. Neurocutaneous syndromes. Radiology 1971; 99:87–94.
504. Adams RD, Victor M, Ropper AH. Principles of Neurology. 6th ed. New York: McGraw-Hill, 1997:1011–1014.
505. Stillwell TJ, Gomez MR, Kelalis PP. Renal lesions in tuberous sclerosis. J Urol 1987; 138:477–481.
506. Webb DW, Thomas RD, Osborne JP. Cardiac rhabdomyomas and their association with tuberous sclerosis. Arch Dis Child 1993; 68:367–370.
507. Latif F, Kalman T, Gnarra J, et al. Identification of the von Hippel–Landau disease tumor suppressor gene. Science 1993; 260:1317–1320.
508. Lamiell JM, Salazar FG, Hsia YE. Von Hippel–Lindau disease affecting 43 members of a single kindred. Medicine 1989; 68:1–29.
509. Filling-Katz MR, Choyke PL, Oldfield E, etal. Central nervous system involvement in von Hippel–Lindau disease. Neurology 1991; 41:41–46.
510. Melmon KL, Rosen SW. Lindau's disease. Review of the literature and study of a large kindred. Am J Med 1964; 36:595–616.
511. Maher ER, Kaelin WG Jr. von Hippel–Lindau disease. Medicine 1997; 76:381–391.
512. Lyon G, Adams RD, Kolodny EH. Neurology of Hereditary Metabolic Diseases of Children. New York: McGraw-Hill, 1996.
513. Mosser J, Douar AM, Sande CO, et al. Putative X-linked adrenoleukodystrophy gene shares unexpected homology with ABC transporters. Nature 1993; 361:726–730.
514. Moser H, Moser A, Singh I, O'Neill BP. Adrenoleukodystrophy: survey of 303 cases: biochemistry, diagnosis, and therapy. Ann Neurol 1984; 16:628–641.
515. Kumar AJ, Kohler W, Kruse B, et al. MR findings in adult-onset adrenoleukodystrophy. AJNR 1995; 16:1227–1237.
516. Goldfischer S, Moore CL, Johnson AB, et al. Peroxisomal and mitochondrial defects in the cerebro-hepato-renal syndrome. Science 1973;182:62–64.
517. Kelley RI. The cerebro-hepato-renal syndrome of Zellweger: morphologic and metabolic aspects. Am J Med Genet 1983; 503–517.
518. Guttmacher AE, Marchuk DA, White RI. Hereditary hemorrhagic telangiectasia. N Engl J Med 1995; 333:918–924.
519. Fullbright RK, Chaloupka JC, Putman CM, et al. MR of hemorrhagic telangiectasia: prevalence and spectrum of cerebrovascular malformations. AJNR 1998; 19:477–484.
520. Adams HP, Subbiah B, Bosch EP. Neurologic aspects of hereditary hemorrhagic telangiectasia. Arch Neurol 1977; 34:101–104.
521. Moyer JH, Glantz G, Brest AN. Pulmonary arteriovenous fistulas: physiological and clinical considerations. Am J Med 1962; 32:417–435.
522. Dines DE, Arms RA, Bernatz PE, et al. Pulmonary arteriovenous fistulas. Mayo Clin Proc 1974; 49:460–465.

523. Roman G, Fisher M, Perl D, Poser C. Neurological manifestations of hereditary hemorrhagic telangiectasia (Rendu-Osler-Weber disease): report of 2 cases and review of the literature. Ann Neurol 1978; 4:130–144.
524. Menkes J. Textbook of Child Neurology. 5th ed. Baltimore: Williams & Wilkins, 1995.
525. Wang CH. Genetic diseases of the central nervous system: chromosomal diseases. Trisomy 21 (Down syndrome). In: Rowland LP, ed. Merritt's Textbook of Neurology. 9th ed. Baltimore: Williams & Wilkins, 1995:535–536.
526. Adams RD, Victor M, Ropper AH. Principles of Neurology. 6th ed. New York: McGraw-Hill, 1997:1008–1009.
527. Lai F, Williams RS. A prospective study of Alzheimer disease in Down syndrome. Arch Neurol 1989; 46:849–853.
528. Schupf N, Kapell D, Nightingale B, et al. Earlier onset of Alzheimer's disease in men with Down syndrome. Neurology 1998; 50:991–995.
529. Nugent EW, Plauth WH, Edwards JE, Williams WH. The pathology, pathophysiology, recognition, and treatment of congenital heart disease. In: Schlant RC, Alexander RW, eds. Hurst's The Heart. 8th ed. New York: McGraw-Hill, 1994:1761–1854.
530. Jones KL. Smith's Recognizable Patterns of Human Malformation. 5th ed. Philadelphia: WB Saunders, 1997.
531. Baty BJ, Blackburn BL, Carey JC. Natural history of trisomy 18 and trisomy 13. I. Growth, physical assessment, medical histories, survival, and recurrence risk. Am J Med Genet 1995; 49:175–188.
532. Bergin A, McManus SP, Clarke TA, Moloney M. Trisomy 18: a nine year review. Irish J Med Sci 1988; 157:5–7.
533. Patau K, Therman E, Smith DW, Inhorn SL, Wagner HP. Multiple congenital anomaly caused by an extra chromosome. Lancet 1960; 1:790–793.
534. Lemieux BG, Wright FS, Swaiman KF. Genetic and congenital structural defects of the brain and spinal cord. In: Swaiman KF, Wright FS, eds. The Practise of Pediatric Neurology. St. Louis: CV Mosby, 1982:344–471.
535. Inagaki M, Ando Y, Mito T, et al. Comparison of brain imaging and neuropathology in cases of trisomy 18 and 13. Neuroradiology 1987; 29:474–479.
536. Gregg N. Congenital cataract following German measles in the mother. Trans Ophthalmol Soc Aust 1941; 3:35–46.
537. Weil ML, Levin M. Infections of the nervous system. In: Menkes J, ed. Textbook of Child Neurology. 5th ed. Baltimore: Williams & Wilkins, 1995:379–509.
538. Miller E, Craddock-Watson JE, Pollock TM. Consequences of confirmed maternal rubella at successive stages of pregnancy. Lancet 1982; 2:781–784.
539. Allanson JE. Noonan syndrome. J Med Genet 1987; 24:9–13.
540. Money J, Kalus ME Jr. Noonan's syndrome: IQ and specific disabilities. Am J Dis Child 1979; 133:846–850.
541. O'Rourke RA, Silverman ME, Schlant RC. General examination of the patient. In: Schlant RC, Alexander RW, eds. Hurst's the Heart. 8th ed. New York: McGraw-Hill, 1994: 217.
542. Lin AE, Perloff JK. Upper limb malformations associated with congenital heart disease. Am J Cardiol 1985; 55:1576–1583.

543. Rubinstein JH, Taybi H. Broad thumbs and toes and facial abnormalities: a possible mental retardation syndrome. Am J Dis Child 1963; 105:588–608.
544. Breuning MH, Dauwerse HG, Fugazza G, et al. Rubinstein-Taybi syndrome caused by submicroscopic deletions within 16p13.3. Am J Hum Genet 1993; 52:249–254.
545. Shprintzen RJ, Goldberg RB, Lewis ML, et al. A new syndrome involving cleft palate, cardiac anomalies, typical facies, and learning disabilities, velo-cardio-facial syndrome. Cleft Palate J 1978; 15:56–62.
546. Shprintzen RJ, Goldberg RB, Young D, Wolford L. The velo-cardio-facial syndrome. A clinical and genetic analysis. Pediatrics 1981; 67:167–172.
547. Young D, Shprintzen RJ, Goldberg RB. Cardiac malformations in the velo-cardio-facial syndrome. Am J Cardiol 1980; 46:643–648.
548. Kelley RI, Zackai EH, Emanuel BS, et al. The association of the DiGeorge anomalad with partial monosomy of chromosome 22. J Pediatr 1982; 101:197–200.
549. Greenberg F, Crowder WE, Paschall V, et al. Familial DiGeorge syndrome and associated partial monosomy of chromosome 22. Hum Genet 1984; 65:317–319.
550. Freedom RM, Rosen FS, Nadas AS. Congenital cardiovascular disease and anomalies of the third and fourth pharyngeal pouch. Circulation 1972; 46:165–172.
551. Hutchinson J. Congenital absence of hair and mammary glands with atrophic conditions of the skin and its appendages in a boy whose mother had been almost wholly bald from alopecia areata from the age of six. Med Chir Trans 1886; 69:473–477.
552. Gilford H. Progeria: a form of senilism. Practitioner 1904; 73:188–217.
553. Herrero FA. Neurological manifestations of hereditable connective tissue disorders. In: Vinken PJ, Bruyn GW, Klawans HL, eds. Neurological Manifestations of Systemic Diseases. Part II. Handbook of Clinical Neurology. Vol. 39. Amsterdam: North-Holland, 1980:379–418.
554. Feingold M. Progeria (Hutchinson-Gilford syndrome). In: Vinken PJ, Bruyn GW, Klawans HL, eds. Neurogenetic Directory. Part II. Handbook of Clinical Neurology. Vol. 43. Amsterdam: North-Holland, 1980:465–466.
555. Brown WT. Progeria. Adv Exp Med Biol 1985; 190:239–244.
556. DeBusk FL. The Hutchinson-Gilford progeria syndrome. J Pediatr 1972; 80:697–724.
557. Werner O. Uber Katarakt in Verbindung mit Sklerodermis. Thesis. Kiel, Germany: Kiel, Schmidt, und Klaunig, 1904.
558. Tokunaga M, Mori S, Sato K, Nakamura K, Wakamatsu E. Postmortem study of a case of Werner's syndrome. J Am Geriat-Soc 1976; 24:407–411.
559. Mudd SH. Vascular disease and homocysteine metabolism. In: Smith U, Eriksson S, Lingarde F, eds. Genetic Susceptibility to Environmental Factors—A Challenge for Public Intervention. Stockholm: Almqvist & Wiksell, 1988:11–24.
560. Welch GN, Loscalzo J. Homocysteine and atherothrombosis. N Engl J Med 1998; 338:1042–1050.
561. Ueland PM, Refsum H, Stabler SP, Malinow MR, Andersson A, Allen RH. Total homocysteine in plasma or serum; methods and clinical applications. Clin Chem 1993; 39: 1764–1769.
562. Finkelstein JD, Martin JJ, Harris BJ. Methionine metabolism in mammals: the methionine-sparing effect of cystine. J Biol Chem 1988; 263:11750–11754.

563. Mudd SH, Skovby F, Levy HL, et al. The natural history of homocystinuria due to cystathione-beta-synthase deficiency. Am J Hum Genet 1985; 37:1–31.
564. Vermaak WJ, Ubbink JB, Barnard HC, Potgeiter GM, van Jaarsveld H, Groenwald AJ. Vitamin B_6 nutrition status and cigarette smoking. Am J Clin Nutr 1990; 51: 1058–1061.
565. Clarke R, Daly L, Robinson K, et al. Hyperhomocysteinemia: an independent risk factor for vascular disease. N Engl J Med 1991; 324:1149–1155.
566. Evers S, Koch H-G, Grotemeyer K-H, et al. Features, symptoms, and neurophysiological findings in stroke associated with hyperhomocysteinemia. Arch Neurol 1997; 54:1276–1282.
567. Harker LA, Slichter SJ, Scott CR. Homocystinemia: vascular injury and arterial thrombosis. N Engl J Med 1974; 291:537–543.
568. Harker LA, Ross R, Slichter SJ, Scott CR. Homocystine-induced arteriosclerosis: the role of endothelial cell injury and platelet response in its genesis. J Clin Invest 1976; 58:731–741.
569. Tsai J-C, Perrella MA, Yoshizumi M, et al. Promotion of vascular smooth muscle cell growth by homocysteine: a link to atherosclerosis. Proc Natl Acad Sci USA 1994; 91:6369–6373.
570. Stampfer MJ, Malinow MR, Willett WC, et al. A prospective study of plasma homocyst(e)ine and risk of myocardial infarction in US physicians. JAMA 1992; 268: 877–881.
571. Selhub J, Jacques PF, Bostom AG, et al. Association between plasma homocysteine concentrations and extracranial carotid-artery stenosis. N Engl J Med 1995; 332: 286–291.
572. Nygard O, Nordrehaug JE, Refsum HM, et al. Plasma homocysteine levels and mortality in patients with coronary artery disease. N Engl J Med 1997; 337:230–236.
573. Boushey CJ, Beresford SA, Omenn GS, Motulsky AG. A quantitative assessment of plasma homocysteine as a risk factor for vascular diasease: probable benefits of increasing folic acid intakes. JAMA 1995; 274:1049–1057.
574. Hagler DJ. Lentiginosis-deafness-cardiopathy syndrome. In: Gomez MR, ed. Neurocutaneous Disease. A Practical Approach. Boston: Butterworths, 1987:80–84.
575. Polani PE, Moynahan EJ. Progressive cardiomyopathic lentiginosis. Q J Med 1972; 41:205–239.
576. Moynahan EJ, Polani P. Progressive Profuse lentiginosis, progressive cardiomyopathy, short stature with delayed puberty, mental retardation or psychic infantilism, and other development anomalies: a new familial syndrome. In: Jadassohn W, Schirren CG, eds. 13th Congressus Internationalis Dermatologiae. Vol. 2. Berlin: Springer-Verlag, 1968:1543.
577. Gorlin RJ, Anderson RC, Blaw M. Multiple lentigenes syndrome: complex comprising multiple lentigenes, electrocardiographic conduction abnormalities, ocular hypertelorism, pulmonary stenosis, abnormalities of genitalia, retardation of growth, sensorineural deafness, and autosomal dominant hereditary pattern. Am J Dis Child 1969; 117:652–662.
578. Pena EA, Marshall JJ. Hypertrophic cardiomyopathy. In: Hurst JW, ed. Medicine for the Practicing Physician. 4th ed. Stamford, CT: Appleton & Lange 1996:1260–1264.

579. Jervell A, Lange-Nielsen F. Congenital deaf mutism, functional heart disease with prolongation of the QT interval, and sudden death. Am Heart J 1947; 54:59–68.
580. Fraser GR, Froggart P, Murphy T. Genetic aspects of the cardioauditory syndrome of Jervell and Lange-Nielsen (congenital deafness and electrocardiographic abnormalities). Am Hum Genet 1964; 28:133–156.
581. Romano C, Gemme G, Pongiglione R. Arithmie cardiache rare dell'eta pediatrica. Clin Pediatr 1963; 45:656–683.
582. Ward OC. A new familial cardiac syndrome in children. J Irish Med Assoc 1964; 54:103–106.
583. Schwartz PJ, Bonazzi O, Locati E, Napolitano C, Sala S. Pathogenesis and therapy of the idiopathic long QT syndrome. In: Hashiba K, Moss AJ, Schwartz PJ, eds. QT Prolongation and Ventricular Arrhythmias. Ann NY Acad Sci 1992; 644:112–141.
584. Schwartz PJ, Stramba-Badiale M, Seganti A, et al. Prolongation of the QT interval and the sudden infant death syndrome. N Engl J Med 1998; 338:1709–1714.
585. Towbin JA, Friedman RA. Prolongation of the QT interval and the sudden infant death syndrome. N Engl J Med 1998; 338:1760–1761.

About the Authors

Louis R. Caplan is a Neurologist at Beth Israel Deaconess Medical Center, Boston, Massachusetts, and a Professor of Neurology at Harvard Medical School, Boston, Massachusetts. He is the author, coauthor, editor, or coeditor of over 570 original reports, conference proceedings, clinical reviews, abstracts, and books. A Fellow of the American College of Physicians, the American Academy of Neurology, the American Neurological Association, and the Royal Society of Medicine (London), he is a member of numerous societies, including the American College of Physicians, the American Heart Association, and the American Society of Neuroimaging. Dr. Caplan received the B.A. degree (1958) from Williams College, Williamstown, Massachusetts, and the M.D. degree (1962) from the University of Maryland School of Medicine, College Park.

J. Willis Hurst is currently Consultant to the Division of Cardiology at the Emory University School of Medicine, Atlanta, Georgia. He was a cardiology fellow at the Massachusetts General Hospital under Paul Dudley White. He was Candler Professor of Medicine and Chairman of the Department of Medicine at Emory University from 1957 to 1986, former President of the American Heart Association; former member of the Advisory Council to the National Heart, Lung, and Blood Institute; former Chairman of the Subspecialty Board of Cardiology; and former President of the Association of Professors of Medicine. He is a Master of the American College of Physicians and has received numerous teaching awards, including the Distinguished Teaching Award of the American College of Physicians and the Master Teacher Award of the American College of Cardiology. He has edited and contributed to 60 books and written 383 articles. He is well known for his creation of the book *The Heart*, which he edited for seven editions.

Marc I. Chimowitz is an Associate Professor and Director of the Cerebrovascular Program, Emory University School of Medicine, Atlanta, Georgia. The author or coauthor of over 100 journal articles, proceedings, abstracts, and book chapters, he is a Fellow of the American Heart Association Stroke Council and a member of the American Academy of Neurology and the American Medical Association. Dr. Chimowitz received the B.Sc. degree (1975) in mathematics and the B.Sc. (Honours) degree (1979) in applied mathematics from the University of Cape Town, South Africa, and the M.B.Ch.B. (1981) degree from the University of Cape Town School of Medicine, South Africa.